The Neurobiology of Pain

(Molecular and Cellular Neurobiology)

The Neurobiology of Pain
(Molecular and Cellular Neurobiology)

Edited by

Stephen P. Hunt
Department of Anatomy and Developmental
Biology, University College
London

Martin Koltzenburg
Institute of Child Health, University College
London

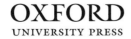

OXFORD
UNIVERSITY PRESS

OXFORD

UNIVERSITY PRESS

Great Clarendon Street, Oxford OX2 6DP

Oxford University Press is a department of the University of Oxford.
It furthers the University's objective of excellence in research, scholarship,
and education by publishing worldwide in

Oxford New York

Auckland Cape Town Dar es Salaam Hong Kong Karachi Kuala Lumpur Madrid
Melbourne Mexico City Nairobi New Delhi Taipei Toronto Shanghai

With offices in

Argentina Austria Brazil Chile Czech Republic France Greece Guatemala Hungary Italy
Japan South Korea Poland Portugal Singapore Switzerland Thailand Turkey Ukraine Vietnam

Oxford is a registered trade mark of Oxford University Press
in the UK and in certain other countries

Published in the United States
by Oxford University Press Inc., New York

A catalogue record for this title is available from the British Library
Library of Congress Cataloging in Publication Data

(Data available)
ISBN 0 19 851561 8 (Hbk)
10 9 8 7 6 5 4 3 2 1

Typeset by Cepha Imaging Pvt. Ltd., Bangalore, India.
Printed in Great Britain
on acid-free paper by Biddles Ltd, King's Lynn

Contents

Contributors

Bandler, Richard
Department of Anatomy
and Histology
Pain Management and Research Centre
Royal North Shore Hospital
University of Sydney
Sydney
NSW 2006
Australia

Bester, Hervé
Département de Neurophysiologie
in vivo
Sanofi-Synthélabo
31 Avenue P. Vaillant Couturier
92225 Bagneaux Cedex
France

Bushnell, M. Catherine
Department of Anaesthesia
Royal Victoria Hospital
687 Pine Avenue
Room F9.12
Montreal
QC H3A 1A1
Canada

Caterina, Michael J.
Department of Biological Chemistry
725 N. Wolfe Street
Baltimore
USA

Dickenson, Anthony H.
Department of Pharmacology
University College London
Gower street
London WC1E 6BT

Ferrari, Michel D.
Department of Neurology
Leiden University Medical Centre
PO Box 9600
2300 RC Leiden
The Netherlands

Fitzgerald, Maria
Department of Anatomy and
Developmental Biology
University College London
Gower Street
London WC1E 6BT

Flor, Herta
Department of Clinical and Cognitive
Neuroscience at the University of
Heidelberg
Central Institute for Mental Health
J5
D-68159 Mannheim
Germany

Gebhart, G.F.
Department of Pharmacology
Roy J. and Lucille A. Carver College of
Medicine
University of Iowa
Iowa City
IA 52242-1109
USA

Goadsby, Peter J.
Institute of Neurology
National Hospital for Neurology and
Neurosurgery
Queen Square
London WC1E 6BT

Gold, M.
Department OCBS
University of Maryland Dental School
666 W. Baltimore Street
Baltimore
MD 21201
USA

Hunt, Stephen P.
Department of Anatomy and
Developmental Biology
University College London
Gower Street
London WC1E 6BT

Koltzenburg, Martin
Institute of Child Health
University College London
30 Guilford Street
London WC1N 1EH

Laird, Jennifer M.A.
Department of Fisiologia
Edificio de Medicina
Universite de Alcala
Alcala de Henares 28871
Madrid Spain

Lovick, Thelma
Department of Physiology
University of Birmingham
The Medical School
Vincent Drive
Birmingham B15 2TJ

MacDermott, Amy
Department of Physiology and Cellular
Biophysics
630 West 168th Street
New York
NY 10032
USA

Mantyh, Patrick W.
Neurosystems Laboratory
University of Minnesota
18-154 Moos Tower
515 Delaware Street
Minneapolis
MN 55455
USA

McMahon, S.B.
Section of Neuroscience
Biomedical Sciences
Centre for Neuroscience Research
King's College London
Hodgin Building
London SE1 1UL

Meyer, R.A.
Department of Neurosurgery
Johns Hopkins University
Meyer 5-109
600 N. Wolfe Street
Baltimore
MD 21287
USA

Priestley, J.V.
Department of Neuroscience
St Bartholomew's and the Royal
London School of Medicine and
Dentistry
Queen Mary University of
London
Mile End Road
London E1 4NS

Proudfit, H.
Department of Pharmacology
Roy J. and Lucille A. Carver College of
Medicine
University of Iowa
Iowa City
IA 52242-1109
USA

Ribeiro-da-Silva, Alfredo
Department of Pharmacology and
Therapeutics
McGill University
3655 Drummond Street
Montreal
Quebec H3G 1Y6
Canada

Salter, Michael W.
Hospital for Sick Children and
University of Toronto Centre for the
Study of Pain
555 University Avenue
Toronto
Ontario M5G 1X8
Canada

Schaible, Hans-Georg
Institut für Physiologie/Neurophysiologie
Teichgraben 8
07740 Jena
Germany

Suzuki, Rie
Department of Pharmacology
University College London
Gower Street
London WC1E 6BT

Todd, Andrew J.
Spinal Cord Group
West Medical Building
University of Glasgow
University Avenue
Glasgow G12 8QQ

Woolf, Clifford J.
Department of Anaesthesia and
Critical Care
Massachusetts General Hospital and
Harvard Medical School
MGH-East
149, 13th Street
Room 4309
Charleston
MA 02129
USA

Yaksh, Tony L.
Department of Anaesthesiology
University of California
9500 Gilman Drive
La Jolla
CA 92093-0818
USA

Chapter 1

Molecular biology of nociceptors

Michael J. Caterina, Michael S. Gold, and
Richard A. Meyer

1.1 Introduction

Pain, like all perceptions, results from a specific spatio-temporal pattern of neurological activity in the cerebral cortex. In most cases, however, pain is initiated by events that occur on the skin, or in deep tissues such as viscera, bone, or muscles. Specialized primary afferent neurons, called nociceptors, constantly survey the environment surrounding their terminals. These neurons are selectively tuned to respond rapidly to mechanical, thermal, or chemical stimuli that are of a sufficient intensity to cause tissue damage or of a quality that indicates existing tissue damage. Upon activation, they transmit this information, via action potentials and neurotransmitter release, to the spinal cord dorsal horn for further processing and transmission to the brain.

This chapter will begin with a functional classification of primary nociceptive neurons. We will then present our current understanding of the molecules that allow nociceptors to detect noxious chemical, thermal, and mechanical stimuli. Next, we will describe the molecular processes by which this information is converted into action potentials and transmitted to the spinal cord. A diagramatic representation of these molecular events can be found in Fig. 1.1. Finally, we will briefly describe the effects of an inflammatory insult on nociceptor function. For the sake of simplicity, we will focus primarily upon events related to cutaneous nociception. Neurotransmission within the spinal cord and mechanisms of visceral or deep tissue pain will be covered in later chapters.

1.2 Physiological characterization of nociceptors

1.2.1 Classification of afferents

Primary afferent nerve fibers provide information to the central nervous system about the environment and also about the state of the organism itself. These sensory fibers are highly specialized with regard to the stimulus modality and stimulus intensity that elicits a response. Afferents that respond at low stimulus intensities are thought to encode innocuous percepts such as touch, cooling, or warmth. Afferents that respond at high stimulus

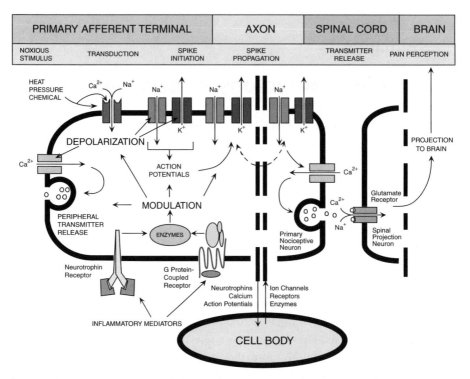

Fig. 1.1 Schematic representation of the processes occurring within a primary afferent nociceptor. Ion channels mediating noxious stimulus detection (dark blue), voltage-gated sodium flux (green), voltage-gated potassium flux (red), voltage-gated calcium flux (light blue), and glutamate-stimulated depolarization of spinal projection neuron (orange) are indicated. Discontinuities in the drawing are represented by the vertical dashed lines. For simplicity, only one terminus is illustrated, although a typical nociceptive neuron contains multiple peripheral terminals. See plate section, Plate 1 (centre of book) for a colour version.

intensities are thought to encode pain sensation. Much of the description of these afferents presented below is based upon studies of human and nonhuman primates. Studies in cats and rodents have revealed analogous, though not entirely identical results.

The sense of touch is signaled by activity in myelinated afferents that are sensitive to slight deformations of the skin. These low threshold cutaneous mechanoreceptors have been differentiated by their response to stepped indentations of the skin and the end-organ structure associated with their terminal. The slowly adapting type 1 afferents end in Merkel cells, whereas the slowly adapting type 2 afferents are thought to terminate in Ruffini corpuscles. Rapidly adapting afferents end in Meissner corpuscles or surround hair follicles. Pacinian afferents end in Pacinian corpuscles and respond well to high frequencies of vibration. These low threshold mechanoreceptive afferents encode different aspects of touch sensation such as texture and shape (Johnson, 2001).

A subpopulation of unmyelinated afferents is exquisitely sensitive to gentle warming of their punctate receptive fields. These afferents are called warm fibers. Warm fibers are thought to encode the quality and intensity of warmth sensation (Darian–Smith *et al.*, 1979*a,b*; Johnson *et al.*, 1979). Similarly, there is a subpopulation of the thinly myelinated Aδ-fiber (Darian–Smith *et al.*, 1973; Johnson *et al.*, 1973) or unmyelinated C-fiber afferents (Campero *et al.*, 2001) that respond selectively to gentle cooling stimuli and are thought to encode the sense of cooling.

A large population of afferents has a high threshold for activation and responds preferentially to intense, noxious stimuli. These afferents are called nociceptors. Nociceptors are thought to encode the sensation of pain. Unlike the innocuous receptors, nociceptors often respond to multiple stimulus modalities and are therefore polymodal. Any stimulus that can produce pain can activate nociceptors including intense heat, intense mechanical stimuli, and various chemicals.

1.2.2 **Relationship of nociceptor activity to pain sensation**

Nociceptors are often subclassified with respect to three physiological criteria:

1. the conduction velocity of their parent axon (i.e. unmyelinated C-fiber afferents versus myelinated A-fiber afferents)

2. the stimulus modalities that evoke a response (i.e. mechanical, heat, or chemical)

3. the temporal characteristics of their response to a stimulus modality (rapid versus slow response).

1.2.2.1 C-fiber mechano-heat nociceptors

Unmyelinated afferents responsive to mechanical and heat stimuli (CMHs) are probably the most commonly described class of cutaneous nociceptors. Their mechanical thresholds and heat thresholds are substantially higher than the low threshold mechanoreceptors and warm fibers described above. Most CMHs also respond to chemical stimuli and can therefore be considered polymodal. Activity in CMHs is thought to lead to the percept of burning pain.

A number of lines of evidence indicate that CMHs play an important role in heat pain sensation:

1. The response of CMH nociceptors to stimuli over the temperature range of 41–49°C correlate well with human judgments of pain over this range (Meyer and Campbell, 1981*b*). The response thresholds for nociceptor activation and heat pain sensation are around 45°C, and the responses increase in parallel with suprathreshold stimuli.

2. The long latency for heat pain sensation on the glabrous skin of the hand is consistent with the slow conduction velocity of peripheral C-fiber afferents (Campbell and LaMotte, 1983).

3. A selective block of A-fiber function does not eliminate heat pain perception for stimuli near the pain threshold (Sinclair and Hinshaw, 1950; Torebjörk and Hallin, 1973).

4. The marked fatigue in the response of CMHs to repeated presentation of a heat stimulus is correlated with a marked suppression of heat pain ratings to repeated heat stimuli (LaMotte and Campbell, 1978).

1.2.2.2 A-fiber nociceptors

A-fiber nociceptors are thought to evoke pricking pain, sharpness, and perhaps aching pain. Three distinct types of A-fiber nociceptors are apparent (Treede *et al.*, 1998). A summary of their properties is shown in Table 1.1. Type I and type II A-fiber nociceptors are typically responsive to heat, mechanical, and chemical stimuli and may therefore be referred to as AMHs or polymodal nociceptors. Another group of A-fiber nociceptors are unresponsive to heat stimuli and have been called high threshold mechanoreceptors (HTMs) by many investigators (Burgess and Perl, 1967; Perl, 1968).

The heat thresholds for type I A-fiber nociceptors are high (typically >53°C) for short duration (less than 1 sec) heat stimuli and have been mistaken for HTMs in some studies that use only short duration stimuli. However, when long duration temperature stimuli are used, the thresholds are in the mid 40–50°C range (Treede *et al.*, 1998). Type I nociceptors respond vigorously throughout a long, intense heat stimulus (e.g. 53°C for 30 sec), whereas CMHs adapt markedly to such a stimulus. Thus, the maintained pain to long duration heat stimuli is probably mediated by type I A-fiber nociceptors (Meyer and Campbell, 1981*a*). In contrast to their high heat thresholds, type I nociceptors have a relatively low mechanical threshold (5 bars). Type I nociceptors are seen in hairy and glabrous skin and have a mean conduction velocity in monkeys of 25 m/sec.

Table 1.1 Comparison of the three different types of A-fiber nociceptors

Characteristic	Type I	Type II	HTM
Heat threshold to short stimuli	High (>53°C)	Low (<47°C)	No response
Response latency to intense heat	Long (>1 sec)	Short (<1 sec)	
Response to intense heat	Slowly increasing	Rapidly adapting	
Mechanical threshold	Most are MSAs	Most are MIAs	Most are MSAs
Conduction velocity	Aδ and Aβ fibers	Aδ fibers	Aδ and Aβ fibers
Sensitization to heat injury	Yes	No	No
Location	Hairy and glabrous skin	Hairy skin	Hairy and glabrous skin
Role in pain sensation	Hyperalgesia to heat	First pain to heat	Pain to mechanical stimuli
	Pain to long duration heat	Pricking pain	

Type II A-fiber nociceptors respond well to short duration (less than 1 sec) heat stimuli with heat thresholds of around 47°C (Treede *et al.*, 1998). Their response to a maintained heat stimulus adapts quickly. In contrast to their low heat thresholds, type II nociceptors have a relatively high mechanical threshold (15 bars) and many do not respond to mechanical stimuli. Type II nociceptors are seen only in hairy skin and have a mean conduction velocity in monkeys of 14 m/sec.

In hairy skin, stepped heat stimuli evoke a double pain sensation (Lewis and Pochin, 1937; Campbell and LaMotte, 1983) — a sharp pricking sensation followed after a momentary lull by a second burning sensation (Lewis and Pochin, 1937). The latency of response to the first pain is too short to be carried by slowly conducting C-fibers. Type II A-fiber nociceptors are likely responsible for this first pain sensation. The absence of a first pain sensation to heat stimuli applied to the glabrous skin of the human hand (Campbell and LaMotte, 1983) is consistent with the absence of type II A-fiber nociceptors on the glabrous skin.

1.2.2.3 Mechanically insensitive afferents

Recently, a great deal of attention has been focused on a class of nociceptors with very high mechanical thresholds (>6 bars) (Handwerker *et al.*, 1991; Meyer *et al.*, 1991; Schmidt *et al.*, 1995). These mechanically insensitive afferents (MIAs) have also been called 'silent' or 'sleeping' nociceptors due to their propensity to become sensitized after injury (Schaible and Schmidt, 1985). The majority of type II A-fiber nociceptors are MIAs, whereas the majority of type I A-fiber nociceptors are mechanically sensitive nociceptors (MSAs). C-fiber MIAs are more responsive to chemicals than C-fiber MSAs (Davis *et al.*, 1993) and may account for some forms of chemogenice pain (Schmelz *et al.*, 2000b). Some C-fiber MIAs also respond vigorously to applications of histamine leading to the hypothesis that these afferents play an important role in itch sensation (Schmelz *et al.*, 1997). Recent evidence indicates that this population of afferents is responsive to prolonged application of intense mechanical stimuli (Schmidt *et al.*, 2000) indicating that MIAs are not necessarily unresponsive to mechanical stimuli.

1.2.3 Efferent role of nociceptors

A large area of vasodilation or flare often surrounds a cutaneous injury. This flare is thought to be caused by a peripheral axon reflex in nociceptive fibers. Activation of one branch of the nociceptor terminal by the injury leads to orthodromic action potential propagation into the parent axon as well as antidromic propagation into other branches. The antidromic action potentials lead to the release of vasoactive neuropeptides (such as substance P and CGRP) that are found in the terminals of nociceptors. Recent evidence suggests that mechanically insensitive afferents may play a major role in the development of flare, especially after chemical stimuli such as capsaicin or histamine (Schmelz *et al.*, 2000a).

1.3 **Molecular mechanisms of nociceptive signal transduction**

The functional diversity exhibited by nociceptive neurons reflects a corresponding diversity in the mechanisms by which noxious stimuli that impinge upon their terminals are transduced into membrane depolarization. The recent identification of membrane proteins responsive to noxious chemical, thermal, and mechanical stimuli by homology-based cloning or expression cloning methods (Box 1.1), coupled with the behavioral, pharmacological, and electrophysiological analysis of mice genetically engineered to lack these proteins, has allowed biologists to begin to piece together a 'rogue's gallery' of membrane proteins that endow nociceptors with their remarkably specialized sensory capabilities.

1.3.1 **Molecular detection of noxious chemical stimuli**

Tissue injury triggers the production and liberation of a diverse array of ions, nucleotides, lipids, peptides, amino acid derivatives, and proteins capable of activating nociceptors or augmenting nociceptor responses to mechanical and thermal stimuli. Electrophysiological and pharmacological studies of cultured, dissociated nociceptive neurons have revealed that certain agents (e.g. protons and capsaicin) directly depolarize nociceptive neurons by triggering the opening of cation channels permeable to sodium and/or calcium. In contrast, agents such as bradykinin and nerve growth factor act on G protein-coupled receptors and receptor tyrosine kinases, respectively, to trigger intracellular signaling cascades that in turn sensitize depolarizing cation channels to their respective physical or chemical regulators. Still other agents (eg. glutamate, acetylcholine, and adenosine triphosphate) activate both ion channels and G protein-coupled receptors to produce a spectrum of direct and indirect effects on nociceptor membrane potential. This section will describe several common mechanisms underlying the detection of noxious chemical stimuli, with a focus on just two chemical transducers that have received considerable experimental attention — vanilloid receptors and acid-sensing ion channels. For a more comprehensive treatment of this topic, readers are referred elsewhere (Wood and Docherty, 1997; Millan, 1999; McCleskey and Gold, 1999).

1.3.1.1 Ion channels gated by vanilloid compounds

Capsaicin (the hydrophobic compound that lends 'hot' peppers their pungency) is one of a family of structurally related irritant compounds that possess a homovanillic acid moiety (Szallasi and Blumberg, 1999). Upon mucosal or subcutaneous administration, vanilloid compounds bind selectively to receptor sites located on the terminals of mammalian C-fiber nociceptors, trigger the influx of sodium and calcium, and thereby initiate nociceptive transmission and ultimately pain. Following protracted vanilloid exposure, this initial pain sensation is followed by a local reduction in nociceptor sensitivity. In fact, high doses of capsaicin administered topically to human skin result in the reversible degeneration of epidermal nerve fibers (Simone et al., 1998), while in

Box 1.1 **Expression cloning**

The discovery of many ion channels involved in nociceptor signaling, including TRPV1, resulted directly from expression cloning experiments. This technique allows one to isolate the gene encoding a particular molecule with no prior knowledge of the protein's sequences or structure. All that is needed is a reliable assay for protein function and a host cell with little or no endogenous activity in this assay. The general strategy behind expression cloning is as follows:

Identify a readily-assayable function for the protein in question
↓
Identify a host cell line that does not exhibit the function
↓
Isolate sensory neuron mRNA, prepare cDNA library in pools of ~20,000 clones
↓
Express recombinant protein pools in host cells
↓
Identify pools conferring responsiveness to the desired stimulus
↓
Subdivide positive pool, retransfect and reassay
↓
Repeat until a single positive clone is identified

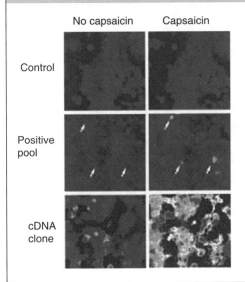

Expression cloning of TRPV1 HEK293 cells were transiently transfected with pools of a dorsal root ganglion- derived plasmid cDNA library. These cells were loaded with a fluorescent calcium-sensing dye, observed microscopically, and stimulated with capsaicin. Capsaicin evokes an increase in free cytoplasmic calcium (brighter colors) in a subset of cells transfected with the positive cDNA pool (arrows). Repeated subdivision and reassay of the positive pool results in a single clone (bottom) that confers capsaicin sensitivity upon a majority of cells in the field. Reproduced with the permission of The Nature Publishing Group.

neonatal rats, high-dose systemic capsaicin treatment produces a lifelong loss of certain small-diameter nociceptive neurons (Jancso *et al.*, 1977). These properties have led to the use of capsaicin in traditional pain therapies, as well as the modern use of vanilloid compounds for the clinical treatment of neuropathic pain (Robbins *et al.*, 1998).

An ion channel activated directly by capsaicin and other vanilloid compounds (TRPV1, previously known as VR1) has been identified and found to be selectively overexpressed in a subset of small to medium diameter nociceptive neurons (Caterina *et al.*, 1997) (see Box 1.1). The functional channel apparently consists of a tetramer of subunits, each with six putative transmembrane domains and cytoplasmic amino and carboxyl termini. Sequence analysis reveals TRPV1 to be part of the TRP family of ion channels, members of which have been implicated in a host of sensory functions in vertebrate and invertebrate species (Montell, 2001). Blockade of the vanilloid receptor with the relatively selective antagonist, capsazepine (Bevan *et al.*, 1992), or targeted deletion of the TRPV1 gene in mice (Caterina *et al.*, 2000; Davis *et al.*, 2000), eliminates vanilloid sensitivity in vitro and in vivo.

Molecular studies have further demonstrated the existence in sensory neurons of multiple TRPV1 splice variants (Schumacher *et al.*, 2000), as well as several ion channel proteins homologous to TRPV1 (Caterina *et al.*, 1999; Liedtke *et al.*, 2000; Peier *et al.*, 2002*b*). While the latter proteins do not appear to be sensitive to capsaicin or other vanilloid compounds, they may play other roles in nociception, as described below.

1.3.1.2 Ion channels gated by acid

Nociceptive neurons can also be activated in vitro or in vivo by reductions in extracellular pH, a circumstance often observed in the context of tissue injury, inflammation, or ischemia (Bevan and Geppetti, 1994). One group of ion channels implicated in acid-evoked nociception is the acid-sensing ion channel (ASIC) family of proteins (Waldmann *et al.*, 1999). At least three homologous isoforms — ASIC1 (aka ASIC, BNaC2), ASIC2 (aka BNC1, mdeg, BNaC1), and ASIC3 (aka DRASIC) — are expressed in nociceptive neurons, and multiple splice variants of ASIC1 and ASIC2 have been identified (Lingueglia *et al.*, 1997; Chen *et al.*, 1998). As their name implies, ASIC channels can be gated by reductions in pH. ASIC subunits have two transmembrane domains and can assemble in different combinations to produce homo- or heteromultimeric channels with distinct acid sensitivities, ion selectivities, and activation/ desensitization kinetics. ASIC family members are also sensitive to inhibition by amiloride, a property shared by a superfamily of related epithelial sodium channel subunits (Waldmann *et al.*, 1999).

One ASIC isoform, ASIC3, appears to be expressed exclusively in sensory neurons (Waldmann *et al.*, 1997*b*). In vitro electrophysiological recordings from isolated cardiac nociceptors indicate that these neurons are rich with ASIC3-containing ion channels (Sutherland *et al.*, 2001). Moreover, the acid sensitivity of ASIC3 can be augmented by lactate ions (Immke and McCleskey, 2001). Together, these findings suggest that ASIC3 activation might be of particular importance for the pain associated with cardiac ischemia. Disruption of the ASIC3 gene in mice results in a loss of large-amplitude, rapidly desensitizing acid-evoked current responses in cultured nociceptive neurons (Price *et al.*, 2001). Mice lacking this protein also exhibit less mechanical hyperalgesia than wild-type mice following the injection of acid into skeletal muscle. However, cutaneous sensitivity to acid appears unaltered in these animals, suggesting the involvement of other ASIC or non-ASIC proton transduction mechanisms.

Another potential site of proton action is the vanilloid receptor, which can be activated directly by protons and whose capsaicin sensitivity can also be augmented by modest reductions in pH (Petersen and LaMotte, 1993; Tominaga *et al.*, 1998). Nociceptive neurons derived from mice lacking TRPV1 exhibit reduced sensitivity to a pH 5 stimulus in both the isolated skin-nerve preparation and in dissociated neuronal cultures (Caterina *et al.*, 2000; Davis *et al.*, 2000). The importance of TRPV1 to acid-evoked nociception in vivo, however, has yet to be determined.

Together, vanilloid receptors and ASICs illustrate several recurring themes in nociceptive signal transduction. First, nociceptors often express multiple members of an ion channel family, with certain members being expressed at much higher levels in these neurons than in other cells of the body. Such specificity might provide a basis for the development of drugs with relative selectivity towards nociceptive neurons. Second, alternative combinations of homologous ion channel subunits produce channels with distinct functional properties. Third, as described in more detail below, stimuli of different modalities can converge upon the same ion channel protein to produce additive or supra-additive responses. Together, these features endow the nociceptor terminal with finely tuned and kinetically controlled responsiveness to its environment and may provide part of the molecular basis for nociceptor heterogeneity and functional plasticity.

1.3.1.3 G protein-coupled receptors (GPCRs) involved in nociceptive signal transduction

As described above, many of the chemical substances that bathe the nociceptor terminal following tissue injury or inflammation modulate neuronal activity through their actions on 'metabotropic' receptors coupled to intracellular, heterotrimeric, guanyl nucleotide regulatory proteins (G proteins). Examples of such substances include the peptide, bradykinin (Steranka *et al.*, 1988); the lipid, prostaglandin E_2 (Ferreira *et al.*, 1978); and even certain proteases (Vergnolle *et al.*, 2001). Occupancy of GPCRs triggers the dissociation of GDP from the alpha subunit of the G protein heterotrimer, the binding of GTP, and the dissociation of the alpha subunit from the beta and gamma subunits (Gilman, 1987). As a consequence, the activated alpha subunit and beta/gamma dimer each go on to interact with a diverse array of downstream target proteins that include ion channels, enzymes such as adenylyl cyclase and phospholipase C, and other signaling molecules. The resulting activation of protein kinases A and C (PKA, PKC) and release of second messengers such as cyclic adenosine monophosphate (cAMP), Ca^{2+} ions, prostaglandin E_2 (PGE_2), and leukotrienes can exert profound effects on the ion channels expressed at nociceptor terminals. Furthermore, it should be noted that while many substances (e.g. bradykinin, PGE_2) increase nociceptor excitability when they bind their respective GPCRs, other substances that act on GPCRs (e.g. opiate peptides, cannabinoids) can inhibit nociceptor excitability and blunt pain sensation (Pasternak, 1993; Calignano et al., 2000).

1.3.1.4 Neurotrophin and cytokine signaling at the nociceptor terminal

Among the most important regulators of nociceptor excitability are the neurotrophin proteins. These polypeptides fall into two main classes — the nerve growth factor (NGF) family (NGF, BDNF, NT3, NT4/5) and the glial cell line-derived neurotrophin (GDNF) family (glial cell line-derived neurotrophic factor, artemein, persephrin, neurturin) (Huang and Reichardt, 2001; Airaksinen and Saarma, 2002). Each of the two classes of neurotrophins binds to a corresponding class of multi-subunit cell-surface neurotrophin receptor proteins. The resulting activation of tyrosine kinase domains on these receptors leads to the coordinate stimulation of several intracellular enzymes, including phospholipase C and phosphatidylinositol 3-kinase. Through these signaling pathways, neurotrophins play critical roles in the development and survival of nociceptive neurons, as described in later chapters. In addition, however, neurotrophins can acutely enhance nociceptor excitability and nociceptive signal transduction (Shu and Mendell, 1999). Cytokines of the interleukin family, whose receptors activate intracellular signaling molecules of the JAK/STAT pathway, can also acutely sensitize nociceptive neurons (Opree and Kress, 2000).

1.3.2 Transduction of painful thermal stimuli

1.3.2.1 Ion channels gated by heat

The characteristic activation thresholds (43–46°C) exhibited by C-fiber nociceptors and the type II A-fiber nociceptors, and the slightly higher threshold (53°C) exhibited by type I A-fiber nociceptors suggest the existence of specific and distinct transduction mechanisms for the detection of noxious heat. Consistent with this prediction, electrophysiological studies of cultured, dissociated nociceptive neurons have revealed the existence of at least two populations of non-selective cationic channels in a subset of these neurons that can be activated by increasing ambient temperature to >43°C and >52°C, respectively (Cesare and McNaughton, 1996; Reichling and Levine, 1997; Nagy and Rang, 1999).

Whole-cell voltage clamp studies have revealed a strong correlation between 'moderate threshold' (~43°C) heat sensitivity and sensitivity to capsaicin (Kirschstein et al., 1997). One likely explanation for this correlation comes from the observation that the vanilloid receptor, TRPV1, can be activated not only by capsaicin or protons, but alternatively by heat at temperatures greater than ~43°C (Caterina et al., 1997; Tominaga et al., 1998). Further evidence for the involvement of TRPV1 in heat nociception comes from studies of mice in which the TRPV1 gene has been disrupted (Caterina et al., 2000). Examination of nociceptors in skin-nerve explants derived from TRPV1 null mice reveals a partial reduction in the proportion of heat-sensitive C-fibers, though not a complete elimination of such units. Similarly, mice lacking TRPV1 exhibit partially reduced behavioral withdrawal responses to heating of the paw or tail. Together, these results suggest that TRPV1 participates in acute thermal nociception, but that additional heat transduction mechanisms must exist in nociceptive neurons.

One protein that might be responsible for some of the 'TRPV1-independent' heat transduction is TRPV2 (previously known as VRL-1 or GRC) — a TRPV1 homolog highly expressed by a subset of medium- to large-diameter neurons that can be activated by temperatures exceeding 52°C (Caterina *et al.*, 1999). Given its anatomical localization and relatively high activation threshold, this molecule might account for the thermal responsiveness of type I AMH nociceptors. While two other TRPV1 homologs — TRPV3 (Peier *et al.*, 2002*b*; Smith *et al.*, 2002; Xu *et al.*, 2002) and TRPV4 (previously known as OTRPC4 or VR-OAC) (Guler *et al.*, 2002) — can also be activated by heat, both exhibit a threshold for activation (~34°C) below the noxious range, making their potential contributions to thermal nociception unclear.

1.3.2.2 Ion channels gated by cold

Cold, like heat, can produce either an innocuous thermal sensation or pain. At present, it remains unclear whether these differences reflect multiple transduction mechanisms or differential expression of the same cold-transducing molecules among classes of primary afferents. Electrophysiological studies of cultured primary afferent neurons have revealed a potentially complex ionic basis for cold transduction; both depolarizing currents that are activated by cold (Reid and Flonta, 2001*b*, 2002) and hyperpolarizing currents that are inhibited by cold (Reid and Flonta, 2001*a*; Viana *et al.*, 2002) have been described.

Several ion channels expressed in sensory neurons are gated by decreases in temperature. Among these are amiloride-sensitive sodium channels of the ENaC family, which can be activated by cold (Askwith *et al.*, 2001); potassium 'leak' channels such as TREK1, whose opening is inhibited by cold (Maingret *et al.*, 2000); and two non-selective cation channels of the TRP family, TRPM8 (CMR-1) (McKemy *et al.*, 2002; Peier *et al.*, 2002a) and TRPA1 (ANKTM1) (Story *et al.*, 2003). Whereas TRPM8 is first activated by temperatures in the innocuous cool range, temperatures below ~22°C are reportedly necessary to activate TRPA1. These findings suggest that TRPM8 and TRPA1 may contribute differentially to the perception of painful versus non-painful cold. However, some investigators have failed to observe cold activation of TRPA1 (Jordt *et al.*, 2004). Both TRPM8 and TRPA1 can alternatively be activated by exposure to certain chemical agents. The cooling mimetic agent menthol can selectively activate TRPM8 (McKemy *et al.*, 2002; Peier *et al.*, 2002*a*). In contrast, two pungent compounds, mustard oil and cinnamon aldehyde, are capable of activating TRPA1 (Bandell *et al.*, 2004; Jordt *et al.*, 2004).

1.3.3 Transduction of painful mechanical stimuli

Intense mechanical stimuli such as pinching or pressing the skin are examples of perhaps the most familiar cause of pain. Despite this fact, relatively little is known about the molecular mechanisms underlying nociceptive mechanotransduction. In a subset of cultured sensory neurons, the direct application of mechanical force evokes non-selective cationic transmembrane currents (McCarter *et al.*, 1999). A number of candidate mechanosensory ion channels have been identified, including members of the ASIC (Garcia–Anoveros and Corey, 1996; Price *et al.*, 2000, 2001), TRP (Strotmann *et al.*, 2000; Birder *et al.*, 2002), and TREK (Maingret *et al.*, 1999) families. The notion that these channels participate in mechanosensation has arisen predominantly from the study of recombinant molecules in heterologous expression systems or from the genetic analysis of touch perception in mice and invertebrate species. It has yet to be determined, however, whether these channels participate in noxious mechanosensation in mammals. Indeed, capsaicin-sensitive neurons exhibit mechanosensory properties distinct from those of capsaicin-insensitive neurons (Drew *et al.*, 2002), suggesting that nociceptive and nonnociceptive neurons might possess distinct mechanosensory machinery.

1.4 Beyond depolarization: spike initiation, action potential propagation, and neurotransmitter release

Neurotransmission by primary afferent nociceptors requires not only that noxious stimuli are converted into an electrical signal (i.e. membrane depolarization), but also that this information is transmitted to the spinal cord. This process requires several additional steps generally referred to as spike initiation, spike propagation, and transmitter release. Each of these steps requires a number of distinct ion channels precisely positioned at discrete sites throughout the plasma membrane. The interrelationship between cytoarchitecture and ion channel composition or properties of nociceptors results in an extraordinary capacity to encode the spatial, temporal, and intensity properties of noxious stimuli. Importantly, the molecules that mediate post-transduction neurotransmission serve as targets both for the accentuation of pain by tissue injury and the pharmacological treatment of such pain.

1.4.1 Spike initiation

Because of the relative inaccessibility of primary afferent nerve endings, our understanding of the processes underlying spike initiation is far from complete. That said, a combination of pharmacological interventions and creative experimental paradigms have shed considerable light on this question in the last several years.

1.4.1.1 The impact of architecture

One of the distinct features of primary afferent nociceptors is that they terminate in 'free' nerve endings with peripheral terminals that are devoid of specialized cell types. Electron micrographic reconstruction of peripheral terminals indicates that these nerve endings are free of even perineurium for up to 300 mm and terminate in small arbors with a number of discrete termination sites (Heppelmann *et al.*, 1990).

These arbors may spread over an area of 150 mm. Furthermore, the branches of these arbors appear 'beaded'. The presence of mitochondria and vesicles in the 'beads' suggests that they serve as sites for transmitter release and/or initiation of generator potentials.

1.4.1.2 Active or passive conduction in peripheral terminals

It is generally assumed that generator potentials are passively conducted along peripheral processes towards sites of spike initiation. Such a separation between sites of stimulus transduction and spike initiation has been demonstrated for other sensory neurons (Lowenstein, 1959; Firestein et al., 1990). However, several factors suggest the existence of active conduction at nociceptor terminals. First, the peculiar geometry of nociceptor terminals greatly limits the theoretical distance over which passive conduction would be expected to occur. Second, focal stimulation within the receptive field of a single neuron may result in a relatively large area of flare. One explanation for this phenomenon, termed the axon reflex, is discussed above (Lewis, 1937). The existence of the axon reflex implies that there are multiple spike initiation zones within a single peripheral arbor. Third, detailed mapping of peripheral receptive fields indicate that a single nociceptive afferent may have several discrete receptive fields or areas of sensitivity within a receptive field. One of the most extreme examples of multiple spike initiation sites in a single peripheral arbor is found in the Aδ-fibers that innervate the cornea (Tanelian and Brunson, 1994). These fibers terminate in processes that run in parallel to the surface of the cornea and have receptive fields that encompass the length of the terminal process suggesting that virtually the entire peripheral process is capable of supporting active conduction. Elegant studies involving the direct recording of spontaneous and antidromically evoked activity in the peripheral terminals of corneal afferents have revealed that this is indeed the case (Brock et al., 1998; Carr et al., 2002).

1.4.1.3 Ion channels mediating spike initiation

There are two main classes of ion channels that underlie spike initiation and propagation: voltage-gated Na^+ channels and voltage-gated Ca^{2+} channels. The association of voltage-gated Na^+ channels with spike initiation has been demonstrated in species across several phyla. Voltage-gated Na^+ channels consist of an α-subunit which contains the voltage sensor, inactivation gate, and channel pore (Cantrell and Catterall 2001) and two β-subunits which influence the biophysical properties of the channel, density, and distribution of the channels in the plasma membrane (Isom 2001). Ten α-subunits and four β-subunits have been identified (Cantrell and Catterall 2001; Yu et al., 2003).

The different α-subunits have different biophysical and pharmacological properties and are differentially expressed throughout the body. One of the most common ways to distinguish among different Na^+ channels is on the basis of their sensitivity to the toxin tetrodotoxin (TTX). Two of the α-subunits, $Na_V1.8$ (previously known as SNS, PN3) and $Na_V1.9$ (previously known as SNS2, PN5), are resistant to TTX at concentrations as high as 10 mM; one of the α-subunits is relatively insensitive to TTX ($Na_V1.5$ is blocked with an IC50 that ranges between 0.1 and 1 mM TTX); the remaining α-subunits are exquisitely sensitive to TTX (IC_{50s} in the low nM range). Sensory neurons express at least six of the ten α-subunits (Black et al., 1996).

Voltage-gated Na^+ channel α-subunits and β-subunits are differentially distributed both within and among sensory neurons. For example, TTX-resistant channels are present in the cell bodies of a subpopulation of sensory neurons at densities sufficient to underlie spiking, while in the same neurons, TTX will completely prevent axonal propagation of action potentials (Ritter and Mendell 1992). The TTX-resistant channels $Na_V1.8$ and $Na_V1.9$ are preferentially expressed among sensory neurons with a small cell body diameter, a property of sensory neurons that tend to give rise to slowly conducting axons. The $\beta1$-subunit is expressed in higher densities among neurons with an intermediate to large cell body diameter (Oh et al., 1995).

The precise anatomical distribution of Na^+ channel subunits in the peripheral terminals of nociceptive afferents is far from clear. That said, it is known that $Na_V1.7$ is preferentially expressed in the terminals of sprouting axons (Toledo et al., 1995), that $Na_V1.8$ is detectable in the terminals' afferents innervating skin (Coward et al., 2000), and that $Na_V1.9$ is distributed throughout putative nociceptive afferents (Fjell et al., 2000).

The intrathecal (IT) administration of antisense oligodeoxynucleotides (ODNs) to reduce the expression of channels of interest also has been used to assess the presence and function of specific channels in nociceptive afferent terminals. Evidence based on this approach indicates that $Na_V1.8$ is present and functional in the peripheral terminals of nociceptive afferents, that this channel is likely to be involved in spike initiation, and that it contributes to the determination of nociceptor mechanical threshold (Khasar et al., 1998).

Further insight into the roles of voltage-gated sodium channel subtypes in nociceptor spike initiation has come from the direct corneal afferent recording studies of Brock and colleagues (1998). In their preparation, action potentials were recorded with suction electrodes as nerve terminal impulses from the terminal fibres innervating the cornea following antidromic electrical stimulation. Locally applied TTX had a small influence on the shape of nerve terminal impulses (NTIs), suggesting a small contribution of TTX-sensitive channels to NTIs; spontaneously evoked NTIs were largely resistant to TTX, even at relatively high concentrations. This observation suggests that TTX-resistant channels underlie spike initiation in corneal nociceptive afferents (Brock et al., 1998). Of note, there is also evidence for spike initiation in the central terminals of nociceptive afferents (Sluka et al., 1995), which also appears to depend, at least in part, on TTX-resistant Na^+ channels (Gu and MacDermott, 1997).

The second major class of ion channel known to underlie spike initiation is that of voltage-gated Ca^{2+} channels. However, while activation of voltage-gated Ca^{2+} channels appears to underlie peripheral transmitter release from nociceptive afferents, indirect evidence suggests these channels do not underlie spike initiation. The line of reasoning behind this suggestion is as follows. First, while there is evidence that opioids influence excitable membrane properties through an action on two classes of ion channel (voltage-gated Ca^{2+} channels and inwardly rectifying K^+ channels (K_{ATP} and K_{IR})), they appear to only inhibit voltage-gated Ca^{2+} channels in sensory neurons (Schroeder *et al.*, 1991). Second, opioid receptor expression among sensory neurons is, in general, restricted to putative nociceptive afferents (Taddese *et al.*, 1995). Third, it is possible to induce neurogenic inflammation following antidromic activation of afferent axons. And fourth, it is possible to inhibit neurogenic inflammation with peripherally administered opioids (Shakhanbeh and Lynn, 1993). Importantly, peripherally administered opioids have no influence on mechanical or thermal threshold in the absence of inflammation suggesting that activation of voltage-gated Ca^{2+} channels, while present in peripheral terminals, have little influence on spike initiation (Shakhanbeh and Lynn, 1993). Consistent with this suggestion, non-specific block of voltage-gated Ca^{2+} channels with Cd^{2+} has little influence on spontaneously evoked and/or antidromically conducting action potentials in peripheral terminals of nociceptive afferents in the cornea (Brock *et al.*, 1998).

In summary, while a number of different voltage-gated Na^+ and Ca^{2+} channels are present in the peripheral terminals of nociceptive afferents, TTX-resistant voltage-gated Na^+ channels, most likely $Na_V1.8$, are primarily responsible for spike initiation.

1.4.1.4 Modulation of spike initiation

The modulation of spike initiation is quite complex. This complexity reflects the multitude of channels present in sensory neurons and the number of ways in which these channels influence one another. A detailed list of the various voltage- and Ca^{2+}-gated channels present in sensory neurons may be found elsewhere (Gold 2001). This list includes a number of isoforms of voltage-gated K^+ channels, Ca^{2+}-gated K^+ and Cl^- channels, anamolous rectification channels I_{KIR} and I_h, and leak channels such as the two pore K^+ channels TRAAK and TREK-1, in addition to those discussed above. Specific channel subtypes involved in the modulation of spike initiation have yet to be identified. However, pharmacological experiments have implicated several broad classes of channel.

Both 4-aminopyradine (4-AP) and tetraethyamonium (TEA) sensitive ion channels appear to control spike initiation (Kirchhoff *et al.*, 1992) as both compounds, applied to peripheral arbors in the skin nerve preparation (Box 1.2), induced spontaneous activity in a subpopulation of isolated units. This observation suggests that tonic activity in members of both channel types are involved in establishing the resting membrane potential. Biophysical properties of members of both channel types indicate that these channels are active over a voltage range corresponding to the resting membrane potential (Gold *et al.*, 1996a). Furthermore, inflammatory mediator-induced increases in neuronal excitability appear to reflect, at least in part, suppression of a delayed rectifier type of K^+ current (Nicol *et al.*, 1997).

A major limitation of these observations, however, is that neither 4-AP, nor TEA are very specific. That is, 4-AP blocks at least two types of inactivating or A-type of voltage-gated K^+ channel in sensory neurons (Gold *et al.*, 1996b), while TEA not only blocks delayed rectifier types of voltage-gated K^+ channels, but it also blocks one class of

Box 1.2 **Single unit recordings**

Investigators have studied cutaneous sensibility by recording from single nerve fibers in different species, including man. Stimuli are applied to the receptive field (i.e. area of the tissue responsive to the applied stimulus) of single fibers, and the characteristics of the neural response are noted. This analysis is particularly powerful when combined with correlative psychophysical studies, in which identical stimuli are rated by human subjects.

Teased fiber technique in anesthetized animals. The peripheral nerve innervating the tissue of interest is dissected from connective tissue and the epineurium and perineurium opened longitudinally over a distance of about 1 cm. A small bundle of nerve fibers is cut at the proximal end of this opening and rotated onto a dissection platform. Under a dissection microscope, the bundle is teased apart using jewelers' forceps, and small filaments containing 1–20 viable axons are placed onto an electrode for extracellular recordings. Neural signals are differentially amplified and filtered. High-quality recordings from single C-fiber afferents can be maintained for hours (Campbell *et al.*, 1979).

Microneurography in awake humans. Insulated tungsten microelectrodes are inserted through the skin into the peripheral nerve of interest to obtain multi-unit recordings from afferents innervating the skin (Torebjörk, 1974). Light pinching of the skin is used to identify the region on the skin over which receptive fields of the multiple units are located. Since the action potential waveforms from the multiple units are quite similar in shape for this preparation, a 'marking' technique is used to evaluate the response properties of single fibers. Two electrodes are inserted about 1 cm apart into the skin within the area of the receptive fields and stimulated at a low frequency (e.g. 0.25 Hz) to obtain a stable latency of the C-fiber afferents. When stimulation of the receptive field with mechanical, heat, or chemical stimuli leads to an evoked response in the fiber, the latency in response to the electrical stimulation increases.

An example of the use of the marking technique to identify a response of C-fiber afferents is shown in Fig. 1.2. The top panel shows the response to electrical stimulation via a pair of intracutaneous electrodes. The three C-fibers (labeled *a, b, c*) that exceeded the upper (u.t.) and lower (l.t.) threshold levels are highlighted. In the bottom panel the response of these three C-fibers to successive electrical stimulation at 3-second intervals is shown (ordered from top to bottom). Mechanical stimulation of the skin with von Frey probes (at time indicated by the horizontal arrows on the left) produced a marked increase in latency for fiber *b* at 15 mN force and fiber *c* at 30 mN force. The amount of latency shift is proportional to the magnitude of the response, and thus a more intense stimulus (e.g. 2.6 N) produced a greater latency shift. Fiber *a* did not respond to the mechanical stimuli. (Reproduced with permission from Schmidt *et al.*, 1995.)

Box 1.2 **Single unit recordings** *(continued)*

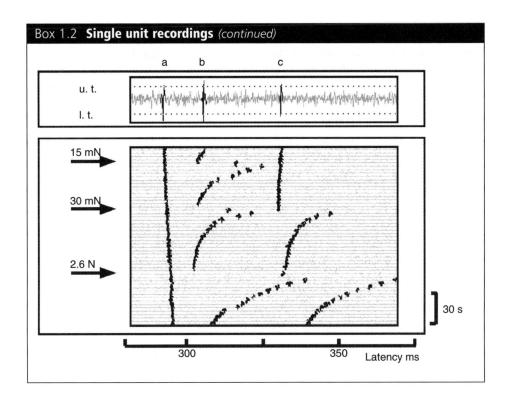

Ca^{2+}-dependent K$^+$ channel, K$_{ATP}$ channels, and I$_{KIR}$ channels. Thus, considerably more work is needed to identify which of the many 4-AP and TEA sensitive channels are involved in the modulation of spike initiation.

Indirect evidence based on nerve injury induced changes in excitability implicates two other channel types in the modulation of spike initiation. One channel is a K$^+$ leak channel and the second is an anomolously rectifying non-selective cation channel (I$_h$). The leak channel is thought to drive the hyperpolarizing phase of action potential inducing membrane oscillations that develop following nerve injury (Amir *et al.*, 1999) suggesting that, at least under certain conditions, this channel is involved in the determination of action potential threshold. Evidence for I$_h$ channels comes from the observation that at least two of the four channel subtypes known to underlie I$_h$ (i.e. HCN channels) are up-regulated following nerve injury (Chaplan *et al.*, 2001). More importantly, application of the I$_h$ channel blocker ZD 7288 to spontaneously active injured neurons abolishes spontaneous activity. Because I$_h$ is normally activated following membrane hyperpolarizing below resting membrane potential, it is generally believed that this current plays a larger role in determination of inter-spike interval than it does in determination of action potential threshold. However, the nerve injury results suggest that this channel may contribute to spike threshold under certain conditions.

1.4.2 **Spike propagation/action potential conduction**

There are two channel types necessary for spike propagation under 'normal' conditions — TTX-sensitive voltage-gated Na$^+$ channels and a delayed rectifier type of K$^+$ channel. Na$^+$ channels drive membrane depolarization and K$^+$ channels drive membrane hyperpolarization of sufficient magnitude and duration to enable the Na$^+$ channel to recover from inactivation and thereby enable subsequent spike propagation (Hille, 1992). 'Normal' is emphasized here because recent observations indicate that under pathophysiological conditions, axonal conduction may become dependent on TTX-resistant voltage-gated Na$^+$ channels (Gold, *et al.*, 2003). Because axonal conduction velocity is not a static property and may change in the presence of inflammation (see below) or simply as a function of the timing between successive action potentials (a phenomena utilized by single unit electrophysiologists in receptive field mapping of isolated units) (see Box 1.2), it is also clear that there are channels involved in the modulation of spike propagation. Thus, as with spike initiation, there are ion channels that are necessary and sufficient to mediate spike propagation and there are channels involved in the modulation of various aspects of this process.

1.4.2.1 Channels necessary for spike propagation

Researchers have employed both anatomical and pharmacological approaches in order to identify specific Na$^+$ and K$^+$ channels involved in spike propagation. As stated above, conduction in a 'normal' axon is dependent on TTX-sensitive voltage-gated Na$^+$ channels. The limited data available indicates that the specific Na$^+$ channels present in peripheral axons include Na$_V$1.6 in myelinated axons (Caldwell *et al.*, 2000), Na$_V$1.9 in unmyelinated axons (Fjell *et al.*, 2000), and a few thinly myelinated axons and Na$_V$1.7 in both myelinated and unmyelinated axons. Na$_V$1.6 is located in the nodal region of myelinated axons and is therefore likely to underlie salutatory conduction in these afferents. The voltage-gated K$^+$ currents that have been demonstrated in axonal membranes include K$_V$1.1 and K$_V$1.2 (Rasband *et al.*, 1998; Fjell *et al.*, 2000). These channels are localized to the juxtanodal region of myelinated axons, and are therefore likely to contribute to membrane repolarization following the action potential. Interestingly, these K$^+$ channel subtypes are of the A-type, or inactivating, variety, and therefore are more likely to be involved in the control in inter-spike interval (see below) than the more slowly activating, delayed rectifier type of channel traditionally believed to control membrane repolarization (Rudy, 1988). The delayed rectifier type of channels driving the downstroke of the axonal action potential have yet to be identified.

1.4.2.2 Modulation of spike propagation

Electrophysiological evidence indicates that at least two channel types influence axonal conduction — a 4-AP sensitive channel and a channel underlying the non-selective anamolous rectifier current, Ih. The 4-AP sensitive channels appear to mediate a prolonged hyperpolarization that follows the action potential, consistent with a role in establishing the inter-spike interval (Honmou *et al.*, 1994). The Ih channels, which are selectively blocked by ZD 7288, appear to influence conduction velocity such that activation of these channels mitigates use-dependent slowing of axonal conduction velocity (Takigawa *et al.*, 1998).

Indirect evidence suggests roles for several other channels in the modulation of axonal conduction. For example, anatomical evidence indicates the Ca^{2+}-activated K^+ channels, SK1 and SK4, are present in peripheral axons (Boettger *et al.*, 2002). Because these channels normally limit action potential burst duration, their presence is likely to be involved in sculpting the specific pattern out of activity arising from the afferents in which they are present. Single-channel recording from isolated peripheral nerves indicates that high threshold voltage-gated Ca^{2+} channels are present in axonal membranes (Quasthoff *et al.*, 1995). Furthermore, Ca^{2+} imaging studies indicate that the density of these channels is sufficient to produce significant elevations in axonal concentration of intracellular Ca^{2+} (Mayer *et al.*, 1999). Thus, while the direct contribution of these channels to spike initiation and propagation is minimal, high threshold voltage-gated Ca^{2+} channels may influence conduction indirectly through their influence on Ca^{2+}-dependent K^+ channels. A Ca^{2+}-independent Cl^- channel is also present in sensory neurons, although the function of this channel has yet to be determined (Strupp and Grafe, 1991).

Finally, TTX-resistant Na^+ channels also appear to be present in peripheral nerves under normal conditions (Quasthoff *et al.*, 1995). While these channels are not present in densities high enough to support axonal conduction directly, they may effect conduction indirectly through an influence on Ca^{2+} influx and, subsequently, Ca^{2+}-dependent K channels.

1.4.3 Transmitter release

The last critical step for afferents in the rapid transmission of nociceptive information is the release of neurotransmitter at central synapses. The importance of this step is highlighted by the fact that pre-synaptic inhibition of transmitter release is a mechanism critical for both endogenous and exogenous pain inhibition. Furthermore, given the relatively recent appreciation for the importance of the peripheral release of transmitter both in physiological and pathophysiological processes (Sluka *et al.*, 1995), identification of the ion channels mediating such release is also an important line of investigation. Finally, it should be understood that whilst there is a growing list of receptor/transmitter systems that appear to influence the release of transmitter from primary afferent neurons (Huang *et al.*, 2003; Lao and Marvizon, 2005), discussion of these pathways is beyond the scope of this book.

1.4.3.1 Necessary channels for transmitter release

Release of transmitter from neuronal terminals requires an increase in the concentration of free cytosolic Ca^{2+}. Voltage-gated Ca^{2+} channels are a major source of this Ca^{2+} in many neurons, including sensory neurons. Like voltage-gated Na^+ channels, voltage-gated Ca^{2+} channels consist of a large α1-subunit that contains the machinery necessary for activation and ion permeation, and three or four ancillary subunits that influence expression and gating (Ertel *et al.*, 2000). These subunits include an intracellular β-subunit, a transmembrane disulfide-linked α2δ-subunit, and, in skeletal muscle, a γ-subunit. Voltage-gated Ca^{2+} channels are critical for transmitter release from primary afferent neurons (see below). RT-PCR analysis indicates that at least eight of the ten known α1-subunits are present in sensory ganglia as well as the α2δ- and β3-subunits (Martin *et al.*, 2002).

Functionally, this translates to four major currents that can be distinguished on the basis of pharmacological sensitivity and biophysical properties. The conotoxin sensitive (or N-type) current is, in general, the most prevalent in sensory neurons, accounting for ~50% of the high threshold current in sensory neurons (Scroggs and Fox, 1992). Dihydropyridine sensitive (or L-type) currents account for another ~27% of high threshold current. The remainder is either sensitive to agitoxin (P-type) or insensitive to any of the three primary channel blockers (R/Q type). Low threshold, T-type currents are also present in sensory neurons, and while not directly implicated in spike initiation, propagation, or transmitter release, these channels have been shown to underlie after-depolarizations (White *et al.*, 1989), and therefore may contribute to burst activity.

Each of these channel types is differentially distributed among subpopulations of sensory neurons such that in some subpopulations, L-type currents predominate, while in others, T-type currents are present in an exceptionally high density (Scroggs and Fox, 1992). While it is generally believed that N-type Ca^{2+} channels constitute the channel subtype primarily responsible for transmitter release, one intriguing observation indicates that the channel mediating transmitter release may vary depending on the mode of stimulation. That is, agonist evoked transmitter release may utilize N-type channels, while generic depolarization, with high extracellular K^+-evoked release depends on the activation of L-type channels (Evans *et al.*, 1996).

1.4.3.2 Modulation of transmitter release

As with spike initiation and propagation, the mechanisms controlling transmitter release are also subject to modulation. As mentioned above, TTX-resistant Na^+ channels may contribute to the modulation (i.e. facilitation) of transmitter release under certain conditions (Gu and MacDermott, 1997). There is also evidence for the involvement of Ca^{2+}-dependent K^+ channels in the control of transmitter release. Activation of these channels results in the inhibition of transmitter release in CNS neurons (Hu *et al.*, 2001).

What is clear from the preceding discussion is that targeting of ion channels to specific membrane regions is highly controlled. Channels involved in spike initiation must be located close to sites of stimulus transduction. The density and distribution of channels involved in spike propagation is critical to the successful conduction of action potentials. And the density and distribution of voltage-gated Ca^{2+} channels is critical to the adequate and appropriate release of transmitter. While many of the molecules involved in the process of shuttling ion channels to specific sites and anchoring them in the membrane at those sites have been identified (Peles and Salzer, 2000), a discussion of this topic is beyond the scope of the present chapter.

1.4.4 Spike invasion in the cell body

Our discussion of the mechanisms underlying spike initiation, propagation, and transmitter release lead us past a discussion of an interesting, yet poorly understood phenomena — spike invasion of the cell body. Given the anatomy of the sensory ganglia with the presence of the T-junction, there is no need for spike invasion of the cell body. Indeed, there are examples in which high levels of afferent activity result in the failure of spike invasion. Two lines of evidence, however, suggest that spike invasion is important for the control of neuronal excitability. First, spike invasion may result in the activation of other neurons within the ganglia (Amir and Devor, 2000). Such co-activation (referred to as cross-talk) seems to involve a diffusible messenger that has yet to be identified. Tackykinins do not appear to underlie this phenomenon, although there is evidence for both the release of substance P within sensory ganglia (Matsuka et al., 2001) and the activation of sensory neurons in response to the application of this mediator (Hutcheon et al., 1993). Second, an increase in the concentration of intracellular Ca^{2+} has been shown to couple to transcriptional changes (Fields et al., 1997). Thus, spike invasion of the cell body may be another mechanism whereby nociceptive afferents obtain information from and respond to changes in their environment (see Fig. 1.1).

1.5 Molecular mechanisms of inflammatory hyperalgesia

1.5.1 Hyperalgesia and sensitization

An injury to tissue and subsequent inflammation leads to an enhanced pain state called hyperalgesia. Hyperalgesia is characterized by a leftward shift of the stimulus–response function that relates magnitude of pain to stimulus intensity. The threshold for pain is lowered and the pain to suprathreshold stimuli is increased. Allodynia corresponds to the lowering of pain threshold such that a stimulus modality which normally does not produce pain (e.g. light touch) becomes painful. The neurophysiological correlate of hyperalgesia is sensitization. Sensitization is characterized by a leftward shift of the stimulus–response function that relates magnitude of response to stimulus intensity. Sensitization of primary afferent nociceptors is thought to account for the primary hyperalgesia that occurs at and near the site of injury. Sensitization in the central nervous system is thought to account for the secondary hyperalgesia that occurs in the uninjured tissue surrounding the site of injury (Raja et al., 1999).

Primary hyperalgesia appears to be principally due to sensitization of primary afferent nociceptors. For example, a marked hyperalgesia to heat stimuli develops within minutes of a burn injury to the skin. A burn injury also produces marked sensitization of A-fiber and C-fiber nociceptors to heat (Meyer and Campbell, 1981a; LaMotte et al., 1983). Both A-fiber and C-fiber nociceptors become sensitized to mechanical stimuli after injection of inflammatory mediators into their receptive field. The greatest changes in threshold are seen for mechanically insensitive afferents (MIAs), which can be unresponsive to mechanical stimuli before inflammation but markedly sensitized to mechanical stimuli afterwards (Davis et al., 1993).

1.5.2 Inflammation alters the chemical milieu of the nociceptor terminal

As described above, inflammation leads to the dynamic production, release, and destruction of numerous chemical substances capable of producing spontaneous nociceptor firing, shifting the thresholds for nociceptor activation and increasing the responsiveness of these neurons to normally noxious thermal and mechanical stimuli. Examples include the release of protons by infiltrating leukocytes undergoing anaerobic metabolism (Bevan and Geppetti, 1994), the production and release of prostaglandins from membrane phospholipids following injury-mediated induction of cyclooxygenase (Ferreira et al., 1978), and the injury-induced cleavage of the peptide, bradykinin, from its circulating precursor, kininogen (Steranka et al., 1988). The importance of chemical mediators to inflammatory hyperalgesia has been illustrated by numerous studies demonstrating that genetic or pharmacological elimination or antagonism of these substances reduces hyperalgesia produced in response to chemically distinct initiators of inflammation such as carrageenan (Van Arman et al., 1970; Koltzenburg et al., 1999) or uric acid (Van Arman et al., 1970; Steranka et al., 1988). The study of inflammatory hyperalgesia has been facilitated by the fact that the early events in this process can be recapitulated in vitro via the administration of individual chemical substances or a cocktail of such substances to either the isolated skin-nerve preparation (Handwerker and Reeh, 1991) or cultured nociceptive neurons (Baccaglini and Hogan, 1983).

1.5.3 Inflammation augments nociceptive signal transduction

Changes in the subcellular localization, expression level, or excitability of ion channels involved in nociceptive signal transduction represent a major mechanism underlying inflammatory thermal and mechanical hyperalgesia. One particularly instructive example of how inflammation can augment nociceptive ion channels comes from studies of TRPV1. The thermal hyperalgesia that typically follows the subcutaneous administration of complete Freund's adjuvant, carrageenan, NGF, mustard oil, or bradykinin to the mouse hindpaw is essentially abolished in mice lacking TRPV1 (Caterina et al., 2000; Davis et al., 2000; Chuang et al., 2001), suggesting its intimate involvement in this phenomenon. Mechanistic studies conducted in vivo and in vitro have revealed that inflammation affects TRPV1 activity in multiple, distinct ways:

1. Protons interact directly with TRPV1, and thereby allosterically sensitize this molecule to heat. Interestingly, this effect appears to be independent of the direct gating of TRPV1 by protons (Tominaga et al., 1998; Jordt et al., 2000).

2. PGE_2 binds to a G protein-coupled receptor to trigger the activation of adenylyl cyclase and cAMP production. The consequent activation of PKA results in phosphorylation of the cytoplasmic domains of TRPV1, rendering the channel more sensitive to vanilloid compounds and other noxious stimuli (Pitchford and Levine, 1991; Bhave et al., 2002).

3. Agents like bradykinin, glutamate, ATP, and NGF bind to their respective receptors, stimulating phospholipase C to cleave membrane-bound phosphatidyl inositol 4,5 bisphosphate to yield diacylglycerol and inositol trisphosphate. Evidence has accumulated for four distinct (but not mutually exclusive) mechanisms by which this enzymatic step might lead to TRPV1 sensitization:

   (a) Diacylglycerol and intracellular calcium activate PKC, which directly phosphorylates TRPV1 (Premkumar and Ahern, 2000; Numazaki et al., 2002).

   (b) Arachidonic acid, which is cleaved from diacylglycerol, is converted to the leukotriene, HPETE, that in turn binds and sensitizes TRPV1 (Hwang et al., 2000).

   (c) Arachidonic acid is converted to PGE_2, which exits the cell and acts in an autocrine fashion to activate PKA, as described above (Hu et al., 2002).

   (d) The cleavage of phosphatidylinositol bisphosphate relieves the direct inhibitory effects of this phospholipid on TRPV1 (Chuang et al., 2001).

4. Within hours following the injection of complete Freund's adjuvant into the rat hindpaw, one can observe increased levels of TRPV1 protein in nociceptor cell bodies and terminals — an effect that is independent of mRNA expression and depends upon the activation of the intracellular protein kinase, p38 (Ji et al., 2002).

While the relative importance of these distinct mechanisms remains unclear, one common consequence that they share is a shift in the temperature response threshold of TRPV1 towards lower temperatures. This phenomenon may explain ongoing pain associated with inflammation, as a sensitized TRPV1 may become active at body temperature, resulting in the generation of spontaneous nociceptor firing.

1.5.4 Inflammation induces changes in the ion channels underlying spike initiation, propagation and transmitter release

A second major way in which inflammation can augment nociception is through the facilitation of those steps of neurotransmission that follow membrane depolarization by nociceptive stimuli. A number of ion channels have been identified that are likely to contribute in one form or another to inflammation-induced sensitization and hyperalgesia. These channels include voltage-gated Na^+, K^+, and Ca^{2+} channels, Ca^{2+}-gated K^+ channels, and I_h channels (Gold, 2001). While the specific contribution of each of these channels to nociceptor sensitization varies according to their role in the control of neuronal excitability (Gold, 2001), space limitations preclude a discussion of each of these channels here. Therefore, we will illustrate what appear to be general principles governing the contribution of ion channels to nociceptor sensitization with a discussion of one class of ion channel — the TTX-resistant voltage-gated Na$^+$ channel. We have chosen to focus on this Na$^+$ channel for two reasons. First, it is only expressed in sensory neurons and primarily in nociceptive afferents. Second, it is involved in both the initiation and maintenance of inflammatory hyperalgesia (Gold, 1999). As with TRPV1, the augmentation of TTX-resistant sodium channel function by inflammation appears to result from several distinct modulatory processes.

1.5.4.1 TTX-resistant sodium channels and initiation of hyperalgesia

The application of inflammatory mediators such as PGE$_2$, serotonin, and adenosine to isolated sensory neurons results in the modulation of TTX-resistant Na$^+$ channels in a manner consistent with an underlying mechanism of nociceptor sensitization: the maximal conductance is increased, the rate of channel activation is increased, and there is a hyperpolarizing shift in the voltage-dependence of activation (Gold, 1999). These changes will result in an increase in the amount of inward or depolarizing current that occurs in response to membrane depolarizing, which will both lower the action potential threshold and decrease the magnitude of the generator potential necessary to evoke an action potential.

Modulation of Na$^+$ channels in dissociated neurons studied in culture develops within 15 seconds of the application of an inflammatory mediator and is usually fully manifest within 2 minutes. This time frame is consistent with a phosphorylation/dephosphorylation event and evidence suggests that the inflammatory mediator-induced modulation of TTX-resistant Na$^+$ channels reflects a direct phosphorylation of the channel α-subunit: inflammatory mediator-induced sensitization and modulation of TTX-resistant Na$^+$ channels depend on the activation of cyclic AMP- dependent protein kinase (PKA) and/or PKC (Gold, 1999); Na$_V$1.8 contains several consensus sequences for phosphorylation by PKA (Fitzgerald et al., 1999); activation of PKA results in an increase in the phosphorylation of Na$_V$1.8 (Fitzgerald et al., 1999); and genetically manipulating the channel in order to delete the five phosphorylation sites that are present in the linker between domains I and II prevents PKA-induced modulation (Fitzgerald et al., 1999). Importantly, opioids block inflammatory mediator-induced modulation of TTX-resistant Na$^+$ currents (Gold, 1999). Furthermore, as mentioned above, knocking-down Na$_V$1.8 in the peripheral terminals of nociceptive afferents with antisense oligodeoxynucleotides blocks the initiation of inflammatory hyperalgesia (Gold, 1999) and nociceptor sensitization (Yoshimura et al., 2001).

1.5.4.2 TTX-resistant sodium channels and maintenance of hyperalgesia

An increase in the expression of TTX-resistant Na$^+$ channels contributes to the maintenance of inflammatory hyperalgesia and nociceptor sensitization. An increase in the expression of Na$^+$ channels will have the same influence on nociceptor excitability as that associated with a phosphorylation-induced increase in Na$^+$ conductance. An inflammation-induced increase in the expression of mRNA encoding Na$_V$1.8

is detectable within 3 days of inducing inflammation (Tanaka *et al.*, 1998). This change in expression appears to reflect the actions of several mediators released in the presence of inflammation and transported back to the neuronal cell body. The most extensively studied of these is NGF. As described above, this neurotrophin induces both transcriptional and non-transcriptional changes in nociceptive and non-nociceptive afferents. Expression of Na$_V$1.8 is in part regulated by NGF such that increases and decreases in NGF result in increases and decreases, respectively, in the expression of Na$_V$1.8 (Waxman *et al.*, 1999). Importantly, Na$_V$1.8 antisense oligodeoxynucleotides significantly attenuate persistent inflammatory hyperalgesia (Porreca *et al.*, 1999).

It should be noted that results obtained with a Na$_V$1.8 null mutant mouse suggest the channel is involved in neither the initiation nor maintenance of inflammatory hyperalgesia (Akopian *et al.*, 1999; Kerr *et al.*, 2001): inflammatory mediator-induced hyperalgesia develops normally and the magnitude of hyperalgesia associated with persistent inflammation, while delayed, is similar to that observed in wild-type mice. We suggest that the differences between results obtained with the Na$_V$1.8 knock-out mouse and those from the studies described above might result from compensatory changes in the mutant animals, At least one of the compensatory changes observed in the Na$_V$1.8 knock-out mouse is an increase in the expression of TTX-sensitive Na$^+$ currents. Exactly how this compensatory change occludes detection of a role for Na$_V$1.8 in inflammatory hyperalgesia has yet to be determined, but it is worth noting that such changes are not observed following the relatively short-term administration of antisense oligodeoxynucleotides in rats (Lai *et al.*, 2002).

1.6 Summary

Nociception involves the activation of a diverse population of specialized sensory neurons that are quantitatively and qualitatively tuned to noxious chemical, thermal, and mechanical stimuli. By directly activating ion channel proteins located on the nociceptor terminal, or by activating G protein-coupled or neurotrophin receptors that indirectly modulate ion channel activity, these stimuli evoke nociceptor depolarization. The subsequent initiation of action potentials, their transmission to the spinal cord and the release of glutamate and other neurotransmitters within the spinal cord dorsal horn is mediated by another diverse group of sodium, potassium, and calcium channel proteins, many of which are voltage-gated.

References

Airaksinen MS and Saarma M (2002). The GDNF family: signalling, biological functions and therapeutic value. *Nature Reviews Neuroscience* **3**, 383–394.

Akopian AN, Souslova V, England S, *et al.* (1999). The tetrodotoxin-resistant sodium channel SNS has a specialized function in pain pathways. *Nature Neuroscience* **2**, 541–548.

Amir R and Devor M (2000). Functional cross-excitation between afferent A- and C-neurons in dorsal root ganglia. *Neuroscience* **95**, 189–195.

Amir R, Michaelis M, and Devor M (1999). Membrane potential oscillations in dorsal root ganglion neurons: role in normal electrogenesis and neuropathic pain. *Journal of Neuroscience* **19**, 8589–8596.

Askwith CC, Benson CJ, Welsh MJ, and Snyder PM (2001). DEG/ENaC ion channels involved in sensory transduction are modulated by cold temperature. *Proceedings of the National Academy of Sciences USA* **98**, 6459–6463.

Baccaglini PI and Hogan PG (1983). Some rat sensory neurons in culture express characteristics of differentiated pain sensory cells. *Proceedings of the National Academy of Sciences USA* **80**, 594–598.

Bandell M, Story GM, Hwang SW, *et al.* (2004). Noxious cold ion channel TRPA1 is activated by pungent compounds and bradykinin. *Neuron* **41**, 849–857.

Bevan S and Geppetti P (1994). Protons: small stimulants of capsaicin-sensitive sensory nerves. *Trends in Neuroscience* **17**, 509–512.

Bevan S, Hothi S, Hughes G, *et al.* (1992). Capsazepine: a competitive antagonist of the sensory neuron excitant capsaicin. *British Journal of Pharmacology* **107**, 544–552.

Bhave G, Zhu W, Wang H, Brasier DJ, Oxford GS, and Gereau RW (2002). cAMP-dependent protein kinase regulates desensitization of the capsaicin receptor (VR1) by direct phosphorylation. *Neuron* **35**, 721–731.

Birder LA, Nakamura Y, Kiss S, *et al.* (2002). Altered urinary bladder function in mice lacking the vanilloid receptor TRPV1. *Nature Neuroscience* **5**, 856–860.

Black JA, Dib–Hajj S, McNabola K, *et al.* (1996). Spinal sensory neurons express multiple sodium channel alpha-subunit mRNAs. *Brain Research and Molecular Brain Research* **43**, 117–131.

Boettger MK, Till S, Chen MX, *et al.* (2002). Calcium-activated potassium channel SK1- and IK1-like immunoreactivity in injured human sensory neurones and its regulation by neurotrophic factors. *Brain* **125**, 252–263.

Brock JA, McLachlan EM, and Belmonte C (1998). Tetrodotoxin-resistant impulses in single nociceptor nerve terminals in guinea-pig cornea. *Journal of Physiology (London)* **512**, 211–217.

Burgess PR and Perl ER (1967). Myelinated afferent fibres responding specifically to noxious stimulation of the skin. *Journal of Physiology (London)* **190**, 541–562.

Caldwell JH, Schaller KL, Lasher RS, Peles E, and Levinson SR (2000). Sodium channel Na(v)1.6 is localized at nodes of ranvier, dendrites, and synapses. *Proceedings of the National Academy of Sciences USA* **97**, 5616–5620.

Calignano A, La Rana G, Loubet–Lescoulie P, and Piomelli D (2000). A role for the endogenous cannabinoid system in the peripheral control of pain initiation. *Progress in Brain Research* **129**, 471–482.

Campbell JN and LaMotte RH (1983). Latency to detection of first pain. *Brain Research* **266**, 203–208.

Campbell JN, Meyer RA, and LaMotte RH (1979). Sensitization of myelinated nociceptive afferents that innervate monkey hand. *Journal of Neurophysiology* **42**, 1669–1679.

Campero M, Serra J, Bostock H, and Ochoa JL. (2001). Slowly conducting afferents activated by innocuous low temperature in human skin. *Journal of Physiology* **535**, 855–865.

Cantrell AR and Catterall WA (2001). Neuromodulation of Na$^+$ channels: an unexpected form of cellular plasticity. *Nature Reviews Neuroscience* **2**, 397–407.

Carr RW, Pianova S, and Brock JA (2002). The effects of polarizing current on nerve terminal impulses recorded from polymodal and cold receptors in the guinea-pig cornea. *Journal of General Physiology* **120**, 395–405.

Caterina MJ, Leffler A, Malmberg AB, *et al.* (2000). Impaired nociception and pain sensation in mice lacking the capsaicin receptor. *Science* **288**, 306–313.

Caterina MJ, Rosen TA, Tominaga M, Brake AJ, and Julius D (1999). A capsaicin receptor homologue with a high threshold for noxious heat. *Nature* **398**, 436–441.

Caterina MJ, Schumacher MA, Tominaga M, Rosen TA, Levine JD, and Julius D (1997). The capsaicin receptor: a heat-activated ion channel in the pain pathway. *Nature* **389**, 816–824.

Cesare P and McNaughton P (1996). A novel heat-activated current in nociceptive neurons and its sensitization by bradykinin. *Proceedings of the National Academy of Sciences USA* **93**, 15435–15439.

Chaplan SR, Guo HQ, Lee DH, Butler MP, Velumian A, and Dubin AE (2001). Markedly increased DRG IH and HCN mRNA accompany neuropathic pain in the rat. *Society of Neuroscience Abstracts* **27**, 54.11.

Chen CC, England S, Akopian AN, and Wood JN (1998). A sensory neuron-specific, proton gated ion channel. *Proceedings of the National Academy of Sciences USA* **95**, 10240–10245.

Chuang H, Prescott ED, Kong H, *et al.* (2001). Bradykinin and nerve growth factor release the capsaicin receptor from PtdIns(4,5)P2-mediated inhibition. *Nature* **411**, 957–962.

Coward K, Plumpton C, Facer P, *et al.* (2000). Immunolocalization of SNS/PN3 and NaN/SNS2 sodium channels in human pain states. *Pain* **85**, 41–50.

Darian–Smith I, Johnson KO, and Dykes R (1973). Cold fiber population innervating palmar and digital skin of the monkey: responses to cooling pulses. *Journal of Neurophysiology* **36**, 325–346.

Darian–Smith I, Johnson KO, LaMotte C, Shigenaga Y, Kenins P, and Champness P (1979). Warm fibers innervating palmar and digital skin of the monkey: responses to thermal stimuli. *Journal of Neurophysiology* **42**, 1297–1315.

Davis JB, Gray J, Gunthorpe MJ, *et al.* (2000). Vanilloid receptor-1 is essential for inflammatory thermal hyperalgesia. *Nature* **405**, 183–187.

Davis KD, Meyer RA, Campbell JN (1993). Chemosensitivity and sensitization of nociceptive afferents that innervate the hairy skin of monkey. *Journal of Neurophysiology* **69**, 1071–1081.

Drew LJ, Wood JN, and Cesare P (2002). Distinct mechanosensitive properties of capsaicin-sensitive and -insensitive sensory neurons. *Journal of Neuroscience* **22**, RC228.

Ertel EA, Campbell KP, Harpold MM, *et al.* (2000). Nomenclature of voltage-gated calcium channels. *Neuron* **25**, 533–535.

Evans AR, Nicol GD, and Vasko MR (1996). Differential regulation of evoked peptide release by voltage-sensitive calcium channels in rat sensory neurons. *Brain Research* **712**, 265–273.

Ferreira SH, Nakamura M, and de Abreu Castro MS (1978). The hyperalgesic effects of prostacyclin and prostaglandin E2. *Prostaglandins* **16**, 31–37.

Fields RD, Eshete F, Stevens B, and Itoh K (1997). Action potential-dependent regulation of gene expression: temporal specificity in ca2+, cAMP-responsive element binding proteins, and mitogen-activated protein kinase signaling. *Journal of Neuroscience* **17**, 7252–7266.

Firestein S, Shepherd GM, and Werblin FS (1990). Time course of the membrane current underlying sensory transduction in salamander olfactory receptor neurones. *Journal of Physiology* **430**, 135–158.

Fitzgerald EM, Okuse K, Wood JN (1999). cAMP-dependent phosphorylation of the tetrodotoxin-resistant voltage-dependent sodium channel SNS. *Journal of Physiology (London)* **516**, 433–446.

Fjell J, Hjelmstrom P, Hormuzdiar W, *et al.* (2000). Localization of the tetrodotoxin-resistant sodium channel NaN in nociceptors. *Neuroreport* **11**, 199–202.

Garcia–Anoveros J and Corey DP (1996). Touch at the molecular level. Mechanosensation. *Current Biology* **6**, 541–543.

Gilman AG (1987). G proteins: transducers of receptor-generated signals. *Annual Reviews in Biochemistry* **56**, 615–649.

Gold MS (1999). Tetrodotoxin-resistant Na$^+$ currents and inflammatory hyperalgesia. *Proceedings of the National Academy of Sciences USA* **96**, 7645–7649.

Gold MS (2001). *Membrane properties: ion channels. Methods in pain research* (ed. L Kruger). New York, CRC Press: 169–186.

Gold MS, Dastmalchi S, and Levine JD (1996). Co-expression of nociceptor properties in dorsal root ganglion neurons from the adult rat in vitro. *Neuroscience* **71**, 265–275.

Gold MS, Shuster MJ, and Levine JD (1996). Characterization of six voltage-gated K^+ currents in adult rat sensory neurons. *Journal of Neurophysiology* **75**, 2629–2646.

Gold MS, Weinreich D, Kim CS, *et al.* (2003). Redistribution of $Na_V1.8$ in uninjured axons enables neuropathic pain. *Journal of Neuroscience*, 23, 158–166.

Gu JG and MacDermott AB (1997). Activation of ATP P2X receptors elicits glutamate release from sensory neuron synapses. *Nature* **389**, 749–53.

Guler AD, Lee H, Iida T, Shimizu I, Tominaga M, and Caterina M (2002). Heat-evoked activation of the ion channel, TRPV4. *Journal of Neuroscience* **22**, 6408–6414.

Handwerker HO and Reeh PW (1991). Pain and Inflammation. In *Proceedings of the VIth World Congress on Pain* (ed. MR Bond, CJE Woolf, and CJ Woolf). Elsevier: 59–70.

Handwerker HO, Kilo S, and Reeh PW (1991). Unresponsive afferent nerve fibres in the sural nerve of the rat. *Journal of Physiology* **435**, 229–242.

Heppelmann B, Messlinger K, Neiss WF, and Schmidt RF (1990). Ultrastructural three-dimensional reconstruction of group III and group IV sensory nerve endings ('free nerve endings') in the knee joint capsule of the cat: evidence for multiple receptive sites. *Journal of Comparative Neurology* **292**, 103–116.

Hille B (1992). *Ionic Channels of Excitable Membranes* (2nd ed). Sinauer, Sunderland, MA: 59–82.

Honmou O, Utzschneider DA, Rizzo MA, Bowe CM, Waxman SG, and Kocsis JD (1994). Delayed depolarization and slow sodium currents in cutaneous afferents. *Journal of Neurophysiology* **71**, 1627–1637.

Hu HJ, Bhave G, and Gereau RW (2002) Prostaglandin and protein kinase A-dependent modulation of vanilloid receptor function by metabotropic glutamate receptor 5: potential mechanism for thermal hyperalgesia. *Journal of Neuroscience* **22**, 7444–7452.

Hu H, Shao LR, Chavoshy S, *et al.* (2001). Presynaptic Ca^{2+}-activated K^+ channels in glutamatergic hippocampal terminals and their role in spike repolarization and regulation of transmitter release. *Journal of Neuroscience* **21**, 9585–97.

Huang EJ and Reichardt LF (2001). Neurotrophins: roles in neuronal development and function. *Annual Reviews in Neuroscience* **24**, 677–736.

Huang H, Wu X, Nicol GD, *et al.* (2003). ATP augments peptide release from rat sensory neurons in culture through activation of PzY receptors. *Journal of Pharmacology and Experimental Therapeutics* **306**, 1137–44.

Hutcheon B, Puil E, and Spigelman I (1993). Histamine actions and comparison with substance P effects in trigeminal neurons. *Neuroscience* **55**, 521–529.

Hwang SW, Cho H, Kwak J, *et al.* (2000). Direct activation of capsaicin receptors by products of lipoxygenases: endogenous capsaicin-like substances. *Proceedings of the National Academy of Sciences USA* **97**, 6155–6160.

Immke DC and McCleskey EW (2001). Lactate enhances the acid-sensing Na+ channel on ischemia-sensing neurons. *Nature Neuroscience* **4**, 869–870.

Isom LL (2001). Sodium channel beta subunits: anything but auxiliary. *Neuroscientist* **7**, 42–54.

Jancso G, Kiraly E, and Jancso–Gabor A (1977). Pharmacologically induced selective degeneration of chemosensitive primary sensory neurons. *Nature* **270**, 741–743.

Ji R, Samad T, Jin S, Schmoll R, and Woolf C (2002). p38 MAPK activation by NGF in primary sensory neurons after inflammation increases TRPV1 levels and maintains heat hyperalgesia. *Neuron* **36**, 57.

Johnson KO (2001). The roles and functions of cutaneous mechanoreceptors. *Current Opinions in Neurobiology* **11**, 455–461.

Johnson KO, Darian–Smith I, LaMotte C (1973). Peripheral neural determinants of temperature discrimination in man: a correlative study of responses to cooling skin. *Journal of Neurophysiology* **36**, 347–370.

Johnson KO, Darian–Smith I, LaMotte C, Johnson B, and Oldfield S (1979). Coding of incremental changes in skin temperature by a monkey: correlation with intensity discrimination in man. *Journal of Neurophysiology* **42**, 1332–1353.

Jordt SE, Bautista DM, Chuang HH, *et al.* (2004). Mustard oils and cannabinoids excite sensory nerve fibres through the TRP channel ANKTM1. *Nature* **427**, 260–265.

Jordt SE, Tominaga M, and Julius D (2000). Acid potentiation of the capsaicin receptor determined by a key extracellular site. *Proceedings of the National Academy of Sciences USA* **97**, 8134–8139.

Kerr BJ, Souslova V, McMahon SB, and Wood JN (2001). A role for the TTX-resistant sodium channel Nav 1.8 in NGF-induced hyperalgesia, but not neuropathic pain. *Neuroreport* **12**, 3077–3080.

Khasar SG, Gold MS, and Levine JD (1998). A tetrodotoxin-resistant sodium current mediates inflammatory pain in the rat. *Neuroscince Letters* **256**, 17–20.

Kirchhoff C, Leah JD, Jung S, and Reeh PW (1992). Excitation of cutaneous sensory nerve endings in the rat by 4-aminopyridine and tetraethylammonium. *Journal of Neurophysiology* **67**, 125–131.

Kirschstein T, Busselberg D, and Treede RD (1997). Coexpression of heat-evoked and capsaicin-evoked inward currents in acutely dissociated rat dorsal root ganglion neurons. *Neuroscience Letters* **231**, 33–36.

Koltzenburg M, Bennett DL, Shelton DL, and McMahon SB (1999). Neutralization of endogenous NGF prevents the sensitization of nociceptors supplying inflamed skin. *European Journal of Neuroscience* **11**, 1698–1704.

Lai J, Gold MS, Kim CS, *et al.* (2002). Inhibition of neuropathic pain by decreased expression of the tetrodotoxin-resistant sodium channel, NaV1.8. *Pain* **95**, 143–152.

LaMotte RH, Campbell JN (1978). Comparison of responses of warm and nociceptive C-fiber afferents in monkey with human judgements of thermal pain. *Journal of Neurophysiology* **41**, 509–528.

LaMotte RH, Thalhammer JG, Robinson CJ (1983). Peripheral neural correlates of magnitude of cutaneous pain and hyperalgesia: a comparison of neural events in monkey with sensory judgements in human. *Journal of Neurophysiology* **50**, 1–26.

Lao L and Marvizon JC (2005). GABA(A) receptor facilitation of neurokinin release from primary afferent terminals in the rat spinal cord. *Neuroscience* **130**, 1013–27.

Lewis T (1937). The nocifensor system of nerves and its reactions. *British Medical Journal* 431–435.

Lewis T and Pochin EE (1937). The double pain response of the human skin to a single stimulus. *Clinical Science* **3**, 67–76.

Liedtke W, Choe Y, Marti–Renom MA, *et al.* (2000). Vanilloid receptor-related osmotically activated channel (VR-OAC), a candidate vertebrate osmoreceptor. *Cell* **103**, 525–535.

Lingueglia E, de Weille JR, Bassilana F, *et al.* (1997). A modulatory subunit of acid sensing ion channels in brain and dorsal root ganglion cells. *Journal of Biological Chemistry* **272**, 29778–29783.

Lowenstein WR (1959). Generation of electrical activity in a nerve ending. *Annals of the New York Academy of Sciences* **81**, 367–387.

Maingret F, Fosset M, Lesage F, Lazdunski M, and Honore E (1999). TRAAK is a mammalian neuronal mechano-gated K+ channel. *Journal of Biological Chemistry* **274**, 1381–1387.

Maingret F, Lauritzen I, Patel AJ, *et al.* (2000). TREK-1 is a heat-activated background K(+) channel. *EMBO Journal* **19**, 2483–2491.

Martin DJ, McClelland D, Herd MB, *et al.* (2002). Gabapentin-mediated inhibition of voltage-activated Ca2+ channel currents in cultured sensory neurones is dependent on culture conditions and channel subunit expression. *Neuropharmacology* **42**, 353–366.

Matsuka Y, Neubert JK, Maidment NT, and Spigelman I (2001). Concurrent release of ATP and substance P within guinea pig trigeminal ganglia in vivo. *Brain Research* **915**, 248–255.

Mayer C, Quasthoff S, and Grafe P (1999). Confocal imaging reveals activity-dependent intracellular Ca2+ transients in nociceptive human C fibres. *Pain* **81**, 317–322.

McCarter GC, Reichling DB, and Levine JD (1999). Mechanical transduction by rat dorsal root ganglion neurons in vitro. *Neuroscience Letters* **273**, 179–182.

McCleskey EW and Gold MS (1999). Ion channels of nociception. *Annual Reviews in Physiology* **61**, 835–856.

McKemy DD, Neuhausser VM, and Julius D (2002). Identification of a cold receptor reveals a general role for TRP channels in thermosensation. *Nature* **416**, 52–58.

Meyer RA, Campbell JN (1981*a*). Myelinated nociceptive afferents account for the hyperalgesia that follows a burn to the hand. *Science* **213**, 1527–1529.

Meyer RA, Campbell JN (1981*b*). Peripheral neural coding of pain sensation. *Johns Hopkins Applied Physics Laboratory Technical Digest* **2**, 164–171.

Meyer RA, Davis KD, Cohen RH, Treede R–D, Campbell JN (1991). Mechanically insensitive afferents (MIAs) in cutaneous nerves of monkey. *Brain Research* **561**, 252–261.

Millan MJ (1999). The induction of pain: an integrative review. *Progress in Neurobiology* **57**, 1–164.

Montell C (2001). Physiology, phylogeny, and functions of the TRP superfamily of cation channels. *Science Signal Transduction Knowledge Environment* 2001, RE1.

Nagy I and Rang H (1999). Noxious heat activates all capsaicin-sensitive and also a sub-population of capsaicin-insensitive dorsal root ganglion neurons. *Neuroscience* **88**, 995–997.

Nicol GD, Vasko MR, and Evans AR (1997). Prostaglandins suppress an outward potassium current in embryonic rat sensory neurons. *Journal of Neurophysiology* **77**, 167–176.

Numazaki M, Tominaga T, Toyooka H, and Tominaga M (2002). Direct phosphorylation of capsaicin receptor VR1 by protein kinase Cepsilon and identification of two target serine residues. *Journal of Biological Chemistry* **277**, 13375–13378.

Oh Y, Sashihara S, Black JA, and Waxman SG (1995). Na+ channel beta 1 subunit mRNA: differential expression in rat spinal sensory neurons. *Brain Research and Molecular Brain Research* **30**, 357–361.

Opree A and Kress M (2000). Involvement of the proinflammatory cytokines tumor necrosis factor-alpha, IL-1 beta, and IL-6 but not IL-8 in the development of heat hyperalgesia: effects on heat-evoked calcitonin gene-related peptide release from rat skin. *Journal of Neuroscience* **20**, 6289–6293.

Pasternak GW (1993). Pharmacological mechanisms of opioid analgesics. *Clinical Neuropharmacology* **16**, 1–18.

Peier AM, Moqrich A, Hergarden AC, *et al.* (2002*a*). A TRP channel that senses cold stimuli and menthol. *Cell* **108**, 705–715.

Peier AM, Reeve AJ, Andersson DA, *et al.* (2002*b*). A heat-sensitive TRP channel expressed in keratinocytes. *Science* **296**, 2046–2049.

Peles E and Salzer SL (2000). *Current Opinions in Neurobiology* **10**, 558–65.

Perl ER (1968) Myelinated afferent fibres innervating the primate skin and their response to noxious stimuli. *Journal of Physiology (London)* **197**, 593–615.

Petersen M and LaMotte RH (1993). Effect of protons on the inward current evoked by capsaicin in isolated dorsal root ganglion cells. *Pain* **54**, 37–42.

Pitchford S and Levine JD (1991). Prostaglandins sensitize nociceptors in cell culture. *Neuroscience Letters* **132**, 105–108.

Porreca F, Lai J, Bian D, *et al.* (1999). A comparison of the potential role of the tetrodotoxin-insensitive sodium channels, PN3/SNS and NaN/SNS2, in rat models of chronic pain. *Proceedings of the National Academy of Sciences USA* **96**, 7640–7644.

Premkumar LS and Ahern GP (2000). Induction of vanilloid receptor channel activity by protein kinase C. *Nature* **408**, 985–990.

Price MP, Lewin GR, McIlwrath SL, *et al.* (2000). The mammalian sodium channel BNC1 is required for normal touch sensation. *Nature* **407**, 1007–1011.

Price MP, McIlwrath SL, Xie J, *et al.* (2001). The DRASIC cation channel contributes to the detection of cutaneous touch and acid stimuli in mice. *Neuron* **32**, 1071–1083.

Quasthoff S, Grosskreutz J, Schroder JM, Schneider U, and Grafe P (1995). Calcium potentials and tetrodotoxin-resistant sodium potentials in unmyelinated C fibres of biopsied human sural nerve. *Neuroscience* **69**, 955–965.

Raja SN, Meyer RA, Ringkamp M, and Campbell JN (1999). Peripheral neural mechanisms of nociception. In *Textbook of Pain* (eds. PD Wall and P Melzack), pp. 11–57. Edinburgh: Churchill Livingstone.

Rasband MN, Trimmer JS, Schwarz TL, *et al.* (1998). Potassium channel distribution, clustering, and function in remyelinating rat axons. *Journal of Neuroscience* **18**, 36–47.

Reichling DB and Levine JD (1997). Heat transduction in rat sensory neurons by calcium-dependent activation of a cation channel. *Proceedings of the National Academy of Sciences USA* **94**, 7006–7011.

Reid G and Flonta M (2001*a*). Cold transduction by inhibition of a background potassium conductance in rat primary sensory neurones. *Neuroscience Letters* **297**, 171–174.

Reid G and Flonta ML (2001*b*). Cold current in thermoreceptive neurons. *Nature* **413**, 480.

Reid G and Flonta ML (2002). Ion channels activated by cold and menthol in cultured rat dorsal root ganglion neurones. *Neuroscience Letters* **324**, 164–168.

Ritter AM and Mendell LM (1992). Somal membrane properties of physiologically identified sensory neurons in the rat: effects of nerve growth factor. *Journal of Neurophysiology* **68**, 2033–2041.

Robbins WR, Staats PS, Levine J, *et al.* (1998). Treatment of intractable pain with topical large-dose capsaicin: preliminary report. *Anesthesiology and Analgesia* **86**, 579–583.

Rudy B (1988). Diversity and ubiquity of K channels. *Neuroscience* **25**, 729–749.

Schaible HG and Schmidt RF (1985). Effects of an experimental arthritis on the sensory properties of fine articular afferent units. *Journal of Neurophysiology* **54**, 1109–1122.

Schmelz M, Michael K, Weidner C, Schmidt R, Torebjörk HE, and Handwerker HO (2000*a*). Which nerve fibers mediate the axon reflex flare in human skin? *Neuroreport* **11**, 645–648.

Schmelz M, Schmidt R, Handwerker HO, and Torebjörk HE (2000*b*). Encoding of burning pain from capsaicin-treated human skin in two categories of unmyelinated nerve fibres. *Brain* **123**, 560–571.

Schmelz M, Schmidt R, Bickel A, Handwerker HO, and Torebjörk HE (1997). Specific C-receptors for itch in human skin. *Journal of Neuroscience* **17**, 8003–8008.

Schmidt R, Schmelz M, Forster C, Ringkamp M, Torebjörk E, and Handwerker H (1995). Novel classes of responsive and unresponsive C nociceptors in human skin. *Journal of Neuroscience* **15**, 333–341.

Schmidt R, Schmelz M, Torebjörk HE, and Handwerker HO (2000). Mechano-insensitive nociceptors encode pain evoked by tonic pressure to human skin. *Neuroscience* **98**, 793–800.

Schroeder JE, Fischbach PS, Zheng D, and McCleskey EW (1991). Activation of mu opioid receptors inhibits transient high- and low-threshold Ca2+ currents, but spares a sustained current. *Neuron* **6**, 13–20.

Schumacher MA, Moff I, Sudanagunta SP, and Levine JD (2000). Molecular cloning of an N-terminal splice variant of the capsaicin receptor. Loss of N-terminal domain suggests functional divergence among capsaicin receptor subtypes. *Journal of Biological Chemistry* **275**, 2756–2762.

Scroggs RS and Fox AP (1992). Calcium current variation between acutely isolated adult rat dorsal root ganglion neurons of different size. *Journal of Physiology* **445**, 639–658.

Shakhanbeh J and Lynn B (1993). Morphine inhibits antidromic vasodilatation without affecting the excitability of C-polymodal nociceptors in the skin of the rat. *Brain Research* **607**, 314–318.

Shu XQ and Mendell LM (1999). Neurotrophins and hyperalgesia. *Proceedings of the National Academy of Sciences USA* **96**, 7693–7696.

Sinclair DC and Hinshaw JR (1950). A comparison of the sensory dissociation produced by procaine and by limb compression. *Brain* **73**, 480–498.

Simone DA, Nolano M, Johnson T, Wendelschafer–Crabb G, and Kennedy WR (1998). Intradermal injection of capsaicin in humans produces degeneration and subsequent reinnervation of epidermal nerve fibers: correlation with sensory function. *Journal of Neuroscience* **18**, 8947–8959.

Sluka KA, Willis WD, and Westlund KN (1995). The role of dorsal root reflexes in neurogenic inflammation. *Pain Forum* **4**, 141–149.

Smith GD, Gunthorpe MJ, Kelsell RE, *et al.* (2002). TRPV3 is a temperature-sensitive vanilloid receptor-like protein. *Nature* **418**, 186–190.

Steranka LR, Manning DC, DeHaas CJ, *et al.* (1988). Bradykinin as a pain mediator: receptors are localized to sensory neurons, and antagonists have analgesic actions. *Proceedings of the National Academy of Sciences USA* **85**, 3245–3249.

Story GM, Peier AM, Reeve AJ, *et al.* (2003). ANKTM1, a TRP-like channel expressed in nociceptive neurons, is activated by cold temperatures. *Cell* **112**, 819–829.

Strotmann R, Harteneck C, Nunnenmacher K, Schultz G, and Plant TD (2000). OTRPC4, a nonselective cation channel that confers sensitivity to extracellular osmolarity. *Nature Cell Biology* **2**, 695–702.

Strupp M and Grafe P (1991). A chloride channel in rat and human axons. *Neuroscience Letters* **133**, 237–240.

Sutherland SP, Benson CJ, Adelman JP, and McCleskey EW (2001). Acid-sensing ion channel 3 matches the acid-gated current in cardiac ischemia-sensing neurons. *Proceedings of the National Academy of Sciences USA* **98**, 711–716.

Szallasi A and Blumberg PM (1999). Vanilloid (Capsaicin) receptors and mechanisms. *Pharmacological Reviews* **51**, 159–212.

Taddese A, Nah SY, and McCleskey EW (1995). Selective opioid inhibition of small nociceptive neurons. *Science* **270**, 1366–1369.

Takigawa T, Alzheimer C, Quasthoff S, and Grafe P (1998). A special blocker reveals the presence and function of the hyperpolarization-activated cation current IH in peripheral mammalian nerve fibres. *Neuroscience* **82**, 631–634.

Tanaka M, Cummins TR, Ishikawa K, Dib–Hajj SD, Black JA, and Waxman SG (1998). SNS Na+ channel expression increases in dorsal root ganglion neurons in the carrageenan inflammatory pain model. *Neuroreport* **9**, 967–972.

Tanelian DL and Brunson DB (1994). Anatomy and physiology of pain with special reference to ophthalmology. *Investigative Ophthalmology and Visual Science* **35**, 759–763.

Toledo AJ, Brehm P, Halegoua S, and Mandel G (1995). A single pulse of nerve growth factor triggers long-term neuronal excitability through sodium channel gene induction. *Neuron* **14**, 607–611.

Tominaga M, Caterina MJ, Malmberg AB, *et al.* (1998). The cloned capsaicin receptor integrates multiple pain-producing stimuli. *Neuron* **21**, 1–20.

Torebjörk HE (1974). Afferent C units responding to mechanical, thermal and chemical stimuli in human non-glabrous skin. *Acta Physiologica Scandanavia* **92**, 374–390.

Torebjörk HE and Hallin RG (1973). Perceptual changes accompanying controlled preferential blocking of A and C fibre responses in intact human skin nerves. *Experimental Brain Research* **16**, 321–332.

Treede RD, Meyer RA, and Campbell JN (1998). Myelinated mechanically insensitive afferents from monkey hairy skin: heat-response properties. *Journal of Neurophysiology* **80**, 1082–1093.

Van Arman CG, Carlson RP, Risley EA, Thomas RH, and Nuss GW (1970). Inhibitory effects of indomethacin, aspirin and certain other drugs on inflammations induced in rat and dog by carrageenan, sodium urate and ellagic acid. *Journal of Pharmacology and Experimental Therapeutics* **175**, 459–468.

Vergnolle N, Wallace JL, Bunnett NW, and Hollenberg MD (2001). Protease-activated receptors in inflammation, neuronal signaling and pain. *Trends in Pharmacological Sciences* **22**, 146–152.

Viana F, de la Pena E, and Belmonte C (2002). Specificity of cold thermotransduction is determined by differential ionic channel expression. *Nature Neuroscience* **5**, 254–260.

Waldmann R, Bassilana F, Weille J, *et al.* (1997). Molecular cloning of a non-inactivating proton-gated Na+ channel specific for sensory neurons. *Journal of Biological Chemistry* **272**, 20975–20978.

Waldmann R, Champigny G, Lingueglia E, De Weille JR, Heurteaux C, and Lazdunski M (1999). H(+)-gated cation channels. *Annals of the New York Academy of Sciences* **868**, 67–76.

Waxman SG, Dib–Hajj S, Cummins TR, and Black JA (1999). Sodium channels and pain. *Proceedings of the National Academy of Sciences USA* **96**, 7635–7639.

White G, Lovinger DM, and Weight FF (1989). Transient low-threshold Ca2+ current triggers burst firing through an afterdepolarizing potential in an adult mammalian neuron. *Proceedings of the National Academy of Sciences USA* **86**, 6802–6806.

Wood JN and Docherty R (1997). Chemical activators of sensory neurons. *Annual Reviews in Physiology* **59**, 457–482.

Xu H, Ramsey IS, Kotecha SA, *et al.* (2002). TRPV3 is a calcium-permeable temperature-sensitive cation channel. *Nature* **418**, 181–186

Yoshimura N, Seki S, Novakovic SD, *et al.* (2001). The involvement of the tetrodotoxin-resistant sodium channel $Na_V1.8$ (PN3/SNS) in a rat model of visceral pain. *Journal of Neuroscience* **21**, 8690–8696.

Yu FH, Westenbroek RE, Silos-Santiago I, *et al.* (2003). *Journal of Neuroscience* **23**, 7577–7585.

Chapter 2

Nociceptor plasticity

S.B. McMahon and J.V. Priestley

2.1 Introduction

Dorsal root ganglion (DRG) neurons have traditionally been characterized based primarily on their anatomy and physiology, but in recent years neurochemical studies have revealed additional and remarkable heterogeneity. In addition, it has become apparent that DRG phenotype is relatively plastic, changing in response to nerve and/or tissue damage. This plasticity is regulated by various target and/or injury derived growth factors. In this chapter we will review published studies on DRG subpopulations and their dependence on neurotrophic factors, with a special emphasis on nociceptive neurons. We will also describe the changes that take place after nerve injury and inflammation and how these relate to chronic pain conditions.

2.2 Biochemical neuroanatomy of dorsal root ganglion cells

2.2.1 DRG subpopulations

DRG cells can be divided into various subpopulations based on their neurochemistry, anatomy and physiology (Priestley *et al.*, 2002) (Fig 2.1). Most information has come from rat studies and this summary is therefore derived from that data. However, it appears that a similar organization applies in other species, although there are many differences in detail (see for example, Del Fiacco and Priestley, 2001; Zwick *et al.*, 2002).

First, large- and medium-sized neurons form a group that can be distinguished by their content of phosphorylated heavy chain (200kDa) neurofilament and that comprises approximately 40% of lumbar DRG cells. These cells have mostly myelinated axons that conduct in the Aα/β range and receive input from peripheral mechanoreceptors. The second major group of DRG cells (about 40% of cells) constitutively express neuropeptides, and for these the best marker is calcitonin gene-related peptide (CGRP). These neurones are mostly small with unmyelinated axons (C fibres) and innervate mainly polymodal nociceptors. DRG cells that utilize substance P fall in this category. An intermediate group between these two major populations comprises CGRP cells that are medium sized with finely myelinated axons (Aδ fibres). Most of these cells are

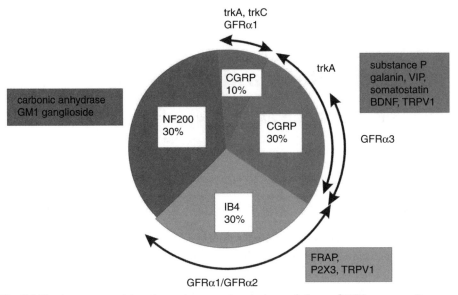

Fig. 2.1 Pie-chart summarizing the main neurochemical populations of DRG neurons. One population comprises large cells which give rise to myelinated axons and have high levels of neurofilament (NF200). Small cells, which have mainly unmyelinated axons and are predominantly nociceptors, comprise two populations — one of cells that constitutively synthesize the neuropeptide CGRP; the other characterized by cells that bind the lectin *Griffonia simplicifolia* IB4. An overlap between the NF200 and CGRP populations corresponds to Aδ nociceptors. There is also some overlap between the IB4 and CGRP populations. Neurotrophin receptors and GDNF receptors expressed by small- and medium-sized cells (predominantly nociceptors) are indicated around the periphery of the chart, together with molecules found in each major population. For further details see text. (Modified from Priestley *et al.*, 2002.)

nociceptors of the high threshold mechanoreceptor (HTM) type, but CGRP has also been reported in non-nociceptive G2 hair afferents (Lawson *et al.*, 1996). In addition, substance P occurs in a few Aα/β myelinated nociceptors (Lawson *et al.*, 1997).

The final class of neurones, comprising about 30% of DRG cells, can be identified using a variety of markers (Alvarez *et al.*, 1991; Lembo *et al.*, 2002; Zylka *et al.*, 2005) but especially by their binding of the lectin *Griffonia simplicifolia* IB4 or the expression of a non-lysosomal fluoride-resistant acid phosphatase (FRAP) (Silverman and Kruger, 1990). This group (which will be referred to as IB4+) also consists of small-diameter cells with unmyelinated axons (C fibres) which are likely to mediate nociception (see below), but they generally either do not contain neuropeptides (Silverman and Kruger, 1990; Alvarez *et al.*, 1991) or only contain low levels (Kashiba *et al.*, 2001). Note that thermoreceptive afferents are thought to be derived predominantly from small-diameter DRG cells with unmyelinated axons (Iggo, 1969; McKemy *et al.*, 2002) and presumably therefore may include both IB4+ and CGRP immunoreactive cells. However, few studies have directly examined their neurochemical properties.

2.2.2 Transduction molecules and ion channels

One aim of the type of work reviewed above is to establish a 'neurochemical profile' for each physiological class of DRG cell, and to determine the key molecules that determine DRG function in both normal and pathological states. Unfortunately, although a great deal is known about the physiological properties of DRG cells, and about the neurotransmitters and neuropeptides that they express, relatively little is known about the molecules involved in signal transduction. This has made it difficult to unequivocally associate a particular physiological group with the neurochemical subdivisions outlined above. However, much progress has been made recently with the cloning and characterization of a number of molecules involved in sensory neuron signal transduction (Table 2.1). Members of the ASIC/degenerin/epithelial sodium channel family (Garcia-Anoveros et al., 2001; Price *et al.*, 2000, 2001) and of the TRPV family (Suzuki *et al.*, 2003) that may mediate mechanotransduction has been identified but their role remains controversial (Drew *et al.*, 2004). A range of thermoceptors have also been identified (see Patapoutian *et al.*, 2003). In addition, a range of receptors have been identified which respond to inflammatory mediators and/or products of tissue damage and which are implicated in nociception (see Chapter 1). These latter include purinoceptors, bradykinin receptors, serotonin (5-hydroxytryptamine, 5-HT) receptors, acid-sensing ion channels (ASICs), the CB1 cannabinoid receptor, the H1 histamine receptor, prostanoid receptors, and the TRPV family of receptors. Of these, the receptor with the strongest link to nociception is probably TRPV1.

TRPV1 (also known as VR1) responds to noxious chemical and heat stimuli (see Chapter 1) (Caterina *et al.*, 1997; Tominaga *et al.*, 1998), and such cells have traditionally fallen into the category of C fibres known as polymodal nociceptors. TRPV1 localization studies are consistent with this, showing that TRPV1 levels vary between individual DRG cells but that it is expressed by many small- and medium-sized DRG cells (Tominaga *et al.*, 1998; Michael and Priestley, 1999). The thermal responsiveness of these cells probably depends on several different transduction molecules, and recent studies have reported that TRPV1 coexists in many cells with TRPV3 (Smith *et al.*, 2002) — a TRPV1 homologue with heat sensitivity that has been variously reported as greater than 39°C (Smith *et al.*, 2002) or as 22–40°C (Xu *et al.*, 2002).

Interestingly, TRPV1 is expressed by the majority of cells in both the IB4+ (75% of IB4 cells) and the CGRP/IB4- (59–65% of CGRP/trkA cells) populations (Guo *et al.*, 1999; Michael and Priestley, 1999). In the rat, TRPV1 is expressed in only a very small number (3%) of neurofilament immunoreactive cells (Michael and Priestley, 1999), implying that TRPV1 is not present in many myelinated axons. Capsaicin-sensitive A fibre nociceptors have been described in monkey (Ringkamp *et al.*, 2001) but are mechanically insensitive. This raises the question of the identity of the transducing molecules in the finely myelinated Aδ HTM nociceptors, and one possible candidate is TRPV2. TRPV2, which was originally described as a vanilloid receptor homologue (VRL1), is a non-selective cation channel which is not activated by vanilloids or by low

Table 2.1 Receptors and ion channels expressed by dorsal root ganglion cells

Transient receptor potential (TRP) family (Vennekens *et al.*, 2002; Gunthorpe *et al.*, 2002; McKemy *et al.*, 2002; Patapoutian *et al.*, 2003; Jordt *et al.*, 2004)

TRPV1 — non-selective cation channel activated by capsaicin, low pH, and heat >43°C

TRPV2 — non-selective cation channel activated by heat >52°C

TRPV3 — non-selective cation channel activated by heat >39°C (human) or 22–40°C (primate)

TRPV4 — non-selective cation channel activated by heat in 30–44°C range, osmosensor

TRPA1 (ANKTM1) — non-selective cation channel activated by mustard oils and by cold below 17°C

TRPM8 (CMR1) — non-selective cation channel activated by menthol and cold between 8–28°C

Acid-sensing ion channels (ASIC) family (Waldmann and Lazdunski, 1998)

ASIC1a (ASIC-a, BNaC2a) – transient Na currents

ASIC1b (ASIC-b, BNaC2b) – predominantly transient Na^+/K^+ currents, DRG specific

ASIC2a (MDEG1, BNC1, BNaC1a) — mechanoreceptor, mainly large cells

ASIC2b (MDEG2, BNaC1b) — inactive ?

ASIC3 (DRASIC) — transient and sustained $Na+/K^+$ currents, DRG specific

ATP-gated ion channels (Hamilton and McMahon, 2000)

$P2X_2$ — G protein linked, CGRP and IB4 cells

$P2X_3$ — G protein linked, IB4 cells, mechanoreceptor

Cannabinoid receptors (Hohmann and Herkenham, 1999; Ahluwalia *et al.*, 2000)

CB1 — G protein linked; some authors report medium–large cells but others report small cells

Bradykinin receptors (Levy and Zochodne, 2000; Wotherspoon and Winter, 2000; Ma, 2001)

B1 — up-regulated in inflammation, but also constitutively expressed

B2 — constitutively expressed

Histamine receptors (Kashiba *et al.*, 1999)

H1 — IB4+ cells

Prostanoid receptors (Oida *et al.*, 1995)

EP1, EP3, EP4, and IP in DRG cells, including some substance P cells

5-HT receptors (Tecott *et al.*, 1993; Bonaventure *et al.*, 1998; Wotherspoon and Priestley, 2000; Zeitz *et al.*, 2002)

1A, 1B, 1D, 2A, 2C, and 3 present in dorsal root ganglia, 1B and 3 in medium-sized, non-substance P, DRG cells

Na channels (Fang *et al.*, 2002; Amaya *et al.*, 2000)

$Na_V1.3$ (type III) — TTX-sensitive, up-regulated after nerve injury

$Na_V1.7$ (PN1) — TTX-sensitive, all DRG cells

$Na_V1.8$ (SNS, PN3) — TTX-resistant; IB4, trkA, and some NF200 cells

$Na_V1.9$ (NaN, SNS2) — TTX-resistant, nociceptors, IB4 and trkA cells

K channels (Rasband *et al.*, 2001)

Kv1.4 homomer (A-type current) expressed by small cells; Kv1.1/Kv1.2 heteromer in large cells

Ca channels (Yusaf *et al.*, 2001)

α_{1A}, α_{1B}, α_{1C}, α_{1D}, α_{1E}, α_{1I}, α_{1S} expressed in all sizes of DRG cells pH but by temperatures above 52°C. Some HTMs are activated in this temperature range, and TRPV2 is expressed by neurofilament immunoreactive DRG cells (Caterina *et al.*, 1999).

Another receptor with a very striking expression in nociceptors is the P2X$_3$ ATP-gated cation channel. DRG cells express a variety of P2X and P2Y subtypes (Nakamura and Strittmatter, 1996; Vulchanova *et al.*, 1997) but P2X$_3$ is unique in being selectively expressed by IB4+ DRG cells (Bradbury *et al.*, 1998). Functional studies indicate that P2X$_3$ plays a role in inflammatory and neuropathic pain (Hamilton and McMahon, 2000; Barclay *et al.*, 2002) and in certain types of mechanosensation (Cockayne *et al.*, 2000) and this will be discussed further below.

From the material reviewed above, it can be seen that nociceptive DRG cells can therefore be divided into three main populations (Fig. 2.2), namely:

1. Small-diameter TRPV1- and P2X$_3$-expressing IB4+ cells that give rise to unmyelinated axons (C fibres)

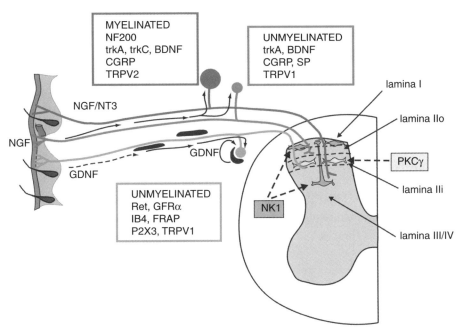

Fig. 2.2 Diagram showing the three main populations of nociceptors, namely: (1) small-diameter IB4+ non-peptide-expressing cells (green) that respond to GDNF and innervate predominantly lamina II inner; (2) small-diameter peptide-expressing (CGRP, substance P) cells (blue) that respond to NGF and innervate predominantly laminae I and II outer; and (3) medium-diameter peptide-expressing (CGRP) cells (red) that have finely myelinated axons, respond to NGF and NT3, and innervate predominantly laminae I and III/IV. For further details see text. (Adapted from Snider and McMahon, 1998; Priestley *et al.*, 2002.) See plate section, Plate 2 (centre of book) for a colour version.

2. Small-diameter TRPV1-expressing peptidergic (CGRP, substance P) cells that give rise to unmyelinated axons (C fibres)

3. Medium-diameter TRPV2-expressing CGRP cells that have finely myelinated (Aδ) axons.

This scheme is derived mainly from correlative studies, but is consistent with the few studies that have directly examined both physiology and neurochemistry. Thus, direct intracellular recording in vivo has shown that substance P-containing afferents are all nociceptors and are predominantly C fibres (Lawson *et al.*, 1997). Studies in vitro have confirmed that both IB4+ and IB4− cells have the properties of nociceptors, but revealed differences in the electrophysiological properties of the two populations (Stucky and Lewin, 1999; Dirajlal *et al.*,2003; Liu *et al.*, 2004).

Amongst cutaneous afferents, all three nociceptive populations have peripheral processes that form free nerve endings in the epidermis (Kruger *et al.*, 1981; Kruger *et al.*, 1989; Simone *et al.*, 1998; Zylka *et al.*, 2005), but peptide-expressing C fibres (population #2) also give rise to perivascular endings in epidermis and dermis. This population also has proportionally more visceral projections than the IB4+ cells (population #1) (Bennett *et al.*, 1996*a*; Perry and Lawson, 1998; Lu *et al.*, 2001). The central projections of these three populations have slightly different termination patterns. The peptide-containing C fibres terminate predominantly in lamina I and outer lamina II (II.) (Priestley *et al.*, 1982); IB4+ fibres terminate mainly in inner lamina II (IIi) (Alvarez *et al.*, 1991); and Aδ fibres terminate predominantly in lamina I and laminae III–V. The detailed organization of the dorsal horn and postsynaptic targets of these three nociceptive populations are discussed in Chapter 3.

2.3 Neurotrophic factors

2.3.1 Target-derived neurotrophins

The development, mature phenotype, and reaction to injury of these DRG subpopulations depends on their response to various growth factors, the most important of which are members of the neurotrophin, glial cell line-derived neurotrophic factor (GDNF), and neuropoetic cytokine families (see Table 2.2). DRG cells show characteristic expression patterns of growth factor receptors, indicative of the fact that the individual DRG subpopulations respond to particular growth factors or combinations of factors (see Fig. 2.1). The distribution of receptors amongst nociceptors is particularly striking, with the CGRP and IB4+ populations each expressing a different family of receptors.

All three high-affinity neurotrophin receptors (trkA, trkB, and trkC) are expressed within dorsal root ganglia (McMahon *et al.*, 1994; Kashiba *et al.*, 1995; Wright and Snider, 1995), but the CGRP-containing population of nociceptors express predominantly trkA. Thus there is extensive overlap (92%) between cells expressing trkA (approximately 40–45% of lumbar DRG cells) and CGRP (Averill *et al.*, 1995). Approximately 20% of these trkA cells are rich in neurofilaments, coexpress trkC, and

Table 2.2 Major neurotrophic factors which support adult dorsal root ganglion cells

Neurotrophins

Actions mediated through three different receptor tyrosine kinases (trks, selectivity indicated below) and a non-selective receptor, p75:

Nerve growth factor (NGF, binds to trkA)

Brain-derived neurotrophic factor (BDNF, binds to trkB)

Neurotrophin-3 (NT-3, binds to trkC)

Neurotrophin-4/5 (NT-4/5, binds to trkB)

GDNF family

Actions mediated through the receptor tyrosine kinase RET and one of four accessory subunits (GFRαs, selectivity indicated below):

Glial cell line-derived neurotrophic factor (GDNF, binds to GFRα1)

Neurturin (binds to GFRα2)

Artemin (binds to GFRα3)

Persephin (binds to GFRα4)

Neuropoeitic cytokines

Actions mediated through the cytoplasmic tyrosine kinase JAK, activated via gp130 and various receptor subunits (selectivity indicated below):

Ciliary neurotrophic factor (CNTF, binds to a complex of gp130, LIFRβ, and CNTFRα)

Oncostatin M (OM, binds to a complex of gp130 and LIFRβ or gp130 and OMRβ)

Leukaemia inhibitory factor (LIF, binds to a complex of gp130 and LIFRβ)

Interleukin-6 (IL6, binds to a complex of gp130 and IL6R

---

probably correspond to the population of Aδ high threshold mechanoreceptors. The rest of the trkA cells have unmyelinated axons and are likely to be polymodal nociceptors. The trkA cells also express the low affinity neurotrophin receptor p75. However, p75 is not a specific marker for nociceptors because it is also coexpressed with trkB and trkC, which are present in many large- and medium-sized cells which have myelinated axons and are predominantly low threshold mechanoreceptors (Kashiba *et al.*, 1995; Wright and Snider, 1995).

The expression of trkA and p75 on CGRP-containing nociceptors suggests that this population responds to NGF, and this is borne out by studies of inflammation and nerve injury (reviewed in sections 2.4 and 2.5 below) and by work on normal animals. Treatment of animals with NGF has a range of direct effects that are mediated by the trkA-expressing DRG cells, including an acute sensitization leading to thermal hyperalgesia (Lewin *et al.*, 1994) and a longer lasting effect on gene expression. Recent studies indicate that the sensitization is partly due to a trkA-mediated activation of phospholipase C (PLCγ) which releases TRPV1 from inhibition by plasma membrane phosphatidylinositol-5,5-bisphosphate (Chuang *et al.*, 2001), although other pathways may also be involved (see section 2.4.1).

The chronic effects are mediated by transcription factors such as ATF2 (Delcroix *et al.*, 1999) and c-fos, which are activated by trkA via various pathways including the extra-cellular signal-regulated protein kinase (ERK) pathway (Segal and Greenberg, 1996; Averill *et al.*, 2001). Proteins upregulated in trkA cells by NGF treatment in vivo include substance P and CGRP (Verge *et al.*, 1995) and P2X$_3$ (Ramer *et al.*, 2001). The increased substance P expression results in increased release from primary afferent terminals in the dorsal horn (Malcangio *et al.*, 1997, 2000*a*) and increased activation of spinal cord neurons (Thompson *et al.*, 1995). In contrast, expression of various proteins expressed by trkA/CGRP cells is decreased by peripheral nerve transection and this decrease can be blocked by exogenous NGF (see section 2.5.2 below).

It thus appears that the adult phenotype of the CGRP-containing nociceptors is maintained by NGF derived from cells in peripheral targets, such as keratinocytes in the epidermis of the skin (Di Marco *et al.*, 1991). This interpretation is supported by studies in which NGF has been sequestered or blocked in normal animals. This produces a thermal and chemical hypoalgesia, a reduction in the sensitivity of individual nociceptors, a downregulation of substance P, CGRP, and Na$_V$1.8 (SNS, TTX-resistant sodium current), and a reduction in the innervation density of the epidermis (McMahon *et al.*, 1995; Bennett *et al.*, 1998*a*; Fjell *et al.*, 1999*c*; Shadiack *et al.*, 2001).

2.3.2 Target-derived GDNF

In contrast to the CGRP cells, the IB4+ population of nociceptors do not normally respond to NGF but do respond to GDNF. IB4+ cells express trkA and respond to NGF in development, but trkA is downregulated in the early postnatal period (Bennett *et al.*, 1996*b*). Over the same period receptor components for the GDNF family are upregulated and become characteristic of the IB4+ cells (Molliver *et al.*, 1997; Bennett *et al.*, 1998*b*). Thus, adult IB4+ cells do not express either p75 or any of the trks (McMahon *et al.*, 1994; Averill *et al.*, 1995; Wright and Snider, 1995), but they virtually all express RET mRNA (95% of IB4+ cells) and approximately 75% express GFRα1, GFRα2, and/or GFRα3 (Bennett *et al.*, 1998*b*, 2000; Orozco *et al.*, 2001).

GDNF treatment in vivo increases expression of proteins such as P2X$_3$ (Ramer *et al.*, 2001) and somatostatin (Issa *et al.*, 2001), which are expressed by IB4+ cells, and protects IB4+ cells from axotomy (see below). GDNF family members may also have effects on other cell populations since many large-diameter (mainly non-nociceptive) DRG cells express GFRα1 and RET (Bennett *et al.*, 1998*b*), and although CGRP cells mainly do not express GFRα1 or GFRα2, many do express GFRα3 (Orozco *et al.*, 2001) and this expression increases after nerve injury (Bennett *et al.*, 2000). However, GDNF effects on these cell populations have not been much studied. The role of endogenous GDNF is also not clear. GDNF (Trupp *et al.*, 1995) is expressed in a number of peripheral tissues and is retrogradely transported by DRG cells following injection into the sciatic nerve (Leitner *et al.*, 1999). It is therefore possible that it acts in a target-derived way to support IB4+ cells, but there is also a strong case for it acting as a local injury-derived factor: GDNF is synthesized by Schwann cells and by DRG satellite glial cells, GDNF levels are higher in peripheral nerve than they are in targets such as muscle or skin, and are increased further by axotomy (Trupp *et al.*, 1995; Hammarberg *et al.*, 1996; Naveilhan *et al.*, 1997; Hoke *et al.*, 2000).

GDNF-treated animals (Boucher *et al.*, 2000) and GDNF-overexpressing mice (Zwick *et al.*, 2002) show normal pain thresholds, but GDNF is analgesic in animal models of neuropathic pain (Boucher *et al.*, 2000; Wang *et al.*, 2003). Similar results have recently been reported for artemin (Gardell *et al.*, 2003) GDNF family members may therefore play a more important role in neuropathic pain states than in normal animals, and this is discussed further below (section 2.6).

2.3.3 Cytokines

Many cytokines are pronociceptive, and have both direct actions on DRG cells as well as actions mediated by bradykinin (Perkins *et al.*, 1995) and NGF (Woolf *et al.*, 1997). In the case of the neuropoietic cytokines, particularly strong evidence for direct effects has come from work showing that the expression of galanin is regulated by LIF (Corness *et al.*, 1996; Sun and Zigmond, 1996; Thompson *et al.*, 1998) and that galanin has both pronociceptive and antinociceptive roles (Kerr *et al.*, 2000; Liu *et al.*, 2001). However, relatively few studies have examined the particular DRG cell types affected by the neuropoietic cytokines or the expression of their receptors by DRG cells. The gp130 signalling component is likely to be expressed by all DRG cells (Mizuno *et al.*, 1997) and LIFRβ mRNA expression and LIF binding by DRG cells has been reported (Qiu *et al.*, 1997; Scott *et al.*, 2000). LIF retrograde transport labels a subgroup of both CGRP and IB4+ cells (Thompson *et al.*, 1997), suggesting some selectivity for nociceptors. However, studies on galanin expression in the LIF knock-out mouse (Corness *et al.*, 1996) suggest that LIF may also affect large-diameter (non-nociceptive) cells.

2.3.4 BDNF synthesis by DRG cells

In addition to retrogradely transporting target or injury-derived neurotrophins, DRG cells are themselves capable of synthesizing BDNF (Wetmore and Olson, 1995; Michael *et al.*, 1997; Cho *et al.*, 1997b). The expression of BDNF appears to be regulated by target-derived factors, being expressed by trkA cells in response to NGF (Michael *et al.*, 1997) and in large-diameter trkB and trkC cells after nerve injury (Cho *et al.*, 1998; Michael *et al.*, 1999). The BDNF is packaged in dense cored vesicles and transported into the central arbors of DRG cells (Zhou and Rush, 1996; Michael *et al.*, 1997) from which it is released (Lever *et al.*, 2001) to control spinal cord excitability (Kerr *et al.*, 1999; Pezet *et al.*, 2002a; Lever *et al.*, 2003). BDNF thus acts as an anterograde trophic messenger, that is synthesized by DFG cells in response to changes in the periphery and that in turn regulates spinal cord activity.

2.4 **Nociceptor plasticity following tissue injury and inflammation**

Although the previous sections have described the organization and neurochemistry of nociceptors, their properties are not stable and can be altered by a large number of factors. The word plasticity is often used to describe these altered properties, although it is worth noting that this term has no formal definition and is taken to mean different things by different authors. In the context of primary afferent nociceptors, functionally relevant forms of plasticity are those that affect the encoding and transmission of pain-related sensory information. There are two broad types of nociceptor plasticity that need to be distinguished. First, rapid onset peripheral sensitization (or desensitization) of nociceptive terminals, arising without altered nociceptor gene expression. And second, slower onset phenotypic change in nociceptor properties as a consequence of altered gene expression. This latter form of plasticity can affect pain signalling in a variety of ways, and both forms of plasticity are discussed in more detail below.

2.4.1 **Peripheral sensitization**

Tissue injury and inflammation and a great many algesic chemicals produce changes in the stimulus–response functions of the primary sensory neurone terminals in peripheral tissues. If the stimulus–response function shows a leftward shift, the nociceptor is sensitized and a greater afferent barrage is generated for a given stimulus. Less studied, but potentially important, nociceptors can be desensitized and show rightward shifts in stimulus–response functions. Chapter 1 of this book reviews in some detail the electrophysiological characteristics of this form of plasticity.

The stimuli that trigger sensitization may activate G-protein coupled receptors in the nociceptor terminal. Stimuli of this type include prostanoids acting at EP receptors (England et al., 1996), ATP acting at P2Y receptors (Tominaga et al., 2001), bradykinin at B2 receptors (Cesare and McNaughton, 1996), glutamate at mGlu5 receptors (Hu et al., 2002), and some agents acting at chemokine receptors (Oh et al., 2001). Alternatively, stimuli may activate ionotropic receptors, such as capsaicin or heat acting on TRPV1 (reviewed in Julius and Basbaum, 2001), or ATP acting at P2X receptors (reviewed in Hamilton and McMahon, 2000). Finally, several trophic factors and cytokines acting at tyrosine kinase receptors may cause sensitization. This has been shown most clearly for NGF, acting at trkA receptors (Shu and Mendell, 1999; Chuang et al., 2001).

These different stimuli recruit a variety of intracellular signalling cascades including PKA (Aley and Levine, 1999) and PKC (Cesare et al., 1999; Khasar et al., 1999; Premkumar and Ahern, 2000; Chuang et al., 2001), or the MAPkinase ERK1/2 (Aley et al., 2001; Dai et al., 2002). The final effector mechanism underlying the sensitization of nociceptors is also quite variable, and can involve the modulation (often by phosphorylation) of Na^+, K^+, or Ca^{++} channels (Gold et al., 1996), or modulation via phosphylation of some receptors such as TRPV1 (Vellani et al., 2001) TRPA1 (Bandell et al., 2004) and P2X (Paukert et al., 2001). Modulation of TRPV1 has been particularly well studied and it is clear that its sensitization can be so large as to lead to activation of the receptor at body temperatures (Premkumar and Ahern, 2000; Tominaga *et al.*, 2001). It is also clear that a great many stimuli are coupled to TRPV1 sensitization and this probably accounts for much of the commonly observed hyperalgesia to heat stimuli. It is interesting that, in contrast to heat sensitization, sensitization to mechanical stimuli has been much less commonly observed, at least for cutaneous nociceptors.

The peripheral sensitization of nociceptors, described above, typically arises within seconds of stimulus application and persists, to a transient stimulus, for a matter of minutes. However, in the presence of ongoing tissue injury or inflammation, sensitization may also be prolonged. In the context of the current chapter, the sensitizing effects of NGF on heat responsiveness of nociceptors is of particular interest. On isolated DRG cells in culture and on nociceptive terminals studied using a skin-nerve preparation (Shu and Mendell, 1999), NGF acutely sensitizes many nociceptive neurones, although the mechanism of sensitization has variously been ascribed to PKA-, PKC-, PIP2- (Chuang *et al.*, 2001), and ERK-dependent mechanisms. Cutaneous nociceptors chronically exposed to elevated NGF levels, in an NGF-overexpressing mouse, showed a marked heat sensitization (Stucky *et al.*, 1999). While the exact mechanism of sensitization is not known in this case, the data nonetheless demonstrate that persistent peripheral sensitization is possible.

2.4.2 Altered gene expression in nociceptors

A second form of nociceptor plasticity involves the regulation of gene expression in DRG cells. There is now a very large body of experimental data that such regulation readily occurs as a consequence of tissue injury, most notably persistent injuries associated with peripheral tissue inflammation. The plasticity of gene expression affects many aspects of nociceptor function including: genes coding for neurotransmitters released with activity from the central terminals of nociceptors; genes coding for receptors which are transported to both the peripheral and central terminals of nociceptors; genes coding for ion channels expressed throughout the neuron and potentially affecting its sensitivity. Genes regulating structural proteins in nociceptors are also affected and this may alter some anatomical features of these neurones.

There are several potentially important signals for this plasticity of gene expression. The most important (and certainly the best studied) is NGF. This molecule is up-regulated in many experimental models of inflammation (including those induced by carrageenan and Freund's adjuvant) and in some clinical inflammatory disorders (Aloe *et al.*, 1992; Donnerer *et al.*, 1992; Woolf *et al.*, 1994; Safieh–Garabedian *et al.*, 1995; Lowe *et al.*, 1997; Oddiah *et al.*, 1998). NGF is internalized following its binding to trkA. In addition to its peripherally sensitizing effects, it is retrogradely transported from peripheral terminals to cell bodies (Miller and Kaplan, 2001). Evidence from several sources suggests that NGF itself cannot initiate signalling in the cell soma, but that the NGF/trkA complex maintains autophosphorylation and activates transcription factors such as CREB and Oct-2 that control gene expression (Kendall *et al.*, 1995; Poo, 2001). The importance of NGF is supported firstly by its ability (when administered exogenously) to induce changes in gene expression (see section 2.3.1 above) and from the many studies which have shown that nociceptor plasticity to inflammation is greatly reduced with strategies that block NGF actions (reviewed in McMahon and Bennett, 1999 and see below).

It is possible that other inflammatory mediators may also drive abnormal gene expression in nociceptors. The cytokines LIF, TNFα, and IL1β are up-regulated in some injury states, alter nociceptor phenotype when administered, and may be necessary for some inflammation-induced plasticity (Woolf *et al.*, 1997; Thompson *et al.*, 1998; Junger and Sorkin, 2000). However, it is not always clear whether these agents act directly. IL1β and TNFα may both lead to the up-regulation of NGF, for instance.

A final possible mechanism for transcriptional regulation of nociceptors is neuronal activity itself. One study reported that electrical stimulation of the peripheral axons of nociceptors at high frequency led to increased expression of BDNF mRNA in DRG cells 2 hours later — a time inconsistent with retrograde transport of signalling molecules such as NGF (Mannion *et al.*, 1999).

2.4.2.1 Neurotransmitter plasticity

The best studied examples are substance P and BDNF. These molecules are constitutively expressed by a modest number of small-diameter DRG neurones (see sections 2.2.1 and 2.3.4 above). However, their expression is dramatically increased in sensory neurones innervating tissues subject to experimental inflammation with either carrageenan or Fruend's adjuvant (Donnerer *et al.*, 1992; Leslie *et al.*, 1995; Safieh–Garabedian *et al.*, 1995; Cho *et al.*, 1997*a,b*; Kerr *et al.*, 1999; Mannion *et al.*, 1999). With inflammation, many more nociceptors, and perhaps some previously non-nociceptive neurones (Neumann *et al.*, 1996; Mannion *et al.*, 1999) begin to express these molecules. Several of these studies have shown that most or all of the inflammation–induced up-regulation of substance P and BDNF depends on peripherally produced NGF. Activity in nociceptors releases substance P and BDNF from central terminals and this activity-dependent release is enhanced in inflammatory conditions (Malcangio *et al.*, 1996, 2000*a*). Since both these molecules exert potent effects on second-order signalling systems within the spinal cord, this form of nociceptor plasticity may contribute to inflammatory pain states (see section 2.6 below).

2.4.2.2 Receptor plasticity

Peripheral inflammation leads to up-regulation of a variety of receptors in primary sensory neurones. These include G-protein coupled receptors such as bradykinin B1 and B2 receptors (the latter of which are normally present at only very low levels), both of which appear to be regulated predominantly by NGF (Petersen *et al.*, 1998; Lee *et al.*, 2002) and the mu opioid receptor (Ji *et al.*, 1995). Some ionotropic receptors such as TRPV1 and P2X3 are also up-regulated in inflammatory conditions (Carlton and Coggeshall, 2001; Xu and Huang, 2002). TRPV1 in particular appears to be strongly regulated by the availability of NGF. VR1 is down-regulated after axotomy, and this can be blocked by NGF treatment (Priestley *et al.*, 2002). However, GDNF can also regulate TRPV1 expression in that proportion of nociceptors that express GDNF receptors (Ogun–Muyiwa *et al.*, 1999; Priestley *et al.*, 2002). Interestingly, expression of the trkA receptor itself is affected by axotomy (Shen *et al.*, 1999), although the extent to which expression is regulated by NGF (Delcroix *et al.*, 1998) or up-regulated in inflammatory conditions (Cho *et al.*, 1996) is unclear.

Since all these different receptors are transported to the peripheral terminals of nociceptors, their up-regulation may increase the sensitivity of peripheral terminals to appropriate ligands, and in the case of the trkA receptor, may establish a positive feedback circuit to maintain this abnormal state. These receptors are also transported to the central terminals of nociceptive neurones, where their presynaptic activation may regulate nociceptor transmitter release. Again, therefore, these phenotypic changes may have functional consequences, for instance contributing to the increased sensitivity to opiates seen in inflammatory conditions.

2.4.2.3 Ion channels

There has been considerable interest in the regulation of TTX-resistant sodium channels in inflammatory as well as neuropathic (considered below) pain states. Much of this interest stems from the observation that these channels can regulate the excitability of afferent nerve terminals (England *et al.*, 1996; Gold *et al.*, 1996) and, since these channels are largely restricted to nociceptors, act as an important peripheral determinant of pain thresholds to all forms of stimulation. Two types of neuronal TTX-resistant sodium channel have been identified, which are formed from $Na_v1.8$ and $Na_v1.9$ α-subunits (formerly known as SNS and NaN). These are expressed in many small-diameter sensory neurones (Amaya *et al.*, 2000; Fang *et al.*, 2002). $Na_v1.8$ is known to be up-regulated under inflammatory conditions (Tanaka *et al.*, 1998; Tate *et al.*, 1998). NGF, which of course is increased in these inflammatory state, is a potent regulator of $Na_v1.8$ expression (Dib–Hajj *et al.*, 1998), but can also regulate other sodium channel subunits (Zur *et al.*, 1995; Fjell *et al.*, 1999*a*). Interestingly, GDNF appears to be an important regulator of $Na_V1.9$ (Fjell *et al.*, 1999*b*; Cummins *et al.*, 2000; Leffler *et al.*, 2002).

The regulation of expression of calcium and potassium currents by inflammatory mediators has been little explored to date, but may prove interesting given that these are known to be important in the control of neuronal excitability and neurotransmitter release.

2.4.2.4 Anatomical plasticity

The growth associated protein GAP43 is up-regulated in sensory neurones supplying an inflamed hindpaw (Leslie *et al.*, 1995), most notably in small-diameter nociceptive neurones. This increase is blocked by administration of neutralizing antiserum to NGF. Thus, the innervation of peripheral structures may undergo some anatomical remodelling in the presence of inflammation. Certainly, there is evidence that some forms of hyperinnervation are secondary to NGF (Constantinou *et al.*, 1994) and conversely,

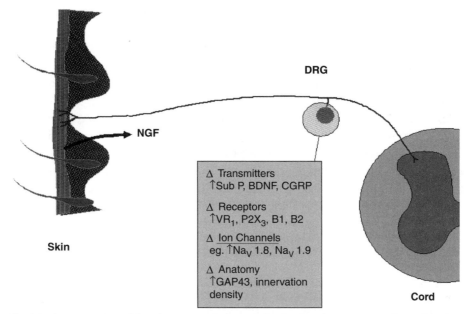

Fig. 2.3 Diagram summarizing the range of phenotypic changes that can occur in nociceptors as a consequence of peripheral tissue injuries that are associated with increased availability of NGF, such as inflammation.

chronic cutaneous deprivation of NGF leads to marked epidermal hypoinnervation and reduced skin sensitivity (Bennett *et al.*, 1998*a*).

Figure 2.3 summarizes the range of phenotypic changes that can occur in nociceptors as a consequence of peripheral tissue injuries and inflammation.

2.5 Nociceptor plasticity following nerve injury

Nerve injuries are frequently associated with abnormal pain sensations, neuropathic pain states. Chapter 5 of this book discusses the features and mechanisms of these states. But a topic of considerable current interest is to what extent nociceptor plasticity contributes to evolution of neuropathic pain, and here we will concentrate on the changes in sensory neurone phenotype that arise following nerve injuries.

2.5.1 Animal models

In humans, nerve injury may be metabolic (e.g. in diabetes), infectious (e.g. following HIV), drug-induced (e.g. some anti-cancer drugs such as taxol), or traumatic. Mechanistic studies in animals have nearly all focused on traumatic injuries, usually in rodents. There are several such animal models in general use. They share the common feature of degeneration of some, but not all, sensory fibres in a major peripheral nerve, so that a peripheral target is partially denervated and conversely, partially innervated. One model involves partial nerve ligation (Seltzer *et al.*, 1990). Typically, a third to a half of the sciatic nerve is tightly ligated with a silk suture. Since sensory fibres in the sciatic exhibit considerable mixing as they travel distally in the nerve, this procedure does not result in total denervation of a confined area, but a partial denervation throughout much of the sciatic innervation territory. A more recent derivative of this approach is to tie off one or more of the branches of the sciatic nerve (Decosterd and Woolf, 2000). The damaged sensory fibres do innervate a more restricted area in this case, but because of the overlap of nerve territories, there are border zones of partial innervation which exhibit neuropathic signs (i.e. altered sensibility to sensory stimuli).

A third, extensively used model is that of chronic nerve constriction (Bennett and Xie, 1988). Here, several chromic ligatures are loosely tied around the sciatic nerve at mid thigh level. The sutures are tight enough to partially restrict blood flow in superficial vessels in the nerve. The nerve swells and a marked constriction results. Anatomical studies show that a substantial fraction, but not all fibres, undergo Wallerian degeneration distal to the ligation site (Coggeshall *et al.*, 1993). This model appears to have a greater inflammatory component than the others. The presence particularly of chromic suture material may exacerbate the inflammatory response. The liberation of cytokines or other factors (e.g. nerve growth factor) from immunocytes at the site of constriction may contribute to the neuropathic symptoms. Indeed, neuropathic symptoms are seen in models of neuritis without direct traumatic injury of nerve (Sorkin *et al.*, 1997).

The most commonly used model today involves the ligation of one or two spinal nerves (usually L5 alone or L5 and L6), just distal to the DRG (Kim and Chung, 1992). Since the sciatic nerve carries large numbers of sensory fibres from the L4 and L5 spinal nerves (and smaller numbers from the L6 nerve), this lesion results in degeneration of about 50% of the fibres in the sciatic nerve, and these project throughout the normal sciatic innervation territory. One advantage of this model for mechanistic studies is that in a particular DRG virtually all sensory neurone cell bodies are either axotomized or intact. This contrasts with other models, where the cell bodies of injured and uninjured neurons are mixed together in one or more DRGs.

In these models there are two different populations of sensory neurones that need to be considered. First, the neurones whose axons are damaged and that are therefore disconnected from peripheral targets. Secondly, the neurones that remain intact but have axons intermingling with those degenerating in the distal nerve. These groups show very marked (and distinct) alterations in phenotype, which are summarized in Fig. 2.4 and described below.

2.5.2 **Plasticity in damaged sensory neurones**

One cause of plasticity is the altered availability of target-derived neurotrophic factors. It is well recognized that sensory neurones during development require an adequate supply of these factors for their survival (see Chapter 9). In adulthood, the survival of

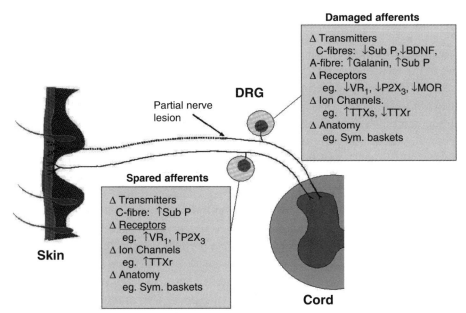

Fig. 2.4 Diagram summarizing the range of phenotypic changes that can occur in both damaged and undamaged (spared) nociceptors as a consequence of a peripheral nerve lesion.

sensory neurones does not depend upon these peripheral factors, but, as reviewed in section 2.3 above, trophic factors such as NGF and GDNF continue to exert powerful effects on nociceptor gene expression. When the axon of a sensory neurone degenerates following injury, the cell loses contact with its peripheral target and loses the supply of target-derived factors such as NGF. Schwann cells in the damaged nerve start to make some of these factors (NGF and GDNF in particular), but this surrogate supply is insufficient to replace that normally derived from the target (Heumann *et al.*, 1987; Naveilhan *et al.*, 1997). It is perhaps therefore not surprising that many of the changes in gene expression in damaged nociceptors are the exact opposite of those occurring with tissue inflammation (when target-derived factors are up-regulated). As illustrated in Fig. 2.4, damaged neurones show alterations in neurotransmitters, receptors, and ion channels.

Many of the neurotransmitters/modulators constitutively expressed by nociceptors (such as substance P, CGRP, somatostatin, and BDNF) are down-regulated in damaged neurones (reviewed in Hokfelt *et al.*, 1994; McMahon and Bennett, 1999; Priestley *et al.*, 2002). These changes develop over a few days and persist for many months. Associated with this down-regulation, there is reduced release of these agents with nociceptor activity (Malcangio *et al.*, 2000*b*). Treatment of the damaged nerves with NGF prevents the down-regulation in the trkA/CGRP population and GDNF prevents the down-regulation in the IB4 population (Verge *et al.*, 1995; Bennett *et al.*, 1998*b*; Wang *et al.*, 2003). Similarly, there is a down-regulation of TRPV1 and P2X3 receptors in damaged nociceptors, which can be reversed or prevented by treating the damaged neurones with

NGF and/or GDNF (Bradbury *et al.*, 1998; Priestley *et al.*, 2002; Wang *et al.*, 2003). As might be expected from the decreased availability of trophic factors, particularly NGF, there is also a down-regulation of TTX-resistant sodium channel subunits $Na_V1.8$ and $Na_V1.9$ (Boucher *et al.*, 2000).

There are, however, some increases in nociceptor gene expression that are rather unexpected on the basis of altered trophic factor availability. One of these is the dramatic up-regulation of the peptide, galanin, in a great number of the damaged afferents, including most of the nociceptive population and many of the large cells (Villar *et al.*, 1989). Interestingly, this up-regulation starts very rapidly, within a day, and well before the down-regulation of transmitters (described above) can be detected. One possibility is that the plasticity in galanin and peptide transcripts have different mechanisms. NGF and GDNF treatment can partially offset galanin up-regulation (Verge *et al.*, 1995; Wang *et al.*, 2003), and NGF deprivation has recently been reported to induce it (Shadiack *et al.*, 2001). In a similar way, NGF and GDNF treatments have been shown to prevent the injury-associated up-regulation of the transcriptor factor ATF 3 (Averill *et al.*, 2004). On the other hand, it is known that some cytokines can induce galanin (Sun and Zigmond, 1996; Thompson *et al.*, 1998). It is possible that in addition to 'negative' factors (i.e. reduced neurotrophic factor support), 'positive' factors (i.e. increased cytokines) may contribute to nociceptor plasticity after damage. Such a mechanism may explain the dynamic pattern of upregulation exhibited by the Schwann cell mitogen, Reg-2, after nerve injury (Averill *et al.*, 2002). Several cytokines are known to be released in damaged nerves (Shamash *et al.*, 2002; Stoll *et al.*, 2002) and may act to induce peptide expression in particular subpopulations of DRG cells.

One transcriptional change that may be of functional importance is altered expression of $Na_V1.3$ (formally brain type III) in damaged neurones. It is not normally expressed in adult DRG but rapidly up-regulated following nerve damage (Boucher *et al.*, 2000). It is not clear which cell types start to express $Na_V1.3$, but the up-regulation can be prevented by GDNF treatment.

2.5.3 Plasticity in 'spared' sensory neurones after nerve injury

While these neurones, by definition, are themselves undamaged, they are still likely to be subject to altered neurotrophic factor support and injury-associated factors. Target-derived trophic factors are usually made in limiting amounts. When a significant number of sensory neurones lose contact with their target, the remaining innervation has less competition for these factors. This is exactly the case with the 'spared' afferents in the models of partial nerve injury that lead to neuropathic states. In one of these models (the so called 'Chung' model), lesion of the L5 spinal nerve results in increased NGF availability and content in the L4 (spared) DRG (Fukuoka *et al.*, 2001). It is less clear what impact 'positive' factors (e.g. cytokines) liberated in damaged nerves will exert. On the one hand, uptake into, and transport by, spared afferents may be much less than in damaged ones (Curtis *et al.*, 1993, 1994). On the other hand, because of the extensive mixing of C-fibre Remak bundles in peripheral nerve, partial injuries lead to major re-organization of the bundles of intact C-fibre axons (Wu *et al.*, 2001).

Several changes in gene expression have been observed in intact nociceptors after partial nerve lesions. These include the up-regulation of substance P, TRPV1 (Hudson *et al.*, 2001), BDNF (Fukuoka *et al.*, 2001), and P2X3 (Tsuzuki *et al.*, 2001). One report (Boucher *et al.*, 2000) demonstrates an increase in $Na_V1.8$ mRNA by PCR in spared afferents, but another recent study found no change in the number of $Na_V1.8$ immunopositive cells in intact axons in several models of partial nerve injury (Decosterd *et al.*, 2002).

2.6 Nociceptor plasticity and chronic pain

The functional consequences of all of the plastic changes described in the preceding sections are not currently known. In some cases, however, we have at least good circumstantial evidence that a particular plastic change contributes to abnormal pain behaviour.

One clear example is the peripheral sensitization of nociceptors to heat stimuli. As described in section 2.4.1, there are several post-translational changes in proteins in nociceptor terminals that make the terminal more sensitive to applied stimuli. Burn injuries lead to nociceptor sensitization that matches closely the altered psychophysical changes that human subjects report with the same injuries (Raja *et al.*, 1999). Changes in the sensitivity of the TRPV1 receptor are most likely to account for the altered heat responsiveness. Mice lacking the TRPV1 receptor show no thermal hyperalgesia to inflammatory stimuli (Caterina *et al.*, 2000). Some forms of heat hyperalgesia may also be mediated by changes in the sensitivity of the sodium channel subunit $Na_V1.8$, since mice with null mutations of this gene show attenuated or delayed heat hyperalgesia in response to NGF and to carrageenan inflammation (Akopian *et al.*, 1999; Kerr *et al.*, 2001).

There is also a body of evidence to suggest that inflammation-induced changes in the neuromodulators, substance P and, particularly, BDNF, may contribute to the hyperalgesia seen in these states. We have recently reviewed this evidence (Pezet *et al.*, 2002*b*). Briefly, BDNF is known to be released with activity from nociceptors (Lever *et al.*, 2001). A variety of forms of noxious stimulation activates post-synaptic trkB receptors and several biochemical, electrophysiological, and behavioural effects of persistent noxious or inflammatory stimuli are reduced in BDNF knock-out mice (MacQueen *et al.*, 2001) or with pharmacological treatments that sequester BDNF in the spinal cord (Kerr *et al.*, 1999; Mannion *et al.*, 1999). The evidence strongly suggests that BDNF is an important mediator of central sensitization (see Chapter 4), and thereby modifies sensory processing.

There is considerable interest and some controversy regarding the relevance of particular changes in gene expression to neuropathic pain. Activity in sensory neurones after injury appears necessary for the elaboration of neuropathic symptoms, since blocking sensory inflow by cutting dorsal roots, or applying local anaesthetics or the sodium channel blocker TTX reportedly prevents the emergence of neuropathic pain in some circumstances in animal models (Sheen and Chung, 1993; Yoon *et al.*, 1996; Liu *et al.*, 2000*a,b*; Lyu *et al.*, 2000). Clinical observations also support the idea that abnormal sensory inputs trigger neuropathic pain (Campbell *et al.*, 1988; Price *et al.*, 1989). Electrophysiological recordings suggest that many large-diameter damaged and intact myelinated fibres become spontaneously active in these models. Somewhat unexpectedly, of the nociceptive neurones, only some of the spared neurones show spontaneous activity, and then at extremely low levels (averaging less than 0.1 Hz).

What are the molecular correlates of this ectopic activity that drives neuropathic pain behaviour? The answer is confused at present. One candidate mechanism is abnormal expression of TTX- resistant sodium channel transcripts. This suggestion comes from experiments with antisense oligonucleotides, given intrathecally to reduce $Na_V1.8$ levels. This manoeuvre is reported to largely abolish or reverse neuropathic pain behaviour (Lai *et al.*, 2002). This protein is normally confined to nociceptive neurones, and it is known to be down-regulated after injury. Thus, it is unlikely to play a role in damaged afferents. However, it is up-regulated in spared afferents (Boucher *et al.*, 2000), presumably in C-fibres (although this is not formally established). It would be expected to increase the excitability of these neurones and could, therefore, account for the low levels of spontaneous activity seen in the spared nociceptors. However, a further confounding factor is the observation that $Na_V1.8$ knock-out mice do not show any appreciable loss of neuropathic pain behaviour (Kerr *et al.*, 2001).

Another candidate mechanism is the up-regulation of $Na_V1.4$, which occurs in damaged sensory neurones. This sodium channel has rapidly repriming characteristics appropriate to maintain high frequency spontaneous activity. There is correlative data in that GDNF treatment largely reverses the up-regulation of $Na_V1.4$ in damaged afferents and also prevents neuropathic pain behaviour (Boucher *et al.*, 2000). However, it is difficult to establish definitively the importance of this transcript in the absence of specific α-subunit antagonists or other tools.

Another somewhat controversial issue relates to the role of galanin, that is dramatically increased (~120-fold) in damaged sensory neurones. This galanin appears to be released from the central terminals of afferent fibres and has the opportunity to affect second-order sensory processes. The initial experiments on the pharmacological effects of galanin observed predominantly inhibitory effects on spinal cord processing of nociceptive information, and the idea emerged that increased galanin expression in neuropathic states might somehow act to check or limit the sensory abnormalities in pain processing associated with neuropathies (Hokfelt *et al.*, 1994). However, it has more recently become clear that there are several different G-protein coupled receptors for galanin and these are coupled to different intracellular signalling cascades, allowing for mixed inhibitory and excitatory actions (Liu *et al.*, 2001). Studies on galanin knock-out mice show that neuropathic pain behaviour is largely abolished in these animals (Kerr *et al.*, 2000), suggesting that the net effect of endogenous galanin is to drive neuropathic behaviour.

Thus, while the nature of plastic changes in nociceptive neurones is undoubtedly complex and may have several causes, this field of study is likely to help elucidate mechanisms of chronic pain.

Acknowledgements

Supported by the Wellcome Trust.

References

Ahluwalia J, Urban L, Capogna M, Bevan S, and Nagy I (2000) Cannabinoid 1 receptors are expressed in nociceptive primary sensory neurons. *Neurosci* **100**, 685–688.

Akopian AN, Souslova V, England S, *et al.* (1999) The tetrodotoxin-resistant sodium channel SNS has a specialized function in pain pathways. *Nat Neurosci* **2**, 541–548.

Aley KO and Levine JD (1999) Role of protein kinase A in the maintenance of inflammatory pain. *J Neurosci* **19**, 2181–2186.

Aley KO, Martin A, McMahon T, Mok J, Levine JD, and Messing RO (2001) Nociceptor sensitization by extracellular signal-regulated kinases. *J Neurosci* **21**, 6933–6939.

Aloe L, Tuveri MA, and Levi–Montalcini R (1992) Studies on carrageenan-induced arthritis in adult rats: presence of nerve growth factor and role of sympathetic innervation. *Rheumatology International* **12**, 213–216.

Alvarez FJ, Morris HR, and Priestley JV (1991) Sub-populations of smaller diameter trigeminal primary afferent neurons defined by expression of calcitonin gene-related peptide and the cell surface oligosaccharide recognized by monoclonal antibody LA4. *J Neurocytol* **20**, 716–731.

Amaya F, Decosterd I, Samad TA, *et al.* (2000) Diversity of expression of the sensory neuron-specific TTX-resistant voltage-gated sodium ion channels SNS and SNS2. *Mol Cell Neurosci* **15**, 331–342.

Averill S, Davis DR, Shortland PJ, Priestley JV, and Hunt SP (2002) Dynamic pattern of Reg-2 expression in rat sensory neurones after peripheral nerve injury. *J Neurosci* **22**, 7493–7501.

Averill S, Delcroix JD, Michael GJ, Tomlinson DR, Fernyhough P, and Priestley JV (2001) Nerve growth factor modulates the activation status and fast axonal transport of ERK1/2 in adult nociceptive neurones. *Mol Cell Neurosci* **18**, 183–196.

Averill S, McMahon SB, Clary DO, Reichardt LF, and Priestley JV (1995) Immunocytochemical localization of trkA receptors in chemically identified subgroups of adult rat sensory neurons. *Eur J Neurosci* **7**, 1484–1494.

Averill S, Michael GJ, Shortland PJ, *et al.* (2004) NGF and GDNF ameliorate the increase in ATF3 expression which occurs in dorsal root ganglion cells in response to peripheral nerve injury. *Eur J Neurosci* **19**, 1437–1445.

Bandell M, Story GM, Hwang SW, *et al.* (2004) Noxious cold ion channel TRPA1 is activated by pungent compounds and bradykinin. *Neuron* **41**, 849–857.

Barclay J, Patel S, Dorn G, *et al.* (2002) Functional downregulation of P2X3 receptor subunit in rat sensory neurons reveals a significant role in chronic neuropathic and inflammatory pain. *J Neurosci* **22**, 8139–8147.

Bennett DLH, Boucher TJ, Armanini MP, *et al.* (2000) The glial cell line-derived neurotrophic factor family receptor components are differentially regulated within sensory neurons after nerve injury. *J Neurosci* **20**, 427–437.

Bennett DLH, Dmietrieva N, Priestley JV, Clary D, and McMahon SB (1996*a*) TrkA, CGRP and IB4 expression in retrogradely labeled cutaneous and visceral primary sensory neurons in the rat. *Neurosci Lett* **206**, 33–36.

Bennett DLH, Averill S, Clary DO, Priestley JV, and McMahon SB (1996*b*) Postnatal changes in the expression of the trkA high-affinity NGF receptor in primary sensory neurons. *Eur J Neurosci* **8**, 2204–2208.

Bennett DLH, Koltzenburg M, Priestley JV, Shelton DL, and McMahon SB (1998a) Endogenous nerve growth factor regulates the sensitivity of nociceptors in the adult rat. *Eur J Neurosci* **10**, 1282–1291.

Bennett DLH, Michael GJ, Ramachandran N, *et al.* (1998b) A distinct subgroup of small DRG cells express GDNF receptor components and GDNF is protective for these neurons after nerve injury. *J Neurosci* **18**, 3059–3072.

Bennett GJ and Xie YK (1988) A painful mononeuropathy in rat produces disorders of pain sensation like those seen in man. *Pain* **33**, 87–107.

Bonaventure P, Voorn P, Luyten WHML, and Leysen JE (1998) 5HT$_{1B}$ and 5HT$_{1D}$ receptor mRNA differential co-localization with peptide mRNA in the guinea pig trigeminal ganglion. *Neuroreport* **9**, 641–645.

Boucher TJ, Okuse K, Bennett DL, Munson JB, Wood JN, and McMahon SB (2000) Potent analgesic effects of GDNF in neuropathic pain states. *Science* **290**, 124–127.

Bradbury EJ, Burnstock G, and McMahon SB (1998) The expression of P2X3 purinoreceptors in sensory neurons: effects of axotomy and glial-derived neurotrophic factor. *Mol Cell Neurosci* **12**, 256–268.

Campbell JN, Raja SN, Meyer RA, and Mackinnon SE (1988) Myelinated afferents signal the hyperalgesia associated with nerve injury. *Pain* **32**, 89–94.

Carlton SM and Coggeshall RE (2001) Peripheral capsaicin receptors increase in the inflamed rat hindpaw: a possible mechanism for peripheral sensitization. *Neurosci Lett* **310**, 53–56.

Caterina MJ, Leffler A, Malmberg AB, *et al.* (2000) Impaired nociception and pain sensation in mice lacking the capsaicin receptor. *Science* **288**, 306–313.

Caterina MJ, Rosen TA, Tominaga M, Brake AJ, and Julius D (1999) A capsaicin-receptor homologue with a high threshold for noxious heat. *Nature* **398**, 436–441.

Caterina MJ, Schumacher MA, Tominaga M, Rosen TA, Levine JD, and Julius D (1997) The capsaicin receptor: a heat-activated ion channel in the pain pathway. *Nature* **389**, 816–824.

Cesare P and McNaughton P (1996) A novel heat-activated current in nociceptive neurons and its sensitization by bradykinin. *Proc Natl Acad Sci USA* **93**, 15435–15439.

Cesare P, Dekker LV, Sardini A, Parker PJ, and McNaughton PA (1999) Specific involvement of PKC-epsilon in sensitization of the neuronal response to painful heat. *Neuron* **23**, 617–624.

Cho HJ, Kim JK, Park HC, Kim DS, Ha SO, and Hong HS (1998) Changes in brain-derived neurotrophic factor immunoreactivity in rat dorsal root ganglia, spinal cord, and gracile nuclei following cut or crush injuries. *Exp Neurol* **154**, 224–230.

Cho HJ, Kim JK, Zhou XF, and Rush RA (1997a) Increased brain-derived neurotrophic factor immunoreactivity in rat dorsal root ganglia and spinal cord following peripheral inflammation. *Brain Res* **764**, 269–272.

Cho HJ, Kim SY, Park MJ, Kim DS, Kim JK, and Chu MY (1997b) Expression of mRNA for brain-derived neurotrophic factor in the dorsal root ganglion following peripheral inflammation. *Brain Res* **749**, 358–362.

Cho HJ, Park EH, Bae MA, and Kim JK (1996) Expression of messenger-RNAs for preprotachykinin and nerve growth factor receptors in the dorsal root ganglion following peripheral inflammation. *Brain Res* **716**, 197–201.

Chuang HH, Prescott ED, Kong H, *et al.* (2001) Bradykinin and nerve growth factor release the capsaicin receptor from PtdIns(4,5)P2-mediated inhibition. *Nature* **411**, 957–962.

Cockayne DA, Hamilton SG, Zhu QM, *et al.* (2000) Urinary bladder hyporeflexia and reduced pain-related behaviour in P2X3- deficient mice. *Nature* **407**, 1011–1015.

Coggeshall RE, Dougherty PM, Pover CM, and Carlton SM (1993) Is large myelinated fiber loss associated with hyperalgesia in a model of experimental peripheral neuropathy in the rat? *Pain* **52**, 233–242.

Constantinou J, Reynolds ML, Woolf CJ, Safieh–Garabedian B, and Fitzgerald M (1994) Nerve growth factor levels in developing rat skin: upregulation following skin wounding. *Neuroreport* **5**, 2281–2284.

Corness J, Shi TJ, Xu ZQ, Brulet P, and Hokfelt T (1996) Influence of leukemia inhibitory factor on galanin/GMAP and neuropeptide Y expression in mouse primary sensory neurons after axotomy. *Exp Brain Res* **112**, 79–88.

Cummins TR, Black JA, Dib–Hajj SD, and Waxman SG (2000) Glial-derived neurotrophic factor upregulates expression of functional SNS and NaN sodium channels and their currents in axotomized dorsal root ganglion neurons. *J Neurosci* **20**, 8754–8761.

Curtis R, Adryan KM, Zhu Y, Harkness PJ, Lindsay RM, and DiStefano PS (1993) Retrograde axonal transport of ciliary neurotrophic factor is increased by peripheral nerve injury. *Nature* **365**, 253–255.

Curtis R, Scherer SS, Somogyi R, *et al.* (1994) Retrograde axonal transport of LIF is increased by peripheral nerve injury: correlation with increased LIF expression in distal nerve. *Neuron* **12**, 191–204.

Dai Y, Iwata K, Fukuoka T, *et al.* (2002) Phosphorylation of extracellular signal-regulated kinase in primary afferent neurons by noxious stimuli and its involvement in peripheral sensitization. *J Neurosci* **22**, 7737–7745.

Decosterd I and Woolf CJ (2000) Spared nerve injury: an animal model of persistent peripheral neuropathic pain. *Pain* **87**, 149–158.

Decosterd I, Ji RR, Abdi S, Tate S, and Woolf CJ (2002) The pattern of expression of the voltage-gated sodium channels Na(v)1.8 and Na(v)1.9 does not change in uninjured primary sensory neurons in experimental neuropathic pain models. *Pain* **96**, 269–277.

Delcroix JD, Averill S, Fernandes K, Tomlinson DR, Priestley JV, and Fernyhough P (1999) Axonal transport of activating transcription factor-2 is modulated by nerve growth factor in nociceptive neurons. *J Neurosci* **0**:RC24, 1–7.

Delcroix JD, Michael GJ, Priestley JV, Tomlinson DR, and Fernyhough P (1998) Effect of nerve growth factor treatment on p75(NTR) gene expression in lumbar dorsal root ganglia of streptozocin-induced diabetic rats. *Diabetes* **47**, 1779–1785.

Del Fiacco M and Priestley JV (2001) Neurotrophins and adult somatosensory neurons. In *Neurobiology of the neurotrophins* (ed. I. Mocchetti), pp. 205–236. Johnson City, TN: F.P. Graham Publishing.

Dib–Hajj SD, Black JA, Cummins TR, Kenney AM, Kocsis JD, and Waxman SG (1998) Rescue of α-SNS sodium channel expression in small dorsal root ganglion neurons after axotomy by nerve growth factor in vivo. *J Neurophysiol* **79**, 2668–2676.

Di Marco E, Marchisio PC, Bondanza S, Franzi AT, Cancedda R, and De Luca M (1991) Growth-regulated synthesis and secretion of biologically active nerve growth factor by human keratinocytes. *J Biol Chem* **266**, 21718–21722.

Dirajlal S, Pauers LE, and Stucky CL (2003) Differential response properties of IB4 –positive and – negative unmyelinated sensory neurons to protons and capsaicin. *J Neurophysiol* **89**, 513–524.

Donnerer J, Schuligoi R, and Stein C (1992) Increased content and transport of substance P and calcitonin gene-related peptide in sensory nerves innervating inflamed tissue: evidence for a regulatory function of nerve growth factor in vivo. *Neurosci* **49**, 693–698.

Drew LJ, Rohrer DK, Prive MP, *et al.* (2004) Acid-sensing ion channels ASIC2 and ASIC3 do not contribute to mechanically activated currents in mammalian sensory neurones. *J Physiol* **556**, 691–710.

England S, Bevan S, and Docherty RJ (1996) PGE2 modulates the tetrodotoxin-resistant sodium current in neonatal rat dorsal root ganglion neurones via the cyclic AMP-protein kinase A cascade. *J Physiol* **495** (**Pt 2**), 429–440.

Fang X, Djouhri L, Black JA, Dib–Hajj SD, Waxman SG, and Lawson SN (2002) The presence and role of the tetrodotoxin-resistant sodium channel Na(v)1.9 (NaN) in nociceptive primary afferent neurons. *J Neurosci* **22**, 7425–7433.

Fjell J, Cummins TR, Davis BM, *et al.* (1999*a*) Sodium channel expression in NGF-overexpressing transgenic mice. *J Neurosci Res* **57**, 39–47.

Fjell J, Cummins TR, Dib–Hajj SD, Fried K, Black JA, and Waxman SG (1999*b*) Differential role of GDNF and NGF in the maintenance of two TTX-resistant sodium channels in adult DRG neurons. *Mol Brain Res* **67**, 267–282.

Fjell J, Cummins TR, Fried K, Black JA, and Waxman SG (1999*c*) In vivo NGF deprivation reduces SNS expression and TTX-R sodium currents in IB4-negative DRG neurons. *J Neurophysiol* **81**, 803–810.

Fukuoka T, Kondo E, Dai Y, Hashimoto N, and Noguchi K (2001) Brain-derived neurotrophic factor increases in the uninjured dorsal root ganglion neurons in selective spinal nerve ligation model. *J Neurosci* **21**, 4891–4900.

Garcia–Anoveros J, Samad TA, Woolf CJ, and Corey DP (2001) Transport and localization of the DEG/ENaC ion channel BNaC1alpha to peripheral mechanosensory terminals of dorsal root ganglia neurons. *J Neurosci* **21**, 2678–2686.

Gardell LR, Wang R, Ehrenfels C, *et al.* (2003) Multiple actions of systemic artemin in experimental neuropathy. *Nat Med* **9**, 1383–1389.

Gold MS, Reichling DB, Shuster MJ, and Levine JD (1996) Hyperalgesic agents increase a tetrodotoxin-resistant Na^+ current in nociceptors. *Proc Natl Acad Sci USA* **93**, 1108–1112.

Gunthorpe MJ, Benham CD, Randall A, and Davis JB (2002) The diversity in the vanilloid (TRPV) receptor family of ion channels. *Trends Pharmacol Sci* **23**, 183–191.

Guo A, Vulchanova L, Wang J, Li X, and Elde R (1999) Immunocytochemical localization of the vanilloid receptor 1 (VR1): relationship to neuropeptides, the P2X3 purinoceptor and IB4 binding sites. *Eur J Neurosci* **11**, 946–958.

Hamilton SG and McMahon SB (2000) ATP as a peripheral mediator of pain. *J Auton Nerv Syst* **81**, 187–194.

Hammarberg H, Piehl F, Cullheim S, Fjell J, Hokfelt T, and Fried K (1996) GDNF mRNA in Schwann cells and DRG satellite cells after chronic sciatic nerve injury. *Neuroreport* **7**, 857–860.

Heumann R, Korsching S, Bandtlow C, and Thoenen H (1987) Changes of nerve growth factor synthesis in nonneuronal cells in response to sciatic nerve transection. *J Cell Biol* **104**, 1623–1631.

Hohmann AG and Herkenham M (1999) Localization of central cannabinoid CB1 receptor messenger RNA in neuronal subpopulations of rat dorsal root ganglia: a double-label in situ hybridization study. *Neurosci* **90**, 923–931.

Hoke A, Cheng C, and Zochodne DW (2000) Expression of glial cell line-derived neurotrophic factor family of growth factors in peripheral nerve injury in rats. *Neuroreport* **11**, 1651–1654.

Hokfelt T, Zhang X, and Wiesenfeld–Hallin Z (1994) Messenger plasticity in primary sensory neurons following axotomy and its functional implications. *Trends Neurosci* **17**, 22–30.

Hu HJ, Bhave G, and Gereau RW (2002) Prostaglandin and protein kinase a-dependent modulation of vanilloid receptor function by metabotropic glutamate receptor 5: potential mechanism for thermal hyperalgesia. *J Neurosci* **22**, 7444–7452.

Hudson LJ, Bevan S, Wotherspoon G, Gentry C, Fox A, and Winter J (2001) VR1 protein expression increases in undamaged DRG neurons after partial nerve injury. *Eur J Neurosci* **13**, 2105–2114.

Iggo A (1969) Cutaneous thermoreceptors in primates and sub-primates. *J Physiol* **200**, 403–430.

Issa PC, Lever IJ, Michael GJ, Bradbury EJ, and Malcangio M (2001) Intrathecally delivered glial cell line-derived neurotrophic factor produces electrically evoked release of somatostatin in the dorsal horn of the spinal cord. *J Neurochem* **78**, 221–229.

Ji R–R, Zhang Q, Law PY, Low HH, Elde R, and Hökfelt T (1995) Expression of mu-opioid, delta-opioid, and kappa-opioid receptor- like immunoreactivities in rat dorsal-root ganglia after carrageenan- induced inflammation. *J Neurosci* **15**, 8156–8166.

Jordt SE, Bautista DM, Chuang HH, *et al.* (2004) Mustard oils and cannabinoids excite sensory nerve fibres through the TRP channel ANKTM1. *Nature* **427**, 260–265.

Julius D and Basbaum AI (2001) Molecular mechanisms of nociception. *Nature* **413**, 203–210.

Junger H and Sorkin LS (2000) Nociceptive and inflammatory effects of subcutaneous TNFalpha. *Pain* **85**, 145–151.

Kashiba H, Fukui H, Morikawa Y, and Senba E (1999) Gene expression of histamine H1 receptor in guinea pig primary sensory neurons: a relationship between H1 receptor mRNA-expressing neurons and peptidergic neurons. *Mol Brain Res* **66**, 24–34.

Kashiba H, Noguchi K, Ueda Y, and Senba E (1995) Coexpression of trk family members and low affinity neurotrophin receptors in rat dorsal root ganglion neurons. *Mol Brain Res* **30**, 158–164.

Kashiba H, Uchida Y, and Senba E (2001) Difference in binding by isolectin B4 to trkA and c-ret mRNA-expressing neurons in rat sensory ganglia. *Mol Brain Res* **95**, 18–26.

Kendall G, Brarrai A, Ensor E, Winter J, Wood JN, and Latchman DS (1995) Nerve growth-factor induces the oct-2 transcription factor in sensory neurons with the kinetics of an immediate-early gene. *J Neurosci Res* **40**, 169–176.

Kerr BJ, Bradbury EJ, Bennett DLH, *et al.* (1999) Brain-derived neurotrophic factor modulates nociceptive sensory inputs and NMDA-evoked responses in the rat spinal cord. *J Neurosci* **19**, 5138–5148.

Kerr BJ, Cafferty WB, Gupta YK, *et al.* (2000) Galanin knockout mice reveal nociceptive deficits following peripheral nerve injury. *Eur J Neurosci* **12**, 793–802.

Kerr BJ, Cafferty WB, Gupta YK, *et al.* (2001) A role for the TTX-resistant sodium channel Nav 1.8 in NGF-induced hyperalgesia, but not neuropathic pain. *Neuroreport* **12**, 3077–3080.

Khasar SG, Lin YH, Martin A, *et al.* (1999) A novel nociceptor signaling pathway revealed in protein kinase C epsilon mutant mice. *Neuron* **24**, 253–260.

Kim SH and Chung JM (1992) An experimental model for peripheral neuropathy produced by segmental spinal nerve ligation in the rat. *Pain* **50**, 355–363.

Kruger L, Perl ER, and Sedivec MJ (1981) Fine structure of myelinated mechanical nociceptor endings in cat hairy skin. *J Comp Neurol* **198**, 137–154.

Kruger L, Silverman JD, Mantyh PW, Sternini C, and Brecha NC (1989) Peripheral patterns of calcitonin-gene-related peptide general somatic sensory innervation: cutaneous and deep terminations. *J Comp Neurol* **280**, 291–302.

Lai J, Gold MS, Kim CS, *et al.* (2002) Inhibition of neuropathic pain by decreased expression of the tetrodotoxin-resistant sodium channel, NaV1.8. *Pain* **95**, 143–152.

Lawson SN, Crepps B, Buck H, and Perl ER (1996) Correlation of CGRP-like immunoreactivity (CGRP-LI) with sensory receptor properties in dorsal root ganglion (DRG) neurons in guinea pigs. *J Physiol* **493P**, P45.

Lawson SN, Crepps BA, and Perl ER (1997) Relationship of substance P to afferent characteristics of dorsal root ganglion neurones in guinea-pig. *J Physiol* **505**, 177–191.

Lee YJ, Zachrisson O, Tonge DA, and McNaughton PA (2002) Upregulation of bradykinin B2 receptor expression by neurotrophic factors and nerve injury in mouse sensory neurons. *Mol Cell Neurosci* **19**, 186–200.

Leffler A, Cummins TR, Dib–Hajj SD, Hormuzdiar WN, Black JA, and Waxman SG (2002) GDNF and NGF reverse changes in repriming of TTX-sensitive Na(+) currents following axotomy of dorsal root ganglion neurons. *J Neurophysiol* **88**, 650–658.

Leitner ML, Molliver DC, Osborne PA, *et al.* (1999) Analysis of the retrograde transport of glial cell line-derived neurotrophic factor (GDNF), neurturin, and persephin suggests that in vivo signaling for the GDNF family is GFRalpha coreceptor-specific. *J Neurosci* **19**, 9322–9331.

Lembo PM, Grazzini E, Groblewski T, *et al.* (2002) Proenkephalin A gene products activate a new family of sensory neuro-specific GPCRs. *Nat Neurosci* **5**, 201–209.

Leslie TA, Emson PC, Dowd PM, and Woolf CJ (1995) Nerve growth factor contributes to the up-regulation of growth-associated protein 43 and preprotachykinin A messenger RNAs in primary sensory neurons following peripheral inflammation. *Neurosci* **67**, 753–761.

Lever IJ, Bradbury EJ, Cunningham JR, *et al.* (2001) Brain-derived neurotrophic factor is released in the dorsal horn by distinctive patterns of afferent fiber stimulation. *J Neurosci* **21**, 4469–4477.

Lever IJ, Pezet S, McMahon SB, and Malcangio M (2003) The signalling components of sensory fiber transmission involved in the activation of ERK MAP kinase in the mouse dorsal horn. *Mol Cell Neurosci* **24**, 259–270.

Levy D and Zochodne DW (2000) Increased mRNA expression of the B1 and B2 bradykinin receptors and antinociceptive effects of their antagonists in an animal model of neuropathic pain. *Pain* **86**, 265–271.

Lewin GR, Rueff A, and Mendell LM (1994) Peripheral and central mechanisms of NGF-induced hyperalgesia. *Eur J Neurosci* **6**, 1903–1912.

Liu CN, Wall PD, Ben Dor E, Michaelis M, Amir R, and Devor M (2000*a*) Tactile allodynia in the absence of C-fiber activation: altered firing properties of DRG neurons following spinal nerve injury. *Pain* **85**, 503–521.

Liu HX, Brumovsky P, Schmidt R, *et al.* (2001) Receptor subtype-specific pronociceptive and analgesic actions of galanin in the spinal cord: selective actions via GalR1 and GalR2 receptors. *Proc Natl Acad Sci USA* **98**, 9960–9964.

Liu M, Willmott NJ, Michael GJ, and Priestley JV (2004) Differential pH and capsaicin responses of Griffonia simplicifolia IB4(IB4)-positive and IB4-negative small sensory neurons. *Neurosci* **127**, 659–672.

Liu X, Eschenfelder S, Blenk KH, Janig W, and Habler H (2000*b*) Spontaneous activity of axotomized afferent neurons after L5 spinal nerve injury in rats. *Pain* **84**, 309–318.

Lowe EM, Anand P, Terenghi G, Williams–Chestnut RE, Sinicropi DV, and Osborne JL (1997) Increased nerve growth factor levels in the urinary bladder of women with idiopathic sensory urgency and interstitial cystitis. *Brit J Urol* **79**, 572–577.

Lu J, Zhou XF, and Rush RA (2001) Small primary sensory neurons innervating epidermis and viscera display differential phenotype in the adult rat. *Neurosci Res* **41**, 355–363.

Lyu YS, Park SK, Chung K, and Chung JM (2000) Low dose of tetrodotoxin reduces neuropathic pain behaviors in an animal model. *Brain Res* **871**, 98–103.

Ma QP (2001) The expression of bradykinin B(1) receptors on primary sensory neurones that give rise to small caliber sciatic nerve fibres in rats. *Neurosci* **107**, 665–673.

MacQueen GM, Ramakrishnan K, Croll SD, *et al.* (2001) Performance of heterozygous brain-derived neurotrophic factor knockout mice on behavioral analogues of anxiety, nociception, and depression. *Behav Neurosci* **115**, 1145–1153.

Malcangio M, Bowery NG, Flower RJ, and Perretti M (1996) Effect of interleukin 1 beta on the release of substance P from rat isolated spinal cord. *Eur J Pharmacol* **299**, 113–118.

Malcangio M, Garrett NE, Cruwys S, and Tomlinson DR (1997) Nerve growth factor and neurotrophin 3 induced changes in nociceptive threshold and the release of substance P from the rat isolated spinal cord. *J Neurosci* **17**, 8459–8467.

Malcangio M, Ramer MS, Boucher TJ, and McMahon SB (2000*a*) Intrathecally injected neurotrophins and the release of substance P from the rat isolated spinal cord. *Eur J Neurosci* **12**, 139–144.

Malcangio M, Ramer MS, Jones MG, and McMahon SB (2000*b*) Abnormal substance P release from the spinal cord following injury to primary sensory neurons. *Eur J Neurosci* **12**, 397–399.

Mannion RJ, Costigan M, Decosterd I, *et al.* (1999) Neurotrophins: peripherally and centrally acting modulators of tactile stimulus-induced inflammatory pain hypersensitivity. *Proc Natl Acad Sci USA* **96**, 9385–9390.

McKemy DD, Neuhausser WM, and Julius D (2002) Identification of a cold receptor reveals a general role for TRP channels in thermosensation. *Nature* **416**, 52–58.

McMahon SB and Bennett DLH (1999) Trophic factors and pain. In *Textbook of Pain* (eds. P.D. Wall and R. Melzack), pp. 105–128. Edinburgh: Churchill Livingstone.

McMahon SB, Armanini MP, Ling LH, and Phillips HS (1994) Expression and coexpression of trk receptors in subpopulations of adult primary sensory neurons projecting to identified peripheral targets. *Neuron* **12**, 1161–1171.

McMahon SB, Bennett DLH, Priestley JV, and Shelton D (1995) The biological effects of endogenous NGF in adult sensory neurons revealed by a trkA-IgG fusion molecule. *Nature* Med **1**, 774–780.

Michael GJ and Priestley JV (1999) Differential expression of the mRNA for the vanilloid receptor subtype 1 in cells of the adult rat dorsal root and nodose ganglia and its downregulation by axotomy. *J Neurosci* **19**, 1844–1854.

Michael GJ, Averill S, Nitkunan A, *et al.* (1997) Nerve growth factor treatment increases brain-derived neurotrophic factor selectively in trkA-expressing dorsal root ganglion cells and in their central terminations within the spinal cord. *J Neurosci* **17**, 8476–8490.

Michael GJ, Averill S, Shortland PJ, Yan Q, and Priestley JV (1999) Axotomy results in major changes in BDNF expression by dorsal root ganglion cells: BDNF expression in large trkB and trkC cells, in pericellular baskets, and in projectons to deep dorsal horn and dorsal column nuclei. *Eur J Neurosci* **11**, 3539–3551.

Miller FD and Kaplan DR (2001) On Trk for retrograde signaling. *Neuron* **32**, 767–770.

Mizuno M, Kondo E, Nishimura *et al.* (1997) Localization of molecules involved in cytokine receptor signaling in the rat trigeminal ganglion. *Mol Brain Res* **44**, 163–166.

Molliver DC, Wright DE, Leitner ML, *et al.* (1997) IB4-binding DRG neurons switch from NGF to GDNF dependence in early postnatal life. *Neuron* **19**, 849–861.

Nakamura F and Strittmatter SM (1996) P2Y(1) purinergic receptors in sensory neurons — contribution to touch-induced impulse generation. *Proc Natl Acad Sci USA* **93**, 10465–10470.

Naveilhan P, ElShamy VM, and Ernfors P (1997) Differential regulation of mRNAs for GDNF and its receptors Ret and GDNFR alpha after sciatic nerve lesion in the mouse. *Eur J Neurosci* **9**, 1450–1460.

Neumann S, Doubell TP, Leslie T, and Woolf CJ (1996) Inflammatory pain hypersensitivity mediated by phenotypic switch in myelinated primary sensory neurons. *Nature* **384**, 360–364.

Oddiah D, Anand P, McMahon SB, and Rattray M (1998) Rapid increase of NGF, BDNF and NT-3 mRNAs in inflamed bladder. *Neuroreport* **9**, 1455–1458.

Ogun-Muyiwa P, Helliwell R, McIntyre P, and Winter J (1999) Glial cell line derived neurotrophic factor (GDNF) regulates VR1 and substance P in cultured sensory neurons. *Neuroreport* **10**, 2107–2111.

Oh SB, Tran PB, Gillard SE, Hurley RW, Hammond DL, and Miller RJ (2001) Chemokines and glycoprotein120 produce pain hypersensitivity by directly exciting primary nociceptive neurons. *J Neurosci* **21**, 5027–5035.

Oida H, Namba T, Sugimoto Y, *et al.* (1995) In situ hybridization studies of prostacyclin receptor mRNA expression in various mouse organs. *Br J Pharmacol* **116**, 2828–2837.

Orozco OE, Walus L, Sah DW, Pepinsky RB, and Sanicola M (2001) GFRalpha3 is expressed predominantly in nociceptive sensory neurons. *Eur J Neurosci* **13**, 2177–2182.

Patapoutian A, Peier AM, Story GM, and Viswanath V (2003) Thermo TRP channels and beyond: mechanisms of temperature sensation. *Nat Rev Neurosci* **4**, 529–539.

Paukert M, Osteroth R, Geisler HS, *et al.* (2001) Inflammatory mediators potentiate ATP-gated channels through the P2X(3) subunit. *J Biol Chem* **276**, 21077–21082.

Perkins MN, Kelly D, and Davis AJ (1995) Bradykinin B1 and B2 receptor mechanisms and cytokine-induced hyperalgesia in the rat. *Can J Physiol Pharmacol* **73**, 832–836.

Perry MJ and Lawson SN (1998) Differences in expression of oligosaccharides, neuropeptides, carbonic anhydrase and neurofilament in rat primary afferent neurons retrogradely labelled via skin, muscle or visceral nerves. *Neurosci* **85**, 293–310.

Petersen M, vonBanchet GS, Heppelmann B, and Koltzenburg M (1998) Nerve growth factor regulates the expression of bradykinin binding sites on adult sensory neurons via the neurotrophin receptor p75. *Neurosci* **83**, 161–168.

Pezet S, Malcangio M, Lever IJ, *et al.* (2002*a*) Noxious stimulation induces Trk receptor and downstream ERK phosphorylation in spinal dorsal horn. *Mol Cell Neurosci* **21**, 684–695.

Pezet S, Malcangio M and McMahon SE (2202*b*) BDNF: a neuromodulator in nociceptive pathways? *Brain Res Rev* **40**, 240–249.

Poo MM (2001) Neurotrophins as synaptic modulators. *Nat Rev Neurosci* **2**, 24–32.

Premkumar LS and Ahern GP (2000) Induction of vanilloid receptor channel activity by protein kinase C. *Nature* **408**, 985–990.

Price DD, Bennett GJ, and Rafii A (1989) Psychophysical observations on patients with neuropathic pain relieved by a sympathetic block. *Pain* **36**, 273–288.

Price MP, Lewin GR, McIlwrath SL, *et al.* (2000) The mammalian sodium channel BNC1 is required for normal touch sensation. *Nature* **407**, 1007–1011.

Price MP, McIlwrath SL, Xie J, *et al.* (2001) The DRASIC cation channel contributes to the detection of cutaneous touch and acid stimuli in mice. *Neuron* **32**, 1071–1083.

Priestley JV, Michael GJ, Averill S, Liu M, and Willmott NJ (2002) Regulation of nociceptive neurons by NGF and GDNF. *Can J Physiol Pharmacol* **80**, 495–505.

Priestley JV, Somogyi P, and Cuello AC (1982) Immunocytochemical localization of substance P in the spinal trigeminal nucleus of the rat: a light and electron microscopic study. *J Comp Neurol* **211**, 31–49.

Qiu L, Towle MF, Bernd P, and Fukada K (1997) Distribution of cholinergic neuronal differentiation factor/leukemia inhibitory factor binding sites in the developing and adult rat nervous system in vivo. *J Neurobiol* **32**, 163–192.

Raja SN, Meyer RA, Ringkamp M, and Campbell JN (1999) Peripheral neural mechanisms of nociception. In *Textbook of Pain* (eds. P.D. Wall and R. Melzack), pp. 11–57. Edinburgh: Churchill Livingstone.

Ramer MS, Bradbury EJ, and McMahon SB (2001) Nerve growth factor induces P2X(3) expression in sensory neurons. *J Neurochem* **77**, 864–875.

Rasband MN, Park EW, Vanderah TW, Lai J, Porreca F, and Trimmer JS (2001) Distinct potassium channels on pain-sensing neurons. *Proc Natl Acad Sci USA* **98**, 13373–13378.

Ringkamp M, Peng YB, Wu G, Hartke TV, Campbell JN, and Meyer RA (2001) Capsaicin responses in heat-sensitive and heat-insensitive A-fiber nociceptors. *J Neurosci* **21**, 4460–4468.

Safieh–Garabedian B, Poole S, Allchorne A, Winter J, and Woolf CJ (1995) Contribution of interleukin-1 beta to the inflammation-induced increase in nerve growth factor levels and inflammatory hyperalgesia. *Br J Pharmacol* **115**, 1265–1275.

Scott RL, Gurusinghe AD, Rudvosky AA, *et al.* (2000) Expression of leukemia inhibitory factor receptor mRNA in sensory dorsal root ganglion and spinal motor neurons of the neonatal rat. *Neurosci Lett* **295**, 49–53.

Segal RA and Greenberg ME (1996) Intracellular signaling pathways activated by neurotrophic factors. *Ann Rev Neurosci* **19**, 463–489.

Seltzer Z, Dubner R, and Shir Y (1990) A novel behavioral model of neuropathic pain disorders produced in rats by partial sciatic nerve injury. *Pain* **43**, 205–218.

Shadiack AM, Sun Y, and Zigmond RE (2001) Nerve growth factor antiserum induces axotomy-like changes in neuropeptide expression in intact sympathetic and sensory neurons. *J Neurosci* **21**, 363–371.

Shamash S, Reichert F, and Rotshenker S (2002) The cytokine network of Wallerian degeneration: tumor necrosis factor-alpha, interleukin-1alpha, and interleukin-1beta. *J Neurosci* **22**, 3052–3060.

Sheen K and Chung JM (1993) Signs of neuropathic pain depend on signals from injured nerve fibers in a rat model. *Brain Res* **610**, 62–68.

Shen H, Chung JM, Coggeshall RE, and Chung KS (1999) Changes in trkA expression in the dorsal root ganglion after peripheral nerve injury. *Exper Brain Res* **127**, 141–146.

Shu XQ and Mendell LM (1999) Neurotrophins and hyperalgesia. *Proc Natl Acad Sci USA* **96**, 7693–7696.

Silverman JD and Kruger L (1990) Selective neuronal glycoconjugate expression in sensory and autonomic ganglia: relation of lectin reactivity to peptide and enzyme markers. *J Neurocytol* **19**, 789–801.

Simone DA, Nolano M, Johnson T, Wendelschafer–Crabb G, and Kennedy WR (1998) Intradermal injection of capsaicin in humans produces degeneration and subsequent reinnervation of epidermal nerve fibers: correlation with sensory function. *J Neurosci* **18**, 8947–8954.

Smith GD, Gunthorpe MJ, Kelsell RE, *et al.* (2002) TRPV3 is a temperature-sensitive vanilloid receptor-like protein. *Nature* **418**, 186–190.

Snider WD and McMahon SB (1998) Tackling pain at the source: new ideas about nociceptors. *Neuron* **20**, 629–632.

Sorkin LS, Xiao WH, Wagner R, and Myers RR (1997) Tumour necrosis factor-alpha induces ectopic activity in nociceptive primary afferent fibres. *Neurosci* **81**, 255–262.

Stoll G, Jander S, and Myers RR (2002) Degeneration and regeneration of the peripheral nervous system: from Augustus Waller's observations to neuroinflammation. *J Peripher Nerv Syst* **7**, 13–27.

Stucky CL, Koltzenburg M, Schneider M, Engle MG, Albers KM, and Davis BM (1999) Overexpression of nerve growth factor in skin selectively affects the survival and functional properties of nociceptors. *J Neurosci* **19**, 8509–8516.

Stucky CL and Lewin GR (1999) Isolectin B(4)-positive and -negative nociceptors are functionally distinct. *J Neurosci* **19**, 6497–6505.

Sun Y and Zigmond RE (1996) Leukemia inhibitory factor-induced in the sciatic-nerve after axotomy is involved in the induction of galanin in sensory neurons. *Eur J Neurosci* **8**, 2213–2220.

Suzuki M, Mizuno A, Kodaira K, and Imai M (2003) Impaired pressure sensation in mice lacking TRPV4. *J Biol Chem* **278**, 22664–22668.

Tanaka M, Cummins TR, Ishikawa K, Dib–Hajj SD, Black JA, and Waxman SG (1998) SNS Na+ channel expression increases in dorsal root ganglion neurons in the carrageenan inflammatory pain model. *Neuroreport* **9**, 967–972.

Tate S, Benn S, Hick C, *et al.* (1998) Two sodium channels contribute to the TTX-R sodium current in primary sensory neurons. *Nature Neuroscience* **1**, 653–655.

Tecott LH, Maricq AV, and Julius D (1993) Nervous system distribution of the serotonin 5-HT3 receptor mRNA. *Proc Natl Acad Sci USA* **90**, 1430–1434.

Thompson SWN, Dray A, Mccarson KE, Krause JE, and Urban L (1995) Nerve growth factor induces mechanical allodynia associated with novel A fiber-evoked spinal reflex activity and enhanced neurokinin 1 receptor activation in the rat. *Pain* **62**, 219–231.

Thompson SWN, Priestley JV, and Southall A (1998) Gp130 cytokines, leukemia inhibitory factor and interleukin-6, induce neuropeptide expression in intact adult rat sensory neurons in vivo: time course, specificity and comparison with sciatic nerve axotomy. *Neurosci* **84**, 1247–1255.

Thompson SWN, Vernallis AB, Heath JK, and Priestley JV (1997) Leukaemia inhibitory factor is retrogradely transported by a distinct population of adult rat sensory neurons: co-localization with trka and other neurochemical markers. *Eur J Neurosci* **9**, 1244–1251.

Tominaga M, Caterina MJ, Malmberg AB, *et al.* (1998) The cloned capsaicin receptor integrates multiple pain-producing stimuli. *Neuron* **21**, 531–543.

Tominaga M, Wada M, and Masu M (2001) Potentiation of capsaicin receptor activity by metabotropic ATP receptors as a possible mechanism for ATP-evoked pain and hyperalgesia. *Proc Natl Acad Sci USA* **98**, 6951–6956.

Trupp M, Ryden M, Jornvall H, *et al.* (1995) Peripheral expression and biological activities of GDNF, a new neurotrophic factor for avian and mammalian peripheral neurons. *J Cell Biol* **130**, 137–148.

Tsuzuki K, Kondo E, Fukuoka T, *et al.* (2001) Differential regulation of P2X(3) mRNA expression by peripheral nerve injury in intact and injured neurons in the rat sensory ganglia. *Pain* **91**, 351–360.

Vellani V, Mapplebeck S, Moriondo A, Davis JB, and McNaughton PA (2001) Protein kinase C activation potentiates gating of the vanilloid receptor VR1 by capsaicin, protons, heat and anandamide. *J Physiol* **534**, 813–825.

Vennekens R, Voets T, Bindels RJ, Droogmans G, and Nilius B (2002) Current understanding of mammalian TRP homologues. *Cell Calcium* **31**, 253–264.

Verge VM, Richardson PM, Wiesenfeld–Hallin Z, and Hokfelt T (1995) Differential influence of nerve growth factor on neuropeptide expression in vivo: a novel role in peptide suppression in adult sensory neurons. *J Neurosci* **15**, 2081–2096.

Villar MJ, Cortes R, Theodorsson E, *et al.* (1989) Neuropeptide expression in rat dorsal root ganglion cells and spinal cord after peripheral nerve injury with special reference to galanin. *Neurosci* **33**, 587–604.

Vulchanova L, Riedl MS, Shuster SJ, *et al.* (1997) Immunohistochemical study of the p2x(2) and p2x(3) receptor subunits in rat and monkey sensory neurons and their central terminals. *Neuropharmacology* **36**, 1229–1242.

Waldmann R and Lazdunski M (1998) H(+)-gated cation channels: neuronal acid sensors in the NaC/DEG family of ion channels. *Curr Opin Neurobiol* **8**, 418–424.

Wang R, Guo W, Ossipov MH, *et al.* (2003) Glial cell line-derived neurotrophic factor normalizes neurochemical changes in injured dorsal root ganglion neurons and prevents the expression of experimental neuropathic pain. *Neurosci* **121**, 815–824.

Wetmore C and Olson L (1995) Neuronal and nonneuronal expression of neurotrophins and their receptors in sensory and sympathetic ganglia suggest new intercellular trophic interactions. *J Comp Neurol* **353**, 143–159.

Woolf CJ, Allchorne A, Safieh–Garabedian B, and Poole S (1997) Cytokines, nerve growth factor and inflammatory hyperalgesia: the contribution of tumour necrosis factor alpha. *Br J Pharmacol* **121**, 417–424.

Woolf CJ, Safieh–Garabedian B, Ma QP, Crilly P, and Winter J (1994) Nerve growth factor contributes to the generation of inflammatory sensory hypersensitivity. *Neurosci* **62**, 327–331.

Wotherspoon G and Priestley JV (2000) Expression of the 5-HT1B receptor by subtypes of rat trigeminal ganglion cells. *Neurosci* **95**, 465–471.

Wotherspoon G and Winter J (2000) Bradykinin B1 receptor is constitutively expressed in the rat sensory nervous system. *Neurosci Lett* **294**, 175–178.

Wright DE and Snider WD (1995) Neurotrophin receptor mRNA expression defines distinct populations of neurons in rat dorsal root ganglia. *J Comp Neurol* **351**, 329–338.

Wu G, Ringkamp M, Hartke TV, *et al.* (2001) Early onset of spontaneous activity in uninjured C-fiber nociceptors after injury to neighboring nerve fibers. *J Neurosci* **21**, RC140.

Xu GY and Huang LY (2002) Peripheral inflammation sensitizes P2X receptor-mediated responses in rat dorsal root ganglion neurons. *J Neurosci* **22**, 93–102.

Xu H, Ramsey IS, Kotecha SA, *et al.* (2002) TRPV3 is a calcium-permeable temperature-sensitive cation channel. *Nature* **418**, 181–186.

Yoon YW, Na HS, and Chung JM (1996) Contributions of injured and intact afferents to neuropathic pain in an experimental rat model. *Pain* **64**, 27–36.

Yusaf SP, Goodman J, Pinnock RD, Dixon AK, and Lee K (2001) Expression of voltage-gated calcium channel subunits in rat dorsal root ganglion neurons. *Neurosci Lett* **311**, 137–141.

Zeitz KP, Guy N, Malmberg AB, *et al.* (2002) The 5-HT3 subtype of serotonin receptor contributes to nociceptive processing via a novel subset of myelinated and unmyelinated nociceptors. *J Neurosci* **22**, 1010–1019.

Zhou XF and Rush RA (1996) Endogenous brain derived neurotrophic factor is anterogradely transported in primary sensory neurons. *Neurosci* **74**, 945–951.

Zur KB, Oh YS, Waxman SG, and Black JA (1995) Differential up-regulation of sodium channel alpha subunit and beta 1 subunit messenger RNAs in cultured embryonic DRG neurons following exposure to NGF. *Mol Brain Res* **30**, 97–105.

Zwick M, Davis BM, Woodbury CJ, *et al.* (2002) Glial cell line-derived neurotrophic factor is a survival factor for isolectin B4-positive, but not vanilloid receptor 1-positive, neurons in the mouse. *J Neurosci* **22**, 4057–4065.

Zylka MJ, Rice FL, and Anderson DJ (2005) Topographically distinct epidermal nociceptive circuits revealed by axonal tracers targeted to Mrgprd. *Neuron* **45**, 17–25.

Chapter 3

Molecular architecture of the dorsal horn

Andrew J. Todd and Alfredo Ribeiro-da-Silva

3.1 Introduction

Rexed (1952) divided the dorsal horn of the cat spinal cord into a series of six parallel laminae, and a similar scheme has since been applied to other species, including rat (Fig. 3.1), monkey, and human. The dorsal horn contains four different neuronal components:

1. the central terminals of primary afferents

2. neurons with long ascending axons that project to the brain (projection neurons)

3. intrinsic spinal neurons (interneurons, many of which have axons that terminate locally)

4. axons that descend from various parts of the brain, including certain monoaminergic nuclei in the brainstem.

Lamina I of the dorsal horn is also known as the marginal layer, and lamina II as the substantia gelatinosa. These two laminae are collectively referred to as the superficial part of the dorsal horn and are of great importance in the spinal processing of pain information, since they are the major target for incoming nociceptive primary afferents. The superficial dorsal horn shows a very complex neurochemical organization: it contains a wide range of neurotransmitters, neuropeptides, and receptors, as well as other compounds such as calcium-binding proteins and enzymes involved in signal transduction. Some of these compounds are associated with the fine primary afferents that arborize in this region, while others are present in the intrinsic neurons. Although this neurochemical complexity suggests that the organization and function of the region are likely to be difficult to unravel, it has provided a means of identifying neuronal populations and investigating their connections.

In this chapter, we review the normal structure of the mammalian dorsal horn, with particular emphasis on neurochemically-defined populations of neurons. We also describe some of the changes that can occur following nerve injury or inflammation, and may therefore contribute to pathological pain states. Much of the recent work on the structure of the spinal cord has been carried out on the rat, we have therefore based

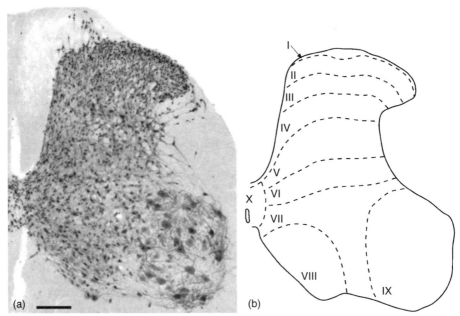

Fig. 3.1 (a) A transverse section of the lumbar spinal cord (L4 segment) of a rat, stained with antibody to NeuN, a neuronal nuclear protein. This results in immunostaining of all neurons in the spinal cord. (b) The positions of Rexed's laminae as applied to the rat lumbar spinal cord. Laminae I–VI make up the dorsal horn. Scale bar = 200 μm. (Modified from *Neuroscience* **85**, Todd AJ *et al.*, A quantitative study of neurons which express neurokinin 1 or somatostatin sst$_{2a}$ receptor in rat spinal dorsal horn, pp 459–473. Copyright 1998, with permission from Elsevier Science.)

our account on this species. We have concentrated on the structure of the superficial dorsal horn, because of its obvious involvement in nociceptive transmission, and also because relatively more is known about its neuronal organization. However, the deeper laminae of the dorsal horn are also important in pain: many cells in the deeper laminae (including projection neurons) respond to acute noxious stimuli, and the low-threshold mechanoreceptive afferents which terminate in this region are responsible for some of the symptoms of neuropathic pain.

3.2 **Primary afferents**

3.2.1 **Central termination and neurochemistry**

Primary afferent axons enter the spinal cord through the dorsal roots. Their subsequent course depends on the type of fibre. Small-diameter afferents either have unmyelinated (C) or thinly myelinated (Aδ) axons: these bifurcate and enter Lissauer's tract, where they travel up and down one or two spinal segments before branching in the dorsal horn (Szentágothai 1964). In contrast, large myelinated (Aβ) afferents enter the dorsal columns and give collateral branches to the spinal grey matter. The distribution of Aβ afferents has been investigated by means of intra-axonal labelling in the cat, and it has been shown that each functional type has a characteristic pattern of termination within the deeper laminae (III–VI) of the dorsal horn (Brown 1981). For example, Aβ hair-follicle afferents form 'flame-shaped' arbors centred on lamina III, whereas Pacinian afferents arborize more widely in laminae III–VI. Many Aβ afferents also project directly to the dorsal column (gracile or cuneate) nuclei.

The central projections of two populations of Aδ afferents have been studied following intra-axonal injection in the cat: those which innervate down hairs (D hair afferents) arborize on either side of the lamina II/III border, while nociceptive Aδ afferents end mainly in laminae I and V (Light and Perl 1979).

Because of technical difficulties, there have been very few studies of individual C afferents, and much of our information comes from indirect approaches. C afferents can be divided into two major neurochemical types: those which contain neuropeptides (e.g. substance P, somatostatin. and calcitonin gene-related peptide) and those which do not (Hunt and Rossi 1985). Although there are species differences, in the rat it appears that all peptidergic primary afferents contain calcitonin gene-related peptide (CGRP), and since this peptide is only found in primary afferents in the dorsal horn, it provides a very useful way of identifying them. While most peptidergic afferents have unmyelinated axons, some are myelinated. Several markers have been used to label C afferents that lack peptides, including fluoride-resistant acid phosphatase (FRAP) activity and binding of *Bandeiraea simplicifolia* isolectin B4 (IB4) (Alvarez and Fyffe 2000). There are differences between the termination regions of these two types of unmyelinated afferent: the peptidergic ones arborize mainly in lamina I and the outer part of lamina II (lamina IIo), whereas those that lack peptides innervate the central part of lamina II (Ribeiro-da-Silva 2002). Sugiura *et al.* (1989) have labelled single C afferents in the guinea pig, and have confirmed that those with somatic receptive fields terminate mainly in laminae I and II, while visceral C afferents arborize more diffusely in the dorsal horn.

The fast synaptic transmitter in most, if not all, primary afferents is glutamate (De Biasi and Rustioni 1988), and as stated above, many also express neuropeptides. There are considerable species differences in the pattern of neuropeptide co-localization in primary afferents. For example, in the rat, but not cat, substance P and somatostatin occur in separate populations. Substance P-immunoreactive afferents can also contain neurokinin A (Dalsgaard *et al.* 1985), galanin (Hökfelt *et al.* 1994), and the opioid peptide, endomorphin-2 (Martin-Schild *et al.* 1997), in addition to CGRP. Somatostatin-containing primary afferents arborize mostly in lamina IIo, while those with substance P are found mainly in laminae I and IIo, but also extend into deeper laminae (III–IV).

Lawson *et al.* (1997) have provided evidence that all substance P-containing primary afferents are nociceptors. However, less is known about the functions of other types of peptidergic C afferents (e.g. those that contain somatostatin). It is likely that the majority of the non-peptidergic C fibres are also nociceptors, since the vanilloid receptor VR1 (the target for capsaicin) is present on many of their central terminals (Guo *et al.* 1999).

3.2.2 **Synaptic arrangements of primary afferents**

In the dorsal horn, primary afferent boutons establish mostly simple axo-dendritic or axo-somatic synapses. However, a significant proportion participate in complex arrangements named synaptic glomeruli, where they form the central terminal (Fig. 2.2). Glomeruli represent 'multiplier systems' (i.e. devices that transmit sensory information to several dorsal horn neurons). They also constitute important modulatory devices, as the primary afferent terminals are often postsynaptic to other neuronal profiles. Since the central terminals of glomeruli are all of primary afferent origin (Ribeiro-da-Silva 2002), they provide a very useful means of identifying these afferents with electron microscopy, without the need for transported or immunocytochemical markers.

The detailed features of synaptic glomeruli have been reviewed by one of us (Ribeiro-da-Silva 2002). Glomeruli can be identified on isolated electron micrographs by the presence of a central bouton with agranular round synaptic vesicles apposed to at least four neuronal profiles (either regular dendrites, vesicle-containing dendrites, or axonal boutons) and at least two visible synaptic contacts between the central and peripheral profiles. The central bouton is presynaptic to dendrites of spinal cord interneurons (Gobel *et al.* 1980) or projection neurons (Maxwell *et al.* 1985), and postsynaptic to both vesicle-containing dendrites (dendro-axonic synapses) and axonal boutons (axo-axonic synapses). Reciprocal synapses, in which the bouton is both pre- and postsynaptic to vesicle-containing dendrites, sometimes occur. Islet cells (see below) are one source of vesicle-containing dendrites in glomeruli (Gobel *et al.* 1980). Complex synaptic arrangements of the triadic type have been described in glomeruli (Knyihár–Csillik *et al.* 1982*a*; Ribeiro-da-Silva *et al.* 1985).

There are significant species differences in the distribution of glomeruli (Ribeiro-da-Silva and Coimbra 1982; Knyihár–Csillik *et al.* 1982*b*). In the rat, glomeruli are virtually absent from lamina I, rare in lamina IIo, but are relatively numerous in the inner part of lamina II (lamina IIi) and in lamina III. They have been divided into two morphological types, I and II (Ribeiro-da-Silva and Coimbra 1982) (see Fig. 3.2). Type I glomeruli have a central bouton that is generally smaller and more scalloped than those of type II glomeruli. They also have darker cytoplasmic matrix and fewer mitochondria. Most type I glomeruli (subtype Ia) have a central bouton that lacks dense-cored vesicles, and these are thought to belong to non-peptidergic C fibres (Ribeiro-da-Silva *et al.* 1989). They are most numerous in the middle third of lamina II and are involved in complex synaptic arrangements, including triads. A small proportion of type I central boutons (subtype Ib) contain dense-cored vesicles and peptide immunoreactivity (CGRP, together with either substance P or somatostatin). These are found in lamina IIo and the dorsal part of lamina IIi, and have a simpler architecture, since they lack axo-axonic and dendro-axonic synapses. In the rat, peptidergic primary afferents are seldom involved in synaptic glomeruli. However, in the cat and monkey these afferents more commonly form glomeruli (Knyihár–Csillik *et al.* 1982*b*; Ribeiro-da-Silva, unpublished observations). Correspondingly, synaptic glomeruli are more often seen in lamina I in these two species.

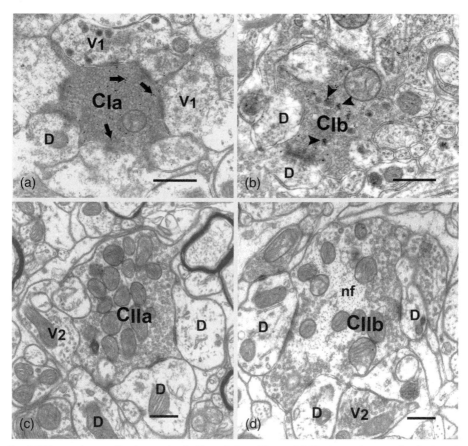

Fig. 3.2 Types of synaptic glomerulus in the rat dorsal horn. (a) Electron micrograph of a type Ia glomerulus. Note the dense cytoplasmic matrix in the central bouton (CIa), which is also devoid of dense-core vesicle and poor in mitochondria. Arrows in the CIa bouton indicate immunogold particles representing glutamate-IR sites. (b) Electron micrograph of a type Ib glomerulus in inner lamina II. Note that the properties of the central bouton (CIb) are similar to those of type Ia, except that the central bouton displays dense-core vesicles (arrowheads) and peptide immunoreactivity (immunogold particles over dense-core vesicles representing substance P). (c) Electron micrograph of a type IIa glomerulus in inner lamina II. Note the large central bouton (CIIa), which is rich in mitochondria and possesses a light cytoplasmic matrix. (d) Electron micrograph of a type IIb glomerulus from lamina III. Note a central bouton (CIIb) that is similar to that of type IIa, but displays bundles of neurofilaments (nf). See text for details. D = dendrites; V1 = presynaptic dendrites; V2 = peripheral axons. Scale bar = 0.5 μm.

In the rat, type II glomeruli occur in laminae IIi–IV. They have been subdivided into two subtypes, IIa and IIb, based on the presence or absence of neurofilament bundles in the central bouton. Type IIa glomeruli are found mostly in lamina IIi and have central boutons that are large, lack neurofilament bundles, and contain numerous mitochondria. Type IIb glomeruli occur predominantly in lamina III, possess bundles of neurofilaments in the central bouton, and have numerous axo-axonic synapses.

Most ultrastructural studies of physiologically identified afferents that have been labelled by intracellular injection have been carried out in cats and primates, and (as stated above) the arrangement of glomeruli differs in these species. In the guinea pig, primary afferents which ended in lamina IIi, and probably originated from non-peptidergic unmyelinated nociceptors, were labelled intracellularly (Sugiura *et al.* 1986) and shown to terminate as glomerular central endings (Light 1992). It is likely that these correspond to central endings in type I glomeruli.

Aδ D-hair (non-nociceptive) afferents terminate in laminae IIi–IV in the cat and monkey as the central element of synaptic glomeruli (Réthelyi *et al.* 1982). Because of their morphological properties and laminar distribution, the central boutons of type IIa glomeruli are likely to represent the termination of D-hair afferents.

The ultrastructure of different classes of cutaneous Aβ afferent in the cat have been studied by several groups (Maxwell and Réthelyi, 1987). These afferents generally form non-glomerular boutons that are presynaptic to one or more profiles and are often postsynaptic to GABA-immunoreactive axon terminals (probably derived from local interneurons) (Todd and Maxwell 2000). It has been reported that boutons belonging to rapidly adapting mechanoreceptors are more often glomerular than other types (Semba *et al.* 1985), and these may correspond to the central axons of type IIb glomeruli.

3.2.3 Receptors on primary afferent terminals

Several receptors have been identified on primary afferent terminals in the spinal dorsal horn. These include neurotransmitter/modulator receptors as well as receptors for neurotrophic factors.

Studies of neurotransmitter/modulator receptors on primary afferents have often been performed on dorsal root ganglia, rather than on the zone of termination of the fibres in the dorsal horn, and detailed anatomical information on the presence of receptors on central terminals is therefore rather limited. Recently, the use of antibodies against receptors has begun to change this situation.

It has been shown that ionotropic glutamate receptors of the AMPA class have a widespread distribution in cells of the dorsal root ganglia (Tachibana *et al.* 1994). NMDA receptors have been demonstrated in sensory fibres using light and electron microscopy (Liu *et al.* 1994), a localization that has also been described for metabotropic glutamate receptors (Ohishi *et al.* 1995). $GABA_A$ receptors have been identified by in situ hybridization in dorsal root ganglia neurons (Persohn *et al.* 1991), supporting a role for GABA in presynaptic inhibition of primary afferents. However, although $GABA_A$ receptor subunits are present throughout the dorsal horn, electron microscopic studies have so far failed to identify them at axo-axonic synapses on primary afferent terminals (Alvarez *et al.* 1996; Todd *et al.* 1996). $GABA_B$ receptor 1 has been identified in dorsal root ganglion neurons and in the central boutons of glomeruli (Poorkhalkali *et al.* 2000; Ribeiro-da-Silva and Shigemoto, unpublished observations).

Opioid receptors are expressed by primary afferents. Both μ and δ-opioid receptor binding are reduced following dorsal rhizotomy (Fields *et al.* 1980), and in situ hybridization cytochemistry has confirmed that mRNA for each of the main opioid receptors (α, δ, and κ) is present in dorsal root ganglion neurons (Minami *et al.* 1995), and should therefore occur in sensory endings in the spinal cord. This has been confirmed for δ-opioid receptors, which have been detected by immunocytochemistry on primary afferent terminals, where they were co-localized with substance P (Zhang *et al.* 1998*a*).

Although there is evidence that the neurokinin 1 (NK1) receptor (the principal receptor for substance P) is present on dorsal root ganglion cells and in peripheral tissues (Ruocco *et al.* 1997; Li and Zhao 1998), it is not seen with immunocyto-chemistry on the central terminals of primary afferents.

Both nicotinic and muscarinic cholinergic receptors have been found on sensory fibres (Flores *et al.* 1996; Haberberger *et al.* 1999). Alpha 2-adrenergic receptors have been localized on dorsal root ganglion neurons and are thought to contribute to the sensitization of the peripheral terminals to noxious stimuli (Kinnman *et al.* 1997). Their role in the central endings is unclear, although it has been reported that α_{2A} receptors are expressed by the central terminals of peptidergic afferents (Stone *et al.* 1998).

Some receptors which are responsible for signal transduction in the periphery are also transported centrally, and are therefore present on primary afferent terminals in the dorsal horn. The vanilloid receptor (VR1), which confers sensitivity to noxious heat and capsaicin, is present in the superficial laminae, although there is controversy concerning which types of primary afferent express the receptor. Michael and Priestley (1999) concluded that it is expressed by the majority of small- and medium-sized dorsal root ganglion neurons which bind the lectin IB4 or express CGRP. However, Guo *et al.* (1999) concluded that VR1 immunoreactivity was mainly associated with the non-peptidergic C afferents. The purinergic receptor $P2X_3$ occurs predominantly in the non-peptidergic population of nociceptive afferents (Bradbury *et al.* 1998; Guo *et al.* 1999). Although most primary afferent neurons express purinergic receptors, the specific localization of the $P2X_3$ receptor on non-peptidergic C afferents suggests a role for ATP in the activation of these fibres.

The expression of trophic factor receptors by primary afferents has recently been reviewed by Priestley *et al.* (2002). The three high-affinity receptors for the neurotrophin family — trkA, trkB, and trkC — have all been identified in dorsal root ganglion neurons. Whereas trkB and trkC have been shown to occur in large-diameter neurons, corresponding to low-threshold mechanoreceptors, trkA is found in peptidergic neurons. The low-affinity neurotrophin receptor, p75, is expressed by dorsal root ganglion cells that have one of the high-affinity neurotrophin receptors. In contrast, the non-peptidergic and somatostatin-containing C fibres do not express any neurotrophin receptor in the adult but rather, components of the GDNF receptor family (Alvarez and Fyffe 2000).

3.3 **Projection neurons**

3.3.1 **Ascending anterolateral system**

Neurons that project to the brain are not uniformly distributed within the dorsal horn: there is a relatively high concentration in lamina I and scattered projection cells are present throughout the deeper laminae (III–VI). However, at least in the lumbar segments, very few lamina II neurons have supraspinal projections. Dorsal horn projection neurons send their axons to several brain regions, including the thalamus and hypothalamus, the midbrain periaqueductal grey matter, the lateral parabrachial area in the pons, various parts of the medullary reticular formation, and the nucleus of the tractus solitarius (Willis and Coggeshall 1991). These projections have common features in terms of the laminar location of their cells of origin (laminae I and III–VI) and the course of their axons, which generally cross the midline and ascend in the ventral and lateral funiculi of the spinal white matter. In addition, many neurons send their axons to more than one of these supraspinal targets. This group of tracts is therefore sometimes referred to as the 'anterolateral system'.

3.3.2 **Neurokinin 1 receptor, substance P, and projection neurons**

There has long been evidence that substance P plays a vital role in nociception, and the development of antibodies against the NK1 receptor has provided important insights into its mechanism of action at the spinal level. Neurons with the NK1 receptor are found throughout the dorsal horn. However, they are most densely packed in lamina I, and around 80% of projection neurons in this lamina express the receptor (Todd *et al.* 2000). Although it has not been directly demonstrated, it is likely that the majority of lamina I neurons with high levels of the NK1 receptor are projection neurons. There is another prominent population of NK1 receptor-immunoreactive neurons with cell bodies in laminae III or IV and dorsally-directed dendrites that enter the superficial laminae. These cells are also projection neurons that belong to the anterolateral system (Todd *et al.* 2000).

Immunocytochemical studies have shown that, following intense noxious stimulation, the NK1 receptor is internalized in many of the dorsal horn neurons which express it, presumably as a result of activation of the receptor by substance P released from nociceptive primary afferents (Mantyh *et al.* 1995). This provides a useful way of assessing the extent to which NK1 receptors have been activated in different situations. Studies of receptor internalization and induction of the immediate early gene, *c-fos*, (Doyle and Hunt 1999; Todd *et al.* 2002) have suggested that most NK1 receptor-immunoreactive projection neurons in lamina I and laminae III/IV respond to acute noxious stimuli. It has also been shown that both types of neuron receive strong monosynaptic innervation from substance P-containing primary afferents (Naim *et al.* 1997; Todd *et al.* 2002) (Fig. 3.3), and that these afferents selectively innervate NK1 receptor-immunoreactive dendrites in the superficial laminae (McLeod *et al.* 1998). Interestingly, not only do many lamina I projection neurons express the NK1 receptor

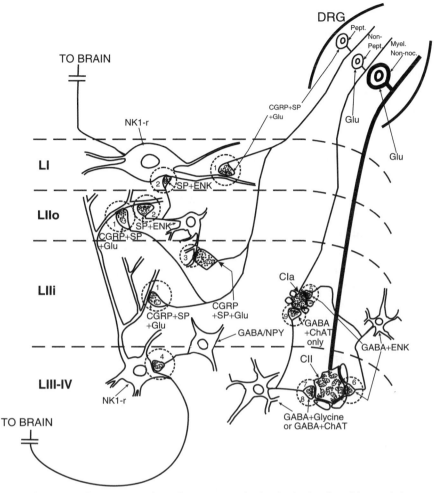

Fig. 3.3 Diagrammatic representation of some synaptic circuits in the dorsal horn of the rat spinal cord. Synaptic contacts are circled and numbered according to the type of cells involved. NK1 receptor-immunoreactive (NK1-r) with cell bodies located in lamina I and laminae III/IV receive primary afferent input from small-diameter, peptidergic (Pept.) fibres co-localizing CGRP, substance P, and glutamate (CGRP+SP+Glu) **(1)**; from interneurons co-localizing substance P and enkephalin (SP+ENK) **(2)**, which are themselves postsynaptic to the peptidergic primary afferents **(3)**. The lamina III/IV NK1-r cells are also postsynaptic to interneurons that contain GABA and NPY (GABA+NPY) **(4)**. Interneurons co-localizing GABA and enkephalin immunoreactivities (GABA+ENK) establish axo-axonic and dendro-axonic (not shown) synapses on the central boutons of synaptic glomeruli of type Ia (CIa) **(5)** and type II (CII) **(6)**. Neurons co-localizing GABA+glycine establish axo-axonic synapses on the CII **(7)** but not on the CIa glomerular boutons. In contrast, neurons co-localizing choline acetyltransferase and GABA (ChAT+GABA) establish axo-axonic synapses on CII **(8)**, and to a lesser extent also on CIa **(9)**, glomerular boutons. The CIa glomerular boutons represent the central termination of non-peptidergic C fibres (Non-Pept.), which are glutamatergic (Glu), have FRAP activity, and bind the lectin IB4. The CII glomerular boutons represent the termination of non-nociceptive myelinated Aδ and Aβ afferents (Myel. Non-noc.), and are glutamatergic (Glu). DRG = dorsal root ganglion.

and receive a strong input from substance P-containing primary afferents, but in addition, some of these cells appear to use substance P as a signalling molecule (Noguchi and Ruda 1992).

In spite of the obvious importance of opioid receptors in analgesia, there is no evidence from anatomical studies that any of these are expressed by spinal projection neurons.

3.3.3 Other ascending pathways from the dorsal horn

There are other ascending tracts from the dorsal horn that are independent of the anterolateral system. These include the postsynaptic dorsal column (PSDC) pathway and the spinocervical tract, with axons that travel to the dorsal column nuclei and the lateral cervical nucleus, respectively. These have been studied most extensively in the cat (Brown 1981), and both have been found to originate mainly from cell bodies in laminae III–IV. The majority of projection neurons in the deeper laminae of the dorsal horn (including PSDC neurons; Polgár *et al.* 1999*b*) do not express the NK1 receptor, and at present there are no suitable immunocytochemical markers which can be used to distinguish these cells from other neurons in the same laminae.

3.4 Interneurons

The great majority of neurons in each lamina of the dorsal horn are interneurons, with axons that remain in the spinal cord. Many of these cells have axons that are restricted to the spinal segment which contains the cell body, and these are sometimes referred to as 'local circuit neurons'. However, there is also evidence that a significant number of dorsal horn interneurons have longer intraspinal connections. For example, although very few lamina II neurons in the lumbar spinal cord project to the brain, it has been reported that 7% of cells in this lamina send their axons as far as the mid-thoracic spinal cord and that approximately half have axons that project at least two segments rostrally and/or caudally (Bice and Beal 1997). Less is known about the intersegmental projections of interneurons in other laminae.

3.4.1 Classification of interneurons

A basic functional distinction can be made between excitatory and inhibitory interneurons. The major inhibitory transmitters in the dorsal horn are GABA and glycine, and there is strong evidence from studies in various parts of the central nervous system that these amino acids are highly enriched in neurons that use them as a neurotransmitter. The most direct way to investigate the anatomy of GABAergic and glycinergic neurons is to use immunocytochemistry with antibodies that recognize the amino acids in fixed tissue.

It has been shown GABA is present in both cell bodies and axon terminals in the upper part of the dorsal horn (particularly laminae I–III), whereas glycine is enriched in relatively few cell bodies and axon terminals in laminae I–II, but in many of those in deeper laminae (III–VI), and in the ventral horn (Todd and Sullivan 1990). GABA is found in approximately one third of the neurons in laminae I and II, and in nearly half of those in lamina III. In these three laminae, glycine enrichment is largely restricted to neurons that are GABA-immunoreactive, and this has led to the suggestion that many neurons in these laminae use GABA and glycine as co-transmitters. In the deeper laminae of the dorsal horn, there are neurons that are GABAergic or glycinergic, as well as cells that appear to use both transmitters. The axons of GABAergic neurons contain the synthetic enzyme glutamic acid decarboxylase (GAD), while those belonging to glycinergic neurons express the neuronal glycine transporter (GLYT2). Antibodies against these compounds can be used as alternative markers for GABAergic and glycinergic axons in immunocytochemical studies (e.g. McLaughlin *et al.* 1975).

Glutamate is the main transmitter used by excitatory interneurons in the spinal cord, as well as by primary afferents and projection neurons, and it is likely that most dorsal horn neurons that do not use GABA or glycine as their transmitter are glutamatergic. Unfortunately, it is not possible to identify a glutamatergic neuron by the level of glutamate in its cell body, and this has proved a major obstacle to the classification of excitatory interneurons in the dorsal horn. Recently, antibodies against vesicular glutamate transporters (VGLUTs) have been developed, and these should prove valuable for identifying axons of spinal glutamatergic neurons. One of these transporters (VGLUT2) is present throughout the dorsal horn (Varoqui *et al.* 2002), and is likely to be expressed by glutamatergic interneurons (Todd *et al.* 2003).

Since the introduction of the 'gate control' theory of pain (Melzack and Wall 1965), there has been a great deal of interest in the interneurons of the superficial laminae, and their role in regulating the flow of somatosensory information through the dorsal horn. In early anatomical studies, attempts were made to classify neurons in this region using morphological criteria (for review, see Todd and Spike 1993). These attempts were partially successful, in that certain distinctive types of neuron were recognized. However, they failed to produce a comprehensive classification scheme that was universally accepted. Gobel (1978) identified two main morphological classes of neuron in lamina II of the cat spinal trigeminal nucleus: islet cells, which were found throughout the lamina had rostrocaudally-orientated dendritic trees and axons that arborized locally; while stalked cells had cell bodies in the outer part of the lamina, dendrites that passed ventrally, and axons that entered lamina I. Another difference between the two types is that the dendrites of islet cells were found to contain vesicles and form synapses with other dendrites and axons, whereas this arrangement was not seen with stalked cells (Gobel *et al.* 1980). Stalked and islet cells have since been found in lamina II of the spinal cord in several species. Gobel concluded that islet cells were inhibitory interneurons and stalked cells were excitatory, and in support of this view we have shown that typical islet cells are GABA-immunoreactive, while stalked cells never contain GABA (Todd and Spike 1993). However, most morphological studies have shown that many lamina II neurons do not belong to either stalked or islet classes. We observed a population of cells that had rostrocaudal dendritic trees but were considerably smaller than typical islet cells, and which (unlike islet cells) were not GABA-immunoreactive (Todd and Spike 1993). In addition, some lamina II neurons that are not islet cells possess presynaptic dendrites and show GABA immunoreactivity.

Overall, these results suggest that the neuronal organization is very complex, even in a single lamina, and that although there is a link between morphology and function, this needs to be interpreted with care. Less is known about the relationship between morphology and transmitter content for neurons in the other laminae of the dorsal horn, although it has been shown that lamina III neurons with rostrocaudally-orientated dendritic trees are often GABA-immunoreactive, whereas cells in this lamina with dorsally-directed dendrites are not (Todd and Spike 1993).

An alternative approach for classifying interneurons in the superficial laminae has been to make use of the neurochemical diversity of the region, by attempting to characterize neurons based on expression of neuropeptides, receptors, enzymes, etc., and then to relate this to the neurotransmitters that they use. This can be carried out most easily with immunocytochemistry and allows investigation of the arrangements of different types of cell in the neuronal circuits of the dorsal horn.

Many peptides are found in axons in the superficial laminae. Some of these (e.g. CGRP) are restricted to primary afferents, some (e.g. neurotensin and neuropeptide Y) are found in axons belonging to dorsal horn neurons, while others (e.g. somatostatin and galanin) are present in both types of cell (Todd and Spike 1993; Ribeiro-da-Silva and Cuello 1995). It has been shown that in the rat dorsal horn certain peptides (e.g. NPY and galanin) are present only in neurons that are GABAergic, while others (e.g. somatostatin and neurotensin) are found exclusively in cells that do not contain GABA (Todd and Spike 1993). The peptides that have been found to coexist with GABA (NPY, galanin, thyrotropin-releasing hormone, and enkephalin), are restricted to those neurons that are not also glycine-immunoreactive. We have recently provided evidence that most axons derived from spinal neurons which synthesise neurotensin or somatostatin have high levels of the vesicular glutamate transporter VGLUT2 (Todd *et al.*, 2003). This suggests that the great majority of neurotensin- and somatostatin-containing cells are glutamatergic excitatory interneurons. One interesting point is that some dorsal horn neurons contain neurochemicals with apparently antagonistic effects: in the rat, substance P-immunoreactive interneurons contain enkephalin immunoreactivity (Ribeiro-da-Silva *et al.* 1991), whereas in the cat (but not the rat), GABA and substance P immunoreactivities are co-localized in the superficial dorsal horn (Ma and Ribeiro-da-Silva 1995). The functional meaning of such co-localizations is not understood but may indicate that some neurons can exert opposite actions on different target neurons. Further studies involving the localization of receptors are required to clarify this issue.

Another group of compounds that have proved useful for anatomical studies in the dorsal horn are proteins that are expressed in a restricted population of neurons, but are present throughout the cytoplasm or else on the plasma membrane of both the cell bodies and dendrites of cells that express them. Immunostaining for these proteins can therefore be used to reveal neuronal morphology and to allow investigation of synaptic inputs to the cells. In this group are the calcium-binding proteins, calbindin D28k and parvalbumin, several enzymes, including nitric oxide synthase (NOS), choline acetyltransferase (ChAT), and the gamma isoform of protein kinase C (PKCγ), as well as certain neuropeptide receptors.

Calbindin-immunoreactive neurons are present throughout the dorsal horn, but are particularly common in laminae I and II. Within these laminae, calbindin is virtually restricted to neurons that are not GABA-immunoreactive (Antal *et al.* 1991). Calbindin-containing cells are a heterogeneous group, including some lamina I projection neurons (Ménétrey *et al.* 1992), as well as lamina II interneurons that contain peptides such as neurotensin or somatostatin (Yoshida *et al.* 1990). Parvalbumin is present in a small number of neurons in laminae II and III, and most of these are GABA- and glycine-immunoreactive (Antal *et al.* 1991; Laing *et al.* 1994). Neurons that contain NOS are widely distributed in the spinal cord, but are most numerous in laminae I–III (Valtschanoff *et al.* 1992). Most NOS-containing cells throughout the dorsal horn are GABA-immunoreactive and many are enriched with glycine (Spike *et al.* 1993). However, even though parvalbumin and NOS can both be present in GABA-immunoreactive islet cells, they are never found in the same neuron (Laing *et al.* 1994).

Cholinergic neurons are scattered throughout the deeper laminae (III–VI) of the dorsal horn (Barber *et al.* 1984; Ribeiro-da-Silva and Cuello 1990*a*), and most contain NOS and GABA (Spike *et al.* 1993; Todd and Spike 1993; Ribeiro-da-Silva 2002). Although each of the neuronal forms of PKC has been found in neurons in the superficial laminae, cells that contain PKCγ have attracted most interest because of the demonstration that mice deficient in this enzyme fail to develop neuropathic pain after peripheral nerve injury (Malmberg *et al.* 1997). Neurons showing high levels of PKCγ are concentrated in the ventral half of lamina II, but are also numerous in lamina III. Most of these cells are not GABAergic, and many contain either neurotensin or somatostatin (Polgár *et al.* 1999*a*).

Since many peptides are present in the superficial laminae of the dorsal horn, it is not surprising that several neuropeptide receptors have been found on neurons in this region. These include the NK1 and NK3 tachykinin receptors; the μ opioid receptor, MOR-1; the somatostatin receptor, sst$_{2a}$; and the Y1 receptor for NPY. Although NK1 receptors are found on a high proportion of projection neurons in the superficial laminae (see section 3.3.2), many cells with this receptor are interneurons, and the other peptide receptors mentioned are present mainly or exclusively on interneurons. These receptors tend to be associated with particular functional types of neuron: both MOR-1 and the NK1 receptor (which are present on different neurons in the superficial dorsal horn) are virtually restricted to cells that are not GABAergic (Kemp *et al.* 1996; Littlewood *et al.* 1995), whereas sst$_{2a}$ is present on neurons that are GABA- and glycine-immunoreactive (Todd *et al.* 1998). NK3 receptors are expressed by NOS-containing neurons (Seybold *et al.* 1997), and the Y1 receptor is found on cells with somatostatin (Zhang *et al.* 1999). Although both MOR-1 and PKCγ are found in non-GABAergic neurons in lamina II, they show very little coexistence (Polgár *et al.* 1999*a*).

This account of the neurochemistry of dorsal horn interneurons indicates that there is a high degree of complexity, particularly in lamina II, where numerous morphological and neurochemical classes can be identified. It is therefore interesting that in a whole-cell recording study in hamster spinal cord slices, Grudt and Perl (2002) have identified at least seven different classes of neuron in lamina II on the basis of combined morphological and physiological criteria. It will be important to determine how the classification scheme of Grudt and Perl is related to the neurochemical classes described here.

3.4.2 Synaptic circuits involving interneurons

Because of technical difficulties associated with the study of small neurons and unmyelinated primary afferents, our knowledge of synaptic circuits in the dorsal horn is still very limited. An additional complicating factor is that there are significant inter-species differences in the neurochemical and anatomical organization of the region. Most studies on physiologically characterized, intracellularly injected neurons have been performed in the cat, whereas tract-tracing and immunocytochemical studies have generally been carried out in the rat.

Before giving an account of some of the circuits involving interneurons, it is important to stress that not all chemical communication involves synapses (Zoli *et al.* 1999). Non-synaptic ('paracrine') transmission is thought to occur particularly with peptides and monoamines, although it probably also occurs for amino acids transmitters at their metabotropic receptors. Under physiological conditions, most chemical communication in the dorsal horn probably takes place either at synapses or close to the site of release, although diffusion of compounds over longer distances cannot be ruled out, particularly in the case of neuropeptides. However, it should be kept in mind that the neuropil represents a significant diffusion barrier, and it is unlikely that even peptides diffuse large distances when released at 'physiological' concentrations. Therefore, a detailed knowledge of the neurochemical anatomy of the circuits of the dorsal horn is of great importance for our understanding of the normal function and changes in pathological conditions.

Unfortunately, little is known about the synaptic inputs to dorsal horn interneurons, since most immunocytochemical markers used to date reveal axons rather than cell bodies and dendritic trees. Studies combining intracellular labelling of interneurons (in vivo or in vitro) with immunocytochemistry would be required to obtain a more complete picture of the afferent and efferent connections of transmitter-specific interneurons. However, such approaches are technically demanding and have seldom been used. Despite these limitations, a pattern is emerging (see Fig. 3.3). At present, more is known about the circuits involving inhibitory interneurons, and this is partly due to the difficulty of identifying glutamatergic neurons.

Since most synapses in the dorsal horn are axo-dendritic, it is not surprising that the majority of interneurons appear to act on their targets through a postsynaptic mechanism. However, some cells clearly participate in presynaptic interactions. GABAergic axons, which are thought to originate from local interneurons, establish axo-axonic synapses on the central boutons of synaptic glomeruli (except for those in peptidergic (type Ib) glomeruli, which are seldom postsynaptic to other profiles). There is a fundamental difference between the types of GABAergic neurons that innervate type Ia and type II glomeruli, since boutons containing GABA and glycine are presynaptic to the central boutons of type II, but not type Ia glomeruli (Todd 1996).

In contrast, neurons co-localizing GABA and enkephalin immunoreactivities seem to innervate central axons of type I and II glomeruli equally (through both axo-axonic and dendro-axonic synapses) (Ribeiro-da-Silva 2002). The population of neurons with GABA and ChAT is relatively small (Todd 1991), but their axons contribute a significant contingent of axo-axonic synapses in type II, and to a lesser extent in type Ib, glomeruli (Ribeiro-da-Silva and Cuello 1990*a*; Ribeiro-da-Silva 2002). The neurons with GABA and ChAT have cell bodies in laminae III and IV, and dendrites that extend superficially, where they receive synaptic input from primary afferents in both type Ia and type II glomeruli. In addition to targeting synaptic glomeruli, their axons also establish axo-dendritic synapses with unidentified dorsal horn neurons (Ribeiro-da-Silva and Cuello 1990*a*). Neurons that co-localize GABA and NPY establish axo-axonic synapses in the cat (Doyle and Maxwell 1993*b*), although it is not yet known whether this arrangement also occurs in the rat.

Most (if not all) of the substance P-containing neurons in superficial laminae are also enkephalin-immunoreactive (Ribeiro-da-Silva *et al.* 1991). They are located in lamina I and II and receive synaptic input from non-peptidergic C fibres in type Ia glomeruli and from substance P-containing afferents outside glomeruli. Interestingly, based on evidence from studies in the cat (Ma *et al.* 1997), these neurons seem to innervate preferentially nociceptive neurons in lamina I and in the deep dorsal horn which probably express the NK1 receptor (see Fig. 3.3).

Dorsal horn neurons that contain somatostatin are particularly numerous, and are mostly located in lamina II. These cells receive primary sensory input from the central boutons of type Ia glomeruli (Ribeiro-da-Silva and Cuello 1990*b*). Interestingly, they are also occasionally presynaptic to the central bouton of such glomeruli via dendro-axonic synapses (Ribeiro-da-Silva and Cuello 1990*b*). The postsynaptic targets of the axons of somatostatin-containing interneurons are not known. Since the axons of most somatostatin-containing neurons in the superficial laminae are VGLUT2-immunoreactive (Todd et al. 2003), it is likely that the great majority of these cells are excitatory interneurons. However, since somatostatin-immunoreactive dendrites are occasionally presynaptic at dendro-axonic synapses, at least some of the cells may be inhibitory.

Knowledge about dorsal horn circuits that involve postsynaptic inhibition is at present very limited. However, it has been shown that axons which contain GABA and NPY (and are presumably derived from local interneurons) selectively target the NK1 receptor-immunoreactive lamina III/IV projection neurons, with which they make numerous axo-dendritic and axo-somatic synapses (Polgár *et al.* 1999*b*) (see Figs. 3.3 and 3.4).

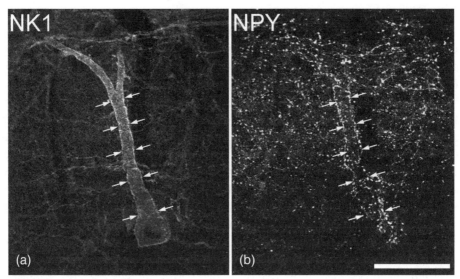

Fig. 3.4 (a) A confocal image from a parasagittal section of the rat spinal cord showing a neuron in lamina III that possesses the neurokinin 1 (NK1) receptor. (b) The cell receives numerous contacts on its dorsal primary dendrite from NPY-immunoreactive axonal varicosities, which are presumably derived from NPY-containing neurons in the superficial dorsal horn. This is an example of selective targeting of axons belonging to a neurochemically defined population of dorsal horn interneurons. Scale bar = 50 μm. (Modified from Polgár *et al.*, 1999, *J Neurosci* 19, 2637–2646. Copyright 1999 by the Society for Neuroscience.)

3.5 **Receptors for glutamate, GABA, and glycine on spinal neurons**

Since most of the studies of receptors for the amino acid transmitters have not distinguished between projection neurons and interneurons, we will deal with them in a separate section.

3.5.1 **Glutamate receptors**

All three types of ionotropic glutamate receptor are present in the dorsal horn, and for most subunits the distribution has been studied with both in situ hybridization and immunocytochemistry. For AMPA receptors, the predominant subunits expressed in dorsal horn are GluR1 and GluR2 (Furuyama *et al.* 1993; Jakowec *et al.* 1995) and the highest levels of expression are seen in laminae I–III. Light microscopic immunocyto-chemistry shows strong labelling of many cell bodies in the dorsal horn, and it has been reported that the GluR1 subunit is particularly associated with inibitory (GABAergic) neurons, while GluR2 is mainly found in cells that lack GABA (Spike *et al.* 1998). This pattern suggests that some GABAergic neurons may express the GluR1 but not the GluR2 subunit, which would imply that these cells possessed Ca^{2+}-permeable AMPA receptors, and there is direct evidence that receptors of this type are present on certain dorsal horn neurons (Engelman *et al.* 1999). A major problem with studying the arrangement of ionotropic receptors at glutamatergic synapses is that access of antibodies is limited by the presence of the postsynaptic density and the synaptic cleft, and for this reason they are best revealed with post-embedding methods. This approach has been used by Popratiloff *et al.* (1996) to demonstrate that AMPA receptors are present at synapses formed by central axons of synaptic glomeruli, which are known to be of primary afferent origin.

There is a high level of expression of the NR1 subunit of the NMDA receptor, and this is probably present on all spinal neurons (Tölle *et al.* 1993; Watanabe *et al.* 1994). However, there is disagreement about the expression of the NR2 subunits, as some authors have identified NR2A and NR2B (Watanabe *et al.* 1994) while others have found only NR2C and NR2D (Tölle *et al.* 1993). Nothing is apparently known about the types of spinal neuron that express particular NR2 subunits. Post-embedding detection has revealed that the NR1 subunit is present at some of the synapses formed by primary afferents in the superficial dorsal horn, including those in synaptic glomeruli (Popratiloff *et al.* 1998*b*).

Much less is known about kainate receptors in the dorsal horn. However, the GluR5, GluR7, KA1, and KA2 subunits have all been found in scattered neurons in the superficial laminae (Furuyama *et al.* 1993; Tölle *et al.* 1993).

Several metabotropic glutamate receptors have been identified in the spinal cord and of these mGluR5 is the most prevalent (Berthele *et al.* 1999; Jia *et al.* 1999). The highest densities of mGluRs 5, 3, and 7 are all found within the superficial dorsal horn, although with slightly different laminar locations. Metabotropic glutamate receptors are present not only on spinal neurons, but also on the central terminals of primary afferents (Ohishi *et al.* 1995).

3.5.2 **GABA and glycine receptors**

$GABA_A$ receptors are probably expressed by all dorsal horn neurons and are found at most (if not all) GABAergic synapses which these cells receive (Todd and Maxwell 2000). The combination of $\alpha3$, $\beta3$, and $\gamma2$ subunits appears to be present in neurons throughout the spinal cord, while $\alpha1$ subunits are also expressed by neurons in deeper laminae. There is extensive evidence that primary afferent terminals are subject to GABAergic presynaptic inhibition, and in situ hybridization studies have shown that dorsal root ganglion cells express $GABA_A$ receptor subunits (particularly $\alpha2$, $\beta3$, and $\gamma2$).

Glycine receptors are also widely distributed, and are probably present on all dorsal horn neurons. Although there are antibodies against the glycine receptor, most immunocytochemical studies have examined the glycine receptor-associated protein, gephyrin (which coexists with the receptor at synapses in the spinal cord). Gephyrin is found at low levels in laminae I and II and in large amounts in the deeper laminae, a distribution that matches that of glycinergic axon terminals, and gephyrin and $GABA_A$ receptors co-localize at some synapses in the dorsal horn (Todd *et al.* 1996). It has been reported that although there is co-release of GABA and glycine at synapses in the superficial laminae, selective distribution of receptors means that individual synapses are effectively either glycinergic or GABAergic (Chéry and De Koninck 1999).

Until recently, GABA$_B$ receptors could only be investigated by radioligand binding, and studies using this approach suggested that high levels of the receptor were present in the superficial part of the dorsal horn, where some were located on primary afferent terminals. A recent study that combined in situ hybridization and immunocytochemistry indicated that GABA$_B$ receptors were widely expressed by primary afferents and dorsal horn neurons (Towers *et al.* 2000).

3.6 Descending inputs

Several pathways project from the brain to the dorsal horn of the spinal cord, and of these, the raphe-spinal serotoninergic system and the noradrenergic projection from the pons have received particular attention because of their involvement in pain mechanisms. Serotonin-containing axons originating from cells in the nucleus raphe magnus are found throughout the dorsal horn, but are concentrated in lamina I and the outer part of lamina II. Because of their wide distribution and diffuse pattern of arborization within the dorsal horn, serotoninergic axons are likely to target several different types of neuron. In the cat, it has been shown that these axons form numerous contacts with some spinothalamic and spinoparabrachial neurons in lamina I (Hylden *et al.* 1986). Miletic *et al.* (1984) reported that in lamina II, stalked cells received many more contacts from serotoninergic axons than islet cells. In a recent study in the rat spinal cord, Stewart and Maxwell (2000) showed that the large NK1 receptor-immunoreactive lamina III/IV cells (all of which are projection neurons) received many contacts from serotonin-immunoreactive axons, and that in some cases these were so numerous that they formed a basket around the cell body. Also in the rat, Polgár *et al.* (2002) reported that NK1 receptor-immunoreactive lamina I projection neurons were often strongly innervated by serotoninergic axons, and received significantly more contacts than did projection cells in this lamina that lacked the NK1 receptor. Since serotonin may act through a non-synaptic mechanism, a lack of direct contacts from serotoninergic axons on a neuron does not rule out the possibility that it is influenced by serotonin, particularly since we have limited information about the distribution of serotonin receptors on dorsal horn neurons. However, the dense and selective innervation of certain dorsal horn neurons (including some projection cells) implies that the descending serotoninergic axons are likely to have a relatively powerful effect on these cells.

Noradrenergic axons can be revealed with antibodies against the synthetic enzyme dopamine-β-hydroxylase. These axons are also widely distributed in the dorsal horn and originate from various brainstem nuclei, including locus coeruleus, nucleus subcoeruleus, and Kölliker–Fuse nucleus. The precise origin appears to vary with species, and even among different strains of rat. Relatively little is known about the targets of noradrenergic neurons in the dorsal horn, although these have been shown to include PSDC cells in the cat (Doyle and Maxwell 1993*a*).

While the importance of monoaminergic systems has been emphasized, other transmitters are also used by descending axons. For example, Antal *et al.* (1996) reported that the dorsal horn is densely innervated by GABAergic axons that originate in the rostral ventromedial medulla (an area that includes the nucleus raphe magnus). It is likely that at least some of these axons use GABA and serotonin as co-transmitters (Maxwell *et al.* 1996). However, it is important to recognize that some of the descending inhibitory effects of brainstem stimulation may occur directly through a GABAergic mechanism.

3.7 Changes following injury or inflammation

There has been a great deal of interest in changes of the neurochemical organization of the dorsal horn which occur in pathological conditions, since these may contribute to chronic pain states. Many neurochemical changes have been demonstrated following nerve injury and in inflammatory pain states. Some of these affect primary afferents, while others involve neurons within the dorsal horn. Here we will review some of the major alterations that have been reported for different groups of chemicals.

3.7.1 Neuropeptides

Although most primary afferent neurons survive following injury to a peripheral nerve, there are dramatic alterations in the expression of neuropeptides in the central terminals of the damaged afferents within the dorsal horn (for review see Hökfelt *et al.* 1994). Most of the peptides that are normally present in fine-diameter afferents, such as substance P, CGRP, and somatostatin, are largely depleted from their central terminals after nerve transection, while galanin is up-regulated. Two further peptides, which are either not expressed by intact primary afferents or are present only in a small number, appear *de novo* after nerve injury — vasoactive intestinal polypeptide (VIP), which is found in terminals of fine-diameter afferents in laminae I and II; and NPY, which is up-regulated in myelinated afferents that terminate in laminae III–V.

The changes of peptide expression in primary afferents that occur as a result of inflammation are more complex. The levels of mRNAs for CGRP, substance P, and galanin in dorsal root ganglion cells are elevated, suggesting that there is an increased rate of synthesis of these peptides by primary afferents. However, NPY and VIP are apparently not up-regulated in primary afferents in this situation (Donaldson *et al.* 1992; Wakisaka *et al.* 1992; Galeazza *et al.* 1995; Calzà *et al.* 1998). The levels of CGRP, substance P, and galanin in axon terminals in the dorsal horn are reduced in the first few days after the induction of inflammation (Galeazza *et al.* 1995; Calzà *et al.* 1998), probably because increased release of these peptides resulting from activity in primary afferents (e.g. Schaible *et al.* 1990) leads to a depletion from their central terminals. A complication in interpreting changes in primary afferent peptide levels in the dorsal horn is that (with the exception of CGRP) the peptides are also present in the axons of some spinal neurons, and these may undergo alterations as well (see below).

There have been reports that substance P, which is normally expressed only by a few Aβ afferents, is up-regulated in many afferents of this class following both nerve section (Noguchi *et al.* 1994) and peripheral inflammation (Neumann *et al.* 1996). Since the great majority of cutaneous Aβ afferents normally function as low-threshold mechanoreceptors, the appearance of substance P in these axons might contribute to abnormal pain sensation. However, although substance P-immunoreactivity was seen in large axons in the dorsal roots in these studies, it has apparently not been possible to demonstrate that the peptide is present in their central terminals in either situation.

Peripheral inflammation also produces changes in the synthesis of peptides in spinal cord neurons: there is a dramatic increase in the level of preprodynorphin mRNA in neurons in lamina I and V, as well as more modest increases in the mRNAs for enkephalin, galanin, and substance P (Dubner and Ruda 1992; Noguchi and Ruda 1992; Calzà *et al.* 1998). Some of the neurons in which substance P is up-regulated are lamina I projection cells (Noguchi and Ruda 1992). There have been reports of both an early increase and a late reduction in the levels of NPY mRNA in the dorsal horn following the induction of inflammation (Ji *et al.* 1994; Calzà *et al.* 1998).

3.7.2 Neuropeptide receptors

NK1 receptor immunoreactivity in the dorsal horn increases as a result of inflammation, peripheral nerve transection, and the chronic constriction injury (CCI) model of painful peripheral neuropathy (Abbadie *et al.* 1996, 1997; Goff *et al.* 1998). This increase apparently results from up-regulation by neurons that normally express the receptor, rather than from an increase in the number of NK1 receptor-expressing neurons.

Inflammation results in a dramatic increase in the internalization of NK1 receptors by dorsal horn neurons in response to peripheral stimulation (Abbadie *et al.* 1997), presumably as a result of increased release of substance P in the dorsal horn (Schaible *et al.* 1990). This is reflected in an increase in the number of neurons that show internalization after a noxious stimulus, as well as by internalization of the receptor on somata and proximal dendrites of cells in laminae III–V and internalization in response to normally innocuous stimuli such as brushing of the skin (neither of which occur in normal animals). NK1 receptor internalisation by dorsal horn neurons resulting from electrical stimulation of the sciatic nerve also increases following both nerve transection and inflammation (Allen *et al.* 1999). However, in neither of these situations was there any internalization if the nerve was stimulated at a strength that would activate only Aβ afferents. This does not, therefore, support the suggestion that up-regulation of substance P in Aβ afferents contributes to neuropathic or inflammatory pain (Noguchi *et al.* 1995; Neumann *et al.* 1996).

Changes have also been reported for the levels of MOR-1 and the Y1 receptor in the dorsal horn. Immunostaining for MOR-1 was increased in the ipsilateral dorsal horn as a result of inflammation and in the CCI model, but reduced after tight ligation of the sciatic nerve (Goff *et al.* 1998). The authors did not determine whether these changes affected lamina II interneurons or the terminals of fine-diameter primary afferents, both of which express MOR-1. Inflammation also causes an increase in MOR-1 immunostaining in dorsal root ganglia (Zhang *et al.* 1998*b*), suggesting that at least some of the increase in dorsal horn may have involved primary afferents. Y1 receptor expression in laminae II and III of the dorsal horn is up-regulated as a result of inflammation (Ji *et al.* 1994).

3.7.3 GABA

It has been reported that the levels of both the synthetic enzyme GAD, and GABA itself are increased in the dorsal horn ipsilateral to a peripheral inflammation (Nahin and Hylden 1991; Castro–Lopes *et al.* 1992). The increases in GAD immunostaining were found throughout the dorsal horn, whereas it was reported that, for GABA, the change was restricted to laminae I–III, where the highest density of GABA immunoreactivity is seen. Since GABA is the major inhibitory transmitter in the dorsal horn, it is thought that the increases may partially compensate for the increased activation of dorsal horn neurons that results from the inflammation.

There have also been reports of a down-regulation of GABAergic systems following nerve injury, and since spinal administration of GABA$_A$ antagonists can produce allodynia which is a feature of neuropathic pain (Yaksh 1989), it has been suggested that reduction in spinal GABAergic inhibition may be a contributory factor in this type of pain. Castro–Lopes *et al.* (1993) found modest reductions of GABA immunoreactivity in the ipsilateral dorsal horn which developed between two and four weeks after sciatic nerve transection, while Ibuki *et al.* (1997) described a dramatic reduction of GABA immunoreactivity in the dorsal horn in the CCI model, with a time-course that matched that of the behavioural signs of pain. The GABA depletion was seen bilaterally, but was more severe on the ipsilateral side. Recently, Moore *et al.* (2001) have reported that there is a selective loss of one of the two GAD isoforms (GAD65) from the dorsal horn in models of peripheral neuropathy. Loss of dorsal horn neurons has also been reported following nerve injury, and it has been suggested that death of GABAergic interneurons in the dorsal horn may contribute to the observed GABA depletion (for review see Woolf 1997).

3.7.4 Glutamate receptors

Changes in AMPA receptors have been found in rats following nerve injury. In the CCI model, immunoreactivity for both GluR1 and GluR2/3 was increased in the medial part of the dorsal horn on the ipsilateral side at two weeks after nerve injury (Harris *et al.* 1996). Popratiloff *et al.* (1998*a*) also reported stronger GluR2/3 immunoreactivity in the ipsilateral dorsal horn two weeks after sciatic nerve transection, and by using post-embedding immunogold electron microscopy, were able to show that there was an increase in the density of GluR2/3 subunits at synapses formed by primary afferent terminals (identified by the presence of glomeruli), but not at synapses formed by other types of axon.

There have been contradictory results regarding changes in ionotropic glutamate receptors from peripheral inflammation. These include reports of reduction in the level of mRNA for GluR1 bilaterally, with no change in those for GluR2 or NMDA (Pellegrini–Giampietro *et al.* 1994), reduction of GluR1 and GluR2/3 immunoreactivity on the ipsilateral side in the spinal trigeminal nucleus (Florenzano and De Luca 1999), and transient up-regulation of individual splice variants of GluR1, GluR2, and GluR3, together with an increase in immunoreactivity for GluR1 and GluR2 in the ipsilateral dorsal horn (Zhou *et al.* 2001). The synaptic distribution of ionotropic glutamate receptors has not been studied in inflammatory models. Boxall *et al.* (1998) have described an increase of mRNA for mGluR3 in the ipsilateral dorsal horn resulting from inflammation.

3.7.5 Other compounds

The level of nitric oxide synthase is reduced in the ipsilateral dorsal horn following nerve injury, but is not altered by peripheral inflammation (Goff *et al.* 1998). PKCγ in the dorsal horn is up-regulated as a result of inflammation, and this is accompanied by a translocation of the enzyme to the plasma membrane (Martin *et al.* 1999). There is apparently no change in PKCγ as a result of nerve injury.

3.7.6 Other changes affecting primary afferents

There are changes in the cell surface molecules expressed by primary afferents following nerve injury that affect the labelling pattern when using tracers. Cholera toxin B subunit (CTb) binds to the GM1 ganglioside, which is normally present on myelinated (but not unmyelinated) axons in somatic peripheral nerves in the rat. If CTb is injected into an intact nerve, it is taken up specifically by myelinated axons and transported to their central terminals. This results in transganglionic labelling in laminae I and III–VI, but not in lamina II which receives very little input from myelinated primary afferents. If CTb is injected into a chronically injured nerve, it is transported to lamina II (as well as the other dorsal horn laminae), and this is taken as evidence that myelinated afferents sprout into lamina II (Woolf *et al.* 1992). However, Tong *et al.* (1999) demonstrated that following nerve injury, CTb is transported into many more dorsal root ganglion cells than normal, including small cells that are likely to give rise to unmyelinated afferents. It therefore appears that, following nerve injury, the GM1 ganglioside is up-regulated in unmyelinated afferents.

Acknowledgements

Work in the authors' laboratories is supported by grants from the Wellcome Trust (AJT) and the Canadian Institutes of Health Research (grant MOP-38093) (AR), which are gratefully acknowledged.

References

Abbadie C, Brown JL, Mantyh PW, and Basbaum AI (1996). Spinal cord substance P receptor immunoreactivity increases in both inflammatory and nerve injury models of persistent pain. *Neuroscience*, **70**, 201–209.

Abbadie C, Trafton J, Liu HT, Mantyh PW, and Basbaum AI (1997). Inflammation increases the distribution of dorsal horn neurons that internalize the neurokinin-1 receptor in response to noxious and non-noxious stimulation. *Journal of Neuroscience*, **17**, 8049–8060.

Allen BJ *et al.* (1999). Primary afferent fibers that contribute to increased substance P receptor internalization in the spinal cord after injury. *Journal of Neurophysiology*, **81**, 1379–1390.

Alvarez FJ and Fyffe RE (2000). Nociceptors for the 21st century. *Current Review of Pain*, **4**, 451–458.

Alvarez FJ, Taylor–Blake B, Fyffe REW, de Blas AL, and Light AR (1996). Distribution of immunoreactivity for the β_2 and β_3 subunits of the GABA$_A$ receptor the mammalian spinal cord. *Journal of Comparative Neurology*, **365**, 392–412.

Antal M, Petko M, Polgar E, Heizmann CW, and Storm–Mathisen J (1996). Direct evidence of an extensive GABAergic innervation of the spinal dorsal horn by fibres descending from the rostral ventromedial medulla. *Neuroscience*, **73**, 509–518.

Antal M *et al.* (1991). Different populations of parvalbumin- and calbindin-D28k-immunoreactive neurons contain GABA and accumulate ^{3}H- D-aspartate in the dorsal horn of the rat spinal cord. *Journal of Comparative Neurology*, **314**, 114–124.

Barber RP *et al.* (1984). The morphology and distribution of neurons containing choline acetyltransferase in the adult rat spinal cord: an immunohistochemical study. *Journal of Comparative Neurology*, **229**, 329–346.

Berthele A *et al.* (1999). Distribution and developmental changes in metabotropic glutamate receptor messenger RNA expression in the rat lumbar spinal cord. *Developmental Brain Research*, **112**, 39–53.

Bice TN and Beal JA (1997). Quantitative and neurogenic analysis of the total population and subpopulations of neurons defined by axon projection in the superficial dorsal horn of the rat lumbar spinal cord. *Journal of Comparative Neurology*, **388**, 550–564.

Boxall SJ *et al.* (1998). Enhanced expression of metabotropic glutamate receptor 3 messenger RNA in the rat spinal cord during ultraviolet irradiation induced peripheral inflammation. *Neuroscience*, **82**, 591–602.

Bradbury EJ, Burnstock G, and McMahon SB (1998). The expression of P2X$_3$ purinoreceptors in sensory neurons: effects of axotomy and glial-derived neurotrophic factor. *Molecular and Cellular Neuroscience*, **12**, 256–268.

Brown AG (1981). *Organization of the spinal cord. The anatomy and physiology of identified neurones.* Springer–Verlag, Berlin, Heildeberg .

Calzà L *et al.* (1998). Peptide plasticity in primary sensory neurons and spinal cord during adjuvant-induced arthritis in the rat: an immunocytochemical and *in situ* hybridization study. *Neuroscience*, **82**, 575–589.

Castro–Lopes JM, Tavares I, and Coimbra A (1993). GABA decreases in the spinal cord dorsal horn after peripheral neurectomy. *Brain Research*, **620**, 287–291.

Castro–Lopes JM, Tavares I, Tölle TR, Coito A, and Coimbra A (1992). Increase in GABAergic cells and GABA levels in the spinal cord in unilateral inflammation of the hindlimb in the rat. *European Journal of Neuroscience*, **4**, 296–301.

Chéry N and De Koninck Y (1999). Junctional versus extrajunctional glycine and GABA(A) receptor-mediated IPSCs in identified lamina I neurons of the adult rat spinal cord. *Journal of Neuroscience*, **19**, 7342–7355.

Dalsgaard CJ, Haegerstrand A, Theodorsson–Norheim E, Brodin E, and Hökfelt T (1985). Neurokinin A-like immunoreactivity in rat primary sensory neurons; coexistence with substance P. *Histochemistry*, **83**, 37–39.

De Biasi S and Rustioni A (1988). Glutamate and substance P coexist in primary afferent terminals in the superficial laminae of spinal cord. *Proceedings of the National Academy of Sciences of the United States of America*, **85**, 7820–7824.

Donaldson LF, Harmar AJ, McQueen DS, and Seckl JR (1992). Increased expression of preprotachykinin, calcitonin gene-related peptide, but not vasoactive intestinal peptide messenger RNA in dorsal root ganglia during the development of adjuvant monoarthritis in the rat. *Molecular Brain Research*, **16**, 143–149.

Doyle CA and Hunt SP (1999). Substance P receptor (neurokinin-1)-expressing neurons in lamina I of the spinal cord encode for the intensity of noxious stimulation: a c-fos study in rat. *Neuroscience*, **89**, 17–28.

Doyle CA and Maxwell DJ (1993*a*). Direct catecholaminergic innervation of spinal dorsal horn neurons with axons ascending the dorsal columns in cat. *Journal of Comparative Neurology*, **331**, 434–444.

Doyle CA and Maxwell DJ (1993*b*). Neuropeptide Y-immunoreactive terminals form axo-axonic synaptic arrangements in the substantia gelatinosa (lamina II) of the cat spinal dorsal horn. *Brain Research*, **603**, 157–161.

Dubner R and Ruda MA (1992). Activity-dependent neuronal plasticity following tissue injury and inflammation. *Trends in Neurosciences*, **15**, 96–103.

Engelman HS, Allen TB, and MacDermott AB (1999). The distribution of neurons expressing calcium-permeable AMPA receptors in the superficial laminae of the spinal cord dorsal horn. *Journal of Neuroscience*, **19**, 2081–2089.

Fields HL, Emson PC, Leigh BK, Gilbert RF, and Iversen LL (1980). Multiple opiate receptor sites on primary afferent fibres. *Nature*, **284**, 351–353.

Florenzano F and De Luca B (1999). Nociceptive stimulation induces glutamate receptor down-regulation in the trigeminal nucleus. *Neuroscience*, **90**, 201–207.

Flores CM, DeCamp RM, Kilo S, Rogers SW, and Hargreaves KM (1996). Neuronal nicotinic receptor expression in sensory neurons of the rat trigeminal ganglion: demonstration of $\alpha 3\beta 4$, a novel subtype in the mammalian nervous system. *Journal of Neuroscience*, **16**, 7892–7901.

Furuyama T *et al.* (1993). Region-specific expression of subunits of ionotropic glutamate receptors (AMPA-type, KA-type, and NMDA receptors) in the rat spinal cord with special reference to nociception. *Molecular Brain Research*, **18**, 141–151.

Galeazza MT *et al.* (1995). Plasticity in the synthesis and storage of substance P and calcitonin gene-related peptide in primary afferent neurons during peripheral inflammation. *Neuroscience*, **66**, 443–458.

Gobel S (1978). Golgi studies of the neurons in layer II of the dorsal horn of the medulla (trigeminal nucleus caudalis). *Journal of Comparative Neurology*, **180**, 395–414.

Gobel S *et al.* (1980). An EM analysis of the synaptic connections of horseradish peroxidase-filled stalked cells and islet cells in the substantia gelatinosa of the adult cat spinal cord. *Journal of Comparative Neurology*, **194**, 781–807.

Goff JR, Burkey AR, Goff DJ, and Jasmin L (1998). Reorganization of the spinal dorsal horn in models of chronic pain: correlation with behaviour. *Neuroscience*, **82**, 559–574.

Grudt TJ and Perl ER (2002). Correlations between neuronal morphology and electrophysiological features in the rodent superficial dorsal horn. *Journal of Physiology*, **540**, 189–207.

Guo A, Vulchanova L, Wang J, Li X, and Elde R (1999). Immunocytochemical localization of the vanilloid receptor 1 (VR1): relationship to neuropeptides, the $P2X_3$ purinoceptor, and IB4 binding sites. *European Journal of Neuroscience*, **11**, 946–958.

Haberberger R, Henrich M, Couraud JY, and Kummer W (1999). Muscarinic M2-receptors in rat thoracic dorsal root ganglia. *Neuroscience Letters*, **266**, 177–180.

Harris JA, Corsi M, Quartaroli M, Arban R, and Bentivoglio M (1996). Upregulation of spinal glutamate receptors in chronic pain. *Neuroscience*, **74**, 7–12.

Hökfelt T, Zhang X, and Wiesenfeld–Hallin Z (1994). Messenger plasticity in primary sensory neurons following axotomy and its functional implications. *Trends in Neurosciences*, **17**, 22–30.

Hunt SP and Rossi J (1985). Peptide- and non-peptide-containing unmyelinated primary sensory afferents: the parallel processing of nociceptive information. *Philosophical Transactions of the Royal Society of London. B:Biological Sciences*, **308**, 283–289.

Hylden JL, Hayashi H, Ruda MA, and Dubner R (1986). Serotonin innervation of physiologically identified lamina I projection neurons. *Brain Research*, **370**, 401–404.

Ibuki T, Hama AT, Wang XT, Pappas GD, and Sagen J (1997). Loss of GABA-immunoreactivity in the spinal dorsal horn of rats with peripheral nerve injury and promotion of recovery by adrenal medullary grafts. *Neuroscience*, **76**, 845–858.

Jakowec MW, Fox AJ, Martin LJ, and Kalb RG (1995). Quantitative and qualitative changes in AMPA receptor expression during spinal cord development. *Neuroscience*, **67**, 893–907.

Ji R–R, Zhang X, Wiesenfeld–Hallin Z, and Hökfelt T (1994). Expression of neuropeptide Y and neuropeptide Y (Y1) receptor mRNA in rat spinal cord and dorsal root ganglia following peripheral tissue inflammation. *Journal of Neuroscience*, **14**, 6423–6434.

Jia H, Rustioni A, and Valtschanoff JG (1999). Metabotropic glutamate receptors in superficial laminae of the rat dorsal horn. *Journal of Comparative Neurology*, **410**, 627–642.

Kemp T, Spike RC, Watt C, and Todd AJ (1996). The μ-opioid receptor (MOR1) is mainly restricted to neurons that do not contain GABA or glycine in the superficial dorsal horn of the rat spinal cord. *Neuroscience*, **75**, 1231–1238.

Kinnman E, Nygårds EB, and Hansson P (1997). Peripheral α-adrenoreceptors involved in the development of capsaicin induced ongoing and stimulus evoked pain in humans. *Pain*, **69**, 79–85.

Knyihár–Csillik E, Csillik B, and Rakic P (1982a). Periterminal synaptology of dorsal root glomerular terminals in the substantia gelatinosa of the spinal cord in the rhesus monkey. *Journal of Comparative Neurology*, **210**, 376–399.

Knyihár–Csillik E, Csillik B, and Rakic P (1982b). Ultrastructure of normal and degenerating glomerular terminals of dorsal root axons in the substantia gelatinosa of the rhesus monkey. *Journal of Comparative Neurology*, **210**, 357–375.

Laing I, Todd AJ, Heizmann CW, and Schmidt HHHW (1994). Subpopulations of GABAergic neurons in laminae I-III of rat spinal dorsal horn defined by coexistence with classical transmitters, peptides, nitric oxide synthase or parvalbumin. *Neuroscience*, **61**, 123–132.

Lawson SN, Crepps BA, and Perl ER (1997). Relationship of substance P to afferent characteristics of dorsal root ganglion neurones in guinea-pig. *Journal of Physiology*, **505**, 177–191.

Li HS and Zhao ZQ (1998). Small sensory neurons in the rat dorsal root ganglia express functional NK-1 tachykinin receptor. *European Journal of Neuroscience*, **10**, 1292–1299.

Light AR (1992). *The initial processing of pain and its descending control: spinal and trigeminal systems*. Karger, Basel .

Light AR and Perl ER (1979). Spinal termination of functionally identified primary afferent neurons with slowly conducting myelinated fibers. *Journal of Comparative Neurology*, **186**, 133–150.

Littlewood NK, Todd AJ, Spike RC, Watt C, and Shehab SAS (1995). The types of neuron in spinal dorsal horn which possess neurokinin-1 receptors. *Neuroscience*, **66**, 597–608.

Liu H *et al.* (1994). Evidence for presynaptic *N*-methyl-D-aspartate autoreceptors in the spinal cord dorsal horn. *Proceedings of the National Academy of Sciences of the United States of America*, **91**, 8383–8387.

Ma W and Ribeiro-da-Silva A (1995). Substance P- and GABA-like immunoreactivities are co-localized in axonal boutons in the superficial laminae of cat but not rat spinal cord. *Brain Research*, **692**, 99–110.

Ma W *et al.* (1997). Substance P and enkephalin immunoreactivities in axonal boutons presynaptic to physiologically identified dorsal horn neurons. An ultrastructural multiple-labelling study in the cat. *Neuroscience*, **77**, 793–811.

Malmberg AB, Chen C, Tonegawa S, and Basbaum AI (1997). Preserved acute pain and reduced neuropathic pain in mice lacking PKCgamma. *Science*, **278**, 279–283.

Mantyh PW *et al.* (1995). Receptor endocytosis and dendrite reshaping in spinal neurons after somatosensory stimulation. *Science*, **268**, 1629–1632.

Martin WJ, Liu H, Wang H, Malmberg AB, and Basbaum AI (1999). Inflammation-induced up-regulation of protein kinase Cγ immunoreactivity in rat spinal cord correlates with enhanced nociceptive processing. *Neuroscience*, **88**, 1267–1274.

Martin–Schild S, Zadina JE, Gerall AA, Vigh S, and Kastin AJ (1997). Localization of endomorphin-2-like immunoreactivity in the rat medulla and spinal cord. *Peptides*, **18**, 1641–1649.

Maxwell DJ and Réthelyi M (1987). Ultrastructure and synaptic connections of cutaneous afferent fibres in the spinal cord. *Trends in Neurosciences*, **10**, 117–123.

Maxwell DJ, Koerber HR, and Bannatyne BA (1985). Light and electron microscopy of contacts between primary sensory fibres and neurones with axons ascending the dorsal columns of the feline spinal cord. *Neuroscience*, **16**, 375–394.

Maxwell L, Maxwell DJ, Neilson M, and Kerr R (1996). A confocal microscopic survey of serotoninergic axons in the lumbar spinal cord of the rat: co-localization with glutamate decarboxylase and neuropeptides. *Neuroscience*, **75**, 471–480.

McLaughlin BJ, Barber RP, Saito K, Roberts E, and Wu J–Y (1975). Immunocytochemical localization of glutamate decarboxylase in rat spinal cord. *Journal of Comparative Neurology*, **164**, 305–322.

McLeod AL, Krause JE, Cuello AC, and Ribeiro-da-Silva A (1998). Preferential synaptic relationships between substance P-immunoreactive boutons and neurokinin 1 receptor sites in the rat spinal cord. *Proceedings of the National Academy of Sciences of the United States of America*, **95**, 15775–15780.

Melzack R and Wall PD (1965). Pain mechanisms: a new theory. *Science*, **150**, 971–979.

Menétrey D, De Pommery J, Thomasset M, and Baimbridge KG (1992). Calbindin-D28K (CaBP28k)-like immunoreactivity in ascending projections. II. Spinal projections to brain stem and mesencephalic areas. *European Journal of Neuroscience*, **4**, 70–76.

Michael GJ and Priestley JV (1999). Differential expression of the mRNA for the vanilloid receptor subtype 1 in cells of the adult rat dorsal root and nodose ganglia and its downregulation by axotomy. *Journal of Neuroscience*, **19**, 1844–1854.

Miletic V, Hoffert MJ, Ruda MA, Dubner R, and Shigenaga Y (1984). Serotoninergic axonal contacts on identified cat spinal dorsal horn neurons and their correlation with nucleus raphe magnus stimulation. *Journal of Comparative Neurology*, **228**, 129–141.

Minami M, Maekawa K, Yabuuchi K, and Satoh M (1995). Double in situ hybridization study on coexistence of μ-, δ- and kappa-opioid receptor mRNAs with preprotachykinin A mRNA in the rat dorsal root ganglia. *Molecular Brain Research*, **30**, 203–210.

Moore KA, Allchorne AJ, Karchewski L, Kohno T, and Woolf CJ (2001). GABAergic disinhibition contributes to pain hypersensitivity in nerve injured rats. *Society for Neuroscience Abstracts*, **27**, 718.11.

Nahin RL and Hylden JL (1991). Peripheral inflammation is associated with increased glutamic acid decarboxylase immunoreactivity in the rat spinal cord. *Neuroscience Letters,* **128,** 226–230.

Naim M, Spike RC, Watt C, Shehab SA, and Todd AJ (1997). Cells in laminae III and IV of the rat spinal cord that possess the neurokinin-1 receptor and have dorsally directed dendrites receive a major synaptic input from tachykinin-containing primary afferents. *Journal of Neuroscience,* **17,** 5536–5548.

Neumann S, Doubell TP, Leslie T, and Woolf CJ (1996). Inflammatory pain hypersensitivity mediated by phenotypic switch in myelinated primary sensory neurons. *Nature,* **384,** 360–364.

Noguchi K and Ruda MA (1992). Gene regulation in an ascending nociceptive pathway: inflammation-induced increase in preprotachykinin mRNA in rat lamina I spinal projection neurons. *Journal of Neuroscience,* **12,** 2563–2572.

Noguchi K, Dubner R, De Leon M, Senba E, and Ruda MA (1994). Axotomy induces preprotachykinin gene expression in a subpopulation of dorsal root ganglion neurons. *Journal of Neuroscience Research,* **37,** 596–603.

Noguchi K, Kawai Y, Fukuoka T, Senba E, and Miki K (1995). Substance P induced by peripheral nerve injury in primary afferent sensory neurons and its effect on dorsal column nucleus neurons. *Journal of Neuroscience,* **15,** 7633–7643.

Ohishi H *et al.* (1995). Presynaptic localization of a metabotropic glutamate receptor, mGluR7, in the primary afferent neurons: an immunohistochemical study in the rat. *Neuroscience Letters,* **202,** 85–88.

Pellegrini–Giampietro DE, Fan S, Ault B, Miller BE, and Zukin RS (1994). Glutamate receptor gene expression in spinal cord of arthritic rats. *Journal of Neuroscience,* **14,** 1576–1583.

Persohn E, Malherbe P, and Richards JG (1991). *In situ* hybridization histochemistry reveals a diversity of $GABA_A$ receptor subunit mRNAs in neurons of the rat spinal cord and dorsal root ganglia. *Neuroscience,* **42,** 497–507.

Polgár E, Fowler JH, McGill MM, and Todd AJ (1999a). The types of neuron which contain protein kinase C gamma in rat spinal cord. *Brain Research,* **833,** 71–80.

Polgár E, Puskár Z, Watt C, Matesz C, and Todd AJ (2002). Selective innervation of lamina I projection neurones that possess the neurokinin 1 receptor by serotonin-containing axons in the rat spinal cord. *Neuroscience,* **109,** 799–809.

Polgár E, Shehab SAS, Watt C, and Todd AJ (1999b). GABAergic neurons that contain neuropeptide Y selectively target cells with the neurokinin 1 receptor in laminae III and IV of the rat spinal cord. *Journal of Neuroscience,* **19,** 2637–2646.

Poorkhalkali N *et al.* (2000). Immunocytochemical distribution of the $GABA_B$ receptor splice variants $GABA_B$ R1a and R1b in the rat CNS and dorsal root ganglia. *Anatomy and Embryology,* **201,** 1–13.

Popratiloff A, Weinberg RJ, and Rustioni A (1998a). AMPA receptors at primary afferent synapses in substantia gelatinosa after sciatic nerve section. *European Journal of Neuroscience,* **10,** 3220–3230.

Popratiloff SA, Weinberg JR, and Rustioni A (1998b). NMDAR1 and primary afferent terminals in the superficial spinal cord. *NeuroReport,* **9,** 2423–2429.

Popratiloff A, Weinberg RJ, and Rustioni A (1996). AMPA receptor subunits underlying terminals of fine-caliber primary afferent fibers. *Journal of Neuroscience,* **16,** 3363–3372.

Priestley JV, Michael GJ, Averill S, Liu M, and Willmott N (2002). Regulation of nociceptive neurons by nerve growth factor and glial cell derived neurotrophic factor. *Canadian Journal of Physiology and Pharmacology,* **80,** 495–505.

Réthelyi M, Light AR, and Perl ER (1982). Synaptic complexes formed by fonctionally defined primary sensory afferent units with fine myelinated fibers. *Journal of Comparative Neurology,* **207,** 381–393.

Rexed B (1952). The cytoarchitectonic organization of the spinal cord in the cat. *Journal of Comparative Neurology,* **96**, 415–495.

Ribeiro-da-Silva A (2002). Substantia gelatinosa of the spinal cord. In *The Rat Nervous System* (ed. G Paxinos). Academic Press, Sydney.

Ribeiro-da-Silva A and Coimbra A (1982). Two types of synaptic glomeruli and their distribution in laminae I–III of the rat spinal cord. *Journal of Comparative Neurology,* **209**, 176–186.

Ribeiro-da-Silva A and Cuello AC (1995). Organization of peptidergic neurons in the dorsal horn of the spinal cord: anatomical and functional correlates. *Progress in Brain Research,* **104**, 41–59.

Ribeiro-da-Silva A and Cuello AC (1990*a*). Choline acetyltransferase-immunoreactive profiles are presynaptic to primary sensory fibers in the rat superficial dorsal horn. *Journal of Comparative Neurology,* **295**, 370–384.

Ribeiro-da-Silva A and Cuello AC (1990*b*). Ultrastructural evidence for the occurrence of two distinct somatostatin-containing systems in the substantia gelatinosa of rat spinal cord. *Journal of Chemical Neuroanatomy,* **3**, 141–153.

Ribeiro-da-Silva A, Pignatelli D, and Coimbra A (1985). Synaptic architecture of glomeruli in superficial dorsal horn of rat spinal cord, as shown in serial reconstructions. *Journal of Neurocytology,* **14**, 203–220.

Ribeiro-da-Silva A, Pioro EP, and Cuello AC (1991). Substance P- and enkephalin-like immunoreactivities are colocalized in certain neurons of the substantia gelatinosa of the rat spinal cord. An ultrastructural double-labeling study. *Journal of Neuroscience,* **11**, 1068–1080.

Ribeiro-da-Silva A, Tagari P, and Cuello AC (1989). Morphological characterization of substance P-like immunoreactive glomeruli in the superficial dorsal horn of the rat spinal cord and trigeminal subnucleus caudalis: a quantitative study. *Journal of Comparative Neurology,* **281**, 497–415.

Ruocco I, Krause JE, and Ribeiro-da-Silva A (1997). Anatomical localization of substance P and the neurokinin-1 receptor in the skin of the rat lower lip: an electron microscopy study. *Society for Neuroscience Abstracts,* **23**, 1490.

Schaible H–G, Jarrott B, Hope PJ, and Duggan AW (1990). Release of immunoreactive substance P in the spinal cord during development of acute arthritis in the knee joint of the cat: a study with antibody microprobes. *Brain Research,* **529**, 214–223.

Semba K *et al.* (1985). An electron microscopic study of terminals of rapidly adapting mechanoreceptive afferent fibers in the cat spinal cord. *Journal of Comparative Neurology,* **232**, 229–240.

Seybold VS *et al.* (1997). Relationship of NK_3 receptor immunoreactivity to subpopulations of neurons in rat spinal cord. *Journal of Comparative Neurology,* **381**, 439–448.

Spike RC, Kerr R, Maxwell DJ, and Todd AJ (1998). GluR1 and GluR2/3 subunits of the AMPA-type glutamate receptor are associated with particular types of neurone in laminae I-III of the spinal dorsal horn of the rat. *European Journal of Neuroscience,* **10**, 324–333.

Spike RC, Todd AJ, and Johnston HM (1993). Coexistence of NADPH diaphorase with GABA, glycine, and acetylcholine in rat spinal cord. *Journal of Comparative Neurology,* **335**, 320–333.

Stewart W and Maxwell DJ (2000). Morphological evidence for selective modulation by serotonin of a subpopulation of dorsal horn cells which possess the neurokinin-1 receptor. *European Journal of Neuroscience,* **12**, 4583–4588.

Stone LS *et al.* (1998). Differential distribution of α_{2A} and α_{2C} adrenergic receptor immunoreactivity in the rat spinal cord. *Journal of Neuroscience,* **18**, 5928–5937.

Sugiura Y, Lee CL, and Perl ER (1986). Central projections of identified, unmyelinated (C) afferent fibers innervating mammalian skin. *Science,* **234**, 358–361.

Sugiura Y, Terui N, and Hosoya Y (1989). Difference in the distribution of central terminals between visceral and somatic unmyelinated (C) primary afferent fibers. *Journal of Neurophysiology,* **62**, 834–840.

Szentágothai J (1964). Neuronal and synaptic arrangement in the substantia gelatinosa Rolandi. *Journal of Comparative Neurology,* **122**, 219–240.

Tachibana M, Wenthold RJ, Morioka H, and Petralia RS (1994). Light and electron microscopic immunocytochemical localization of AMPA-selective glutamate receptors in the rat spinal cord. *Journal of Comparative Neurology,* **344**, 431–454.

Todd AJ (1996). GABA and glycine in synaptic glomeruli of the rat spinal dorsal horn. *European Journal of Neuroscience,* **8**, 2492–2498.

Todd AJ (1991). Immunohistochemical evidence that acetylcholine and glycine exist in different populations of GABAergic neurons in lamina III of rat spinal dorsal horn. *Neuroscience,* **44**, 741–746.

Todd AJ and Maxwell DJ (2000). GABA in the mammalian spinal cord. In *GABA in the Nervous System: The View at Fifty Years* (eds. DL Martin and RW Olsen). Lippincott, Williams & Wilkins.

Todd AJ and Spike RC (1993). The localization of classical transmitters and neuropeptides within neurons in laminae I–III of the mammalian spinal dorsal horn. *Progress in Neurobiology,* **41**, 609–638.

Todd AJ and Sullivan AC (1990). Light microscope study of the coexistence of GABA-like and glycine-like immunoreactivities in the spinal cord of the rat. *Journal of Comparative Neurology,* **296**, 496–505.

Todd AJ *et al.* (2002). Projection neurons in lamina I of rat spinal cord with the neurokinin 1 receptor are selectively innervated by substance P-containing afferents and respond to noxious stimulation. *Journal of Neuroscience,* **22**, 4103–4113.

Todd AJ *et al.* (2003). The expression of vesicular glutamate transporters VGLUT1 and VGLUT2 in neurochemically-defined axonal populations in the rat spinal cord with emphasis on the dorsal horn. *European Journal of Neuroscience,* **17**, 13–27.

Todd AJ, McGill MM, and Shehab SA (2000). Neurokinin 1 receptor expression by neurons in laminae I, III and IV of the rat spinal dorsal horn that project to the brainstem. *European Journal of Neuroscience,* **12**, 689–700.

Todd AJ, Spike RC, and Polgár E (1998). A quantitative study of neurons which express neurokinin-1 or somatostatin sst_{2a} receptor in rat spinal dorsal horn. *Neuroscience,* **85**, 459–473.

Todd AJ, Watt C, Spike RC, and Sieghart W (1996). Colocalization of GABA, glycine, and their receptors at synapses in the rat spinal cord. *Journal of Neuroscience,* **16**, 974–982.

Tölle TR, Berthele A, Zieglgänsberger W, Seeburg PH, and Wisden W (1993). The differential expression of 16 NMDA and non-NMDA receptor subunits in the rat spinal cord and in periaqueductal gray. *Journal of Neuroscience,* **13**, 5009–5028.

Tong YG *et al.* (1999). Increased uptake and transport of cholera toxin B-subunit in dorsal root ganglion neurons after peripheral axotomy: possible implications for sensory sprouting. *Journal of Comparative Neurology,* **404**, 143–158.

Towers S *et al.* (2000). GABAB receptor protein and mRNA distribution in rat spinal cord and dorsal root ganglia. *European Journal of Neuroscience,* **12**, 3201–3210.

Valtschanoff JG, Weinberg RJ, Rustioni A, and Schmidt HH (1992). Nitric oxide synthase and GABA colocalize in lamina II of rat spinal cord. *Neuroscience Letters,* **148**, 6–10.

Varoqui H, Schafer MK, Zhu H, Weihe E, and Erickson JD (2002). Identification of the differentiation-associated Na+/PI transporter as a novel vesicular glutamate transporter expressed in a distinct set of glutamatergic synapses. *Journal of Neuroscience,* **22**, 142–155.

Wakisaka S, Kajander KC, and Bennett GJ (1992). Effects of peripheral nerve injuries and tissue inflammation on the levels of neuropeptide Y-like immunoreactivity in rat primary afferent neurons. *Brain Research,* **598**, 349–352.

Watanabe M, Mishina M, and Inoue Y (1994). Distinct spatiotemporal distributions of the N-methyl-D-aspartate receptor channel subunit mRNAs in the mouse cervical cord. *Journal of Comparative Neurology*, **345**, 314–319.

Willis WD and Coggeshall RE (1991). *Sensory Mechanisms of the Spinal Cord*. Plenum Press, New York.

Woolf CJ (1997). Molecular signals responsible for the reorganization of the synaptic circuitry of the dorsal horn after peripheral nerve injury: the mechanisms of tactile allodynia. In *Molecular Neurobiology of Pain* (ed. D Borsook). IASP Press, Seattle.

Woolf CJ, Shortland P, and Coggeshall RE (1992). Peripheral nerve injury triggers central sprouting of myelinated afferents. *Nature*, **355**, 75–78.

Yaksh TL (1989). Behavioral and autonomic correlates of the tactile evoked allodynia produced by spinal glycine inhibition: effects of modulatory receptor systems and excitatory amino acid antagonists. *Pain*, **37**, 111–123.

Yoshida S *et al.* (1990). Calcium-binding proteins calbindin and parvalbumin in the superficial dorsal horn of the rat spinal cord. *Neuroscience*, **37**, 839–848.

Zhang X, Bao L, Arvidsson U, Elde R, and Hökfelt T (1998*a*). Localization and regulation of the delta-opioid receptor in dorsal root ganglia and spinal cord of the rat and monkey: evidence for association with the membrane of large dense-core vesicles. *Neuroscience*, **82**, 1225–1242.

Zhang X *et al.* (1998*b*). Down-regulation of μ-opioid receptors in rat and monkey dorsal root ganglion neurons and spinal cord after peripheral axotomy. *Neuroscience*, **82**, 223–240.

Zhang X, Tong YG, Bao L, and Hökfelt T (1999). The neuropeptide Y Y1 receptor is a somatic receptor on dorsal root ganglion neurons and a postsynaptic receptor on somatostatin dorsal horn neurons. *European Journal of Neuroscience*, **11**, 2211–2225.

Zhou QQ, Imbe H, Zou S, Dubner R, and Ren K (2001). Selective upregulation of the flip-flop splice variants of AMPA receptor subunits in the rat spinal cord after hindpaw inflammation. *Molecular Brain Research*, **88**, 186–193.

Zoli M, Jansson A, Sykova E, Agnati LF, and Fuxe K (1999). Volume transmission in the CNS and its relevance for neuropsychopharmacology. *Trends in Pharmacological Sciences*, **20**, 142–150.

Chapter 4

Cellular and molecular mechanisms of central sensitization

Michael W. Salter and Clifford J. Woolf

4.1 Introduction

As a sensory and emotional experience generally associated with tissue-damaging or nearly tissue-damaging stimuli, pain might be considered to be a unitary physiological and pathological process. However, a wealth of evidence indicates that multiple mechanisms contribute to pain, each of which is subject to or an expression of neural plasticity (i.e. the capacity of neurons to change their function, chemical profile, or structure). Three principal categories of pain have been identified: physiological, inflammatory, and neuropathic. In this Chapter, we discuss these categories of pain and the mechanisms of pain hypersensitivity using the concepts of activation, modulation, and modification (Woolf and Salter 2000) as applied to integration and processing of sensory inputs by the network of nociceptive neurons in the dorsal horn.

4.1.1 Physiological pain: activation of nociceptive signalling

Physiological pain results from activating a specialized signalling system (the nociceptive system) that alerts the individual to tissue-damaging (i.e. noxious), or potentially tissue-damaging, stimuli in the local environment. This is the type of pain experienced, for example, in response to touching a hot stove or to a needle prick. All organisms need to be able to detect and react to noxious stimuli in their environment and, as such, physiological pain is required for survival. Physiological pain starts by activation of specialized sensory nociceptor primary afferent neurons which innervate peripheral tissues and which are sensitive only to noxious stimuli (described in Chapter 2). The sensory barrage produced by these primary afferent nociceptors activates neurons in the dorsal horn of the spinal cord and the corresponding region of the trigeminal brain stem complex, which project through a thalamic relay to the cortex as the nociceptive transmission system, eliciting pain. Through alternative projections of dorsal horn neurons, the nociceptor input also activates a program of responses consisting of reflex withdrawal, an increase in arousal, as well as emotional, autonomic, and neurohumeral changes. The pain experienced in response to activation of the nociceptive system is powerfully affected by previous experience, context, cultural attitudes, and other cognitive influences.

4.1.2 Clinical pain hypersensitivity: plasticity of nociceptive signalling

Clinical pain may be initiated by tissue damage/inflammation or by lesion of the nervous system. Both inflammatory pain and neuropathic pain are commonly characterized by hypersensitivity at the site of damage and in adjacent normal tissue. Pain may appear to arise spontaneously without cause; stimuli that would not normally provoke pain do so (allodynia) and noxious stimuli evoke pain that is greater and more prolonged than expected (hyperalgesia) (Woolf and Mannion 1999). Inflammatory pain hypersensitivity usually returns to normal if the disease process initiating it is controlled. Neuropathic pain, on the other hand, persists long after the initiating event has healed and indicates pathological operation of the nervous system rather than a reaction to a disease process.

Clinical pain hypersensitivity results from neuronal plasticity mechanisms having two general forms, termed modulation and modification (Woolf and Salter 2000). By modulation we refer to reversible changes mediated by post-translational alterations induced in receptors/ion channels through activation of intracellular signal transduction cascades. By contrast, modification results from persistent alterations in expression of transmitters/receptors/ion channels or in the structure, connectivity, and survival of neurons, such that the system is dramatically modified with grossly distorted stimulus–response characteristics. While modulation and modification occur at every level of the nociceptive system from the peripheral endings of primary afferents to the cortex, the present chapter focuses on the pain processing and transmission modulation network in the dorsal horn of the spinal cord and the changes that underlie what has become known as central sensitization.

4.1.2.1 Nociceptive transmission and modulation network in the dorsal horn

Processing and transmission of nociceptive information at the level of the dorsal horn is through a neuronal network in which the principal output cells have direct synaptic inputs from nociceptive primary sensory afferents and project to thalamus and other supraspinal structures. Nociceptive transmission neurons have two main locations in the dorsal horn: neurons with cell bodies localized in lamina I, and those with cell bodies in lamina V of the dorsal horn (see also Chapter 7). The activity of these transmission neurons is sculpted by local circuit inhibitory and excitatory interneurons, which themselves receive their principal input from sensory afferents, and which may have descending inputs from supraspinal structures.

4.2 Activation of the dorsal horn pain transmission and modulation network

Physiological pain is initiated in the peripheral terminals of nociceptors located in peripheral targets, with the activation by nociceptive transducer receptor/ion channel complexes, which generate depolarizing currents in response to noxious but not lower intensity innocuous stimuli. Transducer proteins that respond to extrinsic or intrinsic irritant chemical stimuli (TRPV, TRPM8, DRASIC, P2X3 are selectively expressed in sensory neurons (Julius and Basbaum 2001; McCleskey and Gold 1999; Tominaga and Caterina 2004). Noxious heat transducers include the vanilloid receptors VR1(Caterina *et al.* 1997), VRL1, and TRPV3 (Peier *et al.* 2002*b*; Smith *et al.* 2002; Xu *et al.* 2002), while the nociceptive cold transducer is the CMR1 receptor (McKemy *et al.* 2002; Peier *et al.* 2002*a*). A transducer for noxious mechanical stimuli has not been definitively identified, although studies in *C. elegans* and DRASIC mouse knockouts suggest it may belong to the mDeg epithelial sodium ion channel (ENAC) family (Price *et al.* 2001; Waldmann and Lazdunski 1998) or it may be TRPA1 (Corey *et al.* 2004).

Transduction is followed, if the receptor current is sufficient, by initiation of action potentials. The action potentials are conducted to the CNS where their invasion of central nociceptor terminals in the spinal cord initiates, after activation of voltage-gated calcium channels, fast excitatory, glutamatergic, synaptic transmission (Fig. 4.1) (Jahr and Jessell 1985; Li *et al.* 1999*b*; Yoshimura and Jessell 1990). The release of transmitter from the primary afferent central terminal is modulated by numerous presynaptic receptors, including opiate (Jessell and Iversen 1977), GABA (Nicoll and Alger 1979), AMPA (Lee *et al.* 2002), and adenosine (Li and Perl 1994) receptors which reduce transmitter release, and by NMDA (Liu *et al.* 1994), P2X3 (Gu and MacDermott 1997), and EP (Vasko 1995) receptors which augment release. Tonic suppression of dynorphin production by the transcription factor DREAM normally permits the excitation of dorsal horn neurons and output of nociceptive signals (Cheng *et al.* 2002). The excitation evoked in the dorsal horn neurons is focused by segmental and descending activation of inhibitory neurons, most of which co-release glycine and GABA (Chery and De Koninck 1999; Narikawa *et al.* 2000; Yoshimura and Nishi 1995).

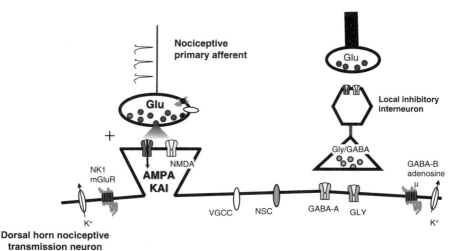

Fig. 4.1 Activation of nociceptive transmission neurons in the dorsal horn I. Fast glutamatergic EPSPs mediated by AMPA and kainite receptors. (Adapted from Woolf and Salter 2000.)

4.2.1 Glutamate mediates fast synaptic transmission at nociceptive primary afferent synapses

Like the vast majority of fast excitatory synapses in the CNS, most presynaptic excitatory terminals in the dorsal horn release glutamate which activates ionotropic glutamate receptors that are strategically localized in the postsynaptic neurons (Dingledine *et al.* 1999). The excitatory postsynaptic potentials (EPSPs) resulting from single presynaptic action potentials are activated primarily by the AMPA and kainate subtypes of ionotropic glutamate receptor, and typically last for only a few milliseconds. The NMDA subtype of glutamate ionotropic receptor, which is also localized at excitatory synapses, contributes little to the responses to single presynaptic action potentials because these receptors are tonically suppressed by extracellular Mg^{2+} which blocks NMDA channels. This type of fast excitatory synaptic transmission occurs even at synapses of 'slow' C-fiber primary afferents which are predominantly nociceptors. With low-frequency activation of nociceptors produced by mild noxious stimuli, these EPSPs signal the onset, duration, intensity, and location of noxious stimuli in the periphery to dorsal horn neurons.

4.2.2 'Windup' versus 'central sensitization'

Discharge of primary afferent nociceptors at high frequencies, produced by more intense or sustained noxious stimuli, results in co-release of peptide neuromodulators such as substance P and CGRP from nociceptor central terminals (Duggan *et al.* 1990; Schaible *et al.* 1994), in turn resulting from dense-core vesicle release in response to a greater influx of calcium. The release of these neuropeptides activates postsynaptic G-protein-coupled receptors, which leads to slow synaptic responses lasting tens of seconds (De Koninck and Henry 1991; Yoshimura and Jessell 1989), as illustrated in Fig. 4.2. These slow EPSPs, each of which lasts for hundreds of minutes, provide substantial opportunities for temporal and spatial summation (Sivilotti *et al.* 1993), and the resultant cumulative depolarization is boosted by the recruitment of NMDA receptor current by inhibiting the Mg^{2+} suppression of the channels (Mayer *et al.* 1984). The sustained depolarization also recruits voltage-gated Ca^{2+} currents, triggering plateau potentials mediated by calcium-activated non-selective cation channels (Morisset and Nagy 1999).

The net effect of these multiple processes in dorsal horn nociceptive transmission neurons is a progressive increase in the action potential discharge elicited by each successive stimulus in a train of low-frequency stimuli — a phenomenon known as 'windup' (Mendell 1966). Windup is thus a form of activity-dependent plasticity that manifests over the course of a stimulus and terminates with the end of stimulation.

Nociceptive dorsal horns show an additional and mechanistically separable form of enhanced responsiveness to nociceptive inputs which is often referred to as 'central sensitization' (Woolf 1983) and is a major component of inflammatory and neuropathic pain (Treede *et al.* 1992). Central sensitization, like windup, is initiated by

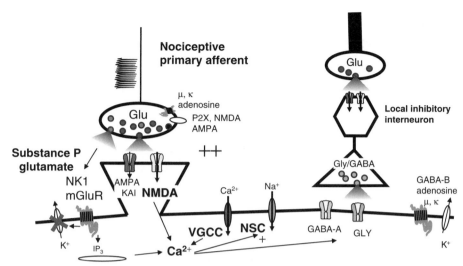

Fig. 4.2 Activation of nociceptive transmission neurons in the dorsal horn II. High-frequency primary-afferent discharges enhance glutamatergic responses through slow EPSPs, plateau potentials, and windup. (Adapted from Woolf and Salter 2000.)

peripheral nociceptor input but not, under normal circumstances at least, by low-threshold peripheral inputs. In contrast to windup, sensitization of central pain pathway neurons outlasts, by up to many hours, the duration of the nociceptor inputs that initiates it. These inputs cause the engagement of multiple intracellular signalling cascades that were dormant before activation, leading to an orchestrated modification of neuronal behaviour consisting of enhanced excitatory postsynaptic responses and depressed inhibition, equivalent to increased excitability or a facilitation of the neurons. The engagement of these signalling cascades functionally increases the gain of pain pathway neurons, resulting in amplified responses to not only noxious but also to innocuous inputs. Most nociceptive transmission neurons have a large excitatory subliminal fringe (Simone *et al.* 1991; Woolf and King 1990), and the increased gain also results in unmasking of subthreshold inputs, causing the neurons to become sensitive to stimuli in surrounding regions of the periphery (Ali *et al.* 1996; Kilo *et al.* 1994). Thus, not only are the responses of individual neurons amplified, but the number of 'pain pathway' neurons activated by any given stimulus is also increased.

Central sensitization is initiated and sustained over the short term primarily through post-translational alterations in the function of the complement of gene products already expressed by pain pathway neurons. However, the signalling cascades activated by nociceptor inputs also produce changes which maintain the increase in gain in the pain pathway in the long term, through altering expression of a repertoire of genes which changes the phenotype of central transmission neurons and may even disrupt or kill inhibitory neurons (Azkue *et al.* 1998; Moore *et al.* 2002; Scholz *et al.* 2005; Sugimoto *et al.* 1990).

4.3 Modulation of the dorsal horn pain transmission and modulation network

Activation of nociceptive pathways is subject to activity-dependent plasticity, which manifests as an increase in the responsiveness of the system persisting long after a conditioning stimulus sufficient to induce central sensitization. The major mechanism responsible for modulation is phosphorylation of receptor/ion channels, or associated regulatory proteins, altering intrinsic functional properties, cell-surface expression, and trafficking of channels in primary sensory and dorsal horn neurons. The intracellular pathways involve interactions of multiple serine/threonine and tyrosine kinase signalling cascades.

4.3.1 Enhancement of excitatory synaptic transmission

Conceptually, the simplest means to sensitize central pain transmission neurons is to increase efficacy at the excitatory primary afferent inputs onto these neurons (Figs. 4.3 and 4.4). In numerous studies, primary afferent-evoked responses of pain pathway neurons have been shown to be enhanced by a wide variety of conditioning stimuli (Liu and Sandkuhler 1998; Lozier and Kendig 1995; Randic *et al.* 1993; Sandkuhler and Liu 1998; Woolf and Thompson 1991). But whether all of these represent enhanced efficacy at primary afferent/second order synapses is unclear because often the neurons studied received long-latency monosynaptic responses that overlap temporally with polysynaptic responses, or the responses were evoked by stimuli producing asynchronous discharge of primary afferents where the requisite timing information is lost.

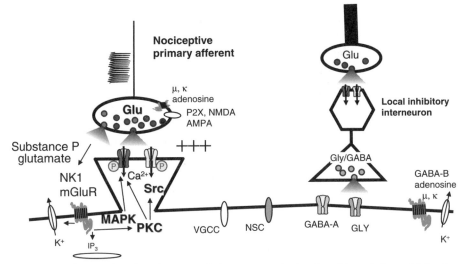

Fig. 4.3 Modulation of nociceptive transmission neurons in the dorsal horn I. A model for the molecular mechanisms producing central sensitization through homosynaptic potentiation of AMPA/kainate receptor function and/or cell-surface expression. (Adapted from Woolf and Salter 2000.)

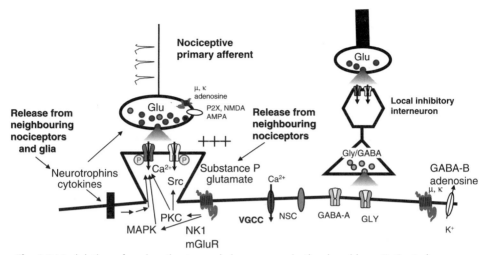

Fig. 4.4 Modulation of nociceptive transmission neurons in the dorsal horn II. Central sensitization through heterosynaptic potentiation of glutamatergic transmission. (Adapted from Woolf and Salter 2000.)

Nevertheless, with the most rigorous studies of monosynaptic responses, which have by necessity been done using superficial dorsal horn neurons, it is clear that brief-duration, high-frequency primary afferent stimulation may induce potentiation of AMPA-receptor-mediated responses at synapses onto second order neurons (Randic *et al.* 1993). The potentiation is prevented by pharmacological blockade of NMDA receptors (Woolf and Thompson 1991), and persists for as long as experimentally observable, up to many hours.

From these properties it is logical to propose that the lasting enhancement of excitatory synaptic responses at primary afferent/second order synapses in pain pathways shares a common signalling cascade with the NMDA receptor-dependent form of long-term potentiation (LTP) of excitatory synaptic transmission that is observed in many regions of the CNS (Ikeda *et al.* 2003; Ji *et al.* 2003). The mechanisms of NMDA receptor-dependent LTP have been examined in most detail for Schaffer collateral synapses onto CA1 neurons in the hippocampus, where a core signalling cascade for initiating LTP in response to tetanic stimulation has been proposed (Malenka and Nicoll 1999; Salter 1998; Salter and Kalin 2004; Soderling and Derkach 2000). This requires calcium influx through NMDA receptors during the tetanic stimulation (Collingridge and Bliss 1987), which is accomplished in part by temporal summation of EPSPs, thereby diminishing Mg^{2+} suppression of NMDA channel activity. Enhancement of NMDA channel function by the tyrosine kinase Src is also necessary (Lu *et al.* 1998), and it has been shown that activation of Src results from stimulation of another tyrosine kinase, CAKß/Pyk2 (Huang *et al.* 2001). The effect of Src activation counters tonic depression of NMDA channel activity by the phosphotyrosine phosphatase, STEP (Pelkey *et al.* 2002). Tetanic stimulation of Schaffer collaterals has been demonstrated to increase the level of tyrosine phosphorylation of the NMDA receptor subunit NR2B in CA1 neurons (Rostas *et al.* 1996), predominantly on Y1472 of NR2B (Nakazawa *et al.* 2001), indicating effects through direct phosphorylation of the NMDA receptor itself. A coincident rise in postsynaptic sodium concentration may additionally contribute to boosting NMDA receptor activity (Yu and Salter 1998).

The multiplicative boost in NMDA receptor function and resultant dramatic enhancement influx of calcium sets off a cascade leading to activation of calcium/ calmodulin dependent kinase II (CAMKII) and phosphorylation of the AMPA receptor subunit protein, GluR1, which causes AMPA channels to open in a high conductance state (Derkach *et al.* 1999). Phosphorylation of AMPA receptors may also cause increased cell surface expression of AMPA receptors and allows conversion of 'silent synapses' (i.e. those lacking AMPA receptors) into active ones (Isaac *et al.* 1995; Liao *et al.* 1995).

The general form of this core signalling cascade — NMDA receptor activation leading to postsynaptic enhancement of AMPA receptor function or cell-surface expression — is likely applicable in spinal pain transmission neurons, as illustrated in Fig. 4.3. It is well known that NMDA receptors are expressed in the dorsal horn and necessary for inducing central sensitization (Woolf and Thompson 1991). The key tyrosine kinases, Src and CAKß/Pyk2, as well as the phosphotyrosine phosphatase, STEP, are all expressed in spinal cord, and are physically associated with spinal NMDA receptors (Huang *et al.* 2001; Pelkey *et al.* 2002; Yu and Salter 1999). The function of NMDA receptors in neurons from the dorsal horn is enhanced by CAKß/Pyk2 – Src signalling and is depressed by STEP. Intraplantar injection of Freund's adjuvant leads to enhanced tyrosine phosphorylation of the NR2B subunit of the NMDAR receptor (Guo *et al.* 2002), and the tyrosine kinase inhibitors, delivered intrathecally, suppress the pain hypersensitivity induced by Freund's adjuvant (Guo *et al.* 2002). Moreover, there is evidence for silent synapses in dorsal horn neurons and for conversion of these to active synapses, a process requiring PDZ-domain interactions of AMPA receptors (Li *et al.* 1999*a*; Li and Zhuo 1998).

As in many regions of the CNS, silent synapses in the dorsal horn are most prominent at early developmental stages, but there may be few, if any, silent synapses in the dorsal horn in the adult. Thus, in the adult dorsal horn LTP may be expressed primarily by enhanced single-channel conductance of AMPA channels or enhanced cell-surface expression of AMPA receptors, although these mechanisms remain to be shown directly in the spinal dorsal horn.

The applicability of the entire signalling cascade described in CA1 is likely limited to a subpopulation of neurons in the dorsal horn. Administering exogenous CAMKII has been shown to enhance AMPA responses of dorsal horn neurons (Kolaj *et al.* 1994), and pharmacological inhibition of CAMKII inhibits neuronal and behavioural responses to intradermal capsaicin (Fang *et al.* 2002) However, expression of endogenous CAMKII is highly restricted within the dorsal horn (Fang *et al.* 2002; Lund and McQuarrie 1997). A protein kinase which is a candidate to substitute for CAMKII is protein kinase C (PKC) which potentiates synaptic transmission in dorsal horn neurons (Zhuo 2000) and elsewhere (Soderling and Derkach 2000). In CA1, PKC has been implicated in initiating LTP, but evidence indicates that it is likely upstream of Src (Ali and Salter 2001) and its effects are mediated via the protein tyrosine kinase CAKß/Pyk2 (Huang *et al.* 2001). In the dorsal horn, PKC could play a dual role, phosphorylating AMPA receptors and stimulating CAKß/Pyk2-Src signalling, or alternatively, phosphorylation of AMPA receptors may be produced by an as yet unidentified serine/threonine kinase.

The lasting potentiation of synaptic transmission at Schaffer collateral synapses onto CA1 neurons in the hippocampus is a form of homosynaptic potentiation (i.e. the potentiation is restricted to synapses that are activated at the time of stimulation). Homosynaptic potentiation of AMPA-receptor responses at synapses on dorsal horn neurons can occur experimentally in response to brief- duration, high-frequency nociceptor stimulation (Randic *et al.* 1993). The potentiation is restricted to the activated synapse, is persistent, and may thus share the common signalling cascade with LTP at Schaffer collateral/CA1 synapses. However, nociceptors do not usually fire at high frequencies, and therefore homosynaptic potentiation may be limited to very intense stimuli producing a spatially and modality constrained, if long-lasting, facilitation.

Heterosynaptic potentiation, by contrast, because it can be initiated by low frequency nociceptor inputs, is the most prominent feature of synaptic modulation in the dorsal horn and enhances synapses not activated by the conditioning input-evoking dispersed hypersensitivity (Simone *et al.* 1989; Woolf *et al.* 1994). Whenever C-fiber nociceptors are activated more than transiently, they induce central sensitization, and this phenomenon is a prominent component both of inflammatory and neuropathic pain (Simone *et al.* 1989). Again, calcium influx through NMDA receptors is a key trigger. Suppression of Mg^{2+} block of NMDA channels occurs during a cumulative depolarization produced by summation of nociceptor-evoked slow synaptic potentials (Sivilotti *et al.* 1993). Also, NMDA-channel gating is increased by through-convergent intracellular signalling cascades downstream of G-protein-coupled receptors, such as the NK1 and metabotropic glutamate receptors which boost channel function without the need for sustained depolarization (Lu *et al.* 1999). Hence, in contrast to homosynaptic potentiation, there is no requirement for high-frequency afferent stimulation.

Calcium influx through the NMDA ion channel is unlikely to be the only way to initiate heterosynaptic potentiation in dorsal horn neurons. Activation of voltage-gated calcium channels is known to enhance excitatory transmission through mechanisms not involving NMDA receptors (Chen *et al.* 1998). Neurotrophins, such as BDNF, acting through their cognate trk receptors, facilitate synaptic transmission in part through a mechanism independent of postsynaptic NMDA receptors (Heppenstall and Lewin 2001). Also, there is emerging evidence for enhancement of synaptic transmission by cytokines, like TNFα, which may be released from glial cells in the dorsal horn (see below).

Another kinase signalling cascade that appears necessary for induction of LTP in CA1 is the mitogen-activated protein kinase (MAPK, also known as ERK) pathway. MAPK is activated upon phosphorylation by MEK and inhibitors of MEK block induction of LTP (English and Sweatt 1997). Importantly, the early phase of LTP is prevented by MEK inhibition at times too early to be accounted for by changes in gene expression known to be induced by MAPK. In the superficial dorsal horn, MAPK phosphorylation increases following nociceptive stimulation, and inhibiting MEK suppresses the second phase of the formalin test, indicative of suppression of central responsiveness (Ji *et al.* 1999). Thus, it has been hypothesized that the MAPK pathway is necessary for amplification in spinal nociceptive pathways (Ji *et al.* 2003). While it is not yet clear what is downstream of ERK activation, it is possible that it interacts with those kinases that phosphorylate or dephosphorylate the NMDA or AMPA receptors.

An additional mechanism for lasting enhancement of excitatory transmission is through activation of AMPA receptors lacking the edited form of the GluR2 subunit (Hollmann and Heinemann 1994). Such GluR2-less AMPA receptors are permeable to Ca^{2+}, which provides the potential to bypass a need for NMDA receptors to initiate synaptic plasticity dependent upon raising postsynaptic Ca^{2+} (MacDermott *et al.* 1999). Neurons expressing Ca^{2+}-permeable AMPA receptors are preferentially localized in the superficial dorsal horn (Albuquerque *et al.* 1999; Engelman *et al.* 1999). Lasting enhancement of synaptic transmission mediated by GluR2-less AMPA receptors by a postsynaptic mechanism has been demonstrated at dorsal horn synapses (Gu *et al.* 1996). Such enhancement may contribute to certain types of amplification of responsiveness of neurons in pain pathways.

In addition to the postsynaptic mechanisms described above, presynaptic increase in the release of glutamate might also result in sustained increase in the gain of pain pathways. This could be produced by direct facilitation of transmitter release or by suppression of tonic presynaptic inhibition. Release of transmitter could be enhanced by stimulating receptors on primary afferent terminals, including P2X3 receptors and NMDA autoreceptors. However, the effects of such receptor stimulation may be relatively short-lived. In contrast, sustained enhancement of the release of glutamate may be produced by the neurotrophin, BDNF, which contributes to the known involvement of BDNF in inflammatory pain hypersensitivity (Kerr *et al.* 1999). The presynaptic effect of BDNF is particularly prominent at low-release probability synapses, and synapses of primary afferent nociceptors may be of this type. Presynaptic facilitation by BDNF is expressed preferentially at excitatory synapses onto excitatory neurons — but only inhibitory neurons (Berninger *et al.* 1999; Schinder and Poo 2000). Such synapse dependency at excitatory–excitatory connections is coupled with postsynaptic suppression of IPSPs. In the dorsal horn such combined effects would amount to a two-pronged attack of pain transmission neurons, which in concert with its increased levels of expression and possible direct postsynaptic excitatory actions, could readily account for the involvement of BDNF in inflammatory pain hypersensitivity.

4.3.2 **Persistent depression of inhibition**

Potentially of equal importance as sustained enhancement of excitatory transmission is depression of spinal inhibitory mechanisms. Long-term depression (LTD) of transmission at primary afferent synapses onto inhibitory dorsal horn neurons is elicited by activation of Aδ primary afferents (Sandkuhler *et al.* 1997). The depression, which requires NMDA-receptor activation and a subsequent rise in postsynaptic Ca^{2+}, is mechanistically similar to LTD in other regions, such as the hippocampus or cerebellum. The molecular basis for LTD in both hippocampus and cerebellum is due to clathrin-mediated endocytosis of synaptically localized AMPA receptors (Man *et al.* 2000; Wang and Linden 2000). Thus, it is likely that LTD at primary afferent synapses onto inhibitory dorsal horn neurons is due to internalization of cell-surface AMPA receptors.

An additional mechanism for suppressing glycine/GABA transmission in pain pathway neurons is down-regulation of postsynaptic receptors. There is little information specifically about control of these receptors in dorsal horn neurons but, by analogy with GABA-receptor regulation in other CNS regions (Moss and Smart 2001; Swope *et al.* 1999), sustained changes in receptor number or function are predicted. Also, there may be a rise in intracellular Cl⁻ concentration, as has been observed in lamina I neurons following peripheral nerve injury (Coull *et al.* 2003). This results in a depolarizing shift in the equilibrium potential for Cl⁻ producing disinhibition and in some neurons net excitation.

Inhibition, rather than being suppressed, might show lasting enhancement under some circumstances (Otis *et al.* 1994), representing a partial compensatory response to excessive excitation. Inhibition may be enhanced through long-term potentiation at primary afferent synapses onto inhibitory neurons, potentially mediated by calcium-permeable AMPA receptors (Albuquerque *et al.* 1999). Alternatively, there may be postsynaptic facilitation at inhibitory synapses onto pain transmission neurons resulting from redistribution of postsynaptic GABA$_A$ receptors towards transmitter release sites.

4.4 Modification of the dorsal horn pain transmission and modulation network

Both inflammation and nerve injury induce transcriptional changes in dorsal horn neurons mainly mediated by activation of the MAPK/pCREB cascade. These include changes in receptors (NK1, TrkB, GABA-R) and transmitters (dynorphin, enkephalin, GABA), and the induction of COX2 (Dubner and Ruda 1992; Ji *et al.* 2002; Mannion *et al.* 1999; McCarson and Krause 1994; Messersmith *et al.* 1998; Samad *et al.* 2001), which by producing PGE2 will create a central prostanoid facilitation of pain transmission (Malmberg and Yaksh 1992). PGE2 can increase transmitter release from primary afferents (Baba *et al.* 2001; Nishihara *et al.* 1995), directly depolarize dorsal horn neurons via a non selective cation channel , and diminish glycine receptor activation (Ahmadi *et al.* 2002; Harvey *et al.* 2003). The transcriptional regulation can be either localized topographically in the spinal cord to the area of afferent input, as for dynorphin (Ji *et al.* 2002), or widely distributed in the CNS, as for COX-2 (Samad *et al.* 2001). The former relates to activity- dependent transcriptional regulation, the latter to a humoral signal originating from inflamed tissue which acts via an elevation in IL-1 beta levels to increase transcription in many neurons in many parts of the CNS.

One prominent pattern of central modification in dorsal horn neurons leads to facilitation of excitation by an increase of the expression of receptors for the transmitters that are increased in primary sensory neurons by peripheral inflammation, such as TrkB, the receptor for BDNF and NK1 the substance P receptor. Moreover, in the spinal cord there is an increase of the enzyme COX-2 whose products modulate synaptic transmission when there is inflammation in peripheral tissues. The system becomes molecularly primed pre- and postsynaptically to produce increased modulation (Woolf and Costigan 1999). A second change is a reduction in inhibitory mechanisms after nerve injury (Fig. 4.5). This occurs in three ways, by a reduction in transmitter levels expressed in dorsal horn neurons, by a reduction in receptors pre and postsynaptically, or by a selective loss of inhibitory interneurons (Woolf and Mannion 1999; Scholz *et al.* 2005). Nerve injury, by virtue of injury discharge, ectopic activity, reduced inhibition, and formation of new connections can lead to excitotoxic cell death in the dorsal horn (Azkue *et al.* 1998; Moore *et al.* 2002; Sugimoto *et al.* 1990). The neuronal loss is prominent in the superficial laminae, where inhibitory interneurons are concentrated, is exacerbated by afferent input, and will produce a permanent disinhibition, which will manifest as facilitated pain transmission.

4.5 Emerging concept — neuron–glia interactions in pain plasticity

Glia, which outnumber neurons in the CNS by about 10:1, have until recently been considered supportive elements in the nervous system, and their functional roles have been largely ignored. However, a growing body of evidence is changing this view of the roles of glia in physiological and pathological processes in the CNS (Araque *et al.* 2001; Bezzi and Volterra 2001). A series of breakthroughs has demonstrated that glia, in particular astrocytes, are intimate partners with neurons at synapses (Araque *et al.* 1999a): astrocytes integrate synaptic activity and modulate synaptic function (Araque *et al.*

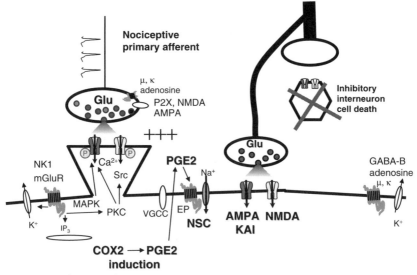

Fig. 4.5 Modification of dorsal horn nociceptive transmission network through altered gene expression, connectivity, and cell death. (Adapted from Woolf and Salter 2000.)

1999*b*, 2000; Haydon 2001; Smith 1994), astrocytes are required for normal synaptogenesis and synaptic stability (Pfrieger and Barres 1997; Ullian *et al.* 2001), and astrocytes can induce neurogenesis from adult neural stem cells (Song *et al.* 2002).

While astrocytes lack the complement of voltage-dependent channels that neurons use for long-range signalling via actions potentials, astrocytes are nevertheless capable of cell–cell communication and long-range signalling via the generation and transmission of intercellular Ca^{2+} waves (Cornell–Bell *et al.* 1990). The principal mechanism for such 'gliotransmission' is through release of ATP (Cotrina *et al.* 2000; Guthrie *et al.* 1999; Hassinger *et al.* 1996) which activates two main subclasses of G-protein-coupled ATP receptors, the P2Y1 and P2Y2 purinoceptors (Fam *et al.* 2000). Through chemical gliotransmission, and in some cases also through direct gap-junctional coupling (Scemes *et al.* 2000), astrocytes communicate in networks which parallel neuronal networks and which have distinctive spatial and temporal neuronal signalling properties.

Astrocyte networks do not just parallel those in neurons; astrocytes release diffusible chemical mediators, in addition to ATP, that regulate neuronal functioning and synaptic transmission (Haydon 2001). Astrocytes can release glutamate which may act on NMDA receptors to excite neurons (Parpura and Haydon 2000). Recently, AMPA-mediated synaptic transmission was found to be potentiated by release of the cytokine, TNFα, from astrocytes which caused enhanced cell-surface expression of AMPA receptors (Beattie *et al.* 2002). Moreover, blocking the action of TNFα reduces synaptic strength, implying that continual exposure to TNFα is necessary for maintaining synaptic strength at excitatory synapses. Thus, neuronal excitability, synaptic efficacy, and synaptic plasticity are all subject to control by astrocytes.

Astrocytes in the dorsal horn are activated by various types of nociceptive stimulation in the periphery, as judged by enhanced expression of the astrocyte-specific intermediate filament, GFAP (Watkins *et al.* 2001*a*,*b*); enhancement of GFAP expression being a downstream consequence of Ca^{2+} waves in astrocytes. Furthermore, ERK becomes activated in dorsal horn astrocytes following peripheral nerve injury and is required for maintaining mechanical allodynia (Zhuang *et al.* 2005). Intrathecally administering cytokines such as TNFα (Reeve *et al.* 2000) or interleukin-1 (Tadano *et al.* 1999) enhances nociceptive behavioural responses, and the endogenous production of these is increased in the dorsal following peripheral noxious stimulation (Ignatowski *et al.* 1999). Finally, depressing astrocyte activation has been found to suppress the enhancement of nociceptive behaviours in models of inflammatory (Meller *et al.* 1994; Watkins *et al.* 1997) and neuropathic (Sweitzer *et al.* 2001) pain.

Another main subtype of CNS glia is the microglia. Microglia activation in the dorsal horn has been observed with peripheral nociceptive stimulation. Activated microglia have been shown to be cellular intermediaries in mechanical allodynia following peripheral nerve injury (Tsuda *et al.* 2003). It is known that activated microglia release a number of cytokines and other neuroactive factors (Tsuda *et al.* 2005). Thus, these findings together suggest roles for astrocytes and microglia in pain hypersensitivity through enhancement of glutamatergic synaptic transmission at nociceptor synapses or suppression of inhibition within the dorsal horn.

4.6 **Overview and conclusions**

One of the key insights in neuroscience over the past decade is that throughout the CNS, synaptic connections between neurons are in a near continual state of change and modification, and this modification is highly dependent upon the activating state of the pre- and postsynaptic neurons. During development, the biasing of these modifications by molecular signals is responsible for such diverse processes as axonal pathfinding and the formation, establishment, and consolidation of synaptic contacts. In the developed nervous system, the continual interplay of modulatory processes subserves to produce synaptic modifications, or plasticity, that underlie physiological processes such as learning and memory. The same molecular signalling cascades that produce these normal forms of plasticity may, if aberrant, lead to pathological excitatory processes including epilepsy, neurodegeneration, and pain.

Central sensitization is a form of synaptic plasticity that is mechanistically similar to persistent enhancement of excitatory synaptic transmission found in most regions of the CNS. The enhancement of excitatory synaptic responses in nociceptive transmission neurons in the dorsal horn is a key active process, which leads to an increased gain of the pain transmission system and to pain hypersensitivity. The molecular mechanisms of pain plasticity in the dorsal horn constitute a continuum encompassing the diverse reactions of neurons to changes in their activity or environment. Pain is an integrative, active process arising in part in the periphery and in part through modulation and modification within the CNS by a diversity of plasticity mechanisms. Our understanding of these plasticity mechanisms is rapidly growing and we anticipate that future advances will provide exciting new insights into the neurobiological basis of pain, laying the groundwork for novel classes of analgesics not now envisaged.

Acknowledgements

The work of the authors is supported by the Canadian Institutes of Health Research and the National Institutes of Health (USA).

References

Ahmadi S, Lippross S, Neuhuber WL, and Zeilhofer HU (2002). PGE(2) selectively blocks inhibitory glycinergic neurotransmission onto rat superficial dorsal horn neurons. *Nat Neurosci*, **5**, 34–40.

Albuquerque C, Lee CJ, Jackson AC, and MacDermott AB (1999). Subpopulations of GABAergic and non-GABAergic rat dorsal horn neurons express Ca2+-permeable AMPA receptors. *Eur J Neurosci*, **11**, 2758–2766.

Ali DW and Salter MW (2001). NMDA receptor regulation by Src kinase signalling in excitatory synaptic transmission and plasticity. *Curr Opin Neurobiol*, **11**, 336–342.

Ali Z, Meyer RA, and Campbell JN (1996). Secondary hyperalgesia to mechanical but not heat stimuli following a capsaicin injection in hairy skin. *Pain*, **68**, 401–411.

Araque A, Carmignoto G, and Haydon PG (2001). Dynamic signaling between astrocytes and neurons. *Ann Rev Physiol*, **63**, 795–813.

Araque A, Li N, Doyle RT, and Haydon PG (2000). SNARE protein-dependent glutamate release from astrocytes. *J Neurosci*, **20**, 666–673.

Araque A, Parpura V, Sanzgiri RP, and Haydon PG (1999a). Tripartite synapses: glia, the unacknowledged partner. *Trends Neurosci*, **22**, 208–215.

Araque A, Sanzgiri RP, Parpura V, and Haydon PG (1999b). Astrocyte-induced modulation of synaptic transmission. *Can J Physiol Pharmacol*, **77**, 699–706.

Azkue JJ, Zimmermann M, Hsieh TF, and Herdegen T (1998). Peripheral nerve insult induces NMDA receptor-mediated, delayed degeneration in spinal neurons. *Eur J Neurosci*, **10**, 2204–2206.

Baba H, Kohno T, Moore KA, and Woolf CJ (2001). Direct activation of rat spinal dorsal horn neurons by prostaglandin E2. *J Neurosci*, **21**, 1750–1756.

Beattie EC, Stellwagen D, Morishita W, et al. (2002). Control of synaptic strength by glial TNFalpha. *Science*, **295**, 2282–2285.

Berninger B, Schinder AF, and Poo MM (1999). Synaptic reliability correlates with reduced susceptibility to synaptic potentiation by brain-derived neurotrophic factor. *Learn Mem*, **6**, 232–242.

Bezzi P and Volterra A (2001). A neuron-glia signalling network in the active brain. *Curr Opin Neurobiol*, **11**, 387–394.

Caterina MJ, Schumacher MA, Tominaga M, Rosen TA, Levine JD, and Julius D (1997). The capsaicin receptor: a heat-activated ion channel in the pain pathway. *Nature*, **389**, 816–824.

Chen HX, Hanse E, Pananceau M, and Gustafsson B (1998). Distinct expressions for synaptic potentiation induced by calcium through voltage-gated calcium and N-methyl-D-aspartate receptor channels in the hippocampal CA1 region. *Neuroscience*, **86**, 415–422.

Cheng HYM, Pitcher GM, Laviolette SR, et al. (2002). Identification of DREAM as a critical transcription repressor for pain modulation. *Cell* **108**, 31–43.

Chery N and De Koninck Y (1999). Junctional versus extrajunctional glycine and GABA(A) receptor-mediated IPSCs in identified lamina I neurons of the adult rat spinal cord. *J Neuroscie*, **19**, 7342–7355.

Collingridge GL and Bliss TVP (1987). NMDA receptors — their role in long-term potentiation. *Trends Neurosci*, **10**, 288–293.

Corey DP, Garcia-Anoveros J, Hold JR, et al. (2004). TRPA1 is a candidate for the mechanosensitive transduction channel of vertebrate hair cells. *Nature* **432**, 723–730.

Cornell–Bell AH, Finkbeiner SM, Cooper MS, and Smith SJ (1990). Glutamate induces calcium waves in cultured astrocytes: long- range glial signaling. *Science*, **247**, 470–473.

Coull JA, Boudreau D, Bachand K, et al. (2003). Trans-synaptic shift in anion gradient in spinal lamina I neurons as a mechanism of neuropathic pain. *Nature* **424**, 938–942.

Cotrina ML, Lin JH, Lopez–Garcia JC, Naus CC, and Nedergaard M (2000). ATP-mediated glia signaling. *J Neurosci*, **20**, 2835–2844.

De Koninck Y and Henry JL (1991). Substance P-mediated slow excitatory postsynaptic potential elicited in dorsal horn neurons in vivo by noxious stimulation. *Proc Natl Acad Sci USA*, **88**, 11344–8.

Derkach V, Barria A, and Soderling TR (1999). Ca2+/calmodulin-kinase II enhances channel conductance of alpha-amino-3- hydroxy-5-methyl-4-isoxazolepropionate type glutamate receptors. *Proc Natl Acad Sci USA*, **96**, 3269–3274.

Dingledine R, Borges K, Bowie D, and Traynelis SF (1999). The glutamate receptor ion channels. *Pharmacol Rev*, **51**, 7–61.

Dubner R and Ruda MA (1992). Activity-dependent neuronal plasticity following tissue injury and inflammation. *Trends Neurosci*, **15**, 96–103.

Duggan AW, Hope PJ, Jarrott B, Schaible HG, and Fleetwood Walker SM (1990). Release, spread and persistence of immunoreactive neurokinin A in the dorsal horn of the cat following noxious cutaneous stimulation. Studies with antibody microprobes. *Neuroscience*, **35**, 195–202.

Engelman HS, Allen TB, and MacDermott AB (1999). The distribution of neurons expressing calcium-permeable AMPA receptors in the superficial laminae of the spinal cord dorsal horn. *J Neurosci*, **19**, 2081–2089.

English JD and Sweatt JD (1997). A requirement for the mitogen-activated protein kinase cascade in hippocampal long term potentiation. *J Biol Chem*, **272**, 19103–19106.

Fam SR, Gallagher CJ, and Salter MW (2000). P2Y(1) purinoceptor-mediated Ca(2+) signaling and Ca(2+) wave propagation in dorsal spinal cord astrocytes. *J Neurosci*, **20**, 2800–2808.

Fang L, Wu J, Lin Q, and Willis WD (2002). Calcium-calmodulin-dependent protein kinase II contributes to spinal cord central sensitization. *J Neurosci*, **22**, 4196–4204.

Gu JG and MacDermott AB (1997). Activation of ATP P2X receptors elicits glutamate release from sensory neuron synapses. *Nature*, **389**, 749–753.

Gu JG, Albuquerque C, Lee CJ, and MacDermott AB (1996). Synaptic strengthening through activation of Ca2+-permeable AMPA receptors. *Nature*, **381**, 793–796.

Guo W, Zou S, Guan Y, *et al.* (2002). Tyrosine phosphorylation of the NR2B subunit of the NMDA receptor in the spinal cord during the development and maintenance of inflammatory hyperalgesia. *J Neurosci*, **22**, 6208–6217.

Guthrie PB, Knappenberger J, Segal M, Bennett MVL, Charles AC, and Kater SB (1999). ATP released from astrocytes mediates glial calcium waves. *J Neurosci*, **19**, 520–528.

Harvey RJ, Depner UB, Wassle H, *et al.* (2004). GlyR alpha3: an essential target for spinal PGE2-mediated inflmmatory pain sensitization. *Science* **304**, 884–887.

Hassinger TD, Guthrie PB, Atkinson PB, Bennett MV, and Kater SB (1996). An extracellular signaling component in propagation of astrocytic calcium waves. *Proc Natl Acad Sci USA*, **93**, 13268–73.

Haydon PG (2001). Glia: listening and talking to the synapse. *Nat Rev Neurosci*, **2**, 185–193.

Heppenstall PA and Lewin GR (2001). BDNF but not NT-4 is required for normal flexion reflex plasticity and function. *Proc Natl Acad Sci USA*, **98**, 8107–8112.

Hollmann M and Heinemann S (1994). Cloned glutamate receptors. *Ann Rev Neurosci*, **17**, 31–108.

Huang Y, Lu W, Ali DW, *et al.* (2001). CAKß/Pyk2 kinase is a signaling link for induction of long-term potentiation in CA1 hippocampus. *Neuron*, **29**, 485–496.

Ignatowski TA, Covey WC, Knight PR, Severin CM, Nickola TJ, and Spengler RN (1999). Brain-derived TNFalpha mediates neuropathic pain. *Brain Res*, **841**, 70–77.

Ikeda H, Heinke B, Ruscheweyh R, and Sandkuhler J. (2003). Synaptic plasticity in spinal lamina I projection neurons that mediate hyperalgesia. *Science* **299**, 1237–1240.

Isaac JT, Nicoll RA, and Malenka RC (1995). Evidence for silent synapses: implications for the expression of LTP. *Neuron*, **15**, 427–434.

Jahr CE and Jessell TM (1985). Synaptic transmission between dorsal root ganglion and dorsal horn neurons in culture: antagonism of monosynaptic excitatory postsynaptic potentials and glutamate excitation by kynurenate. *J Neurosci*, **5**, 2281–2289.

Jessell TM and Iversen LL (1977). Opiate analgesics inhibit substance P release from rat trigeminal nucleus. *Nature*, **268**, 549–551.

Ji RR, Baba H, Brenner GJ, and Woolf CJ (1999). Nociceptive-specific activation of ERK in spinal neurons contributes to pain hypersensitivity. *Nat Neurosci*, **2**, 1114–1119.

Ji RR, Befort K, Brenner GJ, and Woolf CJ (2002). ERK MAP kinase activation in superficial spinal cord neurons induces prodynorphin and NK-1 upregulation and contributes to persistent inflammatory pain hypersensitivity. *J Neurosci*, **22**, 478–485.

Ji RR, Kohno T, Moore KA, and Woolf CJ (2003). Central sensitization and LTP: do pain and memory share similar mechanisms? *Trends Neurosci*, **26**, 696–705.

Julius D and Basbaum AI (2001). Molecular mechanisms of nociception. *Nature*, **413**, 203–210.

Kerr BJ, Bradbury EJ, Bennett DL, *et al.* (1999). Brain-derived neurotrophic factor modulates nociceptive sensory inputs and NMDA-evoked responses in the rat spinal cord. *J Neurosci*, **19**, 5138–48.

Kilo S, Schmelz M, Koltzenburg M, and Handwerker HO (1994). Different patterns of hyperalgesia induced by experimental inflammation in human skin. *Brain*, **117** (**Pt 2**), 385–396.

Kolaj M, Cerne R, Cheng G, Brickey DA, and Randic M (1994). Alpha subunit of calcium/calmodulin-dependent protein kinase enhances excitatory amino acid and synaptic responses of rat spinal dorsal horn neurons. *J Neurophysiol*, **72**, 2525–2531.

Lee CJ, Bardoni R, Tong CK, *et al.* (2002). Functional expression of AMPA receptors on central terminals of rat dorsal root ganglion neurons and presynaptic inhibition of glutamate release. *Neuron*, **35**, 135–146.

Li J and Perl ER (1994). Adenosine inhibition of synaptic transmission in the substantia gelatinosa. *J Neurophysiol*, **72**, 1611–1621.

Li P and Zhuo M (1998). Silent glutamatergic synapses and nociception in mammalian spinal cord. *Nature*, **393**, 695–698.

Li P, Kerchner GA, Sala C, *et al.* (1999*a*). AMPA receptor-PDZ interactions in facilitation of spinal sensory synapses. *Nat Neurosci*, **2**, 972–977.

Li P, Wilding TJ, Kim SJ, Calejesan AA, Huettner JE, and Zhuo M (1999*b*). Kainate-receptor-mediated sensory synaptic transmission in mammalian spinal cord. *Nature*, **397**, 161–164.

Liao D, Hessler NA, and Malinow R (1995). Activation of postsynaptically silent synapses during pairing-induced LTP in CA1 region of hippocampal slice. *Nature*, **375**, 400–404.

Liu H, Wang H, Sheng M, Jan LY, Jan YN, and Basbaum AI (1994). Evidence for presynaptic N-methyl-D-aspartate autoreceptors in the spinal cord dorsal horn. *Proc Natl Acad Sci USA*, **91**, 8383–87.

Liu XG and Sandkuhler J (1998). Activation of spinal N-methyl-D-aspartate or neurokinin receptors induces long-term potentiation of spinal C-fibre-evoked potentials. *Neuroscience*, **86**, 1209–16.

Lozier AP and Kendig JJ (1995). Long-term potentiation in an isolated peripheral nerve-spinal cord preparation. *J Neurophysiol*, **74**, 1001–1009.

Lu WY, Xiong ZG, Lei S, *et al.* (1999). G-protein-coupled receptors act via protein kinase C and Src to regulate NMDA receptors. *Nat Neurosci*, **2**, 331–338.

Lu YM, Roder JC, Davidow J, and Salter MW (1998). Src activation in the induction of long-term potentiation in CA1 hippocampal neurons. *Science*, **279**, 1363–1368.

Lund LM and McQuarrie IG (1997). Calcium/calmodulin-dependent protein kinase II expression in motor neurons: effect of axotomy. *J Neurobiol*, **33**, 796–810.

MacDermott AB, Role LW, and Siegelbaum SA (1999). Presynaptic ionotropic receptors and the control of transmitter release. *Ann Rev Neurosci*, **22**, 443–485.

Malenka RC and Nicoll RA (1999). Long-term potentiation–a decade of progress? *Science*, **285**, 1870–74.

Malmberg AB and Yaksh TL (1992). Antinociceptive actions of spinal nonsteroidal anti-inflammatory agents on the formalin test in the rat. *J Pharmacol Exp Ther*, **263**, 136–146.

Man HY, Lin JW, Ju WH, *et al.* (2000). Regulation of AMPA receptor-mediated synaptic transmission by clathrin- dependent receptor internalization. *Neuron*, **25**, 649–662.

Mannion RJ, Costigan M, Decosterd I, *et al.* (1999). Neurotrophins: peripherally and centrally acting modulators of tactile stimulus-induced inflammatory pain hypersensitivity. *Proc Natl Acad Sci USA*, **96**, 9385–9390.

Mayer ML, Westbrook GL, and Guthrie PB (1984). Voltage-dependent block by Mg2+ of NMDA responses in spinal cord neurones. *Nature*, **309**, 261–263.

McCarson KE and Krause JE (1994). NK-1 and NK-3 type tachykinin receptor mRNA expression in the rat spinal cord dorsal horn is increased during adjuvant or formalin- induced nociception. *J Neurosci*, **14**, 712–720.

McCleskey EW and Gold MS (1999). Ion channels of nociception. *Ann Rev Physiol*, **61**, 835–856.

McKemy DD, Neuhausser WM, and Julius D (2002). Identification of a cold receptor reveals a general role for TRP channels in thermosensation. *Nature*, **416**, 52–58.

Meller ST, Dykstra C, Grzybycki D, Murphy S, and Gebhart GF (1994). The possible role of glia in nociceptive processing and hyperalgesia in the spinal cord of the rat. *Neuropharmacology*, **33**, 1471–8.

Mendell LM (1966). Physiological properties of unmyelinated fiber projection to the spinal cord. *Exper Neurol*, **16**, 316–332.

Messersmith DJ, Kim DJ, and Iadarola MJ (1998). Transcription factor regulation of prodynorphin gene expression following rat hindpaw inflammation. *Mol Brain Res*, **53**, 260–269.

Moore KA, Kohno T, Karchewski LA, Scholz J, Baba H, and Woolf CJ (2002). Partial peripheral nerve injury promotes a selective loss of GABAergic inhibition in the superficial dorsal horn of the spinal cord. *J Neurosci*, **22**, 6724–6731.

Morisset V and Nagy F (1999). Ionic basis for plateau potentials in deep dorsal horn neurons of the rat spinal cord. *J Neurosci*, **19**, 7309–7316.

Moss SJ and Smart TG (2001). Constructing inhibitory synapses. *Nat Rev Neurosci*, **2**, 240–250.

Nakazawa T, Komai S, Tezuka T, *et al.* (2001). Characterization of Fyn-mediated Tyrosine phosphorylation sites on GluRepsilon 2 (NR2B) subunit of the N-Methyl-D-aspartate receptor. *J Biol Chem*, **276** , 693–699.

Narikawa K, Furue H, Kumamoto E, and Yoshimura M (2000). In vivo patch-clamp analysis of IPSCs evoked in rat substantia gelatinosa neurons by cutaneous mechanical stimulation. *J Neurophysiol*, **84**, 2171–2174.

Nicoll RA and Alger BE (1979). Presynaptic inhibition: transmitter and ionic mechanisms. *Int Rev Neurobiol*, **21**, 217–258.

Nishihara I, Minami T, Watanabe Y, Ito S, and Hayaishi O (1995). Prostaglandin E_2 stimulates glutamate release from synaptosomes of rat spinal cord. *Neurosci Let*, **196**, 57–60.

Otis TS, De Koninck Y, and Mody I (1994). Lasting potentiation of inhibition is associated with an increased number of gamma-aminobutyric acid type A receptors activated during miniature inhibitory postsynaptic currents. *Proc Natl Acad Sci USA*, **91**, 7698–7702.

Parpura V and Haydon PG (2000). Physiological astrocytic calcium levels stimulate glutamate release to modulate adjacent neurons. *Proc Natl Acad Sci USA*, **97**, 8629–8634.

Peier AM, Moqrich A, Hergarden AC, *et al.* (2002*a*). A TRP channel that senses cold stimuli and menthol. *Cell*, **108**, 705–715.

Peier AM, Reeve AJ, Andersson DA, *et al.* (2002*b*). A heat-sensitive TRP channel expressed in keratinocytes. *Science*, **296**, 2046–2049.

Pelkey KA, Askalan R, Paul S, *et al.* (2002). Tyrosine phosphatase STEP is a tonic brake on induction of long-term potentiation. *Neuron*, **34**, 127–138.

Pfrieger FW and Barres BA (1997). Synaptic efficacy enhanced by glial cells in vitro. *Science*, **277**, 1684–7.

Price MP, McIlwrath SL, Xie J, *et al.* (2001). The DRASIC cation channel contributes to the detection of cutaneous touch and acid stimuli in mice. *Neuron*, **32**, 1071–1083.

Randic M, Jiang MC, and Cerne R (1993). Long-term potentiation and long-term depression of primary afferent neurotransmission in the rat spinal cord. *J Neurosci*, **13**, 5228–5241.

Reeve AJ, Patel S, Fox A, Walker K, and Urban L (2000). Intrathecally administered endotoxin or cytokines produce allodynia, hyperalgesia and changes in spinal cord neuronal responses to nociceptive stimuli in the rat. *Eur J Pain*, **4**, 247–257.

Rostas JA, Brent VA, Voss K, Errington ML, Bliss TV, and Gurd JW (1996). Enhanced tyrosine phosphorylation of the 2B subunit of the N-methyl-D- aspartate receptor in long-term potentiation. *Proc Natl Acad Sci USA*, **93**, 10452–10456.

Salter MW (1998). Src, N-methyl-D-aspartate (NMDA) receptors, and synaptic plasticity. *Biochem Pharmacol*, **56**, 789–798.

Salter MW and Kalia LV (2004). Src kinases: a hub of synaptic regulation. *Nature Reviews Neuroscience*, **5**, 317–328.

Samad TA, Moore KA, Sapirstein A, *et al.* (2001). Interleukin-1beta-mediated induction of Cox-2 in the CNS contributes to inflammatory pain hypersensitivity. *Nature*, **410**, 471–475.

Sandkuhler J and Liu X (1998). Induction of long-term potentiation at spinal synapses by noxious stimulation or nerve injury. *Eur J Neurosci*, **10**, 2476–2480.

Sandkuhler J, Chen JG, Cheng G, and Randic M (1997). Low-frequency stimulation of afferent Adelta-fibers induces long-term depression at primary afferent synapses with substantia gelatinosa neurons in the rat. *J Neurosci*, **17**, 6483–6491.

Scemes E, Suadicani SO, and Spray DC (2000). Intercellular communication in spinal cord astrocytes: fine tuning between gap junctions and P2 nucleotide receptors in calcium wave propagation. *J Neurosci*, **20**, 1435–1445.

Schaible HG, Freudenberger U, Neugebauer V, and Stiller RU (1994). Intraspinal release of immunoreactive calcitonin gene-related peptide during development of inflammation in the joint in vivo — a study with antibody microprobes in cat and rat. *Neuroscience*, **62**, 1293–1305.

Schinder AF and Poo M (2000). The neurotrophin hypothesis for synaptic plasticity. *Trends Neurosci*, **23**, 639–645.

Scholz J, Broom D, Youn D, *et al.* (2005). Blocking caspase activity prevents transsynaptic neuronal apoptosis and the loss of spinal inhibition following peripheral nerve injury. *Proc Natl Acad Sci USA* In press.

Simone DA, Baumann TK, Collins JG, and LaMotte RH (1989). Sensitization of cat dorsal horn neurons to innocuous mechanical stimulation after intradermal injection of capsaicin. *Brain Res*, **486**, 185–189.

Simone DA, Sorkin LS, Oh U, *et al.* (1991). Neurogenic hyperalgesia: Central neural correlates in responses of spinothalamic tract neurons. *J Neurophysiol*, **66**, 228–246.

Sivilotti LG, Thompson SW, and Woolf CJ (1993). Rate of rise of the cumulative depolarization evoked by repetitive stimulation of small-caliber afferents is a predictor of action potential windup in rat spinal neurons in vitro. *J Neurophysiol*, **69**, 1621–1631.

Smith GD, Gunthorpe MJ, Kelsell RE, *et al.* (2002). TRPV3 is a temperature-sensitive vanilloid receptor- like protein. *Nature*, **418**, 186–190.

Smith SJ (1994). Neural signalling. Neuromodulatory astrocytes. *Curr Biol*, **4**, 807–810.

Soderling TR and Derkach VA (2000). Postsynaptic protein phosphorylation and LTP. *Trends Neurosci*, **23**, 75–80.

Song H, Stevens CF, and Gage FH (2002). Astroglia induce neurogenesis from adult neural stem cells. *Nature*, **417**, 39–44.

Sugimoto T, Bennett GJ, and Kajander KC (1990). Transsynaptic degeneration in the superficial dorsal horn after sciatic nerve injury: effects of a chronic constriction injury, transection, and strychnine. *Pain*, **42**, 205–213.

Sweitzer SM, Schubert P, and DeLeo JA (2001). Propentofylline, a glial modulating agent, exhibits antiallodynic properties in a rat model of neuropathic pain. *J Pharmacol Exp Ther*, **297**, 1210–1217.

Swope SL, Moss SI, Raymond LA, and Huganir RL (1999). Regulation of ligand-gated ion channels by protein phosphorylation. *Adv Second Messenger Phosphoprotein Res*, **33**, 49–78.

Tadano T, Namioka M, Nakagawasai O, *et al.* (1999). Induction of nociceptive responses by intrathecal injection of interleukin-1 in mice. *Life Sci*, **65**, 255–261.

Tominaga M, and Caterina MJ (2004). Thermosensation and pain. *J Neurobiol*, **61**, 3–12.

Treede RD, Meyer RA, Raja SN, and Campbell JN (1992). Peripheral and central mechanisms of cutaneous hyperalgesia. *Prog Neurobiol*, **38**, 397–421.

Tsuda M, Inoue K, and Salter MW (2005). Neuropathic pain and spinal microglia: a big problem from molecules in 'small' glia. *Trends Neurosci*, **28**, 101–107.

Tsuda M, Shigemoto-Mogami Y, Koizumi S, *et al.* (2003). P2X4 receptors induced in spinal microglia gate tactile allodynia after nerve injury. *Nature* **424**, 778–783.

Ullian EM, Sapperstein SK, Christopherson KS, and Barres BA (2001). Control of synapse number by glia. *Science*, **291**, 657–661.

Vasko MR (1995). Prostaglandin-induced neuropeptide release from spinal cord. *Prog Brain Res*, **104**, 367–380.

Waldmann R and Lazdunski M (1998). H(+)-gated cation channels: neuronal acid sensors in the NaC/DEG family of ion channels. *Curr Opin Neurobiol*, **8**, 418–424.

Wang YT and Linden DJ (2000). Expression of cerebellar long-term depression requires postsynaptic clathrin-mediated endocytosis. *Neuron*, **25**, 635–647.

Watkins LR, Martin D, Ulrich P, Tracey KJ, and Maier SF (1997). Evidence for the involvement of spinal cord glia in subcutaneous formalin induced hyperalgesia in the rat. *Pain*, **71**, 225–235.

Watkins LR, Milligan ED, and Maier SF (2001*a*). Glial activation: a driving force for pathological pain. *Trends Neurosci*, **24**, 450–455.

Watkins LR, Milligan ED, and Maier SF (2001*b*). Spinal cord glia: new players in pain. *Pain*, **93**, 201–205.

Woolf CJ (1983). Evidence for a central component of post-injury pain hypersensitivity. *Nature*, **306**, 686–688.

Woolf CJ and Costigan M (1999). Transcriptional and posttranslational plasticity and the generation of inflammatory pain. *Proc Natl Acad Sci USA*, **96**, 7723–7730.

Woolf CJ and King AE (1990). Dynamic alterations in the cutaneous mechanoreceptive fields of dorsal horn neurons in the rat spinal cord. *J Neurosci*, **10**, 2717–2726.

Woolf CJ and Mannion RJ (1999). Neuropathic pain: aetiology, symptoms, mechanisms, and management. *Lancet*, **353**, 1959–1964.

Woolf CJ and Salter MW (2000). Neuronal plasticity: increasing the gain in pain. *Science*, **288**, 1765–1769.

Woolf CJ and Thompson SWN (1991). The induction and maintenance of central sensitization is dependent on *N*-methyl-D-aspartic acid receptor activation; Implications for the treatment of post-injury pain hypersensitivity states. *Pain*, **44**, 293–299.

Woolf CJ, Shortland P, and Sivilotti LG (1994). Sensitization of high mechanothreshold superficial dorsal horn and flexor motor neurones following chemosensitive primary afferent activation. *Pain*, **58**, 141–155.

Xu H, Ramsey IS, Kotecha SA, *et al.* (2002). TRPV3 is a calcium-permeable temperature-sensitive cation channel. *Nature*, **418**, 181–186.

Yoshimura M and Jessell TM (1989). Primary afferent-evoked synaptic responses and slow potential generation in rat substantia gelatinosa neurons in vitro. *J Neurophysiol*, **62**, 96–108.

Yoshimura M and Jessell TM (1990). Amino acid-mediated EPSPs at primary afferent synapses with substantia gelatinosa neurones in the rat spinal cord. *J Physiol (Lond)*, **430**, 315–335.

Yoshimura M and Nishi S (1995). Primary afferent-evoked glycine- and GABA-mediated IPSPs in substantia gelatinosa neurones in the rat spinal cord in vitro. *J Physiol*, **482 (Pt 1)**, 29–38.

Yu XM and Salter MW (1998). Gain control of NMDA-receptor currents by intracellular sodium. *Nature*, **396**, 469–474.

Yu XM and Salter MW (1999). Src, a molecular switch governing gain control of synaptic transmission mediated by N-methyl-D-aspartate receptors. *Proc Natl Acad Sci USA*, **96**, 7697–7704.

Zhuang ZE, Gerner P, Woolf CJ, and Ji RR (2005). ERK is sequentially activated in neurons, microglia and astrocytes by spinal nerve ligation and contributes to mechanical allodynia in this neuropathic pain model. *Pain*, **114**, 149–159.

Zhuo M (2000). Silent glutamatergic synapses and long-term facilitation in spinal dorsal horn neurons. *Prog Brain Res*, **129**, 101–113.

Chapter 5

Mechanisms of peripheral neuropathic pain

Martin Koltzenburg

5.1 Introduction

It is common clinical experience that most lesions of the peripheral PNS or central nervous system do not produce chronic pain. Conditions in which damage of the nervous system does cause pain are a paradox as impairment of nerve fibres carrying nociceptive information in the PNS or CNS should result in a decrease of pain sensibility (hypo- or analgesia). Thus, the presence of pain after neural injury implies qualitative changes of the neurobiological mechanisms encoding pain. In fact, it is one of the puzzles of pain that lesions of peripheral and central pathways normally signalling pain, rather than those subserving non-nociceptive functions, are the culprit of neuropathic pain.

It is the objective of this chapter to review the neural basis that contributes to this altered pain sensibility in peripheral nerve disease. In the past years we have witnessed a surge of major discoveries on the pathophysiology of neuropathic pain stemming from both animal models of nerve injury and from careful detailed examination of patients in neuropathic pain. Much of what has been learnt on the long-term changes of the processing of nociceptive information in painful neuropathies is also derived from the analysis of the commonalties and differences with other chronic pain states, notably inflammatory conditions.

5.2 Neuropathic pains have a heterogeneous clinical presentation

Neuropathies represent one of the most common neurological disorders, with a prevalence of 2.4% in the general population rising to 8% with age (Martyn and Hughes, 1998). Point estimates for neuropathic pain in the general population are 5% (Daousi *et al.*, 2004); estimates of the life-time prevalence of neuropathic pain are as high as 10%. The International Association for the Study of Pain currently defines neuropathic pain as 'pain caused by a primary lesion or dysfunction in the nervous system' (Merskey and Bogduk, 1994). However, this definition has recently come under increasing criticism because of its perceived vagueness and overburdening inclusion of many painful conditions whose relation to a genuine neuropathic process is unclear. An alternative definition could therefore be that neuropathic pain is 'pain arising as a direct consequence of diseases or lesions affecting the somatosensory system'.

Within this framework it is possible to distinguish two major groups of conditions that differ in their clinical presentation as well as in many of their underlying mechanisms:

1. *Peripheral neuropathic pains.* Diseases of the peripheral nervous system, such as traumatic injuries of major peripheral nerves or postherpetic neuralgia.

2. *Central neuropathic pain.* Diseases that affect the CNS such as spinal cord injury or post-stroke pain.

In both peripheral and central neuropathic pains it is useful to make a further distinction between complete and incomplete lesions. The term *deafferentation syndrome is* often used for those diseases in which there is extensive and complete disconnection of peripheral nerves from their target, such as in amputations or interruption of ascending sensory pathways as in spinal cord injury. In these situations the pain is stimulus independent. In contrast, when the connections in the peripheral or CNS are partially retained or at the borders of a completely deafferentated zone, the pain has often stimulus-independent and stimulus-induced components. Because of some overlap in the symptomatic presentation, a third group, *complex regional pain syndrome, type I* (CRPS l; in the past also known as reflex sympathetic dystrophy) is often included under the umbrella term of 'neuropathic pain'. CRPS is a heterogeneous disorder often presenting without demonstrable nerve lesion and thus its inclusion as a neuropathic pain state may in fact be inappropriate. CRPS describes a variety of painful conditions following (often trivial) soft tissue injury which appears regionally and can involve an entire extremity. CRPS has a distal predominance of sensory abnormalities and typically presents with tissue swelling, abnormal pattern of blood flow, and sweating, and trophic changes such as changes in nail growth or demineralization of periarticular bone (Stanton–Hicks *et al.*, 1995).

It is common clinical experience that there are significant comorbidities in patients with neuropathic pain, and these impact significantly on the global pain experience. Psychological factors such as changes in mood, anxiety, and altered sleep patterns have all been identified as significant adjuncts of painful neuropathies. In addition, diseases of the peripheral and CNS commonly cause a variety of secondary painful sequels. For example, patients with incomplete spinal cord injury may suffer from spasticity, which in turn may be a significant secondary source of pain; and in patients with diabetes mellitus, an associated micro- and macroangiopathy may cause exertional ischaemic muscle pain. In individual patients it may be clinically difficult to differentiate between the relative contribution of these secondary factors to the overall burden of pain, and it is the complexity of the clinical diseases that make it difficult to understand the underlying mechanisms and to develop animal models that adequately replicate the clinical condition.

5.3 Anatomical and histopathological classifications

There are different classification schemes for peripheral neuropathic pains. When investigating a patient suspected of having neuropathic pain, clinicians search for the anatomical distribution pattern of the affected nerves as this provides valuable differential diagnostic clues as to possible underlying causes. For example, painful symptoms in the distribution of the orbital division of the trigeminal nerve are only rarely caused by trigeminal neuralgia and would prompt a clinician to seek other causes. It is therefore common clinical practice to group painful neuropathies into symmetrical polyneuropathies (a disease affecting many nerves simultaneously, typically in a glove and stocking distribution) and into asymmetrical mononeuropathies or plexopathies (a disease affecting individual nerves or a nerve plexus). Box 5.1 lists many of the peripheral nerve diseases known to be painful.

Box 5.1 Some causes of painful neuropathies

Diseases causing symmetrical painful neuropathies

Metabolic: diabetes mellitus, pellagra (niacin deficiency), beriberi (thiamine deficiency)

Toxic: ethanol, highly active anti-retroviral drugs, isoniazide, thallium, arsenic, mercury

Immune-mediated: acute inflammatory demyelinating neuropathies (Guillian–Barre syndrome), paraproteinaemic, cryoglobulin-associated, acquired amyloidosis, neuropathy associated with Sjögren's disease, paraneoplastic

Hereditary: sensory and autonomic neuropathy type I (HSAN I), angiokeratoma corporis diffusum (Fabry's disease), hereditary amyloidosis infections: AIDS

Diseases causing asymmetrical and focal painful neuropathies

Cranial neuralgias: trigeminal, glossopharyngeal, laryngeal neuralgia

Nerve compression: post-traumatic, carpal tunnel syndrome and other compression syndromes, meralgia paraesthetic, root compression (herniation of intervertebral disks)

Neuroma: post-traumatic, post-operative, following amputations, Morton's neuralgia

Plexopathies: post-traumatic, idiopathic neuritis, tumour infiltration, radiation-induced, heroin-induced

Diabetic mono-/oligo-neuropathies: acute ophtalmoplegia, acute thoracoabdominal neuropathy, acute diabetic radiculo-/plexo-/neuropathy (diabetic amyotrophy)

Angiopathic neuropathies: inflammatory, occlusive/ischaemic

Infectious/parainfectious: Herpes zoster, postherpetic neuralgia, Herpes simplex, borreliosis, syphilis, AIDS

The diversity of clinical conditions known to produce peripheral neuropathic pain is astonishing and it has been difficult to identify a common denominator for the pains in conditions as diverse as post-traumatic and diabetic neuropathy. A complicating factor is that even within an aetiologic entity such as diabetic polyneuropathy, it is only a minority of patients who develop chronic neuropathic pain. Thus, the point prevalence of chronic painful peripheral neuropathy is only in the order of 10–20% of patients with diabetes mellitus (Daousi *et al.*, 2004). Moreover, it is still unclear why the symptoms within an aetiologically defined population of patients can be extremely diverse. In fact, it is one of the challenges of the field to understand the factors that determine why individuals with apparently identical conditions develop painful symptoms and what determines the range of the presenting symptoms.

If one considers the histological type of nerve pathology, however, it becomes increasingly clear that an axonal injury of a portion of nociceptive fibres in a peripheral nerve emerges as the single most important causal factor for neuropathic pain. There are several painless diseases in which small-diameter sensory neurons are largely spared which strongly endorse this view. This includes (a) most types of Charcot–Marie–Tooth disease (also known as hereditary motor and sensory neuropathy) where demyelination of large myelinated axons features as the dominant pathology, and (b) ataxic neuropathies such as in Friedreich's ataxia where loss of cell bodies and axons of large myelinated fibres is commonly observed. Furthermore, the universal loss of nociceptors as in congenital insensitivity to pain with anhidrosis (also known as hereditary sensory neuropathy type IV) does not cause pain either, and this concurs with the view that severe loss of small-diameter axons in acquired neuropathies can often be painless. Neuropathic pain typically develops only when sensory nerve fibres are affected. Thus, selective axonal or demyelinating lesion of motor fibres, as in motor neuron disease or multifocal motor neuropathy, is generally painless. Furthermore lesions of unmyelinated sympathetic fibres such as in pure autonomic failure or Ross syndrome (segmental anhidrosis) are also not painful. Finally, quantification of unmyelinated fibres in sural nerve biopsies or assessment of epidermal nerve fibre density in skin biopsies revealed substantial damage to unmyelinated fibres in many painful neuropathies (Griffin *et al.*, 2001).

It is also becoming increasingly clear that lesions of central pathways signalling pain, such as the spinothalamic tracts, thalamic relay nuclei, and possibly thalamo-cortical projections, frequently cause neuropathic pain, whereas lesions of pathways subserving non-nociceptive functions do not.

5.4 **Animal models of neuropathic pain**

Much of our knowledge of the mechanisms of neuropathic pain has been derived from animal studies. The models that have been used to investigate nociceptive mechanisms after peripheral nerve injury can be divided into two major groups. One of the first models that was developed was the stump neuroma created by complete transection of a major peripheral nerve and the prevention of regeneration (Wall and Gutnick, 1974; Coderre *et al.,* 1986; Jänig, 1988; Devor, 1994). Rats and mice, but not higher mammals, start to mutilate the denervated limb during the weeks that follow. This behaviour has, not without dispute (Rodin and Kruger, 1984), been taken as behavioural evidence for the presence of pain (Coderre *et al.,* 1986; Blumenkopf and Lipman, 1991). The neuroma model mimics the clinical condition of a phantom limb pain or anaesthesia dolorosa that can develop after amputation or denervation of a limb in humans. Since nerve fibres lose contact with their peripheral targets, the model is not suitable for the study of stimulus-induced pains and, therefore, does not adequately model the situation that is the hallmark of some painful neuropathies.

To overcome these shortcomings, several investigators developed various models of partial injury of the sciatic nerve using a chronic constriction (CCI = chronic constriction injury) (Bennett and Xie, 1988; Sherbourne *et al.,* 1992; Sommer *et al.,* 1993), partial transection (PST = partial sciatic nerve transaction) (Seltzer *et al.,* 1990), ligation of spinal nerves (SNL = spinal nerve ligation) (Kim and Chung, 1992; Carlton *et al.,* 1994), lesions of the tibial and peroneal nerve sparing the sural nerve (SNI = spared nerve injury) (Decosterd and Woolf, 2000), cryoneurolisis (DeLeo *et al.,* 1994), or inflammation (Maves *et al.,* 1992; Eliav and Bennett, 1996) . The common denominator of these models is the combination of a considerable degree of nerve damage and the retention of some innervation of the peripheral tissue that can carry the signals for stimulus-induced pains. In these models animals usually exhibit behavioural signs of ongoing pain (such as licking of the paw in the absence of experimental stimuli) and mechanical hypersensitivity. Hyperalgesia to thermal stimuli seems to be more variable (Fig. 5.1). Some discrepancies may be explained by strain differences, differences in the timing of the investigations after nerve injury, or by different behavioural test paradigms.

5.5 **Symptom-based classification**

Painful symptoms in patients with neuropathic pain are considerably heterogeneous and they often present with a wide range of enigmatic sensory abnormalities that can be broadly separated into two main categories: stimulus-independent ongoing pain, and a wide range of stimulus-induced hyperalgesias. Using careful clinical examination it is often possible to further recognize several distinct sensory abnormalities within each broad category of an hyperalgesic modality (Table 5.1) and patients can often describe different forms of stimulus-independent pain such as burning pain or lancinating pains.

This has led to the development of a symptom-orientated diagnostic approach to neuropathic pain conditions that supplements the aetiology-based classification scheme, recognizing the fact that neuropathic pains are usually a composite of several pain symptoms (Koltzenburg, 1996; Woolf *et al.,* 1998). A symptom-orientated approach does not negate the fact that distinct neuropathies present differently clinically and that some neuropathic disease states may predispose to certain constellations of

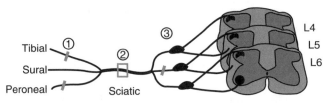

1) Spared nerve injury (SNI)
2) Partial sciatic nerve injuries
   a) Chronic constriction (CCI)
   b) Partial transsection ± ligation (PST)
   c) Inflammation
3) Spinal nerve ligation (SNL)

Symptom	Neuroma	CCI	PST	SNL	SNI
Behavioural evidence for ongoing pain (guarding)	?	+	+	+	+
Heat hyperalgesia	–	+	+	(+)	(+)
Hyperalgesia to cold	–	+	(–)	+	+
Mechanical hyperalgesia	–	+	+	+	+
'Trophic changes'	–	(+)	–	–	–
Autotomy	+	–	–	–	–
Start after operation	Days	24 hours	Hours	12–24 hours	<24 hours
Duration	Months	2–3 months	>7 months	>7 months	>7 months

Fig. 5.1 Behavioural abnormalities indicative of ongoing pain and hyperalgesias in common animal models of neuropathic pain.

pain symptoms (e.g. touch-evoked pain in postherpetic neuralgia). The rationale of this approach recognizes several principles:

1. Clinically distinct pain symptoms such as ongoing stimulus-independent pain may be caused by similar, if not identical, neural mechanisms, even if the underlying diseases differ. For example, nociceptive afferents that develop ongoing activity after axon injury could mediate ongoing pain regardless of the precipitating or sustaining neuropathic event.

2. More than one pain mechanism is usually present in an individual patient. It is not uncommon that patients can clearly differentiate between the different qualities of stimulus-independent and stimulus-induced pains and, as discussed below, these different symptoms are probably caused by diverse neuronal changes.

3. Some symptoms, such as mechanical hypersensitivity, can be explained by several distinct neural mechanisms which may even coexist in an individual patient.

A symptom-based approach to painful neuropathies can be useful for dissecting the underlying neural mechanisms, and this knowledge may be harnessed for the development of novel analgesic drugs that differentially target these mechanisms. For example, a drug reverting some aspects of central sensitization may be beneficial for the reduction

Table 5.1 Stimulus-induced pain*

Modality	Tissue	Location	Afferents involved	Possible mechanisms
Thermal Heat	Injury to skin (common) or cutaneous nerve (rare)	1° zone only	Nociceptors (C-fibres in hairy skin, A-fibres in glabrous skin)	Peripheral sensitization of nociceptors
Cold	Common after nerve injury; nil or rare after skin injury	1° zone	Cold-sensitive nociceptors	Central disinhibition
		1° zone	Cold-sensitive nociceptors	Peripheral sensitization of nociceptors
		1° and 2° zone	Sensitive cold receptors	Central censitization
Chemical Adrenaline; noradrenaline (SMP)	Nerve injury	1° zone	Axotomized and non-axotomized nociceptors. Possibly Aβ fibres when central sensitization is present	Peripheral sensitization
Mechanical Light touch	Injury to skin or cutaneous nerve	1° and 2° zone	Aβ-fibres	Central sensitization initiated and maintained by peripheral nociceptor input
	Trigeminal neuralgia	Trigger zone	Aβ-fibres	Crossed afterdischarges?
Pin prick	Injury to skin or cutaneous nerve	1° and 2° zone	Aδ-fibres	Central sensitization initated, but not maintained by nociceptive input
Blunt pressure	Injury to skin or cutaneous nerve	1° zone	Nociceptors	Peripheral sensitization of nociceptors
Impact	Injury to skin	1° zone	Nociceptors	Peripheral sensitization of nociceptors

*Hyperalgesias (defined as increased pain sensation to a stimulus) of brush-evoked pain, but may be rather ineffective in ameliorating other facets of the pain. In other words, if multiple pain-generating events are operating in an individual patient, a single treatment regimen may not be sufficient for affording global pain relief.

5.6 Persistent stimulus-independent pain is caused by ongoing nociceptor excitation

Although it is clear that changes of central nervous properties are crucial for the development of painful symptoms in peripheral neuropathy, several lines of independent evidence converge to indicate that changes in the excitability of primary nociceptive afferents are the single most important factor in the generation and maintenance of chronic neuropathic pain in humans. First, pain is often abolished or at least significantly reduced by local anaesthetic block of damaged peripheral nerves (Arnér et al., 1990; Fields et al., 1997) or affected skin (Rowbotham and Fields, 1989; Gracely et al., 1992; Rowbotham et al., 1995), indicating that neural activity arising in the nerve or possibly even in the receptive endings contribute to the pain. Second, stimulus-independent pains (and some forms of stimulus-induced pain sensations) persist during a differential nerve fibre block that eliminates conduction in myelinated non-nociceptive afferents (Campbell et al., 1988; Ochs et al., 1989; Ochoa and Yarnitsky, 1993). Third, psychophysical experiments indicate that the magnitude of pain correlates with the levels of nociceptor activity (Gracely et al., 1992; Koltzenburg et al., 1994b). These experimental studies in patients are entirely in agreement with the neuropathological observations mentioned above that implicate small-diameter primary afferent fibres as the primary culprits of peripheral neuropathic pain.

5.7 Factors regulating the sensitivity of nociceptors following nerve injury

Damage of primary afferent neurons produces a large number of changes in gene expression. Using gene microarray technology it is now possible to profile these transcriptional changes on a genome-wide basis. These studies have shown that the expression level of hundreds of genes changes after nerve injury (Costigan et al., 2002; Wang et al., 2002; Xiao et al., 2002). How this multitude of gene changes relates to the generation and maintenance of neuropathic pain is currently an unresolved question. It is known that inbred and hence genetically identical strains of rats and mice have a differential susceptibility to develop neuropathic pain behaviour after nerve injury (Mogil et al., 2000). To narrow the vast number of regulated genes down to those that are specifically involved in pain, one study compared the gene expression changes in two rat strains that have a different susceptibility of developing neuropathic pain. There were more than 200 genes that were regulated after axotomy in both rat strains, but only 15% of those were differentially expressed between the strains. This indicates that only a minority of genes whose expression level changes after nerve lesion are implicated in the generation of neuropathic pain (Valder *et al.*, 2003).

5.8 Electrophysiological studies show profound changes of the properties of damaged primary sensory neurons

There are several microneurographic investigations that have shown abnormal activity and reduced thresholds of nociceptors in patients with chronic painful conditions (Vallbo *et al.*, 1979; Ochoa *et al.*, 1982; Nordin *et al.*, 1984; Cline *et al.*, 1989). One study investigated the properties of unmyelinated nociceptors in patients suffering from erythromelalgia — a condition characterized by painful, red and hot extremities (Ørstavik *et al.*, 2003). The hereditary form of this disease is a channelopathy caused by a mutation of the sodium channel Nav1.7 which leads to the increased excitability (Yang *et al.*, 2004b). The nociceptors in these patients showed slowing of conduction as an indicator of a neuropathic process and ongoing activity which is normally not observed in nociceptors. Some of the findings were consistent with a sensitization of mechanically insensitive afferents to non-painful mechanical stimuli (Ørstavik *et al.*, 2003).

5.8.1 Neurophysiological mechanisms of ectopic impulse generation

There have been a number of neurophysiological studies that have investigated the pattern, source, and mechanism of ectopic action potential generation in various animal models of nerve injury. Together, these studies have shown that ectopic activity can arise at three points along an injured nerve, namely:

1. the site of the neuroma

2. the dorsal root ganglion of damaged and undamaged sensory neurons

3. the receptive terminals of non-axotomized nerve fibres that project into a damaged nerve.

Presently, the relative contribution of the different sources of ectopic discharge to nociceptive behaviour is incompletely understood.

Sprouts that are issued by axotomized afferent fibres are exquisitely sensitive to many stimuli (Jänig, 1988; Lisney, 1989). Many myelinated neurones develop ongoing activity and often respond to a variety of mechanical, thermal, or chemical stimuli (Michaelis *et al.*, 1995; Devor, 2005). The mechanical sensitivity of regenerating myelinated fibres is the basis of the Tinel sign that has been used since the beginning of the last century by neurologists to detect axon tips in focal nerve damage. Most axotomized neurons with ectopic activity are myelinated fibres, although activity in unmyelinated, presumably nociceptive neurons, can also develop (Häbler *et al.*, 1987).

After peripheral nerve lesions, some axotomized afferent neurons develop ongoing discharges that originate in the DRG (Devor, 2005). Most of the neurons with ongoing activity have myelinated axons, and few of them may be nociceptors. The vast majority of these neurons are afferents supplying muscle, probably because of a yet unknown signal in the DRG triggered by axotomy (Michaelis *et al.*, 2000). Using intracellular recordings it was shown that ongoing activity is critically dependent on subthreshold membrane potential oscillations; oscillatory sinusoids that reach threshold trigger low-frequency trains of intermittent spikes. Firing is also maintained by brief regenerative post-spike depolarizing afterpotentials (Amir *et al.*, 2002). Intriguingly, several lines of evidence now indicate that non-axotomized afferent neurons projecting into an injured nerve can change their phenotype (Fukuoka *et al.*, 2000). One feature is the development of low levels of ongoing activity in unmyelinated fibres (Koltzenburg *et al.*, 1994*a*; Ali *et al.*, 1999; Wu *et al.*, 2001; Boucher *et al.*, 2000). Recordings from the SNL models showed extensive changes in intact cell bodies housed in the L4 DRG that were qualitatively similar to changes in the axotomized L5 ganglion and consisted of higher input resistance, lower current, and voltage thresholds (Ma *et al.*, 2003).

5.8.2 What is the cellular and molecular basis of the ectopic excitation of injured and non-injured primary afferent fibres?

One possible explanation for the increased sensitivity is the altered expression or distribution of sodium channels (Waxman, 2001; Waxman *et al.*, 2002; Devor, 2005). On a transcriptional level, there is a decrease of the mRNA, of the tetrodotoxin-resistant (TTX-r) sodium channels Nav1.8 and Nav1.9, as well as of the TTX-sensitive channels Nav1.1, Nav1.6, Nav1.7 (Dib–Hajj *et al.*, 1999; Kim *et al.*, 2002; Lai *et al.*, 2004), but a strong up-regulation and re-expression of the embryonic sodium channels Nav1.3 (Dib–Hajj *et al.*, 1999). This transcriptional regulation corresponds to changes of the corresponding currents recorded from isolated dorsal root ganglion neurons in culture; namely, a reduction in the amplitude of TTX-r and the up-regulation of a rapidly repriming sodium current mediated by Nav1.3 (Cummins and Waxman, 1997). This change in sodium current profile and kinetics in DRG neurons may substantially alter neuronal excitability and could contribute to increased excitability of sensory neurons after injury. Since axotomy-induced changes in sodium conductances are found after lesion of the peripheral, but not the central, branch (Sleeper *et al.*, 2000), it had been suggested that changes in the retrograde supply of neurotrophic factors could account for the altered expression pattern. Moreover, the abnormal regulation of sodium channel expression, sodium channel kinetics, and the ectopic firing of primary afferent neurons was reversed by application of the neurotrophic factors NGF or GDNF (Boucher *et al.*, 2000; Leffler *et al.*, 2002).

Furthermore, studies showed major changes in the subcellular distribution of Nav1.8 protein following nerve transection or in the CCI model. In agreement with mRNA and patch clamp studies, there was a decrease in the intensity of immuno-labelling of the cell bodies of small DRG neurons, but an increased immunoreactivity in sciatic nerve axons at the site of injury (Novakovic *et al.*, 1998). In the SNL model there is little change in Nav1.8 protein or TTX-r currents in the cell bodies of uninjured neurons in L4 ganglia but a striking increase in the axons projecting into the sciatic nerve, primarily in unmyelinated axons (Gold *et al.*, 2003). Thus, there is a redistribution of the

TTX-resistant sodium channel to parts of a sensory neuron that are capable of ectopic impulse generation.

It is also possible that a depression of potassium conductances produce an increased excitability of sensory neurons after injury (Kajander *et al.*, 1992). DRG neurons display complex potassium currents that are composed of distinct kinetic and pharmacological components. Whereas there is no qualitative change of the potassium conductances after nerve injury, there is a significant reduction of the overall outward potassium current in axotomized neurons (Everill and Kocsis, 1999; Abdulla and Smith, 2001). The complexity of potassium channel composition in DRG neurons and their change after nerve injury are only incompletely understood. Amongst the Kv1 family, Kv1.1 and KV1.2 are most abundant, whereas Kv1.3 to Kv1.6 subunits are detected at lower levels. Axotomy reduces the expression level of Kv1.1 to Kv1.4, but leaves that of Kv1.5 and K1.6 unchanged. This suggests that Kv1.1 and Kv1.2 subunits are major components of voltage-gated K+ channels in DRG neurons and that the decreased expression of Kv1-family subunits significantly contributes to the reduction and altered kinetics of Kv current in axotomized neurons (Yang *et al.*, 2004a).

Another factor that could contribute to increased excitability is the increased conductance of the pacemaker current, Ih, that is mediated by hyperpolarization-activated, cyclic nucleotide-modulated channels (HCN). HCN channels, particularly HCN1, are abundantly expressed in primary afferent neurons and, in the SNL model, markedly increase pacemaker currents in axotomized large-diameter dorsal root ganglion neurons. Pharmacological blockade of HCN activity using the specific inhibitor ZD7288 reverses ectopic discharges and also reduces the behavioural hypersensitivity to light touch (Chaplan *et al.*, 2003; Yao *et al.*, 2003).

On the basis of behavioural studies, other compounds have been implicated to change the sensitivity of sensory neurons following focal nerve injury, including inflammatory mediators (Maves *et al.*, 1993; Eliav and Bennett, 1996) and tumour necrosis factor α (TNFα) (Sommer *et al.*, 1998). In agreement, electrophysiological studies have directly shown that intraneural injection of high doses of exogenous TNFα can ectopically excite some sensory neurones (Sorkin *et al.*, 1997; Sommer and Kress, 2004).

5.8.3 **Ephaptic cross-talk**

Neurophysiological studies have identified at least two other mechanisms that could increase the discharge of sensory neurones following focal nerve damage. A common finding in damaged peripheral nerves is electrical cross-talk between axons of all diameters (Jänig, 1988; Lisney, 1989; Devor, 1994). The basis of these short-circuits are so-called 'ephapses', that allow a tight one-to-one coupling between axons. Although rarely present in seemingly normal nerves (Meyer and Campbell, 1987) they are found in up to 20% of the fibres in the stump neuroma of the cat (Blumberg and Jänig, 1982). Ephapses can greatly increase the afferent barrage that impinges on the CNS following activation of few neurones.

5.8.4 **Crossed afterdischarges**

Another mechanism by which afferent activity increases after nerve damage occurs through a mechanism known as 'crossed afterdischarges' within the dorsal root ganglion that contains axotomized neurones. Several days after axotomy, many cells with large myelinated fibres start to discharge spontaneously (Lisney and Devor, 1987; Devor and Wall, 1990). Electrical or adequate natural excitation of neighbouring cells within the ganglion can increase this discharge. The crossed afterdischarges are not tightly locked to the stimulus, like in ephapses, and are probably mediated by an increase of extracellular concentration of potassium and an increase in the neurone's input resistance (Utzschneider *et al.*, 1992; Amir and Devor, 1996).

The interaction is primarily found in axotomized cells with myelinated axons and only rarely in neurones with unmyelinated axons. Interestingly, the electrical or natural excitation of intact nerve cells that have their soma in the same ganglion can evoke the crossed afterdischarge in axotomized, ectopically discharging neurones. The intact neurones capable of inducing the crossed afterdischarge had usually large myelinated fibres and low mechanical threshold. Thus, crossed afterdischarges are predominately an interaction between non-nociceptive sensory neurones that could lead to a temporal and spatial distortion of sensory information in damaged peripheral nerves, although its role in the generation of pain remains unclear.

5.9 **Stimulus-induced pains (hyperalgesias)**

Dating back to the pioneering studies of Lewis (Lewis, 1942), Hardy (Hardy *et al.*, 1952), and their colleagues, two zones of increased pain sensitivity (hyperalgesia) can be distinguished following experimental tissue injury. First, the area of tissue injury (the zone of primary hyperalgesia) in which there is an increased sensitivity for heat and a variety of mechanical and, presumably, chemical stimuli; second, a halo of apparently uninjured tissue (the zone of secondary hyperalgesia) where there is hyperalgesia to mechanical stimuli and possibly to cold. It is also clear that mechanical hyperalgesia can be further differentiated into at least four different subtypes that differ in their temporal and spatial profile, as well as in the relative importance of contributing nociceptive and non-nociceptive primary afferents (see Table 5.1). In neuropathic conditions, the distinction between primary and secondary area is less clearly defined, but probably corresponds to the tissue supplied by a damaged nerve and the area outside this territory.

5.10 **Hyperalgesia to heat is mediated by sensitized nociceptors**

A hallmark of inflammatory pain is the hyperalgesia to heat. Although this symptom occurs only occasionally under neuropathic conditions, the mechanism appears to be similar and is thought to involve sensitized nociceptors. As shown by differential nerve blocks, heat hyperalgesia in hairy skin is signalled by unmyelinated, presumably nociceptive afferents (Cline *et al.*, 1989). When heat hyperalgesia is experimentally induced in healthy volunteers, there is a significant leftward shift of the stimulus–response function that relates the magnitude of pain and the discharge of nociceptive C-fibres to the stimulus energy of a heat stimulus (Meyer *et al.*, 2005). Microneurographic recordings in patients have confirmed directly that chronic sensitization of nociceptors can also occur in patients suffering from neuropathic pain (Torebjörk, 1990; Ørstavik *et al.*, 2003).

Heat hyperalgesia is also a feature of several animal models of neuropathic pain, particularly in the CCI model. The magnitude of the behavioural response is, however, much smaller than in models of inflammatory pain. Animal models also provide evidence that the heat hyperalgesia from nerve injury or inflammation differ on a molecular level. Inflammatory hyperalgesia to heat is abolished in animals lacking TRPV1, whereas it is retained after partial sciatic nerve lesion (Caterina *et al.*, 2000).

5.11 Sensitization of nociceptive afferents to catecholamines could account for sympathetically maintained pain

A special case of chemical hyperalgesia may prevail in sympathetically maintained pain. The importance of the sympathetic nervous system in the generation of pain has been the focus of a long, if controversial, debate. Although there is no hard epidemiological data available, the number of patients with a predominant sympathetically maintained component of their pain is probably small. One group of conditions in which there appears to be frequent involvement of the sympathetic nervous system, at least in the early stages of the disease, is CRPS. Two lines of evidence suggest that the ongoing pain can be caused or maintained by the sympathetic nervous system in selected patients. First, sympatholytic therapy can abolish pain and hyperalgesia (Loh and Nathan, 1978; Bonica, 1990; Campbell *et al.*, 1992). Second, patients in whom sympatholytic therapy had provided pain relief, intracutaneous injection of adrenoceptor agonists can, under certain conditions, rekindle ongoing pain and hyperalgesia (Davis *et al.*, 1991; Torebjörk *et al.*, 1995) and there appears to be an increased density of α-adrenoceptors in hyperalgesic skin (Drummond *et al.*, 1996). Furthermore, injections of catecholamines around a stump neuroma can precipitate pain attacks in humans (Chabal *et al.*, 1992). Since a pain response can be induced during a differential blockade of myelinated fibres, unmyelinated fibres appear to signal sympathetically maintained pain (Torebjörk *et al.*, 1995).

An explanation that is consistent with all these findings is that primary afferents acquire a sensitivity to catecholamines that permits an abnormal excitation by either noradrenaline which is released from postganglionic sympathetic fibres or by circulating catecholamines derived from the adrenal medulla.

5.11.1 Neurophysiological mechanisms of an afferent-sympathetic interaction

Animal studies have shown repeatedly that application of catecholamines or activation of sympathetic postganglionic efferents can only minimally modulate the discharge of non-nociceptive afferents or nociceptors under physiological conditions (Jänig and Koltzenburg, 1992). On the other hand, it has also been shown, beyond doubt, that most types of primary afferents, including nociceptors, can develop a sensitivity to catecholamines and are excited by sympathetic stimulation after peripheral nerve injury (Koltzenburg, 1997; Perl, 1999). The presence of ephapses between unmyelinated axons in damaged peripheral nerves has invited speculation that sympathetic fibres could directly couple to primary afferent neurones. Yet, despite an intensive search, such interaction has never been found in animal models (Blumberg and Jänig, 1982; Meyer and Campbell, 1987; Jänig and Koltzenburg, 1991). By contrast, a chemical interaction has been shown to occur at three sites in a damaged peripheral nerve.

5.11.2 Interaction in the peripheral nerve and target tissue

Sprouts of regenerating sensory neurones that are trapped in a stump neuroma frequently respond to electrical stimulation of postganglionic sympathetic fibres or to systemic or local application of catecholamines (Koltzenburg, 1997). Since the afferents have been disconnected from the periphery, it is not possible to unequivocally determine the receptive function that these neurones might have had. However, primary afferents of all conduction velocities can acquire such responsiveness, including afferent fibres with thin myelinated or unmyelinated axons that are presumably the processes of nociceptors (Devor and Jänig, 1981). The degree of responsiveness varies with species and the time interval after nerve damage. Where tested, the sympathetic effects on nociceptors were usually blocked by application of α-selective adrenoceptor antagonists. It appears that α2-adrenoceptors mediate this excitatory response in rodents (Sato and Perl, 1991; Tracey et al., 1995; Chen et al., 1996), whereas in the monkey (Ringkamp et al., 1996), like in humans (Davis et al., 1991), α1-adrenoceptors have been implicated.

There is also some evidence from animal studies that sympathetic stimulation can excite primary afferent neurones through a non-adrenergic mechanism (de Armentia et al., 2003). Although these excitatory effects have mainly been studied after transection of major nerve trunks, it is reasonable to assume that damage to the terminal branches of a nerve can cause similar consequences. Moreover, in models of partial nerve injury, many axons form a neuroma in-continuity (Carlton et al., 1991; Sommer et al., 1993), and these afferents have, by and large, similar electrophysiological properties as those in a nerve end neuroma (Koltzenburg et al., 1994a; Xie et al., 1995).

An interaction between nociceptors and sympathetic fibres has also been shown to develop in non-transected nerve fibres running in a partially lesioned nerve. Non-axotomized unmyelinated and thin myelinated nociceptive afferents that had either low or no ongoing activity responded with a weak irregular discharge to local applications of catecholamines to the receptive field (Selig et al., 1993; Koltzenburg et al., 1994a; Bossut and Perl, 1995; Ringkamp et al., 1996; O'Halloran and Perl, 1997).

5.11.3 **Interaction in the dorsal root ganglion**

An intriguing interaction between postganglionic sympathetic fibres and the somata of sensory neurones develops in the dorsal root ganglion after axotomy. Several days after axotomy, electrical stimulation of sympathetic fibres or systemic application of adrenaline can modulate the ectopic discharge of cells that had presumably non-nociceptive function prior to their axotomy. Slightly more than half of the responses are excitatory, while the remaining cases display an inhibition of ongoing ectopic activity. Similar effects on dorsal root ganglion cells also appear to occur following partial injury of the sciatic nerve (Xie *et al.*, 1995). There is morphological evidence for a sympathetic-afferent interaction at the level of the dorsal root ganglion. Under normal instances only a few postganglionic fibres innervate blood vessels (Stevens *et al.*, 1983; Risling *et al.*, 1985; McLachlan *et al.*, 1993). However, after axotomy, there is a profuse growth of sympathetic neurones into the dorsal root ganglion and postganglionic sympathetic fibres start to encircle dorsal root ganglion cells to form baskets (McLachlan *et al.*, 1993; Chung *et al.*, 1994). The proliferation of sympathetic fibres occurs within days after axotomy when the spinal nerve is lesioned close to the dorsal root ganglion (Chung *et al.*, 1994), but requires several weeks when the sciatic nerve is damaged at mid-thigh level (McLachlan *et al.*, 1993). The different time course further suggests that changes are related to retrograde changes following axotomy.

Section of the sciatic nerve leads to a progressive reduction of small-diameter sensory neurons (Dreetz–Gjerstadt *et al.*, 2002) projecting to skin, but not to muscle (Hu and McLachlan, 2003). Conversely, p75 is up-regulated in satellite cells around cutaneous but not muscle neurons, and sympathetic baskets form preferentially around cutaneous neurons. Selective lesions of predominantly cutaneous nerves trigger the formation of sympathetic baskets, but none are detected after selective lesions of muscle nerves (Hu and McLachlan, 2003). It seems likely that the damaged sensory neurones, or their surrounding satellite cells, issue growth signals that attract sympathetic fibres. Sprouting of sympathetic fibres can be induced by exogenous application of leukaemia inhibitor factor (LIF) and nerve growth factor (NGF), and the sympathetic sprouting after axotomy can be prevented by application of a neutralizing antibody to the neuro-cytokine receptor component gp130 through which LIF, CNTF, and IL-6 signal to the cut proximal stump of the nerve (Thompson and Majithia, 1998). Moreover, transgenic mice overexpressing NGF in the skin show the same dramatic formation of sympathetic baskets neurones around sensory neurones (Davis *et al.*, 1994). Satellite cells within axotomized DRG have been shown to express mRNA for neurotrophins and for the low-affinity neurotrophin receptor, p75.

One possible scenario for sympathetic sprouting in the DRG that is consistent with many experimental findings involves the activation of satellite cells on the DRG by factors such as NGF, LIF, or IL-6 that are produced during Wallerian degeneration. This is then followed by the generation of a gradient of p75-bound neurotrophins emanating from activated satellite cells that then attract sympathetic fibres

(Ramer *et al.*, 1999). Some morphological studies suggest that the formation of sympathetic baskets can also occur in humans (Shinder *et al.*, 1999). Thus, the dorsal root ganglion is a site for interactions between the soma of sensory neurones and postganglionic sympathetic afferent fibres. However, as mainly neurones with large myelinated axons appear to be excited by sympathetic stimulation, and as sympathetic baskets are usually found around large sensory neurones, the possible clinical importance of this kind of interaction between sympathetic fibres and mainly non-nociceptive afferents for the generation of pain remains to be determined.

5.11.4 Cellular basis of the interaction

Electrophysiological studies have shown that the cell bodies of DRG neurons develop a sensitivity to catecholamines after axotomy (Xie *et al.*, 1995; Chen *et al.*, 1996; Michaelis *et al.*, 1996; Zhang *et al.*, 1997). Patch clamp studies of axotomized sensory neurones have found inward currents (Petersen *et al.*, 1996) following applications of noradrenaline and reduced outward potassium currents (Abdulla and Smith, 1997), both of which contribute to the excitation. Because noradrenaline did not affect total outward current recorded in the presence of Ca 2+ channel blockers, its effects on excitability may result from reduction of Ca 2+-sensitive potassium conductance(s) following suppression of an N-type Ca 2+-channel current (Abdulla and Smith, 1997).

When tested, the adrenergic excitation of nociceptors were quantitatively most prominent two weeks after partial nerve damage and gradually disappeared thereafter. However, nociceptive afferents with moderate or high ongoing activity were either not affected or displayed a slight inhibition of the ongoing activity during application of noradrenaline. This indicates that a high degree of excitability — as judged by the level of ongoing activity — is not the prerequisite for an excitatory sympathetic-afferent interaction, but that other mechanisms may be required. As a proportion of nociceptors develops an adrenergic sensitivity after sympathectomy (Perl, 1994) it has been suggested that factors which induce the typical denervation super sensitivity of autonomic effector organs following sympathetic denervation are responsible. Consistent with this view is the up-regulation of the expression of adrenoceptors on a transcriptional level (Perl, 1999).

In aggregate, the results of these studies now provide experimental support for a number of enigmatic clinical findings:

1. After nerve damage, non-injured nociceptors that innervate partially denervated tissue can develop a sensitivity to catecholamines.

2. The adrenoceptor-mediated excitation can occur distal to a nerve lesion.

3. The contribution of sympathetically maintained pain often decreases with time.

4. The catecholamine sensitivity of nociceptors appears to be present on afferents with no or very low ongoing activity.

Thus, the clinical effectiveness of a sympatholytical procedure may depend on the ratio of responsive and non-responsive fibres at a given moment of time and, therefore, significant relief might only be expected if other factors do not cause a persistent discharge of nociceptors.

5.12 **Mechanical hyperalgesia**

The presentation of mechanical hyperalgesia in humans is diverse and at least four distinct types can be identified after tissue injury (Koltzenburg, 1996), namely:

1. brush-evoked pain

2. pin-prick hyperalgesia

3. hyperalgesia to blunt pressure

4. hyperalgesia to impact stimuli

Brush-evoked pain and pin-prick hyperalgesia are present in the primary and secondary zone, whereas hyperalgesia to blunt pressure and impact stimuli are strictly restricted to the primary zone. With the exception of hyperalgesia to impact stimuli, these mechanical hyperalgesias have been described in neuropathic pain. Microneurographic studies and electrophysiological studies in animals have repeatedly shown that a reduction in the threshold of polymodal nociceptors does not occur under conditions that are clearly producing behavioural or psychophysical evidence for mechanical hyperalgesia (see Chapter 1), and there is consensus that sensitization in the CNS is a major factor. However, presently it is not fully understood which of the many CNS changes that have been described in animal models of neuropathic pain relate to the generation and mainte-nance of the specific subtypes of mechanical hyperalgesia found in humans.

5.12.1 **Brush-evoked pain**

One of the enigmatic painful symptoms, whose neural basis until recently could hardly be explained, is pain evoked by lightly touching the skin, also referred to as dynamic mechanical hyperalgesia or mechanical allodynia. A string of evidence shows that touch-evoked pain in both inflammatory and neuropathic conditions is not mediated by nociceptors, but instead is signalled out of the skin by sensitive mechanoreceptors with large myelinated axons that normally encode non-painful tactile events (see Table 5.1). First, differential blockade of large myelinated non-nociceptive afferents abolishes brush-evoked pain (Campbell *et al.*, 1988; Gracely *et al.*, 1992; Koltzenburg *et al.*, 1994*b*). Second, electrical stimulation (Price *et al.*, 1989; Torebjörk, 1990) of these afferents causes painful dysaesthesias. Third, reaction time measurements indicate that brush-evoked pain is signalled by fast conducting myelinated fibres (Fruhstorfer and Lindblom, 1984). Finally, light punctate mechanical stimuli that can only activate sensitive mechanoreceptors are often called painful in neuralgia (Price *et al.*, 1992; Koltzenburg *et al.*, 1994*b*).

The qualitative change of the Aβ-fibre input implies that there are profound alter-ations in the CNS processes encoding pain. The central sensitization that promotes brush-evoked pain in painful neuropathies requires ongoing excitation of nociceptors

(Gracely *et al.*, 1992; Koltzenburg *et al.*, 1994*b*), and studies in human volunteers have shown that it is the excitation of mechanically insensitive primary afferent neurons that induces this central sensitization (Schmelz *et al.*, 2000; Koppert *et al.*, 2001; Klede *et al.*, 2003).

5.12.2 Pin-prick hyperalgesia

Hyperalgesia to pin-prick stimuli — typically elicited by probing of the skin with a stiff von Frey hair — can be found in the primary and secondary zone of hyperalgesia after experimental tissue injury, and in patients suffering from neuropathy (Pappagallo *et al.*, 2000). It is distinct from brush-evoked pain because of its different spatial and temporal profile (Simone *et al.*, 1989; LaMotte *et al.*, 1991; Koltzenburg *et al.*, 1992; Cervero *et al.*, 1994; Kilo *et al.*, 1994). In contrast to brush-evoked pain, differential nerve block experiments showed that hyperalgesia to punctate stimuli is carried out of the skin by non-sensitized heat-insensitive Aδ nociceptors (Ziegler *et al.*, 1999). Although excitation of mechanically insensitive unmyelinated afferents is important for the initiation of this type of central sensitization, it is not required for sustaining it (LaMotte *et al.*, 1991; Kilo *et al.*, 1994; Koppert *et al.*, 2001).

5.12.3 Hyperalgesia to blunt pressure

Hyperalgesia to blunt pressure can be elicited experimentally by tissue inflammation in normal human volunteers (Koltzenburg *et al.*, 1992; Kilo *et al.*, 1994) and has also been described in patients with neuropathic pain (Ochs *et al.*, 1989; Price *et al.*, 1992; Ochoa and Yarnitsky, 1993). Differential nerve block experiments in models of inflammatory pain indicate that this type of hyperalgesia is signalled by nociceptors. One possible explanation for its generation is the spatial summation of nociceptive input, and this could be brought about by the sensitization of mechanically insensitive nociceptors (Schmidt *et al.*, 2000) and the expansion of the receptive field of mechanosensitive nociceptors (Reeh *et al.*, 1987; Schmelz *et al.*, 1994).

5.13 Changes in the CNS that contribute to neuropathic pain

There are a number of important changes in the CNS following peripheral nerve injury. Ongoing excitation of nociceptors can induce activity dependent plastic changes in the CNS, and these mechanisms are reviewed in Chapter 4.

5.13.1 Changes of neuropeptides in sensory neurons and spinal cord

Peripheral nerve lesions also trigger a large number of transcriptional changes in axotomized cells and non-axotomized neurons projecting into an injured nerve. Transcriptional changes occur also in the spinal cord, but are less pronounced. Changes in neuropeptide expression and their receptors is one of those dramatic consequences. Neuropeptides that are up-regulated are attractive candidates for mediating some of the sensory abnormalities in neuropathic pain conditions and have therefore been studied intensely.

The neuropeptide, galanin, is, under normal circumstances, detectable only in a few DRG neurons, but up to 50% of nociceptive neurons express the peptide after nerve injury (Villar *et al.*, 1989). Galanin appears to have complex pro- and antinociceptive effects on spinal cord level. The pro-nociceptive effects appear to be mediated by presynaptic GalR2 receptors located on DRG neurons, whereas under neuropathic conditions the anti-nociceptive action is exerted via the GalR1 receptor on dorsal horn interneurons (Liu and Hökfelt, 2002).

Neuropeptide Y (NPY) is normally present in few neurons, but it is strongly up-regulated in large-diameter, capsaicin-insensitive sensory neurons following axotomy (Wakisaka *et al.*, 1991; Noguchi *et al.*, 1993). Many of these afferents project via the dorsal columns to the dorsal column nuclei of the brainstem. Surgical disruption of the ipsilateral dorsal columns or administration of lidocaine into the gracile nucleus blocked mechanical allodynia, but not thermal hyperalgesia, in the SNL model (Sun *et al.*, 2001). Whereas spinal application of NPY has anti-nociceptive actions (Hua *et al.*, 1991), NPY microinjection into the gracile nucleus elicits tactile, but not thermal, hypersensitivity in the ipsilateral hindpaw. Administration of function-blocking antibodies of NPY or antagonists of the Y1 receptor reverse the mechanical, but not the thermal hypersensitivity (Ossipov *et al.*, 2002).

An important change in the dorsal horn of the spinal cord for the signalling of neuropathic pain appears to be the up-regulation of the γ isoform of protein kinase C (PKCγ) and correlates with the behavioural manifestations of hyperalgesia (Mao *et al.*, 1995). Mutant mice lacking PKCγ have confirmed its important role, since these mice almost completely failed to develop the behavioural correlates of neuropathic pain behaviour (Malmberg *et al.*, 1997).

There is evidence that dynorphin has a complex role in the maintenance of neuropathic pain. Dynorphin is up-regulated in neurons of the spinal cord with a lag of several days after initiation of the nerve injury (Kajander *et al.*, 1990). Intrathecal administration of dynorphin causes mechanical hyperalgesia, and spinal administration of function-blocking dynorphin antibodies reverse hyperalgesia in models of neuropathic pain (Wang *et al.*, 2001). Animals lacking dynorphin initially develop mechanical hyperalgesia in the SNL model, but, in contrast to wild-type animals, fail to sustain it, suggesting that dynorphin is important for the maintenance, but not the initiation of hyperalgesia (Wang *et al.*, 2001). However, there is also conflicting evidence showing that DREAM (downstream regulatory element antagonistic modulator), a transcriptional repressor of the prodynorphin, is involved in pain modulation. Mice lacking DREAM exhibit reduced responses in most models of pain, including neuropathic pain. This effect is mediated through an increased expression of dynorphin acting through κ-opiate receptors (Cheng *et al.*, 2002).

5.13.2 **Electrophysiological changes**

Dorsal horn neurons develop increased activity after peripheral nerve injury, and this probably reflects both defective inhibitory mechanisms and the ectopic firing of peripheral afferents (Palecek *et al.*, 1992; Laird and Bennett, 1993; Chapman *et al.*, 1998). However, the majority of studies using partial injury models failed to demonstrate increased response of dorsal horn neurons to heat stimuli despite the presence of heat hyperalgesia in these animals (Palecek *et al.*, 1992; Laird and Bennett, 1993), which is small when compared to tissue inflammation.

Changes in the mechanical sensitivity of dorsal horn neurons are subtle. While there is no change of the threshold of these neurons (Laird and Bennett, 1993), responses to innocuous mechanical stimuli represent a larger percentage of the total evoked activity in wide dynamic range spinothalamic tract neurons (Palecek *et al.*, 1992) which have also a larger receptive field size (Suzuki *et al.*, 2000). In addition, afterdischarges are more conspicuous in nerve-injured animals, compared with controls (Palecek *et al.*, 1992), but windup responses are comparable to controls (Chapman *et al.*, 1998). Recording from neurons in the substantia gelatinosa of the spinal cord in slice preparations showed that NMDA receptor currents in the substantia gelatinosa were facilitated in the SNL model (Isaev *et al.*, 2000). In the CCI model, and after complete sciatic nerve transection, there was a decreased threshold for eliciting EPSCs (Kohno *et al.*, 2003) and an increased prevalence of mono- and polysynaptic Aβ-fibre-evoked EPSCs (Kohama *et al.*, 2000; Okamoto *et al.*, 2001).

Transmission of sensory information in the spinal cord is normally subjected to pre- or postsynaptic inhibitory control maintained by activity in sensory afferents, dorsal horn interneurons, and descending pathways. Peripheral nerve lesion precipitates a reduction of spinal inhibition (Wall and Devor, 1981). Primary afferent-evoked IPSCs are substantially reduced in incidence, magnitude, and duration after partial, but not complete nerve injury, and it has been shown that this is the consequence of a reduced GABA release acting on presynaptic GABA A receptors. (Moore *et al.*, 2002).

Behavioural investigations also suggest that descending facilitatory projections from the rostroventromedial medulla (RVM) or periaqueductal grey (PAG) are important for the maintenance of neuropathic pain behaviour. Microinjection of lidocain into these areas attenuated mechanical hyperalgesia in the SNL model, but did not affect nociceptive responses in naïve animals (Pertovaara *et al.*, 1996; Burgess *et al.*, 2002).

5.13.3 **Structural changes are unlikely to contribute to the chronicity of neuropathic pain**

Because of its unrelenting character and resistance to pharmacological interventions, it had been speculated that structural changes in the CNS may perpetuate symptoms in painful neuropathies. One of these proposed mechanisms has been the sprouting of the central terminals of large myelinated mechanosensitive neurons from the deep dorsal horn into the substantia gelatinosa — an area normally receiving the central projections of nociceptors. It has been suggested that novel contacts of Aβ fibres with central pain-signalling neurons could explain persistent brush-evoked pain (Woolf *et al.*, 1992; Woolf and Doubell, 1994). Although clinical investigations on some patients suffering from postherpetic neuralgia are consistent with this possibility (Baron and Saguer, 1993), most clinical studies do not endorse this view and have shown that brush-evoked pain critically depends on a persistent primary afferent input of nociceptors rather than being the result of a rigid structural reorganization after axotomy (Gracely *et al.*, 1992; Treede *et al.*, 1992; Koltzenburg *et al.*, 1994*b*). Much of the evidence for the structural reorganization has come from retrograde-tracing experiments using the sub-unit B of cholera toxin (CTB). This marker normally labels GM1-expressing neurons which are myelinated in naive rats. However, there is now conclusive evidence that there is an up-regulation of GM1 in axotomized, unmyelinated afferents, and because of this, CTB is transported by myelinated and unmyelinated primary afferents. This loss of specificity and the consequent staining of unmyelinated afferents in their normal projection targets masquerades as sprouting (Tong *et al.*, 1999; Bao *et al.*, 2002; Hughes *et al.*, 2003; Shehab *et al.*, 2003). The absence of a structural reorganization does not of course negate the possibility of a functional alteration and an increased A-fibre input into the substantia gelatinosa, as suggested by several electrophysiological investigations.

Histological investigations have also provided evidence for transsynaptic degenerative changes by discovering so-called dark pyknotic cells in the dorsal horn ipsilateral to a chronic constriction injury. Using TUNEL staining, nuclear fragmentation was observed in cells, suggesting apoptotic cell death (Azkue *et al.*, 1998). Complete transection of the sciatic nerve did not result in demonstrable neuronal cell death in the dorsal horn (Coggeshall *et al.*, 2001). The type of cell that undergoes apoptosis has not been unequivocally identified and it is possible that these are neurons or non-neuronal cells or both. Some evidence has implicated death to GABAergic interneurons (Castro–Lopes *et al.*, 1993; Moore *et al.*, 2002). However, unbiased stereological studies have been unable to confirm a loss of GABAergic or glycinergic interneurons in the superficial dorsal horn of the spinal cord (Polgar *et al.*, 2003). The function of the apoptotic cells remains therefore currently elusive.

5.13.4 The potential role of glia cells in neuropathic pain

It has long been recognized that peripheral nerve damage results in activation of glial cells in the spinal cord or brainstem (Streit *et al.*, 1988), but it has only recently been suggested that glia activation could contribute substantially to neuropathic pain (Watkins *et al.*, 2001). In the SNL model there is activation of p38 mitogen-activated protein kinase in the OX-42 positive microglia cells, most prominently in the ipsilateral dorsal horn at the segmental levels that contain the projections of the injured afferents, and application of an p38 inhibitor reduces hyperalgesias (Jin *et al.*, 2003). Release of cytokines from the microglia may contribute to the central sensitization (Watkins *et al.*, 2001). Activated microglia express P2X4 receptors, a subtype of ionotropic ATP receptor, and its pharmacological antagonism reversed mechanical hyperalgesia after peripheral nerve injury without affecting acute pain behaviours in naive animals. Conversely, intraspinal administration of microglia in which P2X4Rs had been induced and stimulated produced tactile allodynia in naive rats (Tsuda *et al.*, 2003).

5.14 Hypersensitivity to cold

Hypersensitivity to cold is particularly prominent after traumatic nerve injury (Wahren and Torebjörk, 1992), but it can also present in painful polyneuropathic conditions (Ochoa and Yarnitsky, 1994) or in postherpetic neuralgia (Pappagallo *et al.*, 2000). Cold hypersensitivity has recently been recognized as one of the major painful, chronic sequels of the so-called trench foot neuropathy (Jensen *et al.*, 2005) which is brought about by non-freezing cold injury of the extremities (Thomas and Holdorff, 1993; Irwin, 1996). Another clinically important condition of cold intolerance is linked with the systemic injection of the chemotherapeutic agent, oxaliplatin, which is associated with paraesthesiae and painful hypersensitivity aggravated by cold (Ibrahim *et al.*, 2004).

Cold hypersensitivity is also prominent in animal models of painful neuropathy. However, most investigations have used behavioural endpoints and there is a dearth of information that directly assesses the functional properties of primary afferent neurons that could contribute to cold hyperalgesia. The behavioural manifestations of cold hyperalgesia in the SNL model do not involve the sympathetic nervous system (Ringkamp *et al.*, 1999), but probably nociceptors (Hama, 2002). Indeed, in the SNL model an increase of cold-sensitive neurons has been found in non-axotomized L4 DRG, but not in the L5 ganglion that contains the cell body of the axotomized neurons (Djouhri *et al.*, 2004).

Currently, there are three hypotheses — central disinhibition, peripheral sensitization, and central sensitization — that have been advanced to explain the generation of cold hyperalgesia in neuropathic pain in humans, although the relative importance of each has not been conclusively established. This involves changes in the main classes of peripheral cold-sensitive afferents, namely cold-sensitive thermoreceptors and nociceptors, as well as changes in their central processing.

5.14.1 Central disinhibition

Because cold stimulation, through excitation of cold-sensitive thermoreceptive afferents, normally suppresses noxious stimuli on a central level (Craig, 2003), the selective loss or dysfunction of these afferents shifts the cold pain threshold to warmer temperatures (Wahren *et al.*, 1989; Yarnitsky and Ochoa, 1990; Ochoa and Yarnitsky, 1994).

5.14.2 Peripheral sensitization

Changes in the excitability of primary afferents have long been established as a mechanism for hyperalgesia to heat. However, whether neurons change their responses to cold has not been systematically investigated. Psychophysical studies of human volunteers strongly suggest that sensitization of cold-sensitive nociceptors by the TRPM8 agonist, menthol, can produce cold hyperalgesia (Wasner *et al.*, 2004). Peripheral sensitization also appears likely for oxaliplatin-induced peripheral neuropathy. Here, studies in patients show an acute hyperexcitability of peripheral nerves (Lehky *et al.*, 2004) and animal studies suggest that this is due to a lengthening of the refractory period and an increase of sodium conductance in subpopulations of peripheral sensory neurons (Adelsberger *et al.*, 2000).

5.14.3 Central sensitization

Central sensitization is an established mechanism for mechanical hyperalgesia in patients suffering from painful neuropathy. Reaction time measurements (Fruhstorfer and Lindblom, 1984; Lindblom, 1994) and differential nerve block experiments (Torebjörk *et al.*, 1995) suggest that thin myelinated cold-sensitive afferents signal pain in some patients with neuropathy. Furthermore, cold hyperalgesia which is probably mediated by myelinated fibres has also been found in the area of secondary hyperalgesia following the injection of capsaicin (Gracely *et al.*, 1993). The qualitative switch from signalling of innocuous cool sensations to cold pain could be analogous to the mechanisms that mediate brush-evoked pain signalled by large myelinated non-nociceptive fibres.

5.15 Conclusion

Neuropathic pain is one of the puzzles of pain and appears to be the result of a disease affecting nociceptive pathways that normally signal pain. Important changes that contribute to this abnormal symptom are changes in the functional properties of primary afferent neurons. This involves abnormal ectopic activity in axotomized and non-axotomized neurons projecting into an injured nerve and are the consequence of an altered expression and distribution of ion channels. This abnormal excitability of sensory neurons is coupled to changes in the neurotransmitter phenotype and this may explain why neuropathic pains are often relatively resistant to conventional analgesic treatments. Major changes in the spinal cord are the loss of inhibitory mechanisms, resulting in an increased activity of interneurons or projection neurons. The relentless persistence of many neuropathic pain conditions cannot be explained by structural reorganization of the central projection pattern of primary afferent neurons, and the relative importance of non-neuronal cells in the peripheral or central nervous system for the generation and maintenance of neuropathic pain remains largely unexplored.

References

Abdulla FA and Smith PA (2001) Axotomy- and autotomy-induced changes in Ca2+ and K+ channel currents of rat dorsal root ganglion neurons. *J Neurophysiol* **85**:644–658.

Abdulla FA and Smith PA (1997) Ectopic α2-adrenoceptors couple to N-type Ca2+ channels in axotomized rat sensory neurons. *J Comp Neurol* **17**:1633–1641.

Adelsberger H, Quasthoff S, Grosskreutz J, Lepier A, Eckel F, and Lersch C (2000) The chemotherapeutic oxaliplatin alters voltage-gated Na(+) channel kinetics on rat sensory neurons. *Eur J Pharmacol* **406**:25–32.

Ali Z, Ringkamp M, Hartke TV, *et al.* (1999) Uninjured C-fiber nociceptors develop spontaneous activity and alpha-adrenergic sensitivity following L6 spinal nerve ligation in monkey. *J Neurophysiol* **81**:455–466.

Amir R and Devor M (1996) Chemically mediated cross-excitation in rat dorsal root ganglia. *J Neurosci* **16**:4733–4741.

Amir R, Michaelis M, and Devor M (2002) Burst discharge in primary sensory neurons: triggered by subthreshold oscillations, maintained by depolarizing afterpotentials. *J Neurosci* **22**:1187–1198.

Arnér S, Lindblom U, Meyerson BA, and Molander C (1990) Prolonged relief of neuralgia after regional anesthetic blocks. A call for further experimental and systematic clinical studies. *Pain* **43**:287–297.

Azkue JJ, Zimmermann M, Hsieh TF, and Herdegen T (1998) Peripheral nerve insult induces NMDA receptor-mediated, delayed degeneration in spinal neurons. *Eur J Neurosci* **10**:2204–2206.

Bao L, Wang HF, Cai HJ, *et al.* (2002) Peripheral axotomy induces only very limited sprouting of coarse myelinated afferents into inner lamina II of rat spinal cord. *Eur J Neurosci* **16**:175–185.

Baron R and Saguer M (1993) Postherpetic neuralgia: are C-nociceptors involved in signalling and maintenance of tactile allodynia? *Brain* **116**:1477–1496.

Bennett GJ and Xie YK (1988) A peripheral mononeuropathy in rat that produces disorders of pain sensation like those seen in man. *Pain* **33**:87–107.

Blumberg H and Jänig W (1982) Activation of fibres via experimentally produced stump neuromas of skin nerves: ephaptic transmission or retrograde sprouting. *Exp Neurol* **76**:468–482.

Blumenkopf B and Lipman JJ (1991) Studies in autotomy: its pathophysiology and usefulness as a model of chronic pain. *Pain* **45**:203–209.

Bonica JJ (1990) Causalgia and other sympathetic reflex dystrophies. In: *The Management of Pain* (Bonica JJ, ed), pp. 220–243. Philadelphia: Lea and Febiger.

Bossut DF and Perl ER (1995) Effects of nerve injury on sympathetic excitation of Aδ mechanical nociceptors. *J Neurophysiol* **73**:1721–1723.

Boucher TJ, Okuse K, Bennett DL, Munson JB, Wood JN, and McMahon SB (2000) Potent analgesic effects of GDNF in neuropathic pain states. *Science* **290**:124–127.

Burgess SE, Gardell LR, Ossipov MH, *et al.* (2002) Time-dependent descending facilitation from the rostral ventromedial medulla maintains, but does not initiate, neuropathic pain. *J Neurosci* **22**:5129–5136.

Campbell JN, Meyer RA, and Raja SN (1992) Is nociceptor activation by alpha-1 adrenoreceptors the culprit in sympathetically maintained pain. *APS Journal* **13**:344–350.

Campbell JN, Raja SN, Meyer RA, and Mackinnon SE (1988) Myelinated afferents signal the hyperalgesia associated with nerve injury. *Pain* **32**:89–94.

Carlton SM, Dougherty PM, Pover CM, and Coggeshall RE (1991) Neuroma formation and numbers of axons in a rat model of experimental peripheral neuropathy. *Neurosci Lett* **131**:88–92.

Carlton SM, Lekan HA, Kim SH, and Chung JM (1994) Behavioral manifestations of an experimental model for peripheral neuropathy produced by spinal nerve ligation in the primate. *Pain* **56**:155–166.

Castro–Lopes JM, Tavares I, and Coimbra A (1993) GABA decreases in the spinal cord dorsal horn after peripheral neurectomy. *Brain Res* **620**:287–291.

Caterina MJ, Leffler A, Malmberg AB, *et al.* (2000) Impaired nociception and pain sensation in mice lacking the capsaicin receptor. *Science* **288**:306–313.

Cervero F, Meyer RA, and Campbell JN (1994) A psychophysical study of secondary hyperalgesia: evidence for increased pain to input from nociceptors. *Pain* **58**:21–28.

Chabal C, Jacobson L, Russell LC, and Burchiel KJ (1992) Pain response to perineuromal injection of normal saline, epinephrine, and lidocaine in humans. *Pain* **49**:9–12.

Chaplan SR, Guo HQ, Lee DH, *et al.* (2003) Neuronal hyperpolarization-activated pacemaker channels drive neuropathic pain. *J Neurosci* **23**:1169–1178.

Chapman V, Suzuki R, and Dickenson AH (1998) Electrophysiological characterization of spinal neuronal response properties in anaesthetized rats after ligation of spinal nerves L5-L6. *J Physiol* **507(Pt 3)**:881–894.

Chen Y, Michaelis M, Jänig W, and Devor M (1996) Adrenoreceptor subtype mediating sympatheticsensory coupling in injured sensory neurons. *J Neurophysiol* **76**:3721–3730.

Cheng HY, Pitcher GM, Laviolette SR, *et al.* (2002) DREAM is a critical transcriptional repressor for pain modulation. *Cell* **108**:31–43.

Chung K, Kim HJ, Na HS, Yoon YW, and Chung JM (1994) Changes in the sympathetic innervation to the sensory ganglia at variable times after a neuropathic nerve injury. *Soc Neurosci Abstr* **20**:760.

Cline MA, Ochoa J, and Torebjörk HE (1989) Chronic hyperalgesia and skin warming caused by sensitized C nociceptors. *Brain* **112**:621–647.

Coderre TJ, Grimes RW, and Melzack R (1986) Deafferentation and chronic pain in animals: an evaluation of evidence suggesting autotomy is related to pain. *Pain* **26**:61–84.

Coggeshall RE, Lekan HA, White FA, and Woolf CJ (2001) A-fiber sensory input induces neuronal cell death in the dorsal horn of the adult rat spinal cord. *J Comp Neurol* **435**:276–282.

Costigan M, Befort K, Karchewski L, *et al.* (2002) Replicate high-density rat genome oligonucleotide microarrays reveal hundreds of regulated genes in the dorsal root ganglion after peripheral nerve injury. *BMC Neurosci* **3**:16.

Craig AD (2003) Pain Mechanisms: labeled lines versus convergence in central processing. *Annu Rev Neurosci* **26**:1–30.

Cummins TR and Waxman SG (1997) Downregulation of tetrodotoxin-resistant sodium currents and upregulation of a rapidly repriming tetrodotoxin-sensitive sodium current in small spinal sensory neurons after nerve injury. *J Neurosci* **17**:3503–3514.

Daousi C, MacFarlane IA, Woodward A, Nurmikko TJ, Bundred PE, and Benbow SJ (2004) Chronic painful peripheral neuropathy in an urban community: a controlled comparison of people with and without diabetes. *Diabet Med* **21**:976–982.

Davis BM, Albers KM, Seroogy KB, and Katz DM (1994) Overexpression of nerve growth factor in transgenic mice induces novel sympathetic projections to primary sensory neurons. *J Comp Neurol* **349**:464–474.

Davis KD, Treede R–D, Raja SN, Meyer RA, and Campbell JN (1991) Topical application of clonidine relieves hyperalgesia in patients with sympathetically maintained pain. *Pain* **47**:309–317.

de Armentia ML, Leeson AH, Stebbing MJ, Urban L, and McLachlan EM (2003) Responses to sympathomimetics in rat sensory neurones after nerve transection. *NeuroReport* **14**:9–13.

Decosterd I and Woolf CJ (2000) Spared nerve injury: an animal model of persistent peripheral neuropathic pain. *Pain* **87**:149–158.

DeLeo JA, Coombs DW, Willenbring S, *et al.* (1994) Characterisation of a neuropathic pain model: sciatic cryoneurolysis in the rat. *Pain* **56**:9–16.

Devor M (in press) Neuropathic pain: response of nerves to injury. In: *Wall and Melzack's Textbook of Pain* (McMahon SB, Koltzenburg M, eds). Edinburgh: Churchill Livingstone.

Devor M (1994) Pathophysiology of injured nerve. In: *Textbook of Pain* (Wall PD, Melzack R, eds), pp. 79–100. Edinburgh: Churchill Livingstone.

Devor M and Jänig W (1981) Activation of myelinated afferents ending in a neuroma by stimulation of the sympathetic supply in the rat. *Neurosci Lett* **24**:43–47.

Devor M and Wall PD (1990) Cross-excitation in dorsal root ganglia of nerve-injured and intact rats. *J Neurophysiol* **64**:1733–1746.

Dib–Hajj SD, Fjell J, Cummins TR, *et al.* (1999) Plasticity of sodium channel expression in DRG neurons in the chronic constriction injury model of neuropathic pain. *Pain* **83**:591–600.

Djouhri L, Wrigley D, Thut PD, and Gold MS (2004) Spinal nerve injury increases the percentage of cold-responsive DRG neurons. *NeuroReport* **15**:457–460.

Dreetz–Gjerstadt M, Tandrup T, Koltzenburg M, and Jakobsen J (2002) Predominant neuronal B-cell loss in L5 DRG of p75 receptor-deficient mice. *J Anat* **200**:81–87.

Drummond PD, Skipworth S, and Finch PM (1996) α1-adrenoceptors in normal and hyperalgesic human skin. *Clin Sci* **91**:73–77.

Eliav E and Bennett GJ (1996) An experimental neuritis of the rat sciatic nerve that produces unilateral allodynia and hyperalgesia in the hind paw. *Abstract 8th World Congress on Pain,* p. 26.

Everill B and Kocsis JD (1999) Reduction in potassium currents in identified cutaneous afferent dorsal root ganglion neurons after axotomy. *J Neurophysiol* **82**:700–708.

Fields HL, Rowbotham MC, and Devor M (1997) Excitability blockers: anticonvulsants and low concentration local anesthetics in the treatment of chronic pain. In: *The Pharmacology of Pain* (Dickenson A and Besson J–M, eds), pp. 93–116. Berlin: Springer–Verlag.

Fruhstorfer H and Lindblom U (1984) Sensibility abnormalities in neuralgic patients studied by thermal and tactile pulse stimulation. In: *Somatosensory Mechanisms* (von Euler U, Franzén O, Lindblom U, and Ottoson D, eds), pp 353–361. London: Macmillan Press.

Fukuoka T, Tokunaga A, Kondo E, and Noguchi K (2000) The role of neighboring intact dorsal root ganglion neurons in a rat neuropathic pain model. In: *Proceedings of the 9th World Congress on Pain* (Devor M, Rowbotham M, and Wiesenfeld–Hallin Z, eds), pp. 137–146. Seattle: IASP Press.

Gold MS, Weinreich D, Kim CS, *et al.* (2003) Redistribution of Na(V)1.8 in uninjured axons enables neuropathic pain. *J Neurosci* **23**:158–166.

Gracely RH, Lynch SA, and Bennett GJ (1993) Evidence for Aβ low threshold mechanoreceptor-mediated mechanoallodynia and cold hyperalgesia following intradermal injection of capsaicin into the foot dorsum. *Abstract of 7th World Congress on Pain*, p. 372.

Gracely RH, Lynch SA, and Bennett GJ (1992) Painful neuropathy: altered central processing, maintained dynamically by peripheral input. *Pain* **51**:175–194.

Griffin JW, McArthur JC, and Polydefkis M (2001) Assessment of cutaneous innervation by skin biopsies. *Curr Opin Neurol* **14**:655–659.

Häbler H–J, Jänig W, and Koltzenburg M (1987) Activation of unmyelinated afferents in chronically lesioned nerves by adrenaline and excitation of sympathetic efferents in the cat. *Neurosci Lett* **82**:35–40.

Hama AT (2002) Capsaicin-sensitive primary afferents mediate responses to cold in rats with a peripheral mononeuropathy. *NeuroReport* **13**:461–464.

Hardy JD, Wolff HG, and Goodell H (1952) *Pain Sensations and Reactions.* Baltimore: Williams & Willkins.

Hu P and McLachlan EM (2003) Selective reactions of cutaneous and muscle afferent neurons to peripheral nerve transection in rats. *J Neurosci* **23**:10559–10567.

Hua XY, Boublik JH, Spicer MA, Rivier JE, Brown MR, and Yaksh TL (1991) The antinociceptive effects of spinally administered neuropeptide Y in the rat: systematic studies on structure- activity relationship. *J Pharmacol Exp Ther* **258**:243–248.

Hughes DI, Scott DT, Todd AJ, and Riddell JS (2003) Lack of evidence for sprouting of A-beta afferents into the superficial laminas of the spinal cord dorsal horn after nerve section. *J Neurosci* **23**:9491–9499.

Ibrahim A, Hirschfeld S, Cohen MH, Griebel DJ, Williams GA, and Pazdur R (2004) FDA drug approval summaries: oxaliplatin. *Oncologist* **9**:8–12.

Irwin MS (1996) Nature and mechanism of peripheral nerve damage in an experimental model of non-freezing cold injury. *Ann R Coll Surg (Engl)* **78**:372–379.

Isaev D, Gerber G, Park SK, Chung JM, and Randik M (2000) Facilitation of NMDA-induced currents and Ca2+ transients in the rat substantia gelatinosa neurons after ligation of L5-L6 spinal nerves. *NeuroReport* **11**:4055–4061.

Jänig W (1988) Pathophysiology of nerve following mechanical injury. In: *Proceedings of the Vth World Congress on Pain* (Dubner R, Gebhart GF, and Bond MR, eds), pp. 89–108. Amsterdam: Elsevier.

Jänig W and Koltzenburg M (1992) Possible ways of sympathetic-afferent interactions. In: *Pathophysiological Mechanisms of Reflex Sympathetic Dystrophy* (Jänig W and Schmidt RF, eds), pp. 213–243. Weinheim: VCH.

Jänig W and Koltzenburg M (1991) Plasticity of sympathetic reflex organization following cross-union of inappropiate nerves in the adult cat. *J Physiol (Lond)* **436**:309–323.

Jensen TS, Koltzenburg M, Wasner G, and Jorum E (in press) Cold allodynia: from molecule to the clinic. *Abstract of 11th World Congress on Pain.*

Jin SX, Zhuang ZY, Woolf CJ, and Ji RR (2003) p38 mitogen-activated protein kinase is activated after a spinal nerve ligation in spinal cord microglia and dorsal root ganglion neurons and contributes to the generation of neuropathic pain. *J Neurosci* **23**:4017–4022.

Kajander KC, Sahara Y, Iadarola MJ, and Bennett GJ (1990) Dynorphin increases in the dorsal spinal cord in rats with a painful peripheral neuropathy. *Peptides* **11**:719–728.

Kajander KC, Wakisaka S, and Bennett GJ (1992) Spontaneous discharge originates in the dorsal root ganglion at the onset of a painful peripheral neuropathy in the rat. *Neurosci Lett* **138**:225–228.

Kilo S, Schmelz M, Koltzenburg M, and Handwerker HO (1994) Different patterns of hyperalgesia induced by experimental inflammation in human skin. *Brain* **117**:385–396.

Kim CH, Oh Y, Chung JM, and Chung K (2002) Changes in three subtypes of tetrodotoxin sensitive sodium channel expression in the axotomized dorsal root ganglion in the rat. *Neurosci Lett* **323**:125–128.

Kim SH and Chung JM (1992) An experimental model for peripheral neuropathy produced by segmental spinal nerve ligation in the rat. *Pain* **50**:355–363.

Klede M, Handwerker HO, and Schmelz M (2003) Central origin of secondary mechanical hyperalgesia. *J Neurophysiol* **90**:353–359.

Kohama I, Ishikawa K, and Kocsis JD (2000) Synaptic reorganization in the substantia gelatinosa after peripheral nerve neuroma formation: aberrant innervation of lamina II neurons by Abeta afferents. *J Neurosci* **20**:1538–1549.

Kohno T, Moore KA, Baba H, and Woolf CJ (2003) Peripheral nerve injury alters excitatory synaptic transmission in lamina II of the rat dorsal horn. *J Physiol* **548**:131–138.

Koltzenburg M (1997) The sympathetic nervous system and pain. In: *The Pharmacology of Pain* (Dickenson A and Besson J–M, eds), pp. 61–91. Berlin: Springer–Verlag.

Koltzenburg M (1996) Afferent mechanisms mediating pain and hyperalgesia in neuralgia. In: *Reflex Sympathetic Dystrophy: A Reappraisal* (Jänig W and Stanton–Hicks M, eds), pp. 123–150. Seattle: IASP Press.

Koltzenburg M, Kees S, Budweiser S, Ochs G, and Toyka KV (1994*a*) The properties of unmyelinated afferents change in a chronic constriction neuropathy. In: *Proceedings of the VIIth World Congress on Pain* (Gebhart GF, Hammond DL, and Jensen TS, eds), pp. 511–522. Seattle: IASP Press.

Koltzenburg M, Lundberg LER, and Torebjörk HE (1992) Dynamic and static components of mechanical hyperalgesia in human hairy skin. *Pain* **51**:207–219.

Koltzenburg M, Torebjörk HE, and Wahren LK (1994*b*) Nociceptor modulated central sensitization causes mechanical hyperalgesia in acute chemogenic and chronic neuropathic pain. *Brain* **117** (Pt 3):579–591.

Koppert W, Dern SK, Sittl R, Albrecht S, Schuttler J, and Schmelz M (2001) A new model of electrically evoked pain and hyperalgesia in human skin: the effects of intravenous alfentanil, S(+)-ketamine, and lidocaine. *Anesthesiology* **95**:395–402.

Lai J, Porreca F, Hunter JC, and Gold MS (2004) Voltage-gated sodium channels and hyperalgesia. *Annu Rev Pharmacol Toxicol* **44**:371–397.

Laird JM and Bennett GJ (1993) An electrophysiological study of dorsal horn neurons in the spinal cord of rats with an experimental peripheral neuropathy. *J Neurophysiol* **69**:2072–2085.

LaMotte RH, Shain CN, Simone DA, and Tsai EF (1991) Neurogenic hyperalgesia: psychophysical studies of underlying mechanisms. *J Neurophysiol* **66**:190–211.

Leffler A, Cummins TR, Dib–Hajj SD, Hormuzdiar WN, Black JA, and Waxman SG (2002) GDNF and NGF reverse changes in repriming of TTX-sensitive Na(+) currents following axotomy of dorsal root ganglion neurons. *J Neurophysiol* **88**:650–658.

Lehky TJ, Leonard GD, Wilson RH, Grem JL, and Floeter MK (2004) Oxaliplatin-induced neurotoxicity: acute hyperexcitability and chronic neuropathy. *Muscle Nerve* 29:387–392.

Lewis T (1942) *Pain*. New York: Macmillan.

Lindblom U (1994) Analysis of abnormal touch, pain, and temperature sensation in patients. In: *Touch, Temperature, and Pain in Health and Disease: Mechanisms and Assessments* (Boivie J, Hansson P, and Lindblom U, eds), pp. 63–84. Seattle: IASP Press.

Lisney SJ (1989) Regeneration of unmyelinated axons after injury of mammalian peripheral nerve. *Q J Exp Physiol* **74**:757–784.

Lisney SJ and Devor M (1987) Afterdischarge and interactions among fibers in damaged peripheral nerve in the rat. *Brain Res* **415**:122–136.

Liu HX and Hökfelt T (2002) The participation of galanin in pain processing at the spinal level. *Trends Pharmacol Sci* **23**:468–474.

Loh L and Nathan PW (1978) Painful peripheral states and sympathetic blocks. *J Neurol Neurosurg Psychiat* **41**:664–671.

Ma C, Shu Y, Zheng Z, *et al.* (2003) Similar electrophysiological changes in axotomized and neighboring intact dorsal root ganglion neurons. *J Neurophysiol* **89**:1588–1602.

Malmberg AB, Chen C, Tonegawa S, and Basbaum AI (1997) Preserved acute pain and reduced neuropathic pain in mice lacking PKC gamma. *Science* **278**:279–283.

Mao J, Price DD, Phillips LL, Lu J, and Mayer DJ (1995) Increases in protein kinase C gamma immunoreactivity in the spinal cord dorsal horn of rats with painful mononeuropathy. *Neurosci Lett* **198**:75–78.

Martyn C and Hughes RAC (1998) Peripheral neuropathies. In: *The Epidemiology of Neurological Disorders* (Martyn CN and Hughes RAC, eds), pp. 96–117. London: BMJ Books.

Maves TJ, Pechman PS, Gebhart GF, and Meller ST (1993) Continuous infusion of acidified saline around the rat sciatic nerve produces a reversible thermal hyperalgesia. *Abstract of 7th World Congress on Pain*, p. 31.

Maves TJ, Pechman PS, Gebhart GF, and Meller ST (1992) Possible chemical contribution from chromic gut sutures produces disorders of pain sensation like those seen in man. *Pain* **54**:57–69.

McLachlan EM, Jänig W, Devor M, and Michaelis M (1993) Peripheral nerve injury triggers noradrenergic sprouting within dorsal root ganglia. *Nature* **363**:543–546.

Merskey H and Bogduk M (1994) *Classification of chronic pain.* Seattle: IASP Press.

Meyer RA and Campbell JN (1987) Coupling between unmyelinated peripheral nerve fibers does not involve sympathetic efferent fibers. *Brain Res* **437**:181–182.

Meyer RA, Ringkamp M, Campbell JN, and Raja SN (2005) Peripheral mechanisms of cutaneous nociception. In: *Wall and Melzack's Textbook of Pain* (McMahon SB and Koltzenburg M, eds). Edinburgh: Churchill Livingstone.

Michaelis M, Blenk KH, Jänig W, and Vogel C (1995) Development of spontaneous activity and mechanosensitivity in axotomized afferent nerve fibers during the first hours after nerve transection in rats. *J Neurophysiol* **74**:1020–1027.

Michaelis M, Devor M, and Jänig W (1996) Sympathetic modulation of activity in rat dorsal root ganglion neurons changes over time following peripheral nerve injury. *J Neurophysiol* **76**:753–763.

Michaelis M, Liu X, and Jänig W (2000) Axotomized and intact muscle afferents but no skin afferents develop ongoing discharges of dorsal root ganglion origin after peripheral nerve lesion. *J Neurosci* **20**:2742–2748.

Mogil JS, Yu L, and Basbaum AI (2000) Pain genes? Natural variation and transgenic mutants. *Annu Rev Neurosci* **23**:777–811.

Moore KA, Kohno T, Karchewski LA, Scholz J, Baba H, and Woolf CJ (2002) Partial peripheral nerve injury promotes a selective loss of GABAergic inhibition in the superficial dorsal horn of the spinal cord. *J Neurosci* **22**:6724–6731.

Noguchi K, De Leon M, Nahin RL, Senba E, and Ruda MA (1993) Quantification of axotomy induced alteration of neuropeptide mRNAs in dorsal root ganglion neurons with special reference to neuropeptide Y mRNA and the effects of neonatal capsaicin treatment. *J Neurosci Res* **35**:54–66.

Nordin M, Nyström B, Wallin U, and Hagbarth K–E (1984) Ectopic sensory discharges and paresthesiae in patients with disorders of peripheral nerves, dorsal roots and dorsal columns. *Pain* **20**:231–245.

Novakovic SD, Tzoumaka E, McGivern JG, *et al.* (1998) Distribution of the tetrodotoxin-resistant sodium channel PN3 in rat sensory neurons in normal and neuropathic conditions. *J Neurosci* **18**:2174–2187.

Ochoa J, Torebjörk HE, Culp WJ, and Schady W (1982) Abnormal spontaneous activity in single sensory nerve fibers in humans. *Muscle Nerve* **5**:S74–S77.

Ochoa JL and Yarnitsky D (1994) The triple cold syndrome: cold hyperalgesia, cold hypoaesthesia and cold skin in peripheral nerve disease. *Brain* **117**:185–197.

Ochoa JL and Yarnitsky D (1993) Mechanical hyperalgesias in neuropathic pain patients: dynamic and static subtypes. *Ann Neurol* **33**:465–472.

Ochs G, Schenk M, and Struppler A (1989) Painful dysaesthesias following peripheral nerve injury: a clinical and electrophysiological study. *Brain Res* **496**:228–240.

O'Halloran KD and Perl ER (1997) Effects of partial nerve injury on the responses of C-fiber polymodal nociceptors to adrenergic agonists. *Brain Res* **759**:233–240.

Okamoto M, Baba H, Goldstein PA, Higashi H, Shimoji K, and Yoshimura M (2001) Functional reorganization of sensory pathways in the rat spinal dorsal horn following peripheral nerve injury. *J Physiol* **532**:241–250.

Ørstavik K, Weidner C, Schmidt R, *et al.* (2003) Pathological C-fibres in patients with a chronic painful condition. *Brain* **126**:567–578.

Ossipov MH, Zhang ET, Carvajal C, *et al.* (2002) Selective mediation of nerve injury-induced tactile hypersensitivity by neuropeptide Y. *J Neurosci* **22**:9858–9867.

Palecek J, Paleckova V, Dougherty PM, Carlton SM, and Willis WD (1992) Responses of spinothalamic tract cells to mechanical and thermal stimulation of skin in rats with experimental peripheral neuropathy. *J Neurophysiol* **67**:1562–1573.

Pappagallo M, Oaklander AL, Quatrano–Piacentini AL, Clark MR, and Raja SN (2000) Heterogenous patterns of sensory dysfunction in postherpetic neuralgia suggest multiple pathophysiologic mechanisms. *Anesthesiology* **92**:691–698.

Perl ER (1999) Causalgia, pathological pain, and adrenergic receptors. *Proc Natl Acad Sci USA* **96**:7664–7667.

Perl ER (1994) Causalgia and reflex sympathetic dystrophy revisited. In: *Touch, Temperature, and Pain in Health and Disease: Mechanisms and Assessments* (Boivie J, Hansson P, and Lindblom U, eds), pp. 231–248. Seattle: IASP Press.

Pertovaara A, Wei H, and Hamalainen MM (1996) Lidocaine in the rostroventromedial medulla and the periaqueductal gray attenuates allodynia in neuropathic rats. *Neurosci Lett* **218**:127–130.

Petersen M, Zhang J, Zhang JM, and LaMotte RH (1996) Abnormal spontaneous activity and responses to norepinephrine in dissociated dorsal root ganglion cells after chronic nerve constriction. *Pain* **67**:391–397.

Polgar E, Hughes DI, Riddell JS, Maxwell DJ, Puskar Z, and Todd AJ (2003) Selective loss of spinal GABAergic or glycinergic neurons is not necessary for development of thermal hyperalgesia in the chronic constriction injury model of neuropathic pain. *Pain* **104**:229–239.

Price DD, Bennett GJ, and Rafii A (1989) Psychophysical observations on patients with neuropathic pain relieved by a sympathetic block. *Pain* **36**:273–288.

Price DD, Long S, and Huitt C (1992) Sensory testing of pathophysiological mechanisms of pain in patients with reflex sympathetic dystrophy. *Pain* **49**:163–173.

Ramer MS, Thompson SW, and McMahon SB (1999) Causes and consequences of sympathetic basket formation in dorsal root ganglia. *Pain* **Suppl 6**:S111–S120.

Reeh PW, Bayer J, Kocher L, and Handwerker HO (1987) Sensitization of nociceptive cutaneous nerve fibers from the rat's tail by noxious mechanical stimulation. *Exp Brain Res* **65**:505–512.

Ringkamp M, Ali Z, Chien HF, Campbell JN, Flavahan NA, and Meyer RA (1996) Alpha-one adrenergic sensitivity in cutaneous C-fiber nociceptors following an L6 nerve ligation in monkey. *Abstract of 8th World Congress on Pain*, p. 349.

Ringkamp M, Eschenfelder S, Grethel EJ, *et al.* (1999) Lumbar sympathectomy failed to reverse mechanical allodynia- and hyperalgesia-like behavior in rats with L5 spinal nerve injury. *Pain* **79**:143–153.

Risling M, Dalsgaard CJ, and Terenius L (1985) Neuropeptide Y-like immunoreactivity in the lumbosacral pia mater in normal cats and after sciatic neuroma formation. *Brain Res* **358**:372–375.

Rodin BE and Kruger L (1984) Deafferentation in animals as a model for the study of pain: an alternative hypothesis. *Brain Res* **319**:213–228.

Rowbotham MC, Davies PS, and Fields HL (1995) Topical lidocaine gel relieves postherpetic neuralgia. *Ann Neurol* **37**:246–253.

Rowbotham MC and Fields HL (1989) Topical lidocaine reduces pain in post-herpetic neuralgia. *Pain* **38**:297–301.

Sato J and Perl ER (1991) Adrenergic excitation of cutaneous pain receptors induced by peripheral nerve injury. *Science* **251**:1608–1610.

Schmelz M, Schmid R, Handwerker HO, and Torebjörk HE (2000) Encoding of burning pain from capsaicin-treated human skin in two categories of unmyelinated nerve fibres. *Brain* **123**:560–571.

Schmelz M, Schmidt R, Ringkamp M, Handwerker HO, and Torebjörk HE (1994) Sensitization of insensitive branches of nociceptors in human skin. *J Physiol (Lond)* **480**:389–394.

Schmidt R, Schmelz M, Torebjörk HE, and Handwerker HO (2000) Mechano-insensitive nociceptors encode pain evoked by tonic pressure to human skin. *Neuroscience* **98**:793–800.

Selig DK, Meyer RA, and Campbell JN (1993) Noradrenaline excitation of cutaneous nociceptors two weeks after ligation of spinal nerve L7 in monkey. *Soc Neurosci Abstr* **19**:326.

Seltzer Z, Dubner R, and Shir Y (1990) A novel behavioral model of neuropathic pain disorders produced in rats by partial sciatic nerve injury. *Pain* **43**:205–218.

Shehab SA, Spike RC, and Todd AJ (2003) Evidence against cholera toxin B subunit as a reliable tracer for sprouting of primary afferents following peripheral nerve injury. *Brain Res* **964**:218–227.

Sherbourne CD, Gonzales R, Goldyne ME, and Levine JD (1992) Norepinephrine-induced increase in sympathetic neuron-derived prostaglandins is independent of neuronal release mechanisms. *Neurosci Lett* **139**:188–190.

Shinder V, Govrin–Lippmann R, Cohen S, *et al.* (1999) Structural basis of sympathetic-sensory coupling in rat and human dorsal root ganglia following peripheral nerve injury. *J Neurocytol* **28**:743–761.

Simone DA, Baumann TK, and LaMotte RH (1989) Dose-dependent pain and mechanical hyperalgesia in humans after intradermal injection of capsaicin. *Pain* **38**:99–107.

Sleeper AA, Cummins TR, Dib–Hajj SD, *et al.* (2000) Changes in expression of two tetrodotoxin-resistant sodium channels and their currents in dorsal root ganglion neurons after sciatic nerve injury but not rhizotomy. *J Neurosci* **20**:7279–7289.

Sommer C, Galbraith JA, Heckman HM, and Myers RR (1993) Pathology of experimental compression neuropathy producing hyperesthesia. *J Neuropathol Exp Neurol* **52**:223–233.

Sommer C and Kress M (2004) Recent findings on how proinflammatory cytokines cause pain: peripheral mechanisms in inflammatory and neuropathic hyperalgesia. *Neurosci Lett* **361**:184–187.

Sommer C, Schmidt C, and George A (1998) Hyperalgesia in experimental neuropathy is dependent on the TNF receptor 1. *Exp Neurol* **151**:138–142.

Sorkin LS, Xiao WH, Wagner R, and Myers RR (1997) Tumour necrosis factor-alpha induces ectopic activity in nociceptive primary afferent fibres. *Neuroscience* **81**:255–262.

Stanton–Hicks M, Jänig W, Hassenbusch S, Haddox JD, Boas R, and Wilson P (1995) Reflex sympathetic dystrophy: changing concepts and taxonomy. *Pain* **63**:127–133.

Stevens RT, Hodge CJ, and Apkarian V (1983) Catecholamine varicosities in cat dorsal root ganglion and spinal ventral roots. *Brain Res* **261**:151–154.

Streit WJ, Graeber MB, and Kreutzberg GW (1988) Functional plasticity of microglia: a review. *GLIA* **1**:301–307.

Sun H, Ren K, Zhong CM, *et al.* (2001) Nerve injury-induced tactile allodynia is mediated via ascending spinal dorsal column projections. *Pain* **90**:105–111.

Suzuki R, Kontinen VK, Matthews E, Williams E, and Dickenson AH (2000) Enlargement of the receptive field size to low intensity mechanical stimulation in the rat spinal nerve ligation model of neuropathy. *Exp Neurol* **163**:408–413.

Thomas PK and Holdorff B (1993) Neuropathy due to physical agents. In: *Peripheral Neuropathy* (Dyck PJ, Thomas PK, Griffin JW, Low P, and Poduslo JF, eds), pp. 990–1013. Philadelphia: Saunders.

Thompson SWN and Majithia AA (1998) Leukemia inhibitory factor induces sympathetic sprouting in intact dorsal root ganglia in the adult rat in vivo. *J Physiol (Lond)* **506**:809–816.

Tong YG, Wang HF, Ju G, Grant G, Hökfelt T, and Zhang X (1999) Increased uptake and transport of cholera toxin B-subunit in dorsal root ganglion neurons after peripheral axotomy: possible implications for sensory sprouting. *J Comp Neurol* **404**:143–158.

Torebjörk E (1990) Clinical and neurophysiological observations relating to pathophysiological mechanisms in reflex sympathetic dystrophy. In: *Reflex Sympathetic Dystrophy* (Stanton–Hicks M, Jänig W, and Boas RA, eds), pp. 71–80. Boston: Kluwer Academic Publishers.

Torebjörk E, Wahren L, Wallin G, Hallin R, and Koltzenburg M (1995) Noradrenaline-evoked pain in neuralgia. *Pain* **63**:11–20.

Tracey DJ, Cunningham JE, and Romm MA (1995) Peripheral hyperalgesia in experimental neuropathy: mediation by alpha 2-adrenoreceptors on post-ganglionic sympathetic terminals. *Pain* **60**:317–327.

Treede R–D, Davis KD, Campbell JN, and Raja SN (1992) The plasticity of cutaneous hyperalgesia during sympathetic ganglion blockade in patients with neuropathic pain. *Brain* **115**:607–621.

Tsuda M, Shigemoto–Mogami Y, Koizumi S, *et al.* (2003) P2X4 receptors induced in spinal microglia gate tactile allodynia after nerve injury. *Nature* **424**:778–783.

Utzschneider D, Kocsis J, and Devor M (1992) Mutual excitation among dorsal root ganglion neurons in the rat. *Neurosci Lett* **146**:53–56.

Valder CR, Liu JJ, Song YH, and Luo ZD (2003) Coupling gene chip analyses and rat genetic variances in identifying potential target genes that may contribute to neuropathic allodynia development. *J Neurochem* **87**:560–573.

Vallbo ÅB, Hagbarth KE, Torebjörk HE, and Wallin BG (1979) Somatosensory, proprioceptive, and sympathetic activity in human peripheral nerves. *Physiol Rev* **59**:919–957.

Villar MJ, Cortes R, Theodorsson E, *et al.* (1989) Neuropeptide expression in rat dorsal root ganglion cells and spinal cord after peripheral nerve injury with special reference to galanin. *Neuroscience* **33**:587–604.

Wahren LK and Torebjörk E (1992) Quantitative sensory tests in patients with neuralgia 11 to 25 years after injury. *Pain* **48**:237–244.

Wahren LK, Torebjörk E, and Jørum E (1989) Central suppression of cold-induced C fibre pain by myelinated fibre input. *Pain* **38**:313–319.

Wakisaka S, Kajander KC, and Bennett GJ (1991) Increased neuropeptide Y (NPY)-like immuno-reactivity in rat sensory neurons following peripheral axotomy. *Neurosci Lett* **124**:200–203.

Wall PD and Devor M (1981) The effect of peripheral nerve injury on dorsal root potentials and on transmission of afferent signals into the spinal cord. *Brain Res* **209**:95–111.

Wall PD and Gutnick M (1974) Properties of afferent nerve impulses originating from a neuroma. *Nature* **248**:740–743.

Wang H, Sun H, Della PK, *et al.* (2002) Chronic neuropathic pain is accompanied by global changes in gene expression and shares pathobiology with neurodegenerative diseases. *Neuroscience* **114**:529–546.

Wang Z, Gardell LR, Ossipov MH, *et al.* (2001) Pronociceptive actions of dynorphin maintain chronic neuropathic pain. *J Neurosci* **21**:1779–1786.

Wasner G, Schwarz K, Schattschneider J, Binder A, Jensen TS, and Baron R (2004) Interaction between histamine-induced itch and experimental muscle pain. *Eur J Pain* **8**:179–185.

Watkins LR, Milligan ED, and Maier SF (2001) Glial activation: a driving force for pathological pain. *Trends Neurosci* **24**:450–455.

Waxman SG (2001) Transcriptional channelopathies: an emerging class of disorders. *Nat Rev Neurosci* **2**:652–659.

Waxman SG, Cummins TR, Black JA, and Dib–Hajj S (2002) Diverse functions and dynamic expression of neuronal sodium channels. *Novartis Found Symp* **241**:34–51.

Woolf CJ and Doubell TP (1994) The pathophysiology of chronic pain – increased sensitivity to low threshold A beta-fibre inputs. *Curr Opin Neurobiol* **4**:525–534.

Woolf CJ, Bennett GJ, Doherty M, *et al.* (1998) Towards a mechansim-based classification of pain? *Pain* **77**:227–229.

Woolf CJ, Shortland P, and Coggeshall RE (1992) Peripheral nerve injury triggers central sprouting of myelinated afferents. *Nature* **355**:75–78.

Wu G, Ringkamp M, Hartke TV, *et al.* (2001) Early onset of spontaneous activity in uninjured C-fiber nociceptors after injury to neighboring nerve fibers. *J Neurosci* **21**:RC140.

Xiao HS, Huang QH, Zhang FX, *et al.* (2002) Identification of gene expression profile of dorsal root ganglion in the rat peripheral axotomy model of neuropathic pain. *Proc Natl Acad Sci USA* **99**:8360–8365.

Xie Y, Zhang J, Petersen M, and LaMotte RH (1995) Functional changes in dorsal root ganglion cells after chronic nerve constriction in the rat. *J Neurophysiol* **73**:1811–1820.

Yang EK, Takimoto K, Hayashi Y, de Groat WC, and Yoshimura N (2004*a*) Altered expression of potassium channel subunit mRNA and alpha-dendrotoxin sensitivity of potassium currents in rat dorsal root ganglion neurons after axotomy. *Neuroscience* **123**:867–874.

Yang Y, Wang Y, Li S, *et al.* (2004*b*) Mutations in SCN9A, encoding a sodium channel alpha subunit, in patients with primary erythermalgia. *J Med Genet* **41**:171–174.

Yao H, Donnelly DF, Ma C, and LaMotte RH (2003) Upregulation of the hyperpolarization-activated cation current after chronic compression of the dorsal root ganglion. *J Neurosci* **23**:2069–2074.

Yarnitsky D and Ochoa JL (1990) Release of cold-induced burning pain by block of cold-specific afferent input. *Brain* **113**:893–902.

Zhang JM, Song XJ, and LaMotte RH (1997) An in vitro study of ectopic discharge generation and adrenergic sensitivity in the intact, nerve-injured rat dorsal root ganglion. *Pain* **72**:51–57.

Ziegler EA, Magerl W, Meyer RA, and Treede RD (1999) Secondary hyperalgesia to punctate mechanical stimuli. Central sensitization to A-fibre nociceptor input. *Brain* **122** (**Pt 12**):2245–2257.

Chapter 6

Targets in pain and analgesia

Anthony Dickenson and Rie Suzuki

6.1 Introduction

For many years, the neurobiological basis for both the understanding of the causes and, therefore, the improvement of the treatment of pain states remained somewhat unclear. The development of a number of animal models of inflammation and nerve injury and, even more recently, of cancer pains, produced by manipulation of either peripheral tissue or nerves, has greatly aided the understanding of the mechanisms of pain. These animal studies have been, to some extent, translated into humans and have pointed out many examples of a marked plasticity in both the signalling and modulation of pain. Although anatomical changes may make a contribution under certain conditions, much of the observed plasticity appears to involve recruitment of different transmitters, receptors, and channels. In the longer term, gene changes may further add to the complexity of the pharmacological changes. Over the past two decades our knowledge of the pharmacology of pain and analgesia has made enormous strides. A long list of interacting mediators, transmitters, and receptors — some peripheral, some central, and some located at both sites — has been established.

Pain provides a model system for examining how the CNS deals with sensory inputs from both the external and internal areas of the body. Not surprisingly, the intensity, duration, and origins of the pain will all have a bearing on the mechanisms underlying the final perception of the patient. There are a number of classifications of pain based on the cause, the duration, and severity. In broad terms, clinically important pains can be classified as those from tissue damage (often involving inflammation), from nerve damage, cancer pains, and headaches. As shown by cancer, surgery, and trauma, different types of pain with different intensities can coexist in an individual patient.

The arrival of activity from peripheral nerves into the spinal cord is the first stage in the processing of pain: changes caused by the balance between excitatory and inhibitory effects within spinal circuits will alter both the motor reflex responses and the messages sent through ascending tracts to higher centres of the brain (Dickenson, 1994, 1996; Hunt and Mantyh, 2001; Yaksh, 1993). The 'gate theory of pain' predicted the importance of interactions at the spinal level (Wall, 1978). However, due to the potential recruitment of different signalling mechanisms as the intensity of the stimulus increases, it is important to note that behavioural studies in animals (and humans) where thresholds are measured, may not provide information on systems brought into play with suprathreshold stimuli. These latter stimuli are those that create clinical pain syndromes and to study these with approaches such as electrophysiology, despite the constraints of anaesthesia, can be useful. Figure 6.1 depicts examples of neuronal responses in vivo.

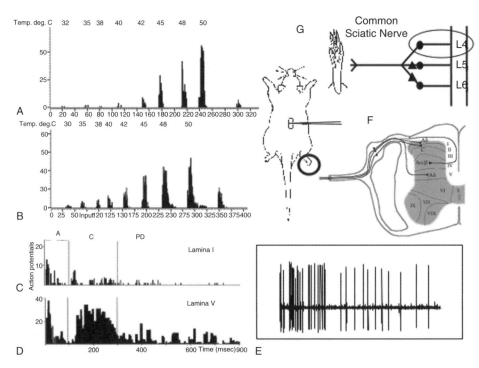

Fig. 6.1 Examples of neuronal activity that can be recorded in anaesthetized animals and related to the processes of pain that occur above the behavioural threshold. **A** and **B** show examples of the neuronal responses to controlled natural stimuli — in this case, thermal. **A** shows the evoked responses of a high-threshold lamina I neurone that only responds in the noxious range to temperatures of 45°C, whereas **B** shows a wide-dynamic range neurone that codes through warm to noxious. **C** and **D** show the electrically evoked responses of these neuronal classes: the high-threshold neurone in **C** has a small evoked constant response to repeated stimuli, whereas the large response of the WDR cell in **D** is due to wind-up of the response. **E** shows an oscilloscope trace of this WDR cell response. The laminae of the spinal cord are shown in **F**. Neurones can be studied in the normal state but also after inflammation or nerve injury as shown in **G**, a schematic diagram of the spinal nerve ligation model.

In broad terms, our other sensations (vision, hearing, taste) are neutral — we make decisions on whether we approve, ignore, or disapprove of these inputs. However, pain is not just a sensation but a spinal reflex motor response, and an affective response which, very importantly, is automatically unpleasant, aversive, and threatening. Thus, the control of pain has to take into account both the sensory and psychological components of the stimulus.

These mechanisms of pain and the ability to control pain may alter in different pain states. This is significant when considering a rational basis for the treatment of both inflammatory and neuropathic pain where the damage to tissue and nerve leads to alterations in both the peripheral and central mechanisms of pain signalling. In terms of existing drug therapies, this plasticity (i.e. the ability of the system to change in the face of a particular pain syndrome) is the reason for the effectiveness of NSAIDs in inflammatory conditions, for the efficacy of anticonvulsants in neuropathic pains, and yet may also be responsible for some of the limitations in the effectiveness of opioids in neuropathic pain (Dickenson and Suzuki, 1999; Dray, 1995; Sindrup and Jensen, 1999).

Acute, everyday pains involve peripheral activation of nociceptors and, as the action potentials invade the spinal terminals, transmitter release (glutamate and peptides) occurs, followed by activation of their receptors. A balance between excitation and inhibition results so that activation of the excitatory receptors for glutamate is controlled by inhibitions such as those induced by GABA. For example, much of the low-threshold, tactile information that enters the spinal cord is controlled by the $GABA_A$ receptor and suppressed under normal conditions. However, given that these amino acids are responsible for most of the fast excitatory and inhibitory transmission in the CNS, manipulation of their receptors is fraught with the problem of unacceptable side-effects (Dickenson, 1996).

6.2 Peripheral events

The first stage in the transmission of acute pain involves activation of specialized sensory receptors on peripheral C-fibres — the nociceptors. These receptors include mechano-, chemo-, and thermoreceptors. The nociceptors associated with C-fibres are often termed polymodal since they can respond to a variety of adequate stimuli (Sorkin and Carlton, 1997). Figure 6.3 depicts some of the sites of action of clinically used drugs at central and peripheral sites. The rationale for their use is discussed in the following sections.

6.2.1 Tissue damage

The peripheral terminals of small-diameter neurones, especially in conditions of tissue damage, may be excited by a number of endogenous chemical mediators that include prostanoids, protons, 5HT, ATP, and bradykinin. These chemical mediators then interact to cause a sensitization of nociceptors so that afferent activity to a given stimulus is increased by the presence of inflammation. This is primary hyperalgesia (Dray, 1997).

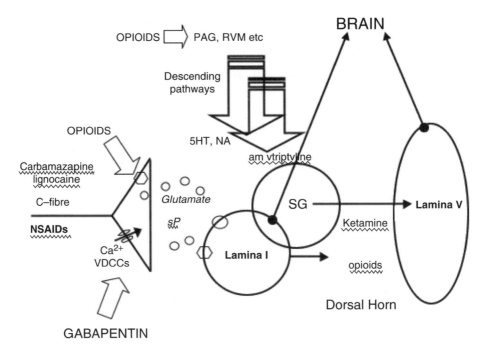

Fig. 6.2 A schematic diagram of a C-fibre synapsing onto the spinal cord circuitry that projects to the brain. The interactions between a number of clinically used drugs and the anatomical and physio-pharmacological substrates are shown.

One of the most important components in inflammation is the production of arachidonic acid metabolites, giving rise to a large number of eicosanoids, the prostaglandins. These chemicals do not normally activate nociceptors directly but, by contrast, reduce the C-fibre threshold and so sensitize them to other mediators and stimuli. Thus, the use of both steroids and the non-steroidal anti-inflammatory (NSAIDs) drugs is based on their ability to block the conversion of arachidonic acid to these mediators. Importantly, a second inducible form of COX, COX-2, has been described. The main action of the NSAIDs is to inhibit COX-1, but as this form is the constitutive enzyme, COX-1 inhibition results in the gastric and other side-effects of the NSAIDs. So, the new generation of selective COX-2 inhibitors have improved therapeutic profiles, as this form of the enzyme is induced at the site of tissue damage. Importantly though, despite the improvements in side-effects, the degree of analgesia is the same as for the older drugs (Camu *et al.*, 2003).

Bradykinin is another chemical with important peripheral actions but, as yet, cannot be manipulated in any direct way by drugs in humans. Hydrogen ions accumulate in damaged tissue and so pH is lowered. The tissue levels of these protons thereby increase in inflammation and ischaemia and may activate nociceptors directly via their

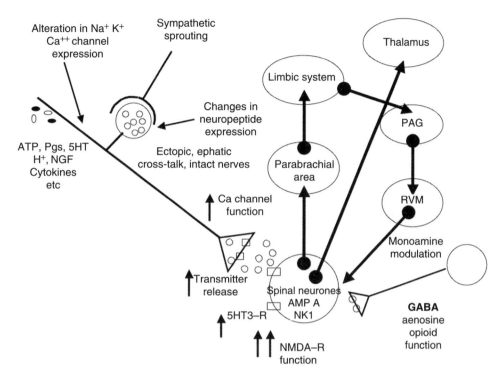

Fig. 6.3 A diagram showing some of the events described in this chapter and how these may be peripheral or central targets for novel pain treatments. A peripheral C-fibre is shown synapsing with spinal neurones that in turn project to various parts of the brain. Some of the changes that accompany nerve injury are shown above the fibre, whereas those that result from inflammation are shown below. Once the fibres terminate in the spinal cord, the increases in transmitter release and peptide and NMDA receptor function appear to be common to both pain states. The excitatory events can be modulated, increased, and decreased by the level of activity in monoamine, GABA, opioid, and other transmitters acting through intrinsic and descending pathways.

own family of ion channels (ASICs) as well as sensitizing them to mechanical stimulation. ATP is an algogen released from damaged cells and has a large number of receptors on sensory fibres. Serotonin, 5-hydroxytrptamine (5HT), can also produce an excitation of nociceptive afferents via the activation of its large number of primary afferent receptors. The key role, but not the exact mechanisms of action, of 5HT in the pain associated with migraine and other headaches is well established, but little is known about the actions of this mediator in other, non-cranial pains (Goadsby, 2002).

Substance P and CGRP released from the peripheral terminals of primary afferents (via the axon reflex) cause a number of effects including vasodilation, plasma extravasation, and mast cell degranulation. Released ATP from mast cells can result in direct nociceptor activation. Other factors such as nerve growth factor (NGF) and cytokines are also important at the peripheral level, and resultant changes in the phenotype of the sensory neurones have been shown (Sommer, 2001). Thus, tissue damage causes complex changes in the transduction of painful stimuli.

But why do C-fibres respond to such a range of peripheral painful stimuli? The answer is that a nociceptor is not a single entity but expresses a number of proteins that function as receptors or channels that sense and respond to thermal and chemical stimuli (Eglen *et al.*, 1999). It has long been known that capsaicin (the hot ingredient in chilli peppers) evokes a sensation of burning pain, but we now know this is because it activates the vanilloid receptors (VR/TRPV family) that act as temperature sensors. The TRPV family of receptors respond to cold and warmth and also to noxious temperatures. They also respond to ATP and other ligands, and so may integrate a number of painful stimuli. At present we are unclear about what mechanical sensors are, but some of the acid-sensing ion channels (ASICs) may have mechanical sensitivity. Thus we have a myriad of channels and receptors that allow peripheral fibres to respond to polymodal painful stimuli and to generate action potentials. In addition, we have cold and warm receptors that may contribute to thermal allodynias in pathological states. All of these receptors and channels are made in the dorsal root ganglion and are transported throughout the nerve. Novel therapies could arise from drugs that block these sensors. A problem is the lack of selective drugs. The role of particular channels and associated proteins has been greatly advanced by the development of transgenic 'gene knock-out' mice, where particular genes have been genetically deleted. This approach has been successful in defining roles for sodium channels and ATP receptors where no blockers are available (Souslova *et al.*, 2000).

Finally, the amount that these 'sensors' are altered by pathology, and their functional roles changed, has to be considered. For example, after nerve injury, the current caused by capsaicin activiation of the VR1 receptor is markedly reduced in the injured cells, whereas that caused by ATP at the P2X3 receptor is upregulated (Fukuoka *et al.*, 2002, Kage *et al.*, 2002).

Thus, the attractive idea of blocking pain where it starts, in the periphery, using drugs that do not have to penetrate the CNS and so are devoid of central side-effects such as sedation and psychomotor effects is complicated by the number of potential targets. NSAIDs have a ceiling effect, but would blocking a particular receptor for ATP or protons have sufficient impact on pain when multiple mediators are being released? These questions can only be answered when selective drugs are developed and tested in patients.

6.2.2 **Nerve damage**

Neuropathic pain states are characterized by both negative symptoms (sensory loss, numbness) and the positive symptoms of allodynia, hyperalgesia, and ongoing pain that are unlike the consequences of damage to our other sensory systems. These positive symptoms strongly suggest changes within the nervous system that are excessive attempts to compensate for sensory loss, since nerve damage should equate with deficits. The initial events of neuropathic pain are thought to be generated in the peripheral sensory neurones within the nerve itself at the site of damage, and so are independent of peripheral nociceptor activation. Following damage to peripheral nerves, a number of changes can be produced in nerves, in terms of activity, properties, and transmitter content. The recent advent of a number of animal models of neuropathic pain states has facilitated understanding of the peripheral mechanisms involved. Damaged nerves may start to generate ongoing ectopic activity due to the accumulation and clustering of sodium channels around the damaged axons, and there is also evidence that mechanoreceptors become highly sensitive to applied stimuli. This aberrant activity can then start to spread rapidly to the cell body in the dorsal root ganglia. In addition to changes within the nerve, sympathetic efferents become able to activate sensory afferents. These peripheral ectopic impulses can cause spontaneous pain and prime the spinal cord to exhibit enhanced evoked responses to stimuli, which themselves have greater effects due to increased sensitivity of the peripheral nerves.

This peripheral activity may be a rational basis for the use of systemic local anaesthetics in neuropathic states, since damaged nerves have been shown to be highly sensitive to systemic sodium channel blockers. This too is probably part of the basis for the effects of established effective anti-convulsants that block sodium channels, such as carbamazepine. The site of actions of antidepressants and other adrenergic agents in the treatment of neuropathic pain are controversial. Recently, it has been clearly shown that C-fibres generate action potentials via both 'normal' and another population of unique sodium channels with very low tetrodotoxin sensitivity (channels that are different from those found in other tissues). These channels may become important targets for drugs since a systemic agent with selectivity for these channels would only block C-fibre activity . However, a downregulation of these channels after nerve injury may be more likely in the control of pain after tissue damage than neuropathy (Baron, 2000; Jensen and Baron, 2003; Suzuki and Dickenson, 2000; Waxman, 1999).

6.3 **Central excitatory systems**

The arrival of action potentials in the dorsal horn of the spinal cord, carrying the sensory information from nociceptors in inflammation or that generated both from nociceptors and intrinsically after nerve damage, add yet greater complexity to pain and analgesia. Within the CNS, not only are excitatory mechanisms vital but, in contrast to much of the peripheral signalling, the role of controlling inhibitory transmitter systems is of paramount importance (see Fig. 6.2).

As peripheral neurones become more active, action potentials arrive in their central terminals and calcium channels open in the membrane. Thus, calcium channels are activated and are critical for transmitter release and important in neuronal excitability. Results with agents that block neuronal voltage-sensitive calcium channels would also suggest that there is an increase in central neuronal excitability after both inflammation and nerve damage that involves the N-, P-, and T-type calcium channels (Vanegas and Schaible, 2000).

Gabapentin is an antiepileptic drug that has analgesic activity in neuropathic pain states from varying origins. Recent randomized controlled trials in patients concluded that gabapentin was effective in the treatment of these pain states (Rowbotham et al., 1998). The mechanism of action of gabapentin is not clearly established but it is thought the drug may interact with calcium channels since it binds to the alpha-2 delta subunit of these channels. How this translates into its clinical actions is unclear, since the subunit is found in all calcium channels — splice variants in DRG have been described. Furthermore, only the N-type channels show changes after nerve injury (Matthews and Dickenson, 2001). Agents that block transmitter release as the afferents enter the spinal cord have potential as a means of interrupting transmission at the first synapse in the polysynaptic pathways from periphery to the highest centres.

The large majority of primary afferents synapsing in the dorsal horn of the spinal cord, regardless of whether they are small or large diameter, contain and release glutamate. Glutamate has an excitatory effect on a number of receptors found on both postsynaptic spinal neurones, leading to a depolarization via three distinct receptor subclasses, the alpha-amino-3-hydroxy 5-methyl-4-isoxazeloproprionic acid (AMPA) receptor, the N-methyl-D-aspartate (NMDA) receptors, and the G-protein-linked metabotropic family of receptors. Also, peptides such as substance P, that acts on the NK1 receptor and CGRP, are co-released (Dickenson, 1997).

Glutamate is released in response to both acute and more persistent noxious stimuli and the AMPA-receptor activation is responsible for setting the baseline level of activity in the responses to both noxious inputs, as well as tactile stimuli. However, if a repetitive and high-frequency stimulation of C-fibres occurs, there is then an amplification and prolongation of the response of spinal dorsal horn neurones, so-called wind-up. This enhanced activity results from the activation of the NMDA receptor. When there are acute or low-frequency noxious or tactile inputs to the spinal cord, the activation of the NMDA receptor is not possible. The reason is that under normal physiological conditions the ion channel of this receptor is blocked by the normal levels of Mg^{++} found in nervous tissues. This unique Mg^{++} plug of the channel requires a repeated depolarization of the membrane to be removed, allowing the NMDA receptor channel to be activated. Here, it is likely that the co-release of the peptides in C-fibres is responsible for a prolonged non-NMDA activation of the neurone and subsequent removal of the block. Large amounts of calcium then enter the neurone, cause high levels of firing, and trigger a number of enzymes that include nitric oxide synthase (NOS). The production of NO, the highly diffusable gas, then leads to further transmitter release, more NMDA activiation, and a positive feedback loop. Furthermore, prostanoids may be produced centrally, particularily as COX-2 is constitutive in the spinal cord (Dickenson, 1997; Meller and Gebhart, 1993).

This NMDA-receptor activation has been clearly shown to play a key role in the hyperalgesia and enhancement of pain signalling and receptive field size seen in more persistent pain states including inflammation and neuropathic conditions . There are a number of antagonists at the multiple regulatory sites found on the NMDA receptor and its channel, including the licensed drug, ketamine, a potent channel blocker. Block of wind-up either by prevention of the peripheral drive needed to maintain activity with such as local anaesthetic or directly, such as with ketamine, can interrupt this central hyperexcitability, and this is known to be important in changed pain states. Thus wind-up can be induced in both volunteers and patients, and this, and pain symptoms, can be reduced by ketamine. Likewise, in patients with arthritis and fibromyalgia, abnormal wind-up can be measured (Staud *et al.*, 2003).

The long-term increase in pain sensitivity frequently seen following injury or peripheral nerve damage is thought to be due to both alterations in synaptic transmission and morphology within the spinal cord and to changes in descending controls from the brainstem. NK1-expressing laminae I–III neurones are the first neurones in the pathways from the periphery to the brain. They are not thought to make extensive local connections within the spinal cord but to be predominantly nociceptive-specific projection neurones that terminate extensively within the parabrachial area of the brainstem, with limited termination in the periaqueductal gray area, thalamus, and reticular formation (Todd, 2002). Importantly, the parabrachial area is thought to access areas of the brain such as the amygdala and hypothalamus that modulate descending serotinergic and noradrenergic inputs from the brainstem that regulate nociceptive processing at spinal levels (Bernard *et al.*, 1996). Selective ablation of laminae I-III NK1-expressing neurones within the spinal cord with substance P-saporin (SP-SAP) conjugate effectively prevented most of the increase in pain sensitivity that follows the establishment of peripheral inflammation and experimental peripheral neuropathy (Mantyh *et al.*, 1997; Nichols *et al.*, 1999).

It was then found that the effects of destruction of the ascending laminae I–III pathway is most readily explained by changes in descending controls. Electrophysiological changes recorded in SP-SAP treated rats include a loss of ability of deep dorsal horn neurones to code thermal, mechanical, and chemical responses. Since these changes are exactly mimicked by block of the excitatory 5HT3 receptor, and since 5HT only originates in the brain, there must be a disruption in descending facilitatory controls from the brainstem. The significant attenuation of chemical activity, wind-up, and receptive field sizes, together with the deficit in the coding of mechanical and thermal stimuli, demonstrates that ablation of the small population of laminae I–III neurones significantly reduces the excitability of the dorsal horn. Thus, a network of spinal and supraspinal circuits interact to allow both a changing spinal sensitivity in the face of peripheral inputs and close regulation of this plasticity by descending pathways from the brain, coupling the level of cord sensitivity to the behavioural and environmental context (Suzuki *et al.*, 2002). It therefore appears that there are differential supraspinal controls of primary afferent input, which could allow the brain to exert modality-dependent regulation of spinal neuronal responses. Under pathological conditions such as neuropathy, descending excitatory controls from the midbrain are likely to be enhanced, and excitatory influences predominate, resulting in yet more central sensitization and contributing to allodynia and hyperalgesia.

It has been shown that block of the RVM, where the serotonergic pathways relay, leads to a reduction in allodynia from nerve injury. Given that the brainstem areas involved in these sensory controls are also implicated in emotions, sleep, and autonomic responses, the state of mind of a patient may well be able to activate these same pathways and provide a basis for alterations in pain as a result of affective changes (Gauriau and Bernard, 2002).

Currently, the main use of 5HT3-receptor antagonists such as ondansetron has been for clinical treatment of postoperative and chemotherapy-induced emesis. Although progress in understanding the pathophysiological mechanisms underlying neuropathy has been considerable, the clinical management remains difficult and drugs such as anticonvulsants, antidepressants, and opioids only produce pain relief in a minority of patients (Sindrup and Jensen, 1999). Further studies are warranted to assess the clinical utility of block of faciltatory effects in the management of various pain states. Interestingly, there are suggestions that block of 5HT3 receptors can be effective in the treatment of fibromyalgias, where the widespread pains indicate the operation of a diffuse non-segmental facilitatory system such as the descending 5HT pathway (Kosek and Hannson, 1997; Lautenbacher and Rollman, 1997; Papadopoulos *et al.*, 2000).

Since pain leads to a number of other changes, including increases and decreases in inhibitory pathways such as those mediated by noradrenaline, 5HT and adenosine further add to the complex links between the sensory, affective, and other components of pain. Thus it appears that a balance between excitatory pathways and inhibitory systems from the brain to spinal cord starts to emerge. In terms of inhibitory systems, tricyclic antidepressants are effective in neuropathic pain and alpha-2 receptor agonists such as clonidine and newer more selective agents are analgesic, although sedation is a major problem (Sindrup and Jensen, 1999).

Overall, these studies indicate that it is likely that aberrant peripheral activity is amplified and enhanced by NMDA receptor-mediated spinal mechanisms in tissue damage and neuropathic pain and that the receptor is critical for both the induction and the maintenance of the pain. Thus, therapy after the initiating damage is still effective. Although there is much good human evidence for effectiveness of agents, especially ketamine, acting at the NMDA receptor complex, it would appear that although some individual patients get good pain relief in nerve injury situations, the majority cannot achieve complete pain control because dose escalation is prevented by the narrow therapeutic window of the existing drugs. These may include drugs acting on subtypes of the receptor such as the NR2B receptor (Carpenter and Dickenson, 2001).

6.4 Central inhibitory systems

Inhibitory systems are important in the control of events following C-fibre stimulation. Opioids are the major inhibitory controls on pain. Almost all clinically used opioid drugs act on the mu receptor (the receptor for morphine), and they can be highly effective analgesics in many patients, unless the complaint is nerve damage. There is no real consensus from clinical studies on the efficacy of morphine in neuropathic pain states (Rowbotham, 2001). Dose escalation with morphine was shown to produce good analgesia in one study and others have reported that, in general, morphine could be effective in a group of patients with neuropathy (Portenoy *et al.*, 1990). Another study concluded that opioids were entirely ineffective and, finally, that opioid analgesia was less in neuropathic pain patients as compared to a group with nociceptive pain. Resolution of this problem has important implications, yet a similar series of discrepant results can be found in the animal literature (Dickenson and Suzuki, 1999).

The mu opiate receptor is the main target for opioid drugs. The receptor is remarkably similar in structure and function in all species studied, so animal studies will be good predictors for clinical applications. Opioids act in the brain and, better understood, within the dorsal horn of the spinal cord. The spinal actions of opioids and their mechanisms of analgesia involve:

1. reduced transmitter release from nociceptive C-fibres. so that spinal neurones are less excited by incoming painful messages

2. postsynaptic inhibitions of neurones conveying information from the spinal cord to the brain.

This dual action of opioids can result in a total block of sensory inputs as they arrive in the spinal cord (Dickenson and Suzuki, 1999).

It would appear unlikely that any new drug acting on the mu opioid receptor would have different effects from the existing drugs, so that advances are being made in formulations and routes (spinal, patches, etc.) rather than different pharmacological agents. However, it may be that drugs acting on the δ and κ opioid receptors and the opioid receptor-like (ORL1) receptors could have different profiles, but progress has been slow and there are no clinically useful agents as yet.

6.5 **Conclusions**

We now have a good understanding of the basic mechanisms of pain transmission and analgesia and can say that hyperexcitability can be set up both peripherally and centrally. The latter means that minor peripheral inputs may cause severe pain. Figure 6.3 summarizes the interactions between the systems discussed here, in terms of how peripheral changes after nerve injury impact upon systems at many levels of the CNS. Table 6.1 lists the potential and existing targets that relate to pain and analgesia. However, there are many areas where our understanding is still inadequate. For example, individual differences in levels of pain, in the transition from acute to chronic pain, differences in susceptibility to neuropathic pain after nerve damage and in analgesic effectiveness may have a genetic basis. There is marked variability in animal genetic strains in terms of the sequelae of tissue and nerve damage and even in their responses to morphine (Wilson *et al.*, 2003). Given the huge range of human phenotypes, this may indicate important individual differences in susceptibility to pain and analgesia, but we

Table 6.1 A list of the receptors and channels that existing and potential novel (denoted by ?) therapeutic agents may act on

TRPV receptors	Peripheral — antagonist	Thermosensation
ASICs	Peripheral — antagonist	Low pH, mechanosensation
Na channels	Peripheral — antagonist	*Broad spectrum pains
TTX-R Na channels	Peripheral — antagonist	Inflammatory, neuropathic pains
K channels	Peripheral — opener	*Pain?
Gabapentinoids	Peripheral — antagonist	Neuropathic pains
Ca channels	Peripheral — antagonist	*N and P type — inflammatory and neuropathic pains
Cannabinoid receptors 1&2	Peripheral — agonist	Pain?
EP prostanoid receptors	Peripheral — antagonist	*Inflammatory pains
P2X receptors	Peripheral — antagonist	Tissue damage pains
P2Y receptors	Peripheral — antagonist	Tissue damage pains
5HT receptors	Peripheral — antagonist/ agonist	Pain? Headache
Bradykinin receptors	Peripheral — antagonist	Inflammatory pains?
NGF	Peripheral — antagonist	*Inflammatory, neuropathic pains?
GDNF, BDNF	Peripheral — antagonist	*Inflammatory, neuropathic pains?
Cytokines	Peripheral — antagonist	*Inflammatory, neuropathic pains?
AMPA receptors	Central — antagonist	*Broad spectrum pains
Kainate receptors	Central — antagonist	Broad spectrum pains
NMDA receptors	Central — antagonist/ subtypes	*Broad spectrum pains
Metabotropic receptors	Central — antagonist	*Broad spectrum pains
NK1 receptors	Central — antagonist	Inflammatory pains?
Other NK receptors	Central — antagonist	Inflammatory pains?
CGRP receptors	Central — antagonist	Pain?
Mu OR	Central — agonist	Broad spectrum pains
Delta OR	Central — agonist	Broad spectrum pains?
Kappa OR	Central — agonist	*Broad spectrum pains?
ORL1 receptor	Central — agonist	Broad spectrum pains?
Alpha–2 NA receptors	Central — agonist	*Broad spectrum pains?
5HT1 receptors	Peripheral/central — agonist	Pain? Headache
5HT3 receptors	Central — antagonist	Broad spectrum pains?
Galanin receptors	Central — R1 agonist	Neuropathic pains?
CCK receptors	Central — A antagonist	Adjuncts to opioids

* Indicates a system where there is good evidence for a role in pain and analgesia but where clinical use may be compromised by adverse effects of drugs acting on these targets.

have no way yet of monitoring this possibility. In order for pain to be better controlled, the knowledge we have of mechanisms needs to be translated into therapy.

Acknowledgements

We are funded by the Wellcome Trust and as part of the London Pain Consortium.

References

Baron, R. (2000) Peripheral neuropathic pain: from mechanisms to symptoms. *Clinical Journal of Pain,* **16,** S12–20.

Bernard, J., Bester, H. and Besson, J. (1996) Involvement of the spino-parabrachio-amygdaloid and hypothalamic pathways in the autonomic and affective emotional aspects of pain. *Progress in Brain Research,* **107,** 243–255.

Camu, F., Shi, L., and Vanlersberghe, C. (2003) The role of COX-2 inhibitors in pain modulation. *Drugs,* **63 (Suppl 1),** 1–7.

Carpenter, K. and Dickenson, A. (2001) Amino acids are still as exciting as ever. *Current opinion in Pharmacology,* **1,** 57–61.

Dickenson, A. (1994) Pharmacology of pain transmission and control. In *Pain 1996— An Updated Review. Refresher Course Syllabus* (ed. J. Campbell). IASP Press, Seattle, pp. 113–122.

Dickenson, A. (1997) Mechanisms of hypersensitivity: excitatory amino acid mechanisms and their control. In *The Pharmacology of Pain* (eds. A. Dickenson and J.–M. Besson). Springer–Verlag, New York/Berlin/Heidelberg, pp. 167–210.

Dickenson, A. and Suzuki, R. (1999) Function and dysfunction of opioid receptors in the spinal cord. In *Opioid Sensitivity of Chronic Noncancer Pain. Progress in Pain Research and Management,* Vol. 14 (eds. E. Kalso, H. McQuay, and Z. and Wiesenfeld–Hallin). IASP Press, Seattle, pp. 17–44.

Dickenson, A.H. (1996) Balances between excitatory and inhibitory events in the spinal cord and chronic pain. *Progress in Brain Research,* **110,** 225–231.

Dray, A. (1995) Inflammatory mediators of pain. *British Journal of Anaesthesia,* **75,** 125–131.

Dray, A. (1997) Pharmacology of peripheral afferent terminals. In *Anesthesia. Biologic Foundations* (eds. T. Yaksh, C. Lynch, W. Zapol, M. Maze, J. Biebuyck, and L. Saidman). Lippincott–Raven, Philadelphia/New York, pp. 543–556.

Eglen, R., Hunter, J., and Dray, A. (1999) Ions in the fire: recent ion-channel research and approaches to pain therapy. *Trends in Pharmacological Sciences,* **20,** 337–342.

Fukuoka, T., Tokunaga, A., Tachibana, T., Dai, Y., Yamanaka, H., and Noguchi, K. (2002) VR1, but not P2X(3), increases in the spared L4 DRG in rats with L5 spinal nerve ligation. *Pain,* **99,** 111–120.

Gauriau, C. and Bernard, J. (2002) Pain pathways and parabrachial circuits in the rat. *Experimental Physiology,* **87,** 251–258.

Goadsby, P. (2002) New directions in migraine research. *Journal of Clinical Neuroscience,* **9,** 368–373.

Hunt, S. and Mantyh, P. (2001) The molecular dynamics of pain control. *Nature reviews,* **2,** 83–91.

Jensen, T. and Baron, R. (2003) Translation of symptoms and signs into mechanisms in neuropathic pain. *Pain,* **102,** 1–8.

Kage, K., Niforatos, W., Zhu, C., Lynch, K., Honore, P., and Jarvis, M. (2002) Alteration of dorsal root ganglion P2X3 receptor expression and function following spinal nerve ligation in the rat. *Experimental Brain Research,* **147,** 511–519.

Kosek, E. and Hannson, P. (1997) Modulatory influence on somatosensory perception from vibration and heterotopic noxious conditioning stimulation (HNCS) in fibromyalgia patients and healthy subjects. *Pain,* **70,** 41–51.

Lautenbacher, S. and Rollman, G. (1997) Modulatory influence on somatosensory perception from vibration and heterotopic noxious conditioning stimulation (HNCS) in fibromyalgia patients and healthy subjects. *Clinical Journal of Pain, 13,* 189–196.

Mantyh, P., Rogers, S., Honore, P., *et al.* (1997) Inhibition of hyperalgesia by ablation of lamina I spinal neurons expressing the substance P receptor. *Science, 278,* 275–279.

Matthews, E. and Dickenson, A. (2001) Effects of spinally delivered N- and P-type voltage-dependent calcium channel antagonists on dorsal horn neuronal responses in a rat model of neuropathy. *Pain, 92,* 235–246.

Meller, S. and Gebhart, G. (1993) Nitric oxide (NO) and nociceptive processing in the spinal cord. *Pain, 52,* 127–136.

Nichols, M., Allen, B., Rogers, S., *et al.* (1999) Transmission of chronic nociception by spinal neurons expressing the substance P receptor. *Science, 286,* 1558–1561.

Papadopoulos, I., Georgiou, P., Katsimbri, P., and Drosos, A. (2000) Treatment of fibromyalgia with tropisetron, a 5HT3 serotonin antagonist, a pilot study. *Clinical Rheumatology, 19,* 6–8.

Portenoy, R.K., Foley, K.M., and Inturrisi, C.E. (1990) The nature of opioid responsiveness and its implications for neuropathic pain: new hypotheses derived from studies of opioid infusions. *Pain, 43,* 273–286.

Rowbotham, M. (2001) Efficacy of opioids in neuropathic pain. In *Neuropathic Pain: Pathophysiology and Treatment,* Vol. 21 (eds. P. Hansson, H. Fields, R. Hill, and P. Marchettini). IASP Press, Seattle, pp. 203–213.

Rowbotham, M., Harden, N., Stacey, B., Bernstein, P., and Magnus–Miller, L. (1998) Gabapentin for the treatment of postherpetic neuralgia: a randomized controlled trial. *The Journal of the American Medical Association, 280,* 1837–1842.

Sindrup, S. and Jensen, T. (1999) Efficacy of pharmacological treatments of neuropathic pain: an update and effect related to mechanism of drug action. *Pain, 83,* 389–400.

Sommer, C. (2001) Cytokines and neuropathic pain. In *Neuropathic Pain: Pathophysiology and Treatment,* Vol. 21 (eds. P. Hansson, H. Fields, R. Hill, and P. Marchettini). IASP Press, Seattle, pp. 37–62.

Sorkin, L. and Carlton, S. (1997) Spinal anatomy and pharmacology of afferent processing. In *Anesthesia. Biologic Foundations* (eds. T. Yaksh, C. Lynch, W. Zapol, M. Maze, J. Biebuyck, and L. Saidman). Lippincott–Raven, Philadelphia/New York, pp. 577–610.

Souslova, V., Cesare, P., Ding, Y., *et al.* (2000) Warm-coding deficits and aberrant inflammatory pain in mice lacking P2X3 receptors. *Nature, 407,* 1015–1017.

Staud, R., Robinson, M., Vierck, C., Cannon, R., Mauderli, A., and Price, D. (2003) Ratings of experimental pain and pain-related negative affect predict clinical pain in patients with fibromyalgia syndrome. *Pain, 105,* 215–222.

Suzuki, R. and Dickenson, A. (2000) Neuropathic pain: nerves bursting with excitement. *Neuroreport, 11,* R17–R21.

Suzuki, R., Morcuende, S., Webber, M., Hunt, S., and Dickenson, A. (2002) NK1 receptors are required for the full sensory coding of deep dorsal horn neurones in mice. *Nature Neuroscience, 5,* 1319–1326.

Todd, A. (2002) Anatomy of primary afferents and projection neurones in the rat spinal dorsal horn with particular emphasis on substance P and the neurokinin 1 receptor. *Experimental Physiolgy, 87,* 245–249.

Vanegas, H. and Schaible, H. (2000) Effects of antagonists to high-threshold calcium channels upon spinal mechanisms of pain, hyperalgesia and allodynia. *Pain, 85,* 9–18.

Wall, P.D. (1978) The gate control theory of pain mechanisms. A re-examination and re-statement. *Brain,* **101,** 1–18.

Waxman, S.G. (1999) The molecular pathophysiology of pain: abnormal expression of sodium channel genes and its contributions to hyperexcitability of primary sensory neurons. *Pain,* **Suppl 6,** S133–140.

Wilson, S., Smith, S., Chesler, E., *et al.* (2003) The heritability of antinociception: common pharmacogenetic mediation of five neurochemically distinct analgesics. *Journal of Pharmacology and Experimental Therapeutics,* **304,** 547–559.

Yaksh, T.L. (1993) New horizons in our understanding of the spinal physiology and pharmacology of pain processing. *Seminars in Oncology,* **20,** 6–18.

Chapter 7

The ascending pain pathways

Stephen P. Hunt and Hervé Bester

7.1 **Introduction**

Pain is an essential survival mechanism, protecting the individual from tissue damage or from further injury to already damaged tissue. However, the relationship of pain to injury is complex and variable, both under normal circumstances and in pathological pain states where anatomical, molecular, and biochemical changes inevitably occur (Wall, 1979).

Noxious stimulation provokes a series of physiological changes in the organism accompanied by a range of affective responses and motivational changes designed to minimize the risk of injury. At the behavioural level, there is usually a rapid withdrawal from the site of stimulation on top of which motor behaviour such as attack or flight and autonomic activity characterized by changes in respiration, heart rate and blood pressure, and muscle tone may occur. This wide range of modulations also prepares the body for emergency and escape. The nature, location, and intensity of the pain will also be registered and the environmental context in which the pain occurred will be stored for future reference.

If noxious stimulation results in injury, then pain sensitivity around the wound usually increases as a result of both local changes in the small diameter nociceptive sensory neurons and alterations in sensory processing within the spinal cord and brain. The increase in pain sensitivity around damaged tissue during healing is also accompanied by motivational changes that encourage rest during recovery. Pain processing at spinal levels is at all times under the control of descending pathways from the brain which registers both the environmental and bodily status (Craig, 2002; Bester *et al.*, 2001, 2000; Hunt and Mantyh, 2001). This contributes to a balance between pain sensitivity and survival after injury. Chronic pain states, particularly when the pain remains after recovery from injury or results from direct injury to the nervous system, have in largely unknown ways, subverted the normal controls that modulate pain sensitivity.

This complex response to noxious stimulation over time implies that nociceptive information is processed at different levels of the brain and spinal cord to deliver an integrated response. Much of the literature on the ascending pain pathways concentrates on different aspects of this processing but it remains unclear as to whether particular pathways can be ascribed a discrete functional role (Treede, 2002; Willis *et al.*, 2002; Lahuerta *et al.*, 1994).

Nociceptive information leaves the spinal cord by a number of distinct pathways and terminates within other areas of the spinal cord and discrete areas of the brainstem including the thalamus. Historically, it had been appreciated that cutting the anterolateral tract or hemisection of the spinal cord in humans led to selective loss of pain, temperature, and itch contralateral and caudal to the lesion (Craig, 2002; Aminoff, 1996; Lahuerta et al., 1994; Denny–Brown, 1979). This approach was exploited neurosurgically to control pain but the (albeit variable) return of pain within a variable period after cord surgery limited the general usefulness of the approach (Bowsher, 1999, 1996). Return of pain implied considerable plasticity within ascending pathways and also suggested that information related to painful sensation could reach the brain through pathways normally not accessed but uncovered in time by spinal lesions. There was also the implication that changes had occurred in the brain that left the potential for re-emergence of a pain state independent of peripheral stimulation (Lenz et al., 1995; Katz and Melzack, 1990). Further experimental work and clinical observation also indicated that the loss, and possibly the return of pain sensation after cordotomy was not simply tied to loss of an ascending pathway but also involved descending pathways from the brainstem. Indeed, pathways known to be essential for the control of spinal excitability were inevitably destroyed by the procedure (Urban and Gebhart, 1999; Aminoff, 1996; Denny–Brown, 1979).

Pain has been described as having affective and discriminative components that, at least in man, have been shown to be dissociable by hypnosis or following cortical lesions (Rainville, 2002; Hofbauer et al., 2001; Price, 2000; Rainville et al., 1999). The discriminative dimension defines the location and describes the feeling of the pain-burning, stabbing, and so on, while the affective dimension attributes an 'unpleasantness' value to the pain. The primary sensory cortex is thought to perform at least the first levels of sensory discriminative analysis — that is, the 'what' and 'where' of the stimulus. The limbic system, including the limbic cortex and subcortical structures such as the amygdala, attribute an affective value to the incoming information based on the past history of the animal and the current behavioural context. Affective behaviours are motor responses that include an integrated autonomic response through activation of brainstem and spinal centres that control sympathetic and parasympathetic outflow to the body.

Many chronic pain states also carry with them a memory of past peripheral injury, for example, with painful events that occurred before amputation of a limb (Katz and Melzack, 1990). Pain memories can also be recovered in the absence of on-going pain by stimulation of particular areas of the thalamus, and retain both a discriminative and affective dimension (Lenz et al., 1995). Pain memories thus may be triggered by peripheral stimulation but do not seem to rely purely on activity within ascending pathways from the spinal cord and may require cortical involvement.

Nociceptive information must gain access to the areas of the spinal cord and brain that are concerned with patterning the fully elaborated and integrated pain response, but how this is achieved remains controversial.

This chapter summarizes and synthesizes recent findings in the field and is intended to complement a number of recent and older reviews (Gauriau and Bernard, 2002; Villanueva and Bernard, 1999; Willis and Coggeshall, 1991; Willis, 1985).

7.2 **The pathways**

7.2.1 **Primary afferent termination within the spinal cord**

Somatosensory information reaches the spinal cord and areas of the brainstem through primary afferent sensory fibres (Hunt and Mantyh, 2001; Snider and McMahon, 1998; Hunt and Rossi, 1985; Nagy and Hunt, 1983). Sensory fibres terminate within the ten designated laminae (I–X) of the spinal cord in a highly reproducible and characteristic fashion depending upon their diameter, biochemical composition, and receptive field properties (Fig. 7.1). Nociceptive information is relayed to spinal cord neurons throughout the dorsal horn, particularly laminae I–II and V–VII (Fig. 7.2) but largely avoids populations of neurons within laminae III and IV which receive, almost exclusively, non-nociceptive projections from Aβ sensory afferents. Neurons within laminae I and II and V and VI receive nociceptive information through unmyelinated C fibres and finely myelinated Aδ sensory afferents. C fibres form the major part of the sensory input to the cord and can be further divided up into almost equal numbers of peptide-containing and non-peptide-expressing neurons that stain for the lectin IB4. Nociceptive information from the skin is distributed between laminae I,II, and V, while

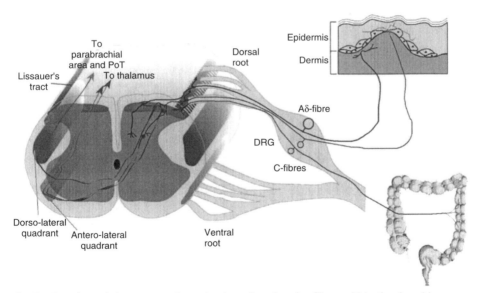

Fig. 7.1 Overview of the pattern of termination of nociceptive fibres within the dorsal horn and the origin and trajectory of the superficial and deep ascending pathways to the brain. See plate section, Plate 3 (centre of book) for a colour version.

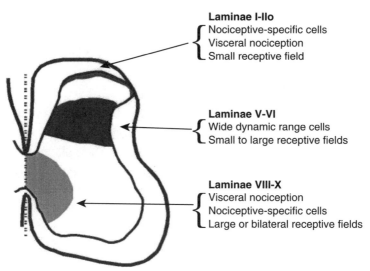

Laminae I-IIo
{ Nociceptive-specific cells
Visceral nociception
Small receptive field

Laminae V-VI
{ Wide dynamic range cells
Small to large receptive fields

Laminae VIII-X
{ Visceral nociception
Nociceptive-specific cells
Large or bilateral receptive fields

Fig. 7.2 Spinal nociceptive regions. Nociceptive neurons are found within different regions of the dorsal horn and have distinct response properties.

visceral input is almost exclusively peptidergic and terminates largely within laminae I and V, avoiding lamina II (Lawson, 2002; Cervero and Laird, 1999; Cervero, 1994; Sharkey *et al.*, 1987; Hunt and Rossi, 1985; Nagy and Hunt, 1983). However, while projection neurons in lamina I receive almost exclusively peptidergic C-fibre input from the body, it should be noted that both lamina I neurons and lamina V neurons — the origins of two of the major ascending pathways — potentially receive all types of nociceptive input.

Neurons that relay nociceptive information to the brain are located primarily in laminae I, III, V–VII, and X (Gauriau and Bernard, 2002; Villanueva and Bernard, 1999; Willis and Coggeshall, 1991). Considerable attention has recently been directed towards the pathway arising largely from lamina I neurons such that many of the functions once ascribed to the deeper pathway are now being reallocated to this pathway arising from the most superficial layer of the dorsal horn. There are a number of reasons for this. Retrograde and anterograde pathway tracing techniques have greatly improved in sensitivity and forced a reappraisal of the connections of spinal projection neurons. Species differences are also important, as well as the level of the spinal cord at which the analysis is made, cervical cord often being very different to the lumbar cord but having traditionally received more attention. However, there has also been a shift in the way that function has been allocated to particular pathways particularly in terms of the affective, discriminative, and homeostatic dimensions of pain (Craig, 2002). Finally, chemical lesioning techniques have been introduced which specifically destroy subpopulations of lamina I neurons and effectively dissociate the lamina I projection from the deeper lying nociceptive pathways that project upon the brainstem *without* disrupting descending pathways (Nichols *et al.*, 1999; Mantyh *et al.*, 1997). This dissociation has permitted the behavioural assessment of the role particular pathways play in nociceptive behaviour and led to a rethinking of the contribution that the different spinal projections make to acute and chronic nociceptive behaviours.

7.2.2 The projection from the superficial dorsal horn

The lamina I pathway has been repeatedly re-described in numerous studies (see below) and in a variety of animals including humans, where it is thought to have reached the highest degree of differentiation. Several sites of termination of the pathway have been described which hint at the function of this pathway in both homeostatic regulation and in supplying information to areas of the brain concerned with discrimination, affect and autonomic regulation (Fig. 7.3).

In a number of recent reports, Craig and his colleagues (Craig, 2002) have made a convincing argument in favour of a role for the lamina I pathway in homeostasis and of being, in one sense, an 'afferent sympathetic' pathway directing both interoceptive and extereoceptive information to areas of the CNS concerned with autonomic regulation and affective expression. In rodents, only a small percentage (~10%) of lamina I neurons have been shown to be projection neurons (Todd *et al.*, 2000). These neurons receive nociceptive information segmentally from all areas of the body and have axons that terminate within the sympathetic preganglionic motor column of the thoracic cord, in the medulla, and throughout other regions of the brainstem as far rostral as the thalamus. These areas of termination can be broken down, somewhat artificially, into areas concerned with sympathetic regulation and affect, motor control, cognition, and sensory discrimination. Obviously, sudden injury is followed by a closely orchestrated sequence of responses in the animal including arousal accompanied by cardiovascular changes, fight or flight responses, and suppression of ongoing pain to aid escape (Keay and Bandler, 2002; Janig and Habler, 2000*a,b*). The success of these survival responses is linked to their close coordination, and this is reflected by substantial interconnections between subsystems within the nervous system.

Recent evidence also supports the view that the lamina I pathway is crucial for the regulation of spinal cord excitability, and therefore pain behaviour, through the activation of descending inhibitory and excitatory pathways from the brainstem (Suzuki *et al.*, 2002; Bester *et al.*, 2001).

Injections of retrograde tracers into brainstem areas known to receive spinal nociceptive input almost tend to label neurons in more than one lamina of the spinal cord. This implies that pathways originating in deep and superficial laminae overlap to some extent at their sites of termination within the brain. This is however not always the case. Indeed, if one considers projections to the parabrachial area, it is now clearly established that lamina I and lamina V neurones send projections to distinct subregions (Gauriau and Bernard, 2002; Bourgeais *et al.*, 2001*b*; Villanueva and Bernard, 1999; Bernard *et al.*, 1996, 1995; Feil and Herbert, 1995; Bernard and Besson, 1990). Lamina I neurons project mainly (80%) to a contralateral parabrachial region centred

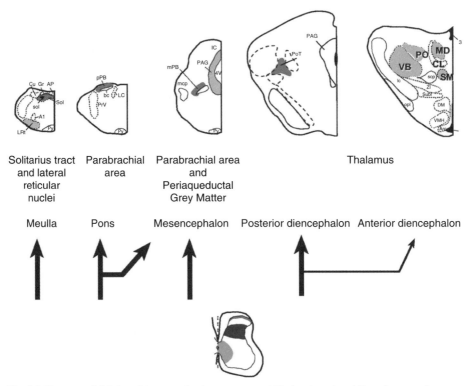

Fig. 7.3 The superficial dorsal horn projection neurons within laminae I and III project to a large number of brainstem areas. Cu: cuneatus nucleus; Gr: gracilis nucleus; AP: area postrema; Sol, solitarius tract nucleus; LRt: lateral reticular nucleus; A1; A1 noradrenergic group; sol: solitarius tract; pyr: pyramidal tract; pPB: pontine division of the parabrachial area; bc: brachium conjunctivum; LC: locus coeruleus; PrV: principal sensory trigeminal nucleus; mPB: mesencephalic division of the parabrachial area; PAG: periaqueductal gray matter; mcp: medial cerebellar pedoncle; IC: inferior colliculus; 4v: forth ventricle; PoT: posterior triangular nucleus of the thalamus (in rodents = Vmpo in the monkey); PO: posterior thalamic nuclei; VB: ventrobasal complex (VPM+VPL); ic: internal capsule; scp: superior cerebellar pedoncle; opt: optic tract; ZI: zona incerta; CL: central lateral thalamic nucleus; SM: submedius nucleus; SubI: subincertal nucleus; DM: dorsomedial hypothalamic nucleus; VMH: ventromedial hypothalamic nucleus; Arc: arcuate nucleus; 3V: third ventricle.

around the external lateral nucleus, whereas lamina V neurones project bilaterally to the internal nucleus (~500 μm medial and dorsal to the ipsilateral external lateral nucleus).

The nociceptive projection pathway originating from the superficial dorsal horn (the 'lamina I pathway') arises from neurons mainly in lamina I (see Bester *et al.*, 2000, 1995) but with a small contribution from laminae III and IV neurons (Todd, 2002;

Todd *et al.*, 2000; Naim *et al.*, 1997; Ding *et al.*, 1995). Strikingly, projection neurons which are only made of 10% of the lamina I neuron population have been shown to be largely nociceptive-specific, receiving input from C and Aδ nociceptors responding to noxious thermal and mechanical stimulation (Lawson, 2002; Bester *et al.*, 2000; Snider and McMahon, 1998). Temperature-specific neurons have been described in primates. Receptive fields are small and the majority (up to 90%) of these projection neurons express the NK1 ('substance P') receptor (Todd *et al.*, 2000). C-Fos histochemistry combined with noxious stimulation at a variety of deep (joints, muscles) and cutaneous sites in the body have indicated that in the rat, lamina I NK1-positive neurons are primarily concerned with the intensity of noxious stimulation rather than the location or tissue of origin of the pain (Doyle and Hunt, 1999*a,b*). Destruction of these neurons with intrathecally delivered saporin–substance P conjugate does not result in obvious changes in behaviourally assessed nociceptive thresholds but does reduce the increased behavioural sensitivity associated with inflammation or neuropathic nociception (Nichols *et al.*, 1999). Axons from superficial projection neurons either cross the spinal cord immediately to ascend in the contralateral ventrolateral and dorsolateral fasciculi or in the dorsolateral fasciculus of the same side.

7.2.2.1 Spinal cord and medulla

Within the spinal cord, ascending fibres terminate around the sympathetic preganglionic motor neurons of the intermediolateral column in thoracic cord segments (Craig, 2002, 2000, 1996) and continue on to terminate in association with discrete areas of the caudal brainstem (see Fig. 7.3). Heavy termination is found in areas concerned with cardiovascular and visceral regulation, particularly the nucleus tractus solitarius (NTS)(Gamboa–Esteves *et al.*, 2001) and ventro lateral medulla (Lima *et al.*, 2002; Bourgeais *et al.*, 2001*a*). Painful stimulation results in responses in the cardiovascular and respiratory systems and afferents from both of these systems terminate within the NTS (Janig and Habler, 2000*a*).

Other areas of termination include the dorsal reticular nucleus, also known as the subnucleus reticularis dorsalis (SRD), and possibly the lateral reticular nucleus and adjacent reticular formation which has motor functions related to the cerebellum. The SRD receives bilateral input from deep and superficial layers of the spinal cord which is largely nociceptive and forms part of a 'pronociceptive' pathway that both projects to the medial thalamus and projects back upon the spinal cord modulating nociceptive transmission (Lima and Almeida, 2002; Monconduit *et al.*, 2002). This is one of many brain areas that both receive nociceptive input from the spinal cord and project back upon the dorsal horn to regulate the flow of pain-related information. Such 'neural loops' connecting the brain and spinal cord appear to be crucial to the ways in which pain sensitivity is regulated in the behaving animal. SRD neurons have extremely large receptive fields, in some cases covering the whole body. The dorsal part of the nucleus receives largely ipsilateral nociceptive input from laminae I and X, and destruction of the nucleus depresses nociceptive responses to acute and inflammatory nociception.

7.2.2.2 Pons and mesencephalon

Further rostrally, axons from the lamina I pathway terminate heavily within the contralateral parabrachial area (PB) (Bernard *et al.*, 1995; Feil and Herbert, 1995) and periaqueductal gray (PAG) (Villanueva and Bernard, 1999). The PB area probably receives the densest set of terminal projections originating in spinal lamina I. Considerable emphasis has recently been placed on the extensive termination of lamina I neurons in the external medial lateral PB. PB is an area that integrates information from the NTS and visceral and somatic information from the body through the spinal cord. Neurons respond almost exclusively to nociceptive stimulation and their receptive fields can be extremely large, including the whole of the body area (see Fig. 7.3) (Bester *et al.*, 1995; Matsumoto *et al.*, 1996; Menendez *et al.*, 1996; Bernard and Besson, 1990) as well as responding to visceral stimulation, such as following colorectal stimulation (Bernard *et al.*, 1992). PB neurons are therefore exquisitely sensitive to intensity of the noxious stimulus rather than location or nature of the stimulus.

PB projects heavily upon areas of the limbic system such as the ventromedial hypothalamus (Bester *et al.*, 1997*a*) and the central nucleus of the amygdala (Bernard *et al.*, 1993), providing the nociceptive input to areas of the brain classically associated with affect (Davis and Shi, 1999; Shi and Davis, 1999; Bester *et al.*, 1995; Bernard and Besson, 1990). The ventromedial hypothalamus has been associated with rage and aggression and projects upon the PAG (Keay and Bandler, 2002). The amygdala regulates autonomic function and is necessary for fear conditioning (Roeling *et al.*, 1994; Adamec and Stark–Adamec, 1983).

Together these areas may be important in regulating pain-related emotional responses, as well as in modulating longer-term functions such as motivational and metabolic states that follow injury. Importantly, these structures give rise to powerful descending projections that modulate nociceptive processing at the level of the spinal cord.

The primary brainstem route for modulating and coordinating pain behaviours is through the PAG of the midbrain (Urban and Gebhart, 1999; Basbaum and Fields, 1984). As would be expected, apart from receiving direct nociceptive inputs from lamina I neurons and neurons of the lateral spinal nucleus, the PAG also receives substantial inputs from PB and the ventromedial hypothalamus (see Chapter 11).

7.2.2.3 Diencephalon

The organization of nociceptive inputs to the thalamus and, therefore, to the cerebral cortex remains controversial (Gariaut and Bernard 2004*a,b*; Craig and Blomquist, 2002; Jones, 2002; Treede, 2002; Willis *et al.*, 2002). Classically, it had been maintained that there were distinct areas in the medial and lateral thalamus that received nociceptive input. The medial pathway terminated within nuclei of the intralaminar and medial thalamic nuclei which projected upon areas of limbic cortex linked to affect and motivation, whereas the lateral thalamic nuclei projected to primary somatosensory cortex concerned with discriminative aspects of pain processing (Melzack and Casey, 1968). Indeed, in the human brain activation of the somatosensory cortex, insula and cingulate corteces have been seen by positron emission tomography following various types of noxious stimulation of the body (see Chapter 13).

However, recent data has blurred this simple mediolateral distinction. Recent anterograde tracing studies following small injections of tracer into lamina I of the spinal cord (which by their nature only label a very small population of neurons in the superficial spinal cord) indicated:

1. input to the ventroposterolateral (VPL) and to the posterior thalamic nuclear group (Po), both of which receive classical non-nociceptive lemniscal input and project upon the somatosensory cortex I and II (SI and SII)

2. afferent termination in the posterior triangular nucleus (PoT) which projects upon SII and insular cortex

3. a projection from lamina I and from the lateral spinal nucleus to the adjacent medial dorsal thalamic nucleus (MD) that projects upon the medial and orbital parts of the frontal cortex and to the cingulate cortex.

That is, there is claimed to be a projection from lamina I to both medial and lateral thalamic territories with access to both limbic and somatosensory cortex (Gauriau and Bernard, 2004a,b, 2002; Craig, 2002; Willis et al., 2001).

PoT has attracted considerable attention. In the rat, this area of the thalamus also receives both superficial and input from SRD, a small input from lamina V spinal neurons, and projects upon SII and insular cortex. PoT and insula together are essential for the acquisition of fear conditioning generated by foot shock (Shi and Davis, 1999). Both nocispecific (NS) and neurons that respond to both noxious and non-noxious stimulation (NNS) have been identified. NS neurons project upon the second somatosensory cortex, while NNS neurons terminate in the insular cortex (Gauriau and Bernard, 2004a), presumably reflecting input from both deep and superficial dorsal horn projection pathways. In primates, a posterior part of the ventromedial nucleus, Vmpo (part of the ventrocaudal nucleus, VMpc, in man) has been identified, which is claimed to receive input only from lamina I nociceptive and temperature-sensitive neurons and to project to insula cortex (Craig, 2002; Craig and Blomquist, 2002; Craig et al., 2000, 1994). The homologue in rodents, if it exists, is unclear.

In a recent series of articles it has been claimed that the projection area of Vmpo within the insula cortex represents a primary sensory representation for pain, temperature, itch, and other feelings from the body and that in humans, stimulation of Vmpo evokes pain and temperature sensation and that 'lesions of Vmpo or its cortical field reduce these sensations specifically' (Craig, 2002). While this idea has been debated and remains controversial (Willis et al., 2002), it re-introduces the possibility of 'hard-wired' pathways (Perl, 1998) uniquely dedicated to the processing of particular types of nociceptive and non-nociceptive sensory information.

7.3 **Deep projections V–VII and X**

Deeper-lying neurons, particularly lamina V and the adjacent laminae IV and VI–VII neurons of the spinal cord, also receive substantial nociceptive input and give rise to a major ascending pathway to the brain (Fig. 7.4). Compared to lamina I neurons however, they generally have a wide dynamic range of response and are rarely nociceptive specific, have larger receptive field sizes, and respond to a variety of noxious and non-noxious stimuli, as well as showing viscero-somatic convergence (Treede, 2002; Willis and Coggeshall, 1991; Maixner *et al.*, 1989; Besson and Chaouch, 1987; Le Bars *et al.*, 1986; Hoffman *et al.*, 1981). This has led to the suggestion that they are well fitted to providing information about the intensity but not the location of the stimulus. Yet they are the most closely studied of spinal nociceptive neurons and give rise to projections that overlap some of the areas of termination of lamina I neurons. Lamina V projections had

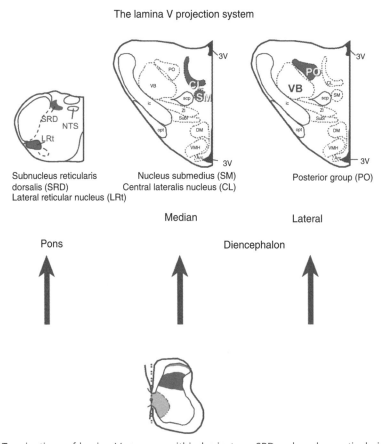

Fig. 7.4 Terminations of lamina V neurons within brainstem. SRD: subnucleus reticularis dorsalis; NTS: nucleus of the tractus solitarius. Other abbreviations, see legend of Fig. 7.3.

not been studied using anterograde tracing until very recently, and these studies only partially agree with previous retrograde tracing studies (Gauriau and Bernard, 2004b).

Nevertheless, within the brainstem, retrograde labelling has identified deep spinal projections to the lateral reticular nucleus and SRD, as well as to areas of the lateral reticular formation and pontine and deep mesencephalic reticular nuclei (Gauriau and Bernard, 2004b; Lima and Almeida, 2002; Bernard et al., 1990). Many of these areas project onto classical motor structures such as the cerebellum and cranial motor nuclei. Terminations are also found in the PB (bilaterally with substantial ipsilateral projections) and adjacent areas. It is clear that many of these areas also receive from lamina I neurons, although the degree of overlap may be restricted. Moreover, certain PB neurons tend to be overwhelmingly nociceptive (Bester et al., 1997b, 1995; Matsumoto et al., 1996; Menendez et al., 1996; Bernard and Besson, 1990), suggesting that at the single-cell level there may well be dedicated nociceptive input from lamina I neurons. This consideration emphasizes the prominent role of the PB area in integrating noxious input from the whole body.

The functional importance of the vast majority of nociceptive information pouring into the reticular formation is unclear. Many reticular nuclei project upon the midline and intralaminar thalamic nuclei, and these nuclei project upon the cortex and also the striatum and globus pallidus, again emphasizing that lamina V neurons seem to terminate largely within areas of the brain considered to have motor and arousal functions. Neurons within the reticular formation and the SRD also project upon the medial and intralaminar nuclei of the thalamus, providing a substantial nociceptive input. Neurons of the intralaminar nuclei, which project to the cingulate cortex, have very large receptive fields, perhaps reflecting input from SRD and PB. The SRD, as described above, receives projections from deep, but also superficial, spinal pathways and projects extensively upon the thalamus, including PoT and areas that are probably homologous to the VMpc of primates. These areas of the reticular formation could therefore be considered nociceptive relays, transferring nociceptive information from the deep spinal cord to the thalamus (Villanueva and Bernard, 1999).

Other midbrain projections of deep neurons include the anterior pretectal nucleus and peripeduncular tegmental areas (Rees and Roberts, 1989). The pretectal area has been implicated in antinociception, and the pedunculo-pontine area is known to be involved in motivational behaviours (Bechara and van der Kooy, 1992), reinforcing the notion that the processing of nociceptive information has to involve many different levels of analysis.

The thalamic connections of deep dorsal horn neurons have recently undergone something of a revision. For many years lamina V neurons were considered to be the major source of the spinothalamic tract, but recent work has begun to suggest that the primary input from deep dorsal horn nociceptive neurons is to the medullary and mesencephalic brainstem, and that nociceptive information is relayed from these sites to the thalamus — for example, from SRD to the intralaminar thalamus and VM (Gauriau and Bernard, 2004b). However, retrograde labelling studies following injections of tracer into the thalamus have reported labelling of deep dorsal horn neurons as well as lamina I–III neurons. Neurons located deep within the dorsal horn have been found in most studies (Kobayashi, 1998; Willis *et al.*, 1979) particularly in the cervical spinal cord. In primates, a strong projection was found from lamina V neurons to the ventrobasal thalamus (VB) which receives non-nociceptive lemniscal projections and projects upon the somatosensory cortex (Willis *et al.*, 2001). However, a recent anterograde tracing study in rodents (and this may reflect a species difference) of lamina V projections by Gauriau and Bernard (2004*b*) has failed to confirm this observation. These authors maintain that the major input to VB comes from lamina I neurons and that the areas of non-nociceptive lemniscal and nociceptive lamina I input are separated within the ventrobasal complex. Thus in the rat, anterograde labelling of deep dorsal horn neuron projections showed very few thalamic sites of termination apart from the centrolateral nucleus (CL), which also receives projections from the lateral spinal nucleus. There were, however, projections to the globus pallidus, the principle output from the striatum. CL projects upon the motor and premotor cortex and to the dorsal striatum underlining the importance of the extrapyramidal motor system in the response to injury and attack.

7.4 **Other ascending pathways**

Recently, lamina X neurons, which lie around the central canal of the spinal cord, have been shown to give rise to an ascending pathway running within the dorsal columns and synapsing within the dorsal column nuclei (Willis and Westlund, 2001; Willis *et al.*, 1999; Al–Chaer *et al.*, 1998). Lamina X neurons respond to noxious stimulation of the viscera, as do neurons within the cuneate nucleus. These project through the medial lemniscus to the ventrobasal complex. Because these ascending fibres run within the most medial aspects of the dorsal columns, it was suggested that the success of midline lesions and commissural myelotomies in relieving pelvic visceral cancer pain might be due to section of these ascending fibres. Functional MRI revealed that changes in blood flow in the thalamus and cortex, following colorectal distention, could be eliminated by midline lesions of the dorsal columns. However, similar visceral pain relief in humans has also been reported following anterolateral cordotomy, although feasibly through a different mechanism such as interruption of descending pathways.

Other ascending nociceptive pathways have been reported which project to the hypothalamus (Burstein *et al.*, 1990) and which are derived from both deep and superficial neurons within the rostral cervical cord or spinal trigeminal nucleus. Anterograde tracing studies have suggested that these projections are modest though, when compared to the density of hypothalamic nociceptive projections originating in the PB area. Overall, these projections are probably involved in direct modulation of hypothalamic mechanisms such as the release of hormones, the regulation of circadian rhythms, and perhaps feeding, drinking, and grooming activity, as well as the generation of aggressive behaviour, and possibly antinociception.

7.5 **Deep and superficial pain pathways — do they subserve different functions?**

Much has been made of the proposed differences between the laminae I–III projection and the pathway that arises from deeper lying laminae V–VII dorsal horn neurons. Essentially, it has been proposed that the superficial pathway carries information more specifically linked to discriminative aspects of pain processing than the deeper lying neurons. Superficial neurons are nocispecific (Christensen and Perl, 1970) with small receptive fields, and subpopulations of neurons also respond to temperature and a range of intense stimuli. Laminae I–III neurons project as far rostrally as the thalamus and terminate in a number of thalamic sites that relay to somatosensory cortex where location and identification of the stimulus would occur. However, there are major inputs from these neurons to the parabrachial nucleus (Bester *et al.*, 2000; Bernard *et al.*, 1995; Feil and Herbert, 1995) and to the SRD (Lima and Almeida, 2002; Villanueva *et al.*, 1996). The neurons in these areas have extremely large receptive fields that can cover the whole body and, in the case of PB, project upon the hypothalamus and amygdala (Bester *et al.*, 1997*b*, 1995; Bernard *et al.*, 1993; Bernard and Besson, 1990) areas of the brain classically associated with affect and motivation rather than discrimination. The receptive field sizes and the fact that most of these neurons respond to all types of noxious stimulation and are exquisitely sensitive to the intensity of the stimulus would also tend to rule out a role in discrimination but reinforce a role in affective and motivational behaviours. Feasibly, it could be argued that there are distinct subpopulations of lamina I neurons that project to different targets and that the superficial nociceptive pathway can concurrently provide information to both somatosensory cortex and limbic cortex through distinct thalamic relay nuclei.

However, this argument effectively relegates the deeper lying lamina V pathway to a non-discriminative role with largely motor and arousal functions. Lamina V neurons respond to both noxious and non-noxious stimuli and possess larger receptive fields. Moreover, the receptive field properties of deep neurons are to an extent dependent on lamina I neurons (Suzuki *et al.*, 2002). Uniquely, there is an extensive zone of termination of lamina V neurons within the brainstem reticular formation where electrical stimulation can elicit escape behaviours (Roberts, 1992; Casey, 1971) and from where there are direct projections to areas of the thalamus and forebrain (PoT, CL, GP) concerned with affect and motor coordination and learning.

Recent data indicates, however, that selective lesioning of laminae I–III neurons did not disturb sensory discrimination (Nichols *et al.*, 1999). In rodents, and probably primates, the vast majority of laminae I–III projection neurons express the NK1 (substance P) receptor. Using saporin-substance P conjugate, it was possible to selectively lesion the laminae I–III ascending pathway (Fig. 7.5). The behaviours of the rats several weeks later were not obviously different. Response to hot plate and noxious mechanical stimulation were not altered, effectively implying that this pathway was not essential for pain perception. However, when inflammatory or neuropathic pain states were established, the degree of increased sensitivity (hyperalgesia and allodynia) were substantially reduced by

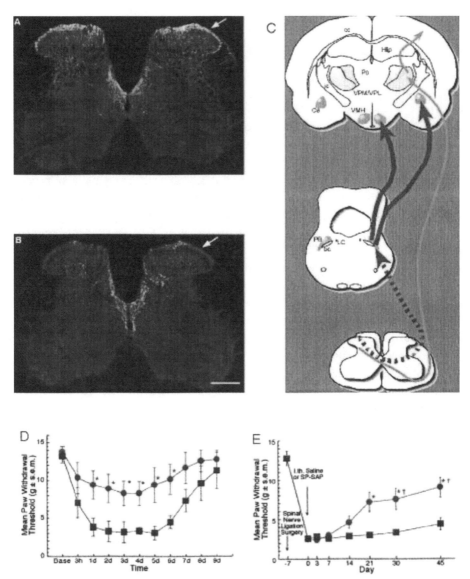

Fig. 7.5 Destruction of lamina I projection neurons with substance P-saporin conjugates
(A, B, C) results in attenuated post-inflammatory hyperalgesia (D) and neuropathic pain (E).
The normal distribution of NK1 immunofluorescence is seen in A, in lumbar cord segment L4.
Saporin substance P conjugates selectively destroy NK1-expressing neurons in lamina I (B) but
do not damage the deeper lamina V pathway (see C). 28 days later there is an attenuation of
inflammatory mechanical hyperalgesia (D). If the procedure is carried out after establishing a
peripheral nerve neuropathy (spinal nerve ligation), mechanical hyperalgesia is reduced (E).
(Adapted from Nichols *et al.*, 1999 and Hunt and Mantyh, 2001.)

destruction of the ascending laminae I–III pathway. To date, no selective lesion of lamina V projection neurons has been made, but it is clear from these experiments that they confer some discriminative capacity, perhaps by virtue of secondary projections to the somatosensory thalamus from sites of termination within the caudal brain stem.

How might these results be explained? It has often been noted that ascending projections from laminae I–III are to areas of the brain that send a reciprocal projection preferentially back to the spinal cord and are closely involved in the control of spinal sensitivity (Hunt and Mantyh, 2001). PAG receives inputs from the hypothalamus, PB, and amygdala and projects upon the rostroventral medulla an area which is in part serotonergic, and projects to spinal cord, both inhibiting and exciting spinal neurons (Suzuki *et al.*, 2002; Basbaum and Fields, 1984). Other areas of the brainstem, such as the SRD, are also reciprocally connected to the dorsal horn, and lateral areas of the reticular formation send descending noradrenergic projections to the spinal cord (Proudfit and Clark, 1991; Sagen and Proudfit, 1984).

These descending controls can be activated following input from spinal neurons as well as from areas of the brain concerned with monitoring the behavioural state of the animal such as the amygdala and hypothalamus. Disconnecting the laminae I–III pathway from the brain would therefore effectively render the brain incapable of modulating spinal sensitivity because there was no longer sufficient information coming from the spinal cord concerning ongoing nociceptive activity (Hunt, 2000). Those parts of the brain that are notably receiving less nociceptive input would be limbic areas associated with affect and motivation. These are parts of the brain that closely monitor the behavioural context of the animal and have considerable influence on spinal processing of nociceptive information alongside autonomic control and modulation.

7.6 **Conclusions**

The detailed anatomy of the ascending pain pathways is still not fully understood, but we can identify projections that terminate in a large number of different areas of the brain associated with autonomic, motor, discriminative, affective, cognitive, and motivational aspects of pain behaviour.

Deep and superficial pathways from the dorsal horn terminate in discrete areas of the brainstem. The superficial laminae I–III pathway, which reaches its highest level of differentiation in primates, seems to have a particular role in delivering nociceptive information to areas of the brain concerned with discrimination, affect, cognition, and motivation and from which extensive descending pathways emerge to modulate activity in many other areas of the brain and spinal cord. Deeper lying dorsal horn neurons can support nociceptive behaviour but the resetting of nociceptive sensitivity following skin or peripheral nerve damage critically requires the laminae I–III pathway and the engagement of descending pathways that regulate spinal sensitivity. How pain is perceived and located is still largely unknown but is assumed to require cortical processing of nociceptive information that could be provided through deep and superficial spinal pathways and from polysynaptic pathways within the brainstem.

References

Adamec, R.E. and Stark–Adamec, C.I. (1983) Limbic control of aggression in the cat. *Prog Neuropsychopharmacol Biol Psychiatry* **7**, 505–512.

Al–Chaer, E.D., Feng, Y., and Willis, W.D. (1998) A role for the dorsal column in nociceptive visceral input into the thalamus of primates. *J Neurophysiol* **79**, 3143–3150.

Aminoff, M.J. (1996) Historical perspective Brown–Sequard and his work on the spinal cord. *Spine* **21**, 133–140.

Basbaum, A.I. and Fields, H.L. (1984) Endogenous pain control systems: brainstem spinal pathways and endorphin circuitry. *Annu Rev Neurosci* **7**, 309–338.

Bechara, A. and van der Kooy, D. (1992) A single brain stem substrate mediates the motivational effects of both opiates and food in nondeprived rats but not in deprived rats. *Behav Neurosci* **106**, 351–363.

Bernard, J.F. and Besson, J.M. (1990) The spino (trigemino) pontoamygdaloid pathway: electrophysiological evidence for an involvement in pain processes. *J Neurophysiol* **63**, 473–490.

Bernard, J.F., Alden, M., and Besson, J.M. (1993) The organization of the efferent projections from the pontine parabrachial area to the amygdaloid complex: a Phaseolus vulgaris leucoagglutinin (PHA-L) study in the rat. *J Comp Neurol* **329**, 201–229.

Bernard, J.F., Bester, H., and Besson, J.M. (1996) Involvement of the spino-parabrachio -amygdaloid and -hypothalamic pathways in the autonomic and affective emotional aspects of pain. *Prog Brain Res* **107**, 243–255.

Bernard, J.F., Dallel, R., Raboisson, P., Villanueva, L., and Le Bars, D. (1995) Organization of the efferent projections from the spinal cervical enlargement to the parabrachial area and periaqueductal gray: a PHA-L study in the rat. *J Comp Neurol* **353**, 480–505.

Bernard, J.F., Huang, G.F., and Besson, J.M. (1992) Nucleus centralis of the amygdala and the globus pallidus ventralis: electrophysiological evidence for an involvement in pain processes. *J Neurophysiol* **68**, 551–569.

Bernard, J.F., Villanueva, L., Carroue, J., and Le Bars, D. (1990) Efferent projections from the subnucleus reticularis dorsalis (SRD): a Phaseolus vulgaris leucoagglutinin study in the rat. *Neurosci Lett* **116**, 257–262.

Besson, J.M. and Chaouch, A. (1987) Peripheral and spinal mechanisms of nociception. *Physiol Rev* **67**, 67–186.

Bester, H., Besson, J.M., and Bernard, J.F. (1997*a*) Organization of efferent projections from the parabrachial area to the hypothalamus: a Phaseolus vulgaris-leucoagglutinin study in the rat. *J Comp Neurol* **383**, 245–281.

Bester, H., Chapman, V., Besson, J.M., and Bernard, J.F. (2000) Physiological properties of the lamina I spinoparabrachial neurons in the rat. *J Neurophysiol* **83**, 2239–2259.

Bester, H., De Felipe, C., and Hunt, S.P. (2001) The NK1 receptor is essential for the full expression of noxious inhibitory controls in the mouse. *J Neurosci* **21**, 1039–1046.

Bester, H., Matsumoto, N., Besson, J.M., and Bernard, J.F. (1997*b*) Further evidence for the involvement of the spinoparabrachial pathway in nociceptive processes: a c-Fos study in the rat. *J Comp Neurol* **383**, 439–458.

Bester, H., Menendez, L., Besson, J.M., and Bernard, J.F. (1995) Spino (trigemino) parabrachiohypothalamic pathway: electrophysiological evidence for an involvement in pain processes. *J Neurophysiol* **73**, 568–585.

Bourgeais, L., Gauriau, C., and Bernard, J.F. (2001a) Projections from the nociceptive area of the central nucleus of the amygdala to the forebrain: a PHA-L study in the rat. *Eur J Neurosci* **14**, 229–255.

Bourgeais, L., Monconduit, L., Villanueva, L., and Bernard, J.F. (2001b) Parabrachial internal lateral neurons convey nociceptive messages from the deep laminas of the dorsal horn to the intralaminar thalamus. *J Neurosci* **21**, 2159–2165.

Bowsher, D. (1996) Central pain of spinal origin. *Spinal Cord* **34**, 707–710.

Bowsher, D. (1999) Central post-stroke ('thalamic syndrome') and other central pains. *Am J Hosp Palliat Care* **16**, 593–597.

Burstein, R., Dado, R.J., and Giesler, G.J. Jr. (1990) The cells of origin of the spinothalamic tract of the rat: a quantitative reexamination. *Brain Res* **511**, 329–337.

Casey, K.L. (1971) Somatosensory responses of bulboreticular units in awake cat: relation to escape-producing stimuli. *Science* **173**, 77–80.

Cervero, F. (1994) Sensory innervation of the viscera: peripheral basis of visceral pain. *Physiol Rev* **74**, 95–138.

Cervero, F. and Laird, J.M. (1999) Visceral pain. *Lancet* **353**, 2145–2148.

Christensen, B.N. and Perl, E.R. (1970) Spinal neurons specifically excited by noxious or thermal stimuli: marginal zone of the dorsal horn. *J Neurophysiol* **33**, 293–307.

Craig, A.D. (1996) An ascending general homeostatic afferent pathway originating in lamina I. *Prog Brain Res* **107**, 225–242.

Craig, A.D. (2000) The functional anatomy of lamina I and its role in post-stroke central pain. *Prog Brain Res* **129**, 137–151.

Craig, A.D. (2002) How do you feel? Interoception: the sense of the physiological condition of the body. *Nat Rev Neurosci* **3**, 655–666.

Craig, A.D. and Blomqvist, A. (2002) Is there a specific lamina I spinothalamocortical pathway for pain and temperature sensation in the thalamus? *J Pain* **3**, 95–101.

Craig, A.D., Bushnell, M.C., Zhang, E.T., and Blomqvist, A. (1994) A thalamic nucleus specific for pain and temperature sensation. *Nature* **372**, 770–773.

Craig, A.D., Chen, K., Bandy, D., and Reiman, E.M. (2000) Thermosensory activation of insular cortex. *Nat Neurosci* **3**, 184–190.

Davis, M. and Shi, C. (1999) The extended amygdala: are the central nucleus of the amygdala and the bed nucleus of the stria terminalis differentially involved in fear versus anxiety? *Ann N Y Acad Sci* **877**, 281–291.

Denny–Brown, D. (1979) The enigma of crossed sensory loss with cord hemisection. In: (Eds: J. J. Bonica, J. C. Liebeskind and D. G. Albe-Fessard) *Advances in Pain Research and Therapy*, pp. 889–895. New York: Raven Press.

Ding, Y.Q., Takada, M., Shigemoto, R., and Mizumo, N. (1995) Spinoparabrachial tract neurons showing substance P receptor-like immunoreactivity in the lumbar spinal cord of the rat. *Brain Res* **674**, 336–340.

Doyle, C.A. and Hunt, S.P. (1999a) A role for spinal lamina I neurokinin-1-positive neurons in cold thermoreception in the rat. *Neuroscience* **91**, 723–732.

Doyle, C.A. and Hunt, S.P. (1999b) Substance P receptor (neurokinin-1)-expressing neurons in lamina I of the spinal cord encode for the intensity of noxious stimulation: a c-Fos study in rat. *Neuroscience* **89**, 17–28.

Feil, K. and Herbert, H. (1995) Topographic organization of spinal and trigeminal somatosensory pathways to the rat parabrachial and Kolliker-Fuse nuclei. *J Comp Neurol* **353**, 506–528.

Gamboa–Esteves, F.O., Tavares, I., Almeida, A., Batten, T.F., McWilliam, P.N., and Lima, D. (2001) Projection sites of superficial and deep spinal dorsal horn cells in the nucleus tractus solitarii of the rat. *Brain Res* **921**, 195–205.

Gauriau, C. and Bernard, J.F. (2002) Pain pathways and parabrachial circuits in the rat. *Exp Physiol* **87**, 251–258

Gauriau, C. and Bernard, J.F. (2004*a*) Posterior thalamic neurons convey nociceptive messages to the second somatosensory and insular cortices in the rat. *J Neuroscience* **24**, 752–761

Gauriau, C. and Bernard, J.F. (2004*b*) A comparative reappraisal of projections from the superficial laminae of the dorsal horn of the rat. *J Comp. Neurol.* **468**, 24–56

Hofbauer, R.K., Rainville, P., Duncan, G.H., and Bushnell, M.C. (2001) Cortical representation of the sensory dimension of pain. *J Neurophysiol* **86**, 402–411.

Hoffman, D.S., Dubner, R., Hayes, R.L., and Medlin, T.P. (1981) Neuronal activity in medullary dorsal horn of awake monkeys trained in a thermal discrimination task. I. Responses to innocuous and noxious thermal stimuli. *J Neurophysiol* **46**, 409–427.

Hunt, S.P. (2000) Pain control: breaking the circuit. *Trends Pharmacol Sci* **21**, 284–287.

Hunt, S.P. and Mantyh, P.W. (2001) The molecular dynamics of pain control. *Nat Rev Neurosci* **2**, 83–91.

Hunt, S.P. and Rossi, J. (1985) Peptide- and non-peptide-containing unmyelinated primary afferents: the parallel processing of nociceptive information. *Philos Trans R Soc Lond B Biol Sci* **308**, 283–289.

Janig, W. and Habler, H.J. (2000*a*) Specificity in the organization of the autonomic nervous system: a basis for precise neural regulation of homeostatic and protective body functions. *Prog Brain Res* **122**, 351–367.

Janig, W. and Habler, H.J. (2000*b*) Sympathetic nervous system: contribution to chronic pain. *Prog Brain Res* **129**, 451–468.

Jones, E.J. (2002) A pain in the thalamus. *J Pain* **3**, 102–104.

Katz, J. and Melzack, R. (1990) Pain 'memories' in phantom limbs: review and clinical observations. *Pain* **43**, 319–336.

Keay, K.A. and Bandler, R. (2002) Distinct central representations of inescapable and escapable pain: observations and speculation. *Exp Physiol* **87**, 275–279.

Kobayashi, Y. (1998) Distribution and morphology of spinothalamic tract neurons in the rat. *Anat Embryol (Berl)* **197**, 51–67.

Lahuerta, J., Bowsher, D., Lipton, S., and Buxton, P.H. (1994) Percutaneous cervical cordotomy: a review of 181 operations on 146 patients with a study on the location of 'pain fibers' in the C-2 spinal cord segment of 29 cases. *J Neurosurg* **80**, 975–985.

Lawson, S.N. (2002) Phenotype and function of somatic primary afferent nociceptive neurones with C-, Adelta- or Aalpha/beta-fibres. *Exp Physiol* **87**, 239–244.

Le Bars, D., Dickenson, A.H., Besson, J.M., and Villanueva, L. (1986) Aspects of sensory processing through convergent neurons. In: *Spinal Afferent Processing*, pp. 467–479. Plenum Press.

Lenz, F.A., Gracely, R.H., Romanoski, A.J., Hope, E.J., Rowland, L.H., and Dougherty, P.M. (1995) Stimulation in the human somatosensory thalamus can reproduce both the affective and sensory dimensions of previously experienced pain. *Nat Med* **1**, 910–913.

Lima, D., Albino–Teixeira, A., and Tavares, I. (2002) The caudal medullary ventrolateral reticular formation in nociceptive cardiovascular integration. An experimental study in the rat. *Exp Physiol* **87**, 267–274.

Lima, D. and Almeida, A. (2002) The medullary dorsal reticular nucleus as a pronociceptive centre of the pain control system. *Prog Neurobiol* **66**, 81–108.

Maixner, W., Dubner, R., Kenshalo, D.R. Jr, Bushnell, M.C., and Oliveras, J.L. (1989) Responses of monkey medullary dorsal horn neurons during the detection of noxious heat stimuli. *J Neurophysiol* **62**, 437–449.

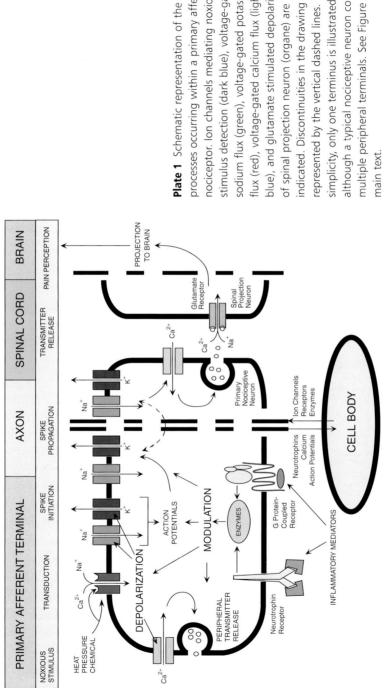

Plate 1 Schematic representation of the processes occurring within a primary afferent nociceptor. Ion channels mediating noxious stimulus detection (dark blue), voltage-gated sodium flux (green), voltage-gated potassium flux (red), voltage-gated calcium flux (light blue), and glutamate stimulated depolarization of spinal projection neuron (organe) are indicated. Discontinuities in the drawing are represented by the vertical dashed lines. For simplicity, only one terminus is illustrated, although a typical nociceptive neuron contains multiple peripheral terminals. See Figure 1.1, main text.

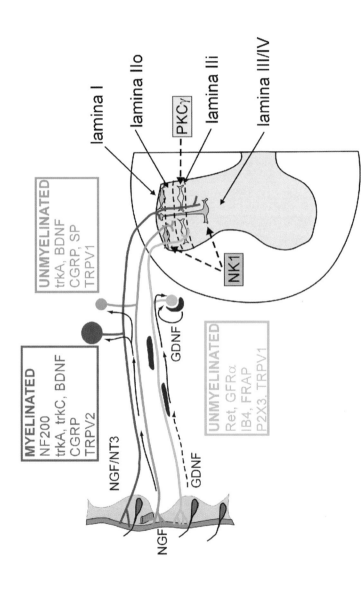

MYELINATED
NF200
trkA, trkC, BDNF
CGRP
TRPV2

UNMYELINATED
trkA, BDNF
CGRP, SP
TRPV1

UNMYELINATED
Ret, GFRα
IB4, FRAP
P2X3, TRPV1

NGF/NT3

NGF

GDNF

GDNF

NK1

PKCγ

lamina I

lamina IIo

lamina IIi

lamina III/IV

Plate 2 Diagram showing the three main populations of nociceptors, namely: (1) small-diameter IB4 non-peptide-expressing cells (green) that respond to GDNF and innervate predominantly limina II inner; (2) small-diameter peptide-expressing (CGRP, substance P) cells (blue) that respond to NGF and innervate predominantly laminae I and II outer; and (3) medium-diameter peptide-expressing (CGRP) cells (red) that have finely myelinated axons, respond to NGF and NT3, and innervate predominantly laminae I and III/IV. For further details see text. (Adapted from Snider and McMahon, 1998; Priestley *et al.*, 2002.) See Figure 2.2, main text.

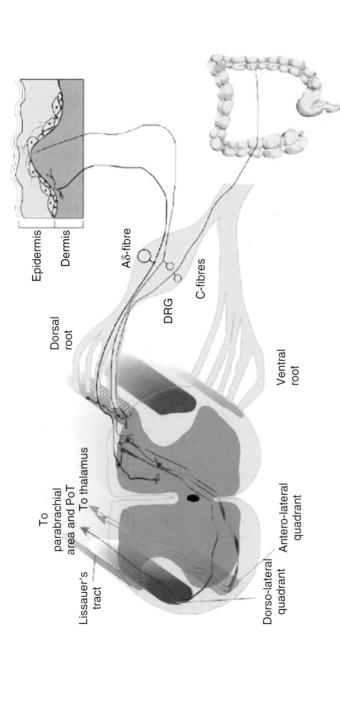

Plate 3 Overview of the pattern of termination of nociceptive fibres within the dorsal horn and the origin and trajectory of the superficial and deep ascending pathways to the brain. See Figure 7.1, main text.

Epidermis

Dermis

Aδ-fibre

DRG

C-fibres

Dorsal root

Ventral root

To parabrachial area and PoT

To thalamus

Lissauer's tract

Antero-lateral quadrant

Dorso-lateral quadrant

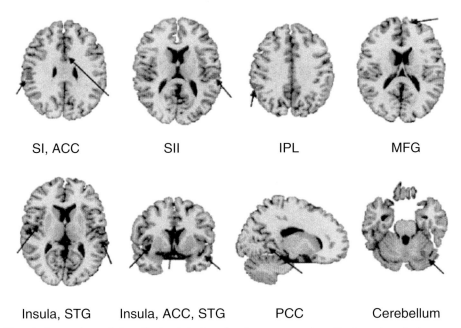

SI, ACC	SII	IPL	MFG

Insula, STG	Insula, ACC, STG	PCC	Cerebellum

Plate 4 Comparison of the effects of similar stimulus pressures in patients and controls. Results of unpaired *t*-tests of the mean difference in signal (arrows) between pain pressure and innocuous touch for each group are shown in standard space superimposed on an anatomic image of a standard brain. Images are shown in radiologic view, with the right brain shown on the left. Regions in which the response in patients was significantly greater than the response in controls are shown in red; regions in which the response in controls was significantly greater than that in patients are shown in green. The level of significance was adjusted for multiple comparisons at $P < 0.05$. Patients showed significant activations that were markedly different from those in the healthy controls in the primary somatosensory cortex (SI), inferior parietal lobe (IPL), insula, posterior cingulate cortex (PCC), secondary somatosensory cortex (SII), superior temporal gyrus (STG), and cerebellum. The peak of the significant difference in anterior cingulate cortex (ACC) is in the right hemisphere, although the activation is near the midline and spreads into both hemispheres. Significant increases in the contralateral STG and in a second region of ipsilateral cerebellum are not shown. In contrast to these regions of greater signal differences in patients, similar stimulus pressures resulted in one region of significantly increased stimulus intensity in control subjects, located in the medial frontal gyrus (MFG). (From Gracely *et al.*, 2002, with permission.) See Figure 13.2, main text.

Mantyh, P.W., Rogers, S.D., Honore, P., *et al.* (1997) Inhibition of hyperalgesia by ablation of lamina I spinal neurons expressing the substance P receptor. *Science* **278**, 275–279.

Matsumoto, N., Bester, H., Menendez, L., Besson, J.M., and Bernard, J.F. (1996) Changes in the responsiveness of parabrachial neurons in the arthritic rat: an electrophysiological study. *J Neurophysiol* **76**, 4113–4126.

Melzack, R. and Casey, K.L. (1968) Sensory, motivational and central control determinants of pain: a new conceptual model. In: (Ed. D. Kenshalo Publisher: Charles C Thomas, Springfield I11) *The Skin Senses*, pp. 423–443.

Menendez, L., Bester, H., Besson, J.M., and Bernard, J.F. (1996) Parabrachial area: electrophysiological evidence for an involvement in cold nociception. *J Neurophysiol* **75**, 2099–2116.

Monconduit, L., Desbois, C., and Villanueva, L. (2002) The integrative role of the rat medullary subnucleus reticularis dorsalis in nociception. *Eur J Neurosci* **16**, 937–944.

Nagy, J.I. and Hunt, S.P. (1983) The termination of primary afferents within the rat dorsal horn: evidence for rearrangement following capsaicin treatment. *J Comp Neurol* **218**, 145–158.

Naim, M., Spike, R.C., Watt, C., Shehab, S.A., and Todd, A.J. (1997) Cells in laminae III and IV of the rat spinal cord that possess the neurokinin-1 receptor and have dorsally directed dendrites receive a major synaptic input from tachykinin-containing primary afferents. *J Neurosci* **17**, 5536–5548.

Nichols, M.L., Allen, B.J., Rogers, *et al.* (1999) Transmission of chronic nociception by spinal neurons expressing the substance P receptor. *Science* **286**, 1558–1561.

Perl, E.R. (1998) Getting a line on pain: is it mediated by dedicated pathways? *Nat Neurosci* **1**, 177–178.

Price, D.D. (2000) Psychological and neural mechanisms of the affective dimension of pain. *Science* **288**, 1769–1772.

Proudfit, H.K. and Clark, F.M. (1991) The projections of locus coeruleus neurons to the spinal cord. *Prog Brain Res* **88**, 123–141.

Rainville, P. (2002) Brain mechanisms of pain affect and pain modulation. *Curr Opin Neurobiol* **12**, 195–204.

Rainville, P., Carrier, B., Hofbauer, R.K., Bushnell, M.C., and Duncan, G.H. (1999) Dissociation of sensory and affective dimensions of pain using hypnotic modulation. *Pain* **82**, 159–171.

Rees, H. and Roberts, M.H. (1989) Antinociceptive effects of dorsal column stimulation in the rat: involvement of the anterior pretectal nucleus. *J Physiol* **417**, 375–388.

Roberts, V.J. (1992) NGC-evoked nociceptive behaviors: I. Effect of nucleus gigantocellularis stimulation. *Physiol Behav* **51**, 65–71.

Roeling, T.A., Veening, J.G., Kruk, M.R., Peters, J.P., Vermelis, M.E., and Nieuwenhuys, R. (1994) Efferent connections of the hypothalamic 'aggression area' in the rat. *Neuroscience* **59**, 1001–1024.

Sagen, J. and Proudfit, H.K. (1984) Effect of intrathecally administered noradrenergic antagonists on nociception in the rat. *Brain Res* **310**, 295–301.

Sharkey, K.A., Sobrino, J.A., and Cervero, F. (1987) Evidence for a visceral afferent origin of substance P-like immunoreactivity in lamina V of the rat thoracic spinal cord. *Neuroscience* **22**, 1077–1083.

Shi, C. and Davis, M. (1999) Pain pathways involved in fear conditioning measured with fear-potentiated startle: lesion studies. *J Neurosci* **19**, 420–430.

Snider, W.D. and McMahon, S.B. (1998) Tackling pain at the source: new ideas about nociceptors. *Neuron* **20**, 629–632.

Suzuki, R., Morcuende, S., Webber, M., Hunt, S.P., and Dickenson, A.H. (2002) Superficial NK1-expressing neurons control spinal excitability through activation of descending pathways. *Nat Neurosci* **5**, 1319–1326.

Todd, A.J. (2002) Anatomy of primary afferents and projection neurones in the rat spinal dorsal horn with particular emphasis on substance P and the neurokinin 1 receptor. *Exp Physiol* **87**, 245–249.

Todd, A.J., McGill, M.M., and Shehab, S.A. (2000) Neurokinin 1 receptor expression by neurons in laminae I, III and IV of the rat spinal dorsal horn that project to the brainstem. *Eur J Neurosci* **12**, 689–700.

Treede, R.–D. (2002) Spinothalamic and thalamocortical nociceptive pathways. *J Pain* **3**, 109–112.

Urban, M.O. and Gebhart, G.F. (1999) Supraspinal contributions to hyperalgesia. *Proc Natl Acad Sci USA* **96**, 7687–7692.

Villanueva, L. and Bernard, J.–F. (1999) The multiplicity of ascending pain pathways. In: *Handbook of Behavioral State Control: Cellular and Molecular Mechanisms*, pp. 569–585. CRC Press.

Villanueva, L., Bouhassira, D., and Le Bars, D. (1996) The medullary subnucleus reticularis dorsalis (SRD) as a key link in both the transmission and modulation of pain signals. *Pain* **67**, 231–240.

Wall, P.D. (1979) On the relation of injury to pain. The John J. Bonica lecture. *Pain* **6**, 253–264.

Willis, W.D. and Coggeshall, R.E. (1991) Sensory mechanisms of the spinal cord. 2nd edn. New York: Plenum Press.

Willis, W.D., Al–Chaer, E.D., Quast, M.J., and Westlund, K.N. (1999) A visceral pain pathway in the dorsal column of the spinal cord. *Proc Natl Acad Sci USA* **96**, 7675–7679.

Willis, W.D., Kenshalo, D.R. Jr. and Leonard, R.B. (1979) The cells of origin of the primate spinothalamic tract. *J Comp Neurol* **188**, 543–573.

Willis, W.D., Zhang, X., Honda, C.N., and Giesler, G.J. Jr. (2002) A critical review of the role of the proposed VMpo nucleus in pain. *J Pain* **3**, 79–94.

Willis, W.D. Jr. (1985) Central nervous system mechanisms for pain modulation. *Appl Neurophysiol* **48**, 153–165.

Willis, W.D. Jr. and Westlund, K.N. (2001) The role of the dorsal column pathway in visceral nociception. *Curr Pain Headache Rep* **5**, 20–26.

Willis, W.D. Jr, Zhang, X., Honda, C.N., and Giesler, G.J. Jr. (2001) Projections from the marginal zone and deep dorsal horn to the ventrobasal nuclei of the primate thalamus. *Pain* **92**, 267–276.

Chapter 8

Spinal delivery of drugs in pain control

Tony L. Yaksh and Patrick W. Mantyh

8.1 Introduction

The development of analgesic therapy has benefited from the growth in our under-standing of the biology of pain processing. A variety of stimuli (thermal, mechanical, and perhaps most importantly, chemical) applied to the skin, muscle, bone, and viscera can evoke a pain report. While the perceptual consequences of these stimuli are clearly organized in the brain, we recognize that the response to the stimulus is largely deter-mined by the nature of the message that is encoded in the afferent traffic flowing into the spinal cord. Thus, the pain relief obtained by blocking that input at the spinal level with local anesthetics, emphasizes that the pain experience usually depends upon the spinal output. The content of this message is determined not just by the stimulus, but by the spinal processes which encode that information. The original gate control formalization of Melzack and Wall (1965) was important not just because it emphasized the dynamic nature of the encoding process, but because it placed a large component of this regulation at the level of the spinal dorsal horn (Yaksh, 1999a). Though not fully appreciated at the time, this emphasis upon spinal processing was to become impor-tant later when it became evident that selective manipulations of spinal pharmacology in unanesthetized, unrestrained animal models could specifically alter pain behavior.

8.2 Evolution of the use of spinal analgesics

The demonstration in animal models with chronic intrathecal catheters (Fig. 8.1) that the spinal delivery of opiates at non-systemically active doses would produce a highly selective block of pain behavior, with no effect upon non-noxious processing or on motor behavior, and with a pharmacology which indicated the effects were mediated by a μ opiate receptor, provided the first indication that the processing of spinal noci-ceptive vs. non-nociceptive input could be differentially regulated by specific spinal receptors (Yaksh and Rudy, 1976). It should be stressed that the demonstration of behavioral selectivity is a crucial component in analgesic drug development. Thus, in the early and mid 1970s, while single unit recording had pointed to a spinal morphine

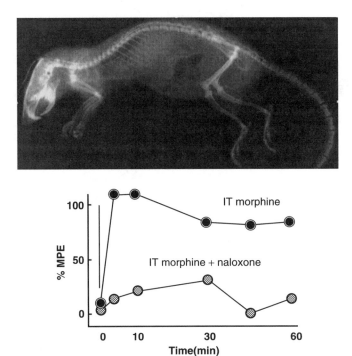

Fig. 8.1 Top: X-ray of intrathecal catheterized rat. **Bottom**: intrathecal delivery of morphine (10 μg) results in a potent, long-lasting elevation in the thermal escape latency (expressed as % of the maximum possible effect (MPE)). These effects were reversed by the IP delivery of naloxone (0.3 mg/kg).

effect, an equal number of observations argued that morphine would suppress both dorsal (sensory) and ventral (motor) horn function (Duggan and North, 1983). The functional specificity of the spinal effect in terms of sensory vs. motor, much less its specificity viz. nociception and light touch, was thus not evident based on such mechanistic, neurophysiological studies.

Importantly, these effects of spinal opiates on behavior and the pharmacology of these actions defined in preclinical studies were soon found to be relevant to the processing of pain in humans suffering from acute and chronic pain states. Thus, some three years later, the potent analgesic effects of intrathecal (Wang *et al.*, 1979) and epidural morphine (Behar *et al.*, 1979) were first described. A quantitative indication of the rapid clinical impact of the use of spinal opiates can be appreciated by noting that the clinical reports regarding the use of neuraxial opiates rose from nil prior to 1978, to 296 for the period 1978–1982, to 669 for 1983–87, and on to 1057 for 1998– 2003. The rapid development of spinal opiate use reflected not only the efficacy of the effects in humans, but also the facility with which anesthesiologists were able to access the spinal canal. Management of certain chronic pain states was addressed by the use of implantable pump and catheter systems. First described as a therapeutic approach in chronic pain in 1981 (Onofrio *et al.*, 1981), it is estimated that at present there are over 13 000 patients receiving chronic intrathecal drug delivery (Bennett *et al.*, 2000).

The development of spinal drugs for the management of pain has depended heavily upon the use of opiates. In the years since the initial report, there has been a growing appreciation of the complexity of the pain state. It is now appreciated that following injury or inflammation of peripheral tissue or nerve, anomalous behavioral pain states (hyperalgesia/allodynia) arise in humans and animals, which are mediated by changes initiated by these injury conditions in the spinal encoding processes. Importantly, current work has pointed to a complex spinal pharmacology underlying this anomalous encoding. The importance of these distinct pharmacological pathways to pain processing have been confirmed by demonstrating that the intrathecal delivery of drugs targeting a variety of signaling pathways specifically attenuate hyperalgesia and allodynia without altering the acute response to the noxious stimulus. Such pharmacological cascades have now provided additional targets where by spinal output initiated by tissue injury and inflammation may be modulated.

8.3 **Overview of the spinal biology of nociception**

Broadly, it is possible to consider spinal systems in terms of the pharmacology of the first order synapse and that of intrinsic systems which enhance the excitability of the spinofugal projections (Fig. 8.2). More detailed discussion of these cascades will be found in other chapters of this book and elsewhere (Yaksh *et al.*, 1999*a*; Ji and Woolf, 2001). The present comments will, however, serve to focus on issues relevant to the actions of spinally delivered analgesics.

At the level of the primary afferents, small high-threshold C-fibers release excitatory amino acid (glutamate) and a variety of peptides (e.g. sP, CGRP) (Todd, 2002). The excitatory amino acid and peptides evoke excitation in second order neurons. Considerable data suggests that the acute primary excitatory drive is largely mediated by glutamate through AMPA/Kainate receptors (Yoshimura and Jessell, 1990; Stanfa and Dickenson, 1999; Kocsis *et al.*, 2003).

In the face of persistent depolarization, as occurs with tissue or nerve injury, populations of dorsal horn neurons display an exaggerated response to afferent input. This exaggerated response is associated with an enhanced response of the neurons to subsequent input (Willis, 2002). This facilitated reactivity reflects a series of intra- and extra-neuronal cascades. Several of these cascades begin with a persistent depolarization initiated by the ongoing afferent input and by the increased release of SP, which through an NK1 receptor leads to prolonged sensitization to subsequent input, including 'wind-up' and long-term potentiation (Ikeda *et al.*, 2003). This persistent membrane depolarization serves to remove the Mg block of the NMDA receptor, allowing activation by extra cellular glutamate (Foster and Fagg, 1987).

Through several mechanisms, there is an increase in intracellular calcium (i.e. via the IP3 pathways of the NK1 receptor and by the movement of extracellular Ca through

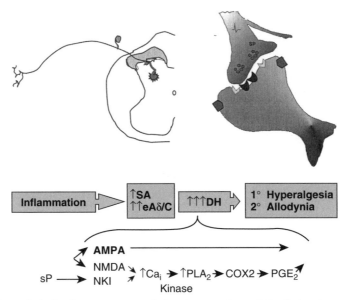

Fig. 8.2 Schematic indicating one aspect of the pharmacology of the first order synapse in the spinal dorsal horn. As indicated, tissue injury and inflammation leads to a sensitization of peripheral afferent terminals and the initiation of ongoing spontaneous activity. This ongoing activity in small afferents leads to a cascade of events as a result of the release of glutamate and peptides such as sP. As shown, the acute activation leads to a second order depolarization mediated by the AMPA receptor. In the face of continued depolarization, there is an activation of NMDA and NK1 receptors. The resulting increase in intracellular calcium leads to a series of cascades, one component of which is activation of MAP kinases, activation of phospholipase A2 (PLA2), which provides arachidonic acid which serves as a substrate for constitutively expressed cyclooxygenbase 2 (COX2). This gives rise to a family of prostanoids that can exert their downstream effects through a variety of prostanoid receptors. The net effect of this cascade is to allow processing through the first order synapse, leading to a facilitated behavioral state. See text for other details.

the NMDA ionophore, and by subclasses of AMPA channels, which are also Ca-permeant (Wollmuth and Sakmann, 1998)). Increased intracellular calcium serves to activate a variety of intracellular kinases, which feed back on cellular excitability. Thus, activation of PKC leads to a phosphorylation of the NMDA receptor and an enhanced activation of that ionophore (MacDonald *et al.*, 2001). Similarly, downstream phosphorylation of MAPKinases (Johnson and Lapadat, 2002) can subsequently activate several enzyme pathways such as PLA2 and nitric oxide synthase (Svensson and Yaksh, 2002). PLA2 activation provides cleavage of arachidonic acid from the cellular membrane (Balsinde *et al.*, 2002). Arachidonic acid can facilitate the activation of the NMDA ionophore (Richards *et al.*, 2003) and provides an essential substrate for cyclooxygenase (COX). Current evidence suggests that the COX2 isozyme constitutively expressed in spinal neurons then leads to the synthesis of a variety of prostaglandins (Svensson and Yaksh, 2002).

Prostaglandins of, for example, the E type, act upon a variety of EP receptors. EP1 receptors located on primary afferent terminals serve to enhance primary afferent transmitter release though an augmentation of the opening of voltage-activated Ca channels necessary for transmitter release. In addition, EP receptors can directly and indirectly activate dorsal horn nociresponsive neurons (Samad *et al.*, 2002). The net effect of these cascades is to enhance the activation of dorsal horn neurons by subsequent afferent input. Components of these events are presented in Fig. 8.2.

In addition to many of the events that occur after tissue injury, as outlined above, additional events are observed to occur after frank mechanical or chemical injury to the nerve. Two examples will be noted. First, after nerve injury, there is evidence to suggest a loss of tonic GABAergic or glycinergic modulation (Ibuki *et al.*, 1997; Moore *et al.*, 2002). GABA/glycinergic terminals are frequently presynaptic to the large central afferent terminal complexes and form reciprocal synapses, while GABAergic axosomatic connections on spinothalamic cells have also been identified (Todd, 2002; Watson, 2003). Accordingly, it is not surprising that these amino acids exert an important tonic or evoked inhibitory control over the activity of Aβ non-nociceptive primary afferent terminals and second order neurons in the spinal dorsal horn (Lin *et al.*, 1996). Secondly, it has been shown that there is a significant increase in activation of spinal microglia and astrocytes in the spinal segments receiving input from the injured nerves (Watkins *et al.*, 2003). Of particular interest is that in the face of pathology such as bone cancer, such up-regulation has been clearly shown (Honore *et al.*, 2000). Astrocytes are activated by a variety of neurotransmitters and growth factors. While the origin of this activation is not clear, it can potentially lead to an increased spinal expression of COX/ NOS/glutamate transporters/proteinases. Recent studies have emphasized that P38 MAPK is present in microglia (Svensson *et al.*, 2003).

8.4 Regulation of spinal nociceptive processing

The above comments relate to mechanisms which are present within the spinal dorsal horn, based on immunohistochemistry and electrophysiological indices. As with the original work with spinal morphine, the relevance of these spinal cascades in spinal pain processing is established by demonstrating that the spinal delivery of these agents in the unanesthetized animal will alter defined aspects of the behavioral response, in well-defined models, to nociception. Pharmacological components that are associated with non-noxious stimuli or with motor function may indeed alter nociceptive processing but, in the absence of specificity, would fail to qualify as analgesic agents.

Given the above, it is not surprising that in the last decade, there has been an explosion in drug candidates and a real expansion in the number of therapeutic targets, which can alter afferent processes and pain behavior. The continuing development of insights into the pharmacology of the spinal cord alone promises a rich source of approaches to managing pain states. At virtually every level, there is potential for controlling the encoding process. The diversity of receptors and the potential association of receptor and channel subtype with specific functions offer broad possibilities of creating approaches with improved therapeutic ratios. Heuristically, pharmacological interventions can be targeted at the processes leading to the release of the primary afferent transmitter and the second order events that arise from the tissue or nerve injury-induced input, as outlined above.

8.5 **Primary afferent terminal excitability**

As outlined above, the first link in afferent processing is the primary afferent synapses which, for small high-threshold afferents, are present in the substantia gelatinosa and marginal layer of the superficial dorsal horn. The pharmacology of this terminal and synapse has been a rich target for selective interventions. Table 8.2 summarizes the spinal actions of several classes of drugs which regulate nociceptive processing.

8.5.1 **Opioids**

The spinal delivery of opioids in mice through to primates will reliably attenuate the response of the animal to a variety of unconditioned somatic and visceral stimuli that otherwise evoke an organized escape behavior in all species thus far examined (Yaksh, 1987, 1997a) (see Table 8.2). Initial work demonstrated that these effects were mediated by spinal μ and δ opioid receptors based on agonist structure, activity relationship, stereospecificity, and antagonist pharmacology.

Table 8.1 Mechanistic organization of pain states*

'Pain state'	Afferent linkage	Spinal linkage	Behavior models
ACUTE	Aδ/C	Stimulus dependent	Hot plate
Focal /transient		Activation of spinal	Tail flick
Mechanical/thermal		nociceptive neuron	Paw Press
stimuli			
TISSUE INJURY	Terminal sensitization:	Facilitation: ↑ receptive field of spinal nociceptive	Formalin (phase 2) Carrageenan inflamed
Spontaneous pain	Aδ/C (SA)	neuron; windup/long-term	Paw incision
1° hyperalgesia	Aδ/C	potentiation	Focal paw burn
2° tactile allodynia	Aβ		
NERVE INJURY		Facilitation: ↑ spontaneous	Bennett (CCI)
Spontaneous pain	Aδ/C (SA)	activity; ↑ stimulus-evoked	Chung (L5/6 ligation)
1° hyperalgesia	Aδ/C	discharge; loss of inhibitory	Shir (sciatic hemiligation)
2° tactile allodynia	Aβ	neurons; ↑ sprouting (Aβ)	IT strychnine
		↑ receptors	

* Yaksh, 1999

Table 8.2 Spinal agents in preclinical pain models

Drug classes	Acute (thermal/ Mechanical)	Tissue injury (thermal/ mechanical	References
Agonists			
Opioid μ/d	+	+	Yaksh, 1993
Alpha₂ adrenergic	+	+	Yaksh et al., 1993
Neuropeptide Y	+	+	Hua et al., 1991
Antagonists/inhibitors			
Glutamate — NMDA	0	+	Chaplan et al., 1997
— AMPA	+	+	Nozaki–Taguchi & Yaksh, 2002
Tachykinin: NK1	0	+	Yamamoto & Yaksh, 1991
P38 MAPKinase	0	+	Svensson et al., 2003
PLA2	0	+	Killerman et al., in press
VDCC: N-type	0	+	Malmberg & Yaksh, 1994
COX (2)	0	+	Malmberg & Yaksh, 1992a,b
PG: EP1	0	+	Malmberg et al., 1994

Subsequent work using receptor autoradiography with opiate ligands or immuno-histochemistry revealed that the binding to receptor protein is limited for the most part to the substantia gelatinosa, the region in which small afferents principally terminate (Besse *et al.*, 1990). Dorsal rhizotomies result in a great reduction in dorsal horn opiate binding, suggesting that a significant proportion is associated with the primary afferents, the remainder of dorsal horn binding presumably being related to the membranes postsynaptic to the primary afferent (Abbadie *et al.*, 2002). This finding is consistent with the presence of opioid receptor protein being synthesized in and transported from small dorsal root ganglion cells. Confirmation of the presynaptic action is provided by the observation that opiates reduce the release of primary afferent peptide transmitters such as substance P contained in small afferents (Yaksh *et al.*, 1980). The presynaptic action corresponds to the ability of opiates to prevent the opening of voltage-sensitive Ca^{++} channels, thereby preventing release (Law *et al.*, 2000). A postsynaptic action was demonstrated by the ability of opiates to block the excitation of dorsal horn neurons evoked by glutamate, reflecting a direct activation of the dorsal horn. The activation of potassium channels, leading to hyperpolarization, is consistent with direct postsynaptic inhibition. The dual ability of spinal opiates to reduce the release of excitatory neurotransmitters from C-fibers as well as decrease the excitability of dorsal horn neurons is believed to account for the powerful and selective effect upon spinal nociceptive processing (Yaksh, 1997*b*).

8.5.2 **Alpha-adrenergic receptors**

The spinal delivery of agents such as clonidine and dexmedetomidine can produce a powerful analgesia in human and animal models. The agonist and antagonist pharmacology emphasizes that these effects are mediated by a spinal alpha 2 receptor (Takano and Yaksh, 1992). This spinal action of alpha 2 is mediated by a mechanism remarkably similar to that employed by spinal opiates:

1. Alpha 2 receptors are present in high concentrations in the DRG and in the substantia gelatinosa (Shi *et al.*, 2000).
2. Significant binding disappears after rhizotomy (Howe *et al.*, 1987).
3. Alpha 2 agonists can depress the release of C-fiber transmitters (Takano *et al.*, 1993; Kawasaki *et al.*, 2003).
4. Alpha 2 agonists can block the opening of voltage-sensitive Ca channels and hyperpolarize dorsal horn neurons through a Gi coupled K channel (Aantaa *et al.*, 1995).

There are three subclasses of alpha 2 receptors, which have been cloned (2A, 2B, and 2C). Pharmacological studies suggest that the analgesic effects may be mediated distinctly at the spinal level by both alpha 2A and non-A subclasses (Takano and Yaksh, 1992).

8.5.3 **Other drug classes**

This regulatory control of afferent terminal excitability suggested by the effects of alpha 2 adrenergic and μ and δ opioid agonists is important in defining spinal targets for antinociception with a significant therapeutic ratio, including receptor systems located presynaptically on C-fibers and postsynaptically on spinal neurons, the block of small afferent peptide release, and the ability to hyperpolarize dorsal horn neurons. Importantly, that rationale led to the specific consideration of the spinal actions of neuropeptide Y (NPY). Spinal receptors for this peptide have been found, and NPY has been shown to alter afferent peptide release and to produce a potent analgesia following spinal delivery (Walker *et al.*, 1988; Duggan *et al.*, 1991; Hua *et al.*, 1993).

8.6 **Postsynaptic processes**

8.6.1 **Postsynaptic primary afferent transmitter action**

Given the identification of primary afferent transmitters such as SP and glutamate, an evident target would appear to be their respective receptors on the second order neuron. The strength of this approach rests on the uniqueness of the role played by the respective transmitter. As noted, the postsynaptic depolarization produced by afferent terminals reflects the concurrent release of several transmitters (e.g. glutamate, several peptides, and perhaps ATP) (Chizh and Illes, 2001). Accordingly, block of a single receptor will be effective only to the degree that the excitatory drive is provided uniquely by those agonists. In this regard, the spinal delivery of NK1 (substance P) receptor or NMDA (glutamate) ionophore antagonists have not been particularly effective in blocking the net postsynaptic depolarization or in altering acute afferent traffic. In contrast, non-NMDA (AMPA) antagonists have been potently effective in blocking terminal- evoked depolarization and altering stimulus-evoked pain behavior. The AMPA receptor is widely distributed on dorsal horn neurons and appears to mediate depolarization secondary to large and small afferent input (Dickenson *et al.*, 1997). Consistent with this scenario, intrathecal AMPA, but not NMDA or NK1 antagonists, diminishes the behavioral response to acute, thermal, or mechanical stimuli (see Table 8.2).

8.6.2 **Facilitated processing**

Aside from altering afferent input and its postsynaptic activation, it is clear that persistent afferent input (as occurs after tissue injury or nerve injury) can induce a strong facilitator state such that there is an enhanced behavioral response to a given non-noxious or mildly aversive stimuli. Consistent with the cascade outlined in Fig. 8.2, underlying facilitated spinal processing, several classes of agents have been identified as altering the behaviorally defined hyperalgesic states otherwise observed following a variety of tissue and nerve injuries.

As outlined in the above sections, these facilitated states represent complex cascades in which there appears to be a net amplification of the spinofugal message generated by a given stimulus (wind-up/LTP) initiated by NK1 and NMDa receptor activation. Behavioral work has indeed confirmed that the spinal delivery of NMDA and NK1 antagonists at doses which have no effect upon acute nocisponsive behavior, prominently diminishes the hyperalgesic states that arise from tissue injury and inflammation. Importantly, blockade of other components of this proposed cascade, including protein kinase C (PKC), P38 mitogen activated protein kinase (MAPK), phospholipase A2 (PLA2), cyclooxygenase 2 (COX2), and E-type prostagandins receptors (EP-r) (see Table 8.2), can diminish prominently the hyperpathia at doses which have little or no effect upon the response to either acute nociceptive stimuli or upon motor function. This list is not meant to be exhaustive, but gives some sense of the breadth of the endeavor. While a major discussion could be targeted at each of these receptors/channels, this is beyond the scope of this chapter. However, for each specific drug class, several points can be made.

There are published preclinical studies that provide support for the ability of representative agents to alter the behavior of the preclinical surrogate in a manner that is indicative of changes in nociceptive responding.

The presumed actions of several classes of drugs accord with our understanding of the biology of the pharmacologically distinct systems that process nociceptive information. Thus, the effects of opiates and alpha 2 agonists are reversed by the respective receptor antagonists. The actions of prostaglandins synthesis inhibitors parallel their ability to block cyclooxygenase, particularly that of the COX2 isozyme (Malmberg and Yaksh, 1992*a*; Dirig *et al.*, 1998). In each case it is possible, based on our understanding of the underlying neurobiology, to hypothesize spinal mechanisms by which the facilitated state is generated. Such facilitated states can be regulated in several specific ways:

1. They may be pre-emptively diminished by pretreatment with spinal drug classes which block the initiating small afferent input (e.g. local anesthetics, opiate and alpha 2 agonists).

2. As reviewed, there are specific pharmacologically defined links in the downstream cascade where the facilitatory components may be blocked. In such cases, the linkages may not be relevant to acute nociceptive processing. Thus, the intrathecal delivery of NMDA antagonists or COX inhibitors will have little effect upon an acute high-intensity stimulus but will block the injury-induced facilitation observed in models of inflammation and tissue injury.

3. The concept of a cascade implies the importance of timing. Thus, to the extent that a given mechanism is believed to trigger the downstream event, pharmacological intervention at that link after the initiation has occurred will be proportionately less effective. Thus, treatment with intrathecal NMDA antagonists after phase 1 of the formalin test is substantially less effective than pretreatment (Yamamoto and Yaksh, 1992).

8.7 Spinal interventions that alter the biology of synaptic transmission

While the classic approach to analgesic therapies have typically involved the delivery of agents which have a pharmacological action at some critical link (e.g. morphine and the opiate receptor, NSAIDs, and cyclooxygenase inhibition), advances have pointed to a variety of mechanistically unique interventions which might be particularly useful when the target is a spinal system. The facility of routinely delivering drugs into this geographically circumscribed region with the blood–brain barrier provides an opportunity to employ unique therapeutic agents.

8.7.1 Antisense

To the degree that the physiologist and pharmacologist can identify the role of specific proteins such as the NK1 receptor, an appropriate antisense sequence may be predictably developed targeted at the respective mRNA to block the expression of that protein (Wagner, 1995). Studies have shown, for example, that the intrathecal delivery of NK1 receptor antisense will reduce the spinal expression of NK1 protein and binding and produce an anti-hyperalgesic profile similar to that resulting from intrathecally delivered NK1 antagonists. (Hua et al., 1998). This approach has been similarly used to target NMDA ionophore channels such as the PN3 sodium channel and enzymes such as cyclooxygenase 2. In each case, the treatment results in down-regulation of the expression of the protein and/or the mRNA and changes in pain processing that are consistent with the effects of the respective drug where available (Table 8.3).

Table 8.3 Intrathecal antisense and nociception

Target	Model	Reference
NK1-r	IT: formalin	Hua et al., 1999
PN3 sodium channel	IT: inflammation, hyperalgesia	Lai et al., 2000
NMDA-r	IT: formalin	Yukhananov et al., 2002
PKCa	IT: formalin	Hua et al., 2002
COX2	IT: NMDA hyperalgesia	Svensson & Yaksh, unpublished

8.7.2 Transfection/cell replacement

Augmenting the functionality of endogenous systems is a potential approach for altering spinal nociceptive transmission. The spinal delivery of vectors that would target local cell populations could result in hypersecretion of a given target transmitter such as enkephalin (Goss et al., 2001) or IL2 (Yao et al., 2003) and could feasibly provide a possible method of long-term management of afferent processing (Pohl et al., 2003). Alternately, the spinal delivery of cells that secrete target agents to modulate spinal processing, such as β endorphin (Saitoh et al., 1995) or enkephalin (Wu et al., 1994), has been demonstrated (Hentall and Sagen, 2000).

8.7.3 Targeted cell death

The observation that the cell may answer a discrete knock at its membrane by opening a specific door may prove to be of particular significance. Activation of the NK1 receptor, for example, is known to be accompanied by an internalization of the receptor protein and its bound ligand. The NK1 receptor for substance P is clearly believed to be on cells that are important to nociceptive processing. Attaching toxins to the SP ligand (and that are otherwise unable to penetrate the cell) has led to the demonstration that the SP-toxin complex can be internalized and destroy that cell (Fig. 8.3) leading to antinociception (Nicols et al., 1999; Khasabov et al., 2002). Internalization systems for different G protein-coupled receptors (e.g. μ opioid) will permit functionally selective alterations in spinal processing by targeting specific populations of neurons.

8.8 Clinical and preclinical correlates

An important issue relates to the comparability of the mechanisms of spinal nociceptive processing defined in preclinical models and those that are at play in humans. While many agents are clearly relevant in preclinical models, their action in humans has, for reasons of safety and toxicity, been less well evaluated. Nevertheless, as noted in Table 8.4, the preclinical observations have in fact been paralleled by corresponding observations of potency in human pain states for many agents. These observations serve to validate the preclinical models and indirectly suggest that in humans, as in animals, post-injury pain states engage complex mechanisms that lead to alterations in the processing otherwise initiated by the acute high-intensity stimulus.

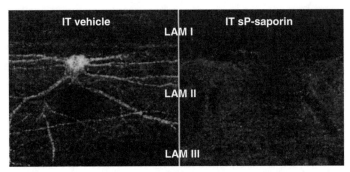

Fig. 8.3 Immunohistochemistry shown in a portion of the dorsal horn taken from a dog receiving the intrathecal injections of a vehicle (left) or 150 μg of sP-saporin (right). At one month, in the vehicle- treated animal, the typical NK1- bearing neurons are observed. In sP-saporin-treated animals there is almost complete loss of the NK1-bearing neurons, with continued preservation of a large proportion of non-NK1-bearing cells as determined by cell counts of NeuN positive cells (not shown).

8.9 Polypharmacy

While the use of a single entity in managing any clinical problem is preferable, there are logical reasons why even at the spinal level, polypharmacy may be necessary or preferred. The first relates to the fact that clinical pain states often possess multiple etiologies. Cancer may be associated with acute tissue distention and erosion as well as nerve compression or toxicity secondary to chemotherapy. Different systems display multiple pharmacological mechanisms. Accordingly, a reasonable theoretical approach is the use of agents that target the several components. Thus, agents that block acute small afferent traffic (e.g. μ and α_2) in combination with agents that alter post nerve-injury states (low concentrations of local anesthetic or gabapentinoids) present as a rational polypharmacy. The second reason for polypharmacy relates to the possibility that the therapeutic advantage of an agent may be enhanced when two or more classes of agents with different side- effect profiles interact in a non-linear fashion with respect to their antinociceptive action. Such interactions have been characterized for several classes of drugs and are typically complex. This has been reviewed elsewhere (Yaksh and Malmberg, 1994). It is important to note that in the management of chronic pain in humans, such intrathecal polypharmacy is the rule rather than the exception (Bennett *et al.*, 2000).

8.10 Issues pertinent to spinal drug delivery

While comments have been targeted at aspects of spinal pharmacology, it should be appreciated that the delivery of agents into the spinal space must also consider the prosaic issue of drug delivery. With systemic delivery, the agent distributes to all areas of the body reached by the circulation and where local tissue concentrations are

Table 8.4 Clinical and preclinical correlates of spinal drug action

Drug classes	Animal models*	Human pain states	Drugs	References
μ opiates	A/P	Post-op Arthritis Cancer	Morphine, methadone fentanyl, sufentanil; dilaudid, meperidine β-endorphin	Yaksh, 1993
δ opiates		Cancer	D-ala-2-d-leu 5 enkephalin (DADL)	Yaksh, 1993 Onofrio & Yaksh, 1983
K opiate	A	Post-op Cancer	Butorphanol	
Alpha 2 adrenergic Agonist	A/P/N	Post-op Cancer Neuropathic	Clonidine	Yaksh et al., 1993 Eisenach et al., 1996
AChase inhibitor	A/P	Post-op Cancer	Neostigmine	Prado & Goncalves, 1997 Naguib & Yaksh, 1994 Naguib & Yaksh, 1997 Hood et al., 1995 Lauretti & Lima, 1996
COX inhibitor	P	Post-op Cancer	Lysine-acetylsalicylate	Malmberg & Yaksh, 1992 Devoghel, 1983
Adenosine A-1 agonist	P/N	Neuropathic	R-PIA adenosine	Poon & Sawynok, 1998 Karlsten & Gordh Jr, 1995 Rane et al., 1998
GABA (GABA-B)	P/N	Neuropathic	Baclofen	Dirig & Yaksh, 1995 Porter, 1997
Ca++ channel blocker, N-type	P/N	Neuropathic Cancer	Ziconotide	Malmberg & Yaksh, 1994 Brose et al., 1997
NMDA antagonist	P/N	Neuropathic	Ketamine, CPP	Chaplan et al., 1997 Abdel–Ghaffar et al., 1998 Kristensen et al., 1992

*Indicates class of pain model. A: acute nociception; P: post-tissue injury; N: neuropathic.

proportional to the total dose delivered into the organism. In contrast, several properties distinguish the spinal delivery of drugs from the systemic route. First, the spinal delivery of drugs targeted at specific receptors/channels/enzymes reflects the local application of the agent into a fluid volume that bathes the external surface of spinal cord. For agents other than local anesthetics, these targets lie up 50 μ from the surface in the rat, 200 μ from the surface in dogs, and 500 μ in humans. The agents must then penetrate the lipid-heavy white matter to reach these sites. The force driving this diffusion depends upon the physical chemical properties of the drug (molecular weight, lipid partition coefficient), the local gradient (injectate concentration).

Second, the spinally delivered drug must reach the receptors that are relevant to the underlying components that are being regulated. Thus, for example, to block the input from the foot and lower leg, a local anesthetic would work at the level of approximately 6 roots (Fig. 8.4). In contrast, with spinal opiates, the intrathecal drug must reach the terminals of the sensory afferent carrying the injury message. It is clear that the spinal terminals for any given root distribute rostrocaudally over an extended number of segments, perhaps as many as 4 or 5 segments rostally and 2 or 3 segments caudally (Wall and Shortland, 1991; Shortland and Wall, 1992; Wilson and Kitchener, 1996) (see Fig. 8.4). Again, unlike the systemic delivery, where the distribution is dependent upon the vascular absorption and flow, CSF kinetics are slow and frequently erratic (Bernards, 2002; Eisenach *et al.*, 2003). Accordingly, achieving such a distribution with the normal catheter may involve using larger doses or volumes. An anesthesiologist may 'barbatoge' the local anesthetic to achieve the appropriate sensory level of block. Accordingly, the effect of a spinal-delivered agent (bolus/infusion) is dependent upon a number of physical parameters such as the volume of the injection or the rate of infusion. Advances in the use of spinal agents may thus depend, in part, upon advances in the delivery systems themselves. For example, the use of catheter systems that uniformly deliver the agent over a length of spinal cord, rather than from a single point, may well serve to diminish the total dose required.

8.11 **Spinal drug safety**

All drugs, no matter by what route they are given, must be considered in the context of their safety. This issue of safety is of particular importance for spinal drug delivery. Here, there is a direct application of the agent into the spinal space at a concentration that frequently exceeds that employed in pharmacological studies (e.g. mg/mL). There is little doubt that such agents merit a particularly robust assessment. The development of well-documented preclinical models using chronically catheterized large animal models have been shown to be of particular significance in achieving some degree of assurance as to the lack of toxicity prior to intrathecal delivery in humans.

It important to stress that long experience with an agent delivered by a systemic route gives only a modest indication of the local toxicity when the higher concentrations required are employed for direct delivery. Moreover, agents such as lidocaine, which

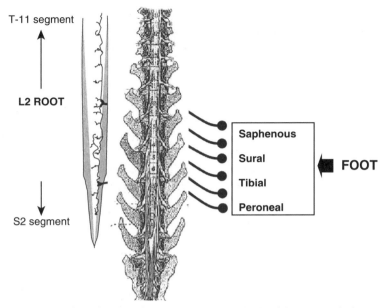

Fig. 8.4 Innervation of the foot and lower extremities is obtained by axons which travel through a variety of peripheral nerves. These nerves are comprised of axons arising from roots ranging in the animal from L7 to L2. It is appreciated that the axons entering the spinal dorsal horn send collaterals both rostrally and caudally to terminals several segments distal to the root of entry. For a local anesthetic to block pain from the foot, it need only block the afferent axons at the level of several roots. In contrast, agents acting to alter the excitability of the central afferent terminal must reach spinal levels that are contiguous with these distal afferent terminals.

have long been used with spinal delivery, have in recent years been discovered to have important local safety issues — lidocaine radiculopathies (Johnson, 2000) and morphine-evoked intrathecal granulomas (Yaksh *et al.*, 2002, 2003; Gradert *et al.*, 2003). These agents, because of their historic precedence, had not been appropriately studied under conditions in which they were ultimately employed. In each case, the problem arose because of the progressively increasing concentrations that were being used to permit smaller volumes and longer infusion pump refill intervals. Importantly, these problems were defined in preclinical models. This unfortunate validation of the ability of the preclinical model to predict human toxicity emphasizes that such models are appropriate indices of human safety (Yaksh *et al.*, 1999; Eisenach *et al.*, 2002).

8.12 **Concluding comments**

The extraordinary development in our understanding of the spinal biology of pain processing has led to an appreciation of the complexity of the underlying systems at the level of the primary afferent and spinal cord. This brief overview emphasizes that spinal systems encode information that is sufficient to engender a pain state. This encoding occurs by multiple mechanisms manifesting a complex pharmacology.

Importantly, these advances in the biology of pain have led to an implementation of several of these insights into clinical pain management. The focus on spinal drug delivery has achieved its goals by virtue of the distinct pharmacology of sensory encoding (e.g. light touch versus tissue injury). As such, it provides validation of the Cartesian assertion that pain at the spinal level has a specific encoding. The routine ability to deliver drugs acutely and chronically into the intrathecal space, along with the multiple targets and methods for intervening in the biology of specific neural nets and the importance of the spinal cord in pain processing, suggest that the continued development of agents for spinal delivery will yield important advances in the control of pain. It should be stressed in conclusion, however, that the movement of these novel therapies into the clinic depends upon the demonstration of their safety in robust preclinical models.

References

Aantaa R, Marjamaki A, Scheinin M (1995) Molecular pharmacology of alpha 2-adrenoceptor subtypes. *Ann Med* **7(4)**:439–49.

Abbadie C, Lombard MC, Besson JM, Trafton JA, Basbaum AI (2002) Mu and delta opioid receptor-like immunoreactivity in the cervical spinal cord of the rat after dorsal rhizotomy or neonatalcapsaicin: an analysis of pre- and postsynaptic receptor distributions. *Brain Res* **930(1–2)**:150–62.

Abdel–Ghaffar ME, Abdulatif MA, al–Ghamdi A, Mowafi H, Anwar A (1998) Epidural ketamine reduces post-operative epidural PCA consumption of fentanyl/bupivacaine. *Can J Anaesth* **45(2)**:103–9.

Balsinde J, Winstead MV, Dennis EA (2002) Phospholipase A(2) regulation of arachidonic acid mobilization. *FEBS Lett* **531(1)**:2–6.

Behar M, Magora F, Olshwang D, Davidson JT (1979) Epidural morphine in treatment of pain. *Lancet* **1(8115)**:527–9.

Bennett G, Serafini M, Burchiel K, *et al.* (2000) Evidence-based review of the literature on intrathecal delivery of pain medication. *J Pain Symptom Manage* **20**: S12–36.

Bernards CM (2002) Understanding the physiology and pharmacology of epidural and intrathecal opioids. *Best Pract Res Clin Anaesthesiol* **16(4)**:489–505.

Besse D, Lombard MC, Zajac M, Roques BP, Besson JM (1990) Pre- and post-synaptic distribution of μ, δ, and κ opioid receptors in the superficial layers of the dorsal horn of the rat spinal cord. *Brain Res* **521(1–2)**:15–22.

Brose WG, Gutlove DP, Luther RR, Bowersox SS, McGuire D (1997) Use of intrathecal SNX-111, novel, N-type, voltage-sensitive, calcium channel blocker, in the management of intractable brachial plexus avulsion pain. *Clin J Pain* **13(3)**:256–9.

Chaplan SR, Malmberg AB, Yaksh TL (1997) Efficacy of spinal NMDA receptor antagonism in formalin hyperalgesia and nerve injury evoked allodynia in the rat. *J Pharmacol Exper Ther* **280**: 829–38.

Chizh BA, Illes P (2001) P2X receptors and nociception. *Pharmacol Rev* **53(4)**:553–68.

Devoghel JC (1983) Small intrathecal doses of lysine-acetylsalicylate relieve intractable pain in man. *J Int Med Res* **11(2)**:90–1.

Dickenson AH, Stanfa LC, Chapman V, Yaksh TL (1997) Response properties of dorsal horn neurons: pharmacology of the dorsal horn. In *Anesthesia: Biologic Foundations* (eds. Yaksh TL, Lynch III C, Zapol WM, Maze M, Biebuyck JF, Saidman LJ). Lippincott–Raven Publishers, Philadelphia, pp. 611–24.

Dirig DM, Yaksh TL (1995) Intrathecal baclofen and muscimol, but not midazolam, are antinociceptive using the rat-formalin model. *J Pharmacol Exper Ther* **275**:219–27.

Dirig DM, Isakson PC, Yaksh TL (1998) Effect of COX-1 and COX-2 inhibition on induction and maintenance of carrageenan-evoked thermal hyperalgesia in rats. *J Pharmacol Exper Ther* **285**:1031–7.

Duggan AW, North RA (1983) Electrophysiology of opioids. *Pharmacol Rev* **35(4)**:219–81.

Duggan AW, Hope PJ, Lang CW (1991) Microinjection of neuropeptide Y into the superficial dorsal horn reduces stimulus-evoked release of immunoreactivesubstance P in the anaesthetized cat. *Neuroscience* **44(3)**:733–40.

Eisenach JC, Yaksh TL (2002) Safety in numbers: how do we study toxicity of spinal analgesics? *Anesthesiology* **97(5)**:1047–9.

Eisenach JC, De Kock M, Klimscha W (1996) *Anesthesiology* **85**:655–74.

Eisenach JC, Hood DD, Curry R, Shafer SL (2003) Cephalad movement of morphine and fentanyl in humans after intrathecal injection. *Anesthesiology* **99(1)**:166–73.

Foster AC, Fagg GE (1987) Neurobiology. Taking apart NMDA receptors. *Nature* **329(6138)**:395–6.

Goss JR, Mata M, Goins WF, Wu HH, Glorioso JC, Fink DJ (2001) Antinociceptive effect of a genomic herpes simplex virus-based vector expressing human proenkephalin in rat dorsalroot ganglion. *Gene Ther* **8(7)**:551–6.

Gradert TL, Baze WB, Satterfield WC, Hildebrand KR, Johansen MJ, Hassenbusch SJ (2003) Safety of chronic intrathecal morphine infusion in a sheep model. *Anesthesiology* **99(1)**:188–98

Hentall ID, Sagen J (2000) The alleviation of pain by cell transplantation. *Prog Brain Res* **127**:535–50.

Honore P, Rogers SD, Schwei MJ, *et al.* (2000) Murine models of inflammatory, neuropathic and cancer pain: each generates a unique set of neurochemical changes in the spinal cord and sensory neurons. *Neuroscience* **98(3)**:585–98.

Hood DD, Eisenach JC, Tuttle R (1995) Phase I safety assessment of intrathecal neostigmine methylsulfate in humans. *Anesthesiology* **82(2)**:331–43.

Howe JR, Yaksh TL, Go VL (1987) The effect of unilateral dorsal root ganglionectomies or ventral rhizotomies on alpha 2-adrenoceptor binding to, and the substance P, enkephalin, and neurotensin content of, the cat lumbar spinal cord. *Neuroscience* **21(2)**:385–9

Hua X–Y, Boublik JH, Spicer MA, Rivier JE, Brown MR, Yaksh TL (1991) The antinociceptive effects of spinally administered neuropeptide Y in the rat: systematic studies on structure-activity relationship. *J Pharmacol Exper Ther* **258**:243–58.

Hua XY, Chen P, Polgar E, *et al.* (1998) Spinal neurokinin NK1 receptor down-regulation and antinociception: effects of spinal NK1 receptor antisense oligonucleotides and NK1 receptor occupancy. *J Neurochem* **70**:688–98.

Hua XY, Moore A, Malkmus S, *et al.* (2002) Inhibition of spinal protein kinase Calpha expression by an antisense oligonucleotide attenuates morphine infusion-induced tolerance. *Neuroscience* **113(1)**:99–107.

Ibuki T, Hama AT, Wang XT, Pappas GD, Sagen J (1997) Loss of GABA-immunoreactivity in the spinal dorsal horn of rats with peripheral nerve injury and promotion of recovery by adrenal medullary grafts. *Neuroscience* **76(3)**:845–58.

Ikeda H, Heinke B, Ruscheweyh R, Sandkuhler J (2003) Synaptic plasticity in spinal lamina I projection neurons that mediate hyperalgesia. *Science* **299(5610)**:1237–40.

Ji RR, Woolf CJ (2001) Neuronal plasticity and signal transduction in nociceptive neurons: implications for the initiation and maintenance of pathological pain. *Neurobiol Dis* **8(1)**:1–10

Johnson GL, Lapadat R (2002) Mitogen-activated protein kinase pathways mediated by ERK, JNK, and p38 protein kinases. *Science* **298(5600)**:1911–2.

Johnson ME (2000) Potential neurotoxicity of spinal anesthesia with lidocaine. *Mayo Clin Proc* **75(9)**:921–32

Karlsten R, Gordh T Jr. (1995) An A1-selective adenosine agonist abolishes allodynia elicited by vibration and touch after intrathecal injection. *Anesth Analg* **80(4)**:844–7.

Kawasaki Y, Kumamoto E, Furue H, Yoshimura M (2003) Alpha 2 adrenoceptor-mediated presynaptic inhibition of primary afferent glutamatergic transmission in rat substantia gelatinosa neurons. *Anesthesiology* **98(3)**:682–9.

Khasabov SG, Rogers SD, Ghilardi JR, Peters CM, Mantyh PW, Simone DA (2002) Spinal neurons that possess the substance P receptor are required for the development of central sensitization. *J Neurosci* **22(20)**:9086–98.

Kocsis P, Tarnawa I, Szombathelyi Z, Farkas S (2003) Participation of AMPA- and NMDA-type excitatory amino acid receptors in the spinal reflex transmission, in rat. *Brain Res Bull* **60(1–2)**:81–91.

Kondo I, Marvizon JC, Song B, Sargado F, Codeluppi S, Hua XY, Yaksh TL (2005) Inhibition by spinal μ- and δ-opioid agonists of afferent evoked substance P release. *J Neurosci* in press.

Kristensen JD, Svensson B, Gordh T Jr. (1992) The NMDA-receptor antagonist CPP abolishes neurogenic 'wind-up pain' after intrathecal administration in humans. *Pain* **51(2)**:249–53.

Lai J, Hunter JC, Ossipov MH, Porreca F (2000) Blockade of neuropathic pain by antisense targeting of tetrodotoxin-resistant sodium channels in sensory neurons. *Methods Enzymol* **314**:201–13.

Lauretti GR, Lima IC (1996) The effects of intrathecal neostigmine on somatic and visceral pain: improvement by association with a peripheral anticholinergic. *Anesth Analg* **82(3)**:617–20.

Law PY, Wong YH, Loh HH (2000) Molecular mechanisms and regulation of opioid receptor signaling. *Annu Rev Pharmacol Toxicol* **40**:389–430.

Lin Q, Peng YB, Willis WD (1996) Inhibition of primate spinothalamic tract neurons by spinal glycine and GABA is reduced during central sensitization. *J Neurophysiol* **6(2)**:1005–14.

Lucas KL, Svensson CI, Hua XY, Yaksh TL, Dennis EA (in press) Spinal phospholipase A$_2$ in inflammatory hyperalgesia: role of group IV cPLA$_2$ and group VI iPLA$_2$. *Brit J Pharmacol* in press.

MacDonald JF, Kotecha SA, Lu WY, Jackson MF (2001) Convergence of PKC-dependent kinase signal cascades on NMDA receptors. *Curr Drug Targets* **2(3)**:299–312.

Malmberg AB, Yaksh TL (1992a) Hyperalgesia mediated by spinal glutamate or substance P receptor blocked by spinal cyclooxygenase inhibition. *Science* **257**:1276–9.

Malmberg AB, Yaksh TL (1992b) Antinociceptive actions of spinal nonsteroidal anti-inflammatory agents on the formalin test in the rat. *J Pharmacol Exper Ther* **263**:136–46.

Malmberg AB, Yaksh TL (1994) Voltage-sensitive calcium channels in spinal nociceptive processing: blockade of N- and P-type channels inhibits formalin-induced nociception. *J Neurosci* **14**:4882–90.

Malmberg AB, Rafferty MF, Yaksh TL (1994) Antinociceptive effect of spinally delivered prostaglandin E receptor antagonists in the formalin test on the rat. *Neurosci Lett* **173**:193–6.

Melzack R, Wall PD (1965) Pain mechanisms: a new theory. *Science* **150**:971–9.

Moore KA, Kohno T, Karchewski LA, Scholz J, Baba H, Woolf CJ (2002) Partial peripheral nerve injury promotes a selective loss of GABAergic inhibition in the superficial dorsal horn of the spinal cord. *J Neurosci* **22(15)**:6724–31.

Naguib M, Yaksh TL (1994) Antinociceptive effects of spinal cholinesterase inhibition and isobolographic analysis of the interaction with μ and α$_2$ receptor systems. *Anesthesiology* **80**: 1338–48.

Naguib M, Yaksh TL (1997) Characterization of muscarinic receptor subtypes that mediate antinociception in the rat spinal cord. *Anesth Analg* **85**:847–53.

Nichols ML, Allen BJ, Rogers SD, *et al.* (1999) Transmission of chronic nociception by spinal neurons expressing the substance P receptor. *Science* **286**:1558–61.

Nozaki–Taguchi N, Yaksh, TL (2002) Pharmacology of spinal glutamatertgic receptors in post-thermal injury-evoked tactile allodynia and thermal hyperalgesia. *Anesthesiology* **96**:617–26.

Onofrio BM, Yaksh TL (1983) Intrathecal delta-receptor ligand produces Analgesia in humans. *Lancet* **1**:1386–7.

Onofrio BM, Yaksh TL, Arnold PG (1981) Continuous low-dose intrathecal morphine administration in the treatment of chronic pain of malignant origin. *Mayo Clin Proc* **56**:516–20.

Pohl M, Meunier A, Hamon M, Braz J (2003) Gene therapy of chronic pain. *Curr Gene Ther* **3(3)**:223–38.

Poon A, Sawynok J (1998) Antinociception by adenosine analogs and inhibitors of adenosine metabolism in an inflammatory thermal hyperalgesiamodel in the rat. *Pain* **74(2–3)**:235–45.

Porter B (1997)A review of intrathecal baclofen in the management of spasticity. *Br J Nurs* **6(5)**:253–60, 262.

Prado WA, Goncalves AS (1997) Antinociceptive effect of intrathecal neostigmine evaluated in rats by two different pain models. *Braz J Med Biol Res* **30(10)**:1225–31.

Rane K, Segerdahl M, Goiny M, Sollevi A (1998) Intrathecal adenosine administration: a phase 1 clinical safety study in healthy volunteers, with additional evaluation of its influence on sensory thresholds and experimental pain. *Anesthesiology* **89(5)**:1108–15.

Richards DA, Bliss TV, Richards CD (2003) Differential modulation of NMDA-induced calcium transients by arachidonic acid and nitric oxide in cultured hippocampal neurons. *Eur J Neurosci* **17(11)**:2323–8.

Saitoh Y, Taki T, Arita N, Ohnishi T, Hayakawa T (1995) Cell therapy with encapsulated xenogeneic tumor cells secreting beta-endorphin for treatment of peripheral pain. *Cell Transplant* **4 (Suppl 1)**:S13–7.

Samad TA, Sapirstein A, Woolf CJ (2002) Prostanoids and pain: unraveling mechanisms and revealing therapeutic targets. *Trends Mol Med* **8(8)**:390–6.

Shi TS, Winzer–Serhan U, Leslie F, Hokfelt T (2000) Distribution and regulation of alpha(2)-adrenoceptors in rat dorsal root ganglia. *Pain* **84(2–3)**:319–30.

Shortland P, Wall PD (1992) Long-range afferents in the rat spinal cord. II. Arborizations that penetrate grey matter. *Philos Trans R Soc Lond B Biol Sci* **337(1282)**:445–55.

Stanfa LC, Dickenson AH (1999) The role of non-N-methyl-D-aspartate ionotropic glutamate receptors in the spinal transmission of nociception in normal animals and animals with carrageenan inflammation. *Neuroscience* **93(4)**:1391–8.

Svensson CI, Yaksh TL (2002) The spinal phospholipase-cyclooxygenase-prostanoid cascade in nociceptive processing. *Annu Rev Pharmacol Toxicol* **42**:553–83.

Svensson CI, Marsala M, Westerlund A, *et al.* (2003) Activation of p38 mitogen-activated protein kinase in spinal microglia is a critical link in inflammation-induced spinal painprocessing. *J Neurochem* **86(6)**:1534–44.

Takano M, Takano Y, Yaksh TL (1993) Release of calcitonin gene-related peptide (CGRP), substance P (SP), and vasoactive intestinal polypeptide (VIP) from rat spinal cord: modulation by ?$_2$ agonists. *Peptides* **14**:371–8.

Takano Y, Yaksh TL (1992) Characterization of the pharmacology of intrathecally administered alpha-2 agonists and antagonists in rats. *J Pharmacol Exper Ther* **261**:764–72.

Todd AJ (2002) Anatomy of primary afferents and projection neurones in the rat spinal dorsal horn with particular emphasis on substance P and the neurokinin 1 receptor. *Exp Physiol* **87(2)**:245–9.

Wagner RW (1995) The state of the art in antisense research. *Nat Med* 1:1116–8.

Walker MW, Ewald DA, Perney TM, Miller RJ (1988) Neuropeptide Y modulates neurotransmitter release and Ca2+ currents in rat sensory neurons. *J Neurosci* 8(7):2438–46.

Wall PD, Shortland P (1991) Long-range afferents in the rat spinal cord. 1. Numbers, distances and conduction velocities. *Philos Trans R Soc Lond B Biol Sci* 334(1269):85–93.

Wang JK, Nauss LA, Thomas JE (1979) Pain relief by intrathecally applied morphine in man. *Anesthesiology* 50:149–51.

Watkins LR, Milligan ED, Maier SF (2003) Glial proinflammatory cytokines mediate exaggerated pain states: implications for clinical pain. *Adv Exp Med Biol* 521:1–2.

Watson AH (2003) GABA- and glycine-like immunoreactivity in axons and dendrites contacting the central terminals of rapidly adapting glabrous skin afferents in rat spinal cord. *J Comp Neurol* 464(4):497–510.

Willis WD (2002) Long-term potentiation in spinothalamic neurons. *Brain Res Brain Res Rev* 40(1–3):202–14.

Wilson P, Kitchener PD (1996) Plasticity of cutaneous primary afferent projections to the spinal dorsal horn. *Prog Neurobiol* 48(2):105–29.

Wollmuth LP, Sakmann B (1998) Different mechanisms of Ca2+ transport in NMDA and Ca2+- permeable AMPA glutamate receptor channels. *J Gen Physiol* 112(5):623–36.

Wu HH, Wilcox GL, McLoon SC (1994) Implantation of AtT-20 or genetically modified AtT-20/hENK cells in mouse spinal cord induced antinociception and opioid tolerance. *J Neurosci* 14(8):4806–14.

Yaksh TL (1987) Spinal opiates: a review of their effect on spinal function with emphasis on pain processing. *Acta Anaesthesiol Scand* 31:25–37.

Yaksh TL (1993) The spinal actions of opioids. In *Handbook of Experimental Pharmacology*, Vol. 104/II (ed. Herz A). Springer–Verlag, Berlin, Heidelberg, pp. 53–90.

Yaksh TL (1997a) Pharmacology and mechanisms of opioid analgesic activity. *Acta Anaesthesiol Scand* 41:94–111.

Yaksh TL (1997b) Preclinical models of nociception. In *Anesthesia: Biologic Foundations* (eds. Yaksh TL, Lynch III C, Zapol WM, Maze M, Biebuyck JF, Saidman LJ). Lippincott–Raven Publishers, Philadelphia, pp. 685–718.

Yaksh TL (1999) Regulation of spinal nociceptive processing: where we went when we wandered onto the path marked by the gate. *Pain* **Suppl. 6**:149–52.

Yaksh TL, Malmberg AB (1994) Interaction of spinal modulatory receptor systems. In *Progress in Pain Research and Management*, Vol. 1 (eds. Fields HL, Liebeskind JC). IASP Press, Seattle, pp. 151–71.

Yaksh TL, Rudy TA (1976) Analgesia mediated by a direct spinal action of narcotics. *Science* 192:1357–8.

Yaksh TL, Hassenbusch S, Burchiel K, Hildebrand KR, Page LM, Coffey RJ (2002) Inflammatory masses associated with intrathecal drug infusion: a review of preclinical evidence and human data. *Pain Med* 3:300–12.

Yaksh TL, Horais KA, Tozier NA, *et al.* (2003) Chronically infused intrathecal morphine in dogs. *Anesthesiology* 99:174–87.

Yaksh TL, Hua X–Y, Kalcheva I, Nozaki–Taguchi N, Marsala M (1999a) The spinal biology in humans and animals of pain states generated by persistent small afferent input. *Proc Natl Acad Sci, USA* 96:7680–6.

Yaksh TL, Jage J, Takano Y (1993) Pharmacokinetics and pharmacodynamics of medullar agents. c. The spinal actions of α_2-adrenergic agonists as analgesics. In *Baillière's Clinical Anaesthesiology*, vol. 7, no. 3 (eds. Aitkenhead AR, Benad G, Brown BR, et al.). Baillière Tindall, London, pp. 597–614.

Yaksh TL, Jessell TM, Gamse R, Mudge AW, Leeman SE (1980) Intrathecal morphine inhibits substance P release from mammalian spinal cord *in vivo*. *Nature* **286**:155–6.

Yaksh TL, Rathbun ML, Provencher JC (1999b) Preclinical safety evaluation for spinal drugs. In *Spinal Drug Delivery* (ed. Yaksh TL). Elsevier Science BV, Amsterdam, pp. 417–37.

Yamamoto T, Yaksh TL (1991) Stereospecific effects of a nonpeptidic NK1 selective antagonist, CP-96,345: antinociception in the absence of motor dysfunction. *Life Sciences* **49**:1955–63.

Yamamoto T, Yaksh TL (1992) Comparison of the antinociceptive effects of pre- and posttreatment with intrathecal morphine and MK801, an NMDA antagonist, on the formalin test in the rat. *Anesthesiology* **77**:757–63.

Yao MZ, Gu JF, Wang JH, Sun LY, Liu H, Liu XY (2003) Adenovirus-mediated interleukin-2 gene therapy of nociception. *Gene Ther* **10(16)**:1392–9.

Yoshimura M, Jessell TM (1990) Amino acid-mediated EPSPs at primary afferent synapses with substantia gelatinosa neurons in the rat spinal cord. *J Physiol* **430**:315–35.

Yukhananov R, Guan J, Crosby G (2002) Antisense oligonucleotides to N-methyl-D-aspartate receptor subunits attenuate formalin-induced nociception in the rat. *Brain Res* **930(1–2)**:163–9.

Chapter 9

The development of pain systems

Maria Fitzgerald and Amy MacDermott

9.1 **Introduction**

The study of pain development provides a fascinating insight into how immature neurons connect to analyse and process sensory information that may threaten the postnatal integrity and survival of the organism. The sensory connections involved go through a series of transient functional stages to achieve the final adult pain system, and these need to be thoroughly understood if we are to assess and treat pain adequately in the newborn. Pain development is also a model for many general fundamental questions in developmental neurobiology, such as the specification of cellular phenotype, the formation of appropriate connections, and organization of circuits and systems in the maturing brain. In this chapter we concentrate upon the development of primary afferent nociceptors and their synaptic connections within the dorsal horn, the development of dorsal horn circuitry, and the maturation of spinal sensory reflex responses to noxious stimulation.

9.2 **The development of pain behaviour**

Reflex muscle contraction to stimulation of the body surface can be observed in rat foetuses from embryonic day (E) 15 onwards and develop in a rostrocaudal gradient. The first reflexes are evoked from the mouth and snout regions, followed by the forelimbs and trunk, and finally the hindlimbs at E17–18 (Narayanan et al., 1971). A feature of cutaneous reflexes in the newborn rat, kitten, and human is that they are exaggerated compared to the adult (Ekholm, 1967; Stelzner, 1971; Issler and Stephens, 1983; Fitzgerald et al., 1988b).

In the neonatal rat, a prick on the hind foot may bring about 'a whole body movement' involving wriggling, rolling, and both fore and hindlimb activity, but the response becomes more individuated and restricted to an isolated leg or foot movement as the rat matures. Ekholm (1967) detected that the elicitation of a flexor reflex response in young kittens often did not require a painful stimulus as in the adult, but only light touch. More recent studies of the flexor reflex in humans and rats have confirmed this (Fitzgerald *et al.*, 1988*b*; Andrews and Fitzgerald, 1994; Andrews *et al.*, 2002). In both preterm infants and newborn rat pups, flexor reflex thresholds are very low and reflex muscle contractions are synchronized and long-lasting. In addition, repeated skin stimulation results in sensitization of the response. Thresholds gradually increase with age and the emergence of specific nociceptive responses that cannot be evoked by low-intensity stimuli occurs postnatally, coinciding with a depression of the overall response.

Thresholds for withdrawal from heat stimuli are also lower in younger animals (Falcon *et al.*, 1996; Hu *et al.*, 1997; Marsh *et al.*, 1999*a*). The responses to more persistent chemical irritants or inflammatory agents administered subcutaneously have also been investigated. Up until day 10, the behavioural responses following application to chemical irritants are predominantly 'non-specific' whole body movements, while the 'specific' flexion reflex and shaking and licking the paw predominates from then on (Guy and Abbot, 1992). The response to formalin was found to have a ten-fold higher sensitivity in neonatal rats compared to weanlings (Teng and Abbott, 1998), although the classic biphasic behavioural response to formalin is not apparent in the rat pup until P15, coinciding with the overall depression in the response. In contrast, the hyperalgesia or drop in mechanical threshold that follows carageenan injection (Marsh *et al.*, 1999*b*) and mustard oil application (Jiang and Gebhart, 1998), is smaller in amplitude in P3 neonates than at P21. This may be a reflection of the high level of background sensitivity of young rats which limits the degree of hypersensitivity that they can display. Nevertheless, it is possible to demonstrate a clear enhancement of amplitude and duration of the flexion reflex with peripheral inflammation.

9.3 Nociceptor development

9.3.1 Birth and specification

Dorsal root ganglion (DRG) neurons, including nociceptors, arise from neural crest cells. Fig. 9.1 (pp. 210–11) summarizes the time course for some of the major events in the birth of DRG cells. These cells become restricted to sensory or autonomic sublineages even before becoming committed to neuronal or glial fates and while they are still migrating into position. A group of mammalian gene transcriptional regulators, the neurogenins, have a critical role in defining sensory neuron lineage. Neurogenins 1 and 2 act via a cascade of transcription factors, which control distinct sublineages for different classes of sensory neurons, to form the progenitors of large and small cutaneous neurons and proprioceptive neurones (Anderson, 1999; Zirlinger *et al.*, 2002). These neuronal groups are therefore specified independently of their peripheral or central targets. The majority of lumbar DRG cells in the rodent are born before birth in a rostrocaudal wave from E12 (embryonic day 12; gestation period of a rat is 21.5 days) onwards, the peak of large A cell birth occurring before that of small C cells (Altman and Bayer, 1984). The final numbers of DRG cells are determined by the balance

Box 9.1 **Neurotrophins and sensory neurone development**

The pattern and density of sensory innervation depends upon access to neurotrophic factors in the skin or other target tissue (Snider 1994; Kirstein and Farinas, 2002). The birth of sensory neurons and outgrowth of peripheral and central axons is accompanied by their programmed cell death. Sensory neuron survival is dependent upon access to neurotrophic factors, nerve growth factor (NGF), neurotrophin-3 (NT-3), NT-4/5, and brain-derived neurotrophic factor (BDNF), which are produced in the target tissue acting via a family of receptor proteins, the trk receptors. TrkA is the primary receptor for NGF, trkB for BDNF and NT-4/5, and trkC for NT-3. Most nociceptor sensory neurons are dependent on NGF produced in the skin and other target cells for survival during early embryonic development (Ruit *et al.*, 1992) and humans that have deletions, mutations, or aberrations of the gene encoding the trkA receptor suffer from a rare sensory and autonomic neuropathy with congenital insensitivity to pain (Indo *et al.*, 1996). However, a subpopulation of nociceptors downregulate trkA expression around birth, lose NGF dependency, and become responsive to glial cell line-derived growth factor (GDNF), a member of the transforming growth factor beta (TGF-b) family. These form the IB4+ve group of nociceptors (Bennett *et al.*, 1996).

In addition to regulating cell survival, neurotrophic factors play a number of other important roles in the development of sensory neurons. They also regulate (i) axon outgrowth (Davies, 2000; Markus *et al.*, 2002); (ii) receptor physiology (e.g. NT3 regulates C fibre nociceptor mechanical thresholds and BDNF regulates mechanoreceptor sensitivity) (Koltzenburg, 1999); and (iii) cutaneous innervation density; access to excess NGF and BDNF leads to skin hyperinnervation (Albers *et al.*, 1994; LeMaster *et al.*, 1999).

between cell birth and subsequent cell death, and the survival of DRG cell populations is regulated by access to neurotrophic factors (see Box 9.1).

9.3.2 **Peripheral and central target innervation**

Outgrowth of peripheral and central fibres begins prenatally, and innervation of the skin occurs in an organized proximo-distal manner, independently of motor axons. The precise timing of target innervation depends upon the maturation of the target rather than the neurons themselves. By birth in the rat, and the second trimester in man, sensory fibres have reached the most distal skin of the foot. A fibres form a cutaneous nerve plexus before the C fibres which follow soon after. Dorsal root fibres reach the lumbar cord soon from E12, but do not penetrate the lumbar grey matter in the rat until E15; A fibres, first followed by C fibres several days later (Reynolds *et al.*, 1991; Mirnics and Koerber, 1995*a,b*; Jackman and Fitzgerald, 2000; Wang and Scott, 2000).

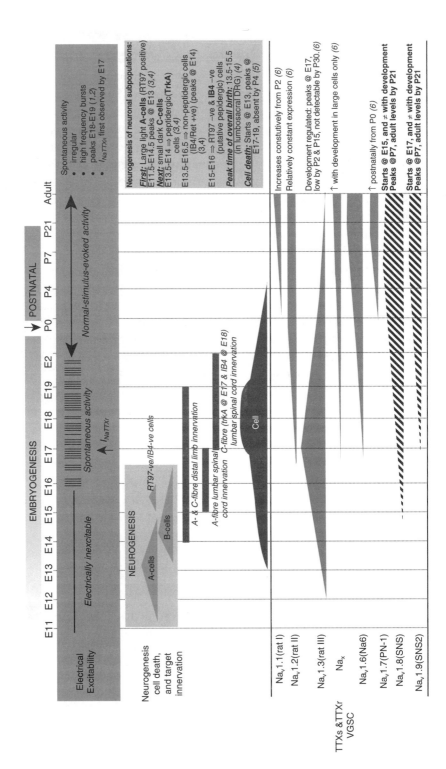

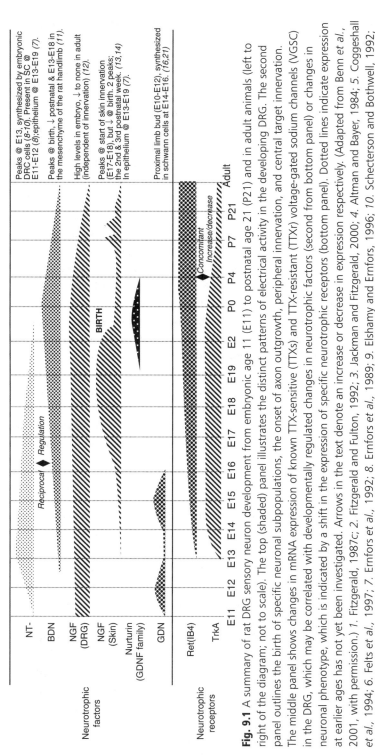

Fig. 9.1 A summary of rat DRG sensory neuron development from embryonic age 11 (E11) to postnatal age 21 (P21) and in adult animals (left to right of the diagram; not to scale). The top (shaded) panel illustrates the distinct patterns of electrical activity in the developing DRG. The second panel outlines the birth of specific neuronal subpopulations, the onset of axon outgrowth, peripheral innervation, and central target innervation. The middle panel shows changes in mRNA expression of known TTX-sensitive (TTXs) and TTX-resistant (TTXr) voltage-gated sodium channels (VGSC) in the DRG, which may be correlated with developmentally regulated changes in neurotrophic factors (second from bottom panel) or changes in neuronal phenotype, which is indicated by a shift in the expression of specific neurotrophic receptors (bottom panel). Dotted lines indicate expression at earlier ages has not yet been investigated. Arrows in the text denote an increase or decrease in expression respectively. (Adapted from Benn et al., 2001, with permission.) 1. Fitzgerald, 1987c; 2. Fitzgerald and Fulton, 1992; 3. Jackman and Fitzgerald, 2000; 4. Altman and Bayer, 1984; 5. Coggeshall et al., 1994; 6. Felts et al., 1997; 7. Ernfors et al., 1992; 8. Ernfors et al., 1989; 9. Elshamy and Ernfors, 1996; 10. Schecterson and Bothwell, 1992; 11. Sebert, 1993; 12. Constantinou et al., 1994; 13. Davies et al., 1987; 14. Rohrer et al., 1988; 15. Molliver et al., 1997b; 16. Alvares and Fitzgerald, 1999; 17. Bennett et al., 1996; 18. Phillips and Armanini, 1996; 19. Farinas et al., 1998; 20. Ehrhard and Otten, 1994; 21. Wright et al., 1996.

Expression of GAP 43 in peripheral axons is high in the perinatal period and then falls rapidly postnatally (Chong *et al.*, 1992). Peripheral axon elongation during development is regulated by neurotrophins (Markus *et al.*, 2002) (see Box 9.1). Sensory axons grow to peripheral and central targets with remarkable precision and from the outset each DRG innervates characteristic skin dermatomes and projects in a precise somatotopic pattern in the dorsal horn. A number of extracellular molecular cues are responsible for this, including the inhibitory growth cone collapsing molecule, semaphorin 3A (Dickson, 2002), although the extensive sensory axon guidance abnormalities observed in semaphorin 3A knockout mice in early embryonic life are largely corrected by birth (White and Behar, 2000), suggesting that powerful correction mechanisms exist for eliminating pathfinding errors.

Limb bud grafting experiments in chick embryos have demonstrated that somatotopic precision is preserved even if inappropriate DRG neurons are innervating the targets. Thus, there is no evidence that DRGs are matched to particular skin targets and, in the spinal cord, while the peripheral target skin influences the pattern of CNS projections, it does not direct cutaneous axons to specific populations of neurons in the dorsal horn (Wang and Scott, 2002). A feature of early skin target innervation is that it is initially hyperinnervated, with the sensory terminal plexus reaching up to the epidermal surface. This subsequently withdraws as the morphologically distinct end organs develop and become innervated, leaving the dermal plexus with occasional epidermal fibres observed in mature skin (Jackman and Fitzgerald, 2000; Peters *et al.*, 2002).

In the rat, both A and C fibres have grown into the spinal cord by birth, but C-fibre terminals are still notably immature in the perinatal period. C-type afferent terminals within synaptic glomeruli are not observed at EM level until P5 (Pignatelli *et al.*, 1989). While the growth of both A and C fibres into the rat cord is somatotopically precise, there is considerable reorganization of A-fibre terminals in the dorsal horn (Beggs *et al.*, 2002). While some A fibres have the characteristics of mature terminals at birth, others extend dorsally right up into laminae I and II to reach the surface of the grey matter, a feature which is not seen in adults (Beggs *et al.*, 2002; Woodbury and Koerber, 2003). Some of these fibres are cutaneous mechanoreceptors, with medium-range touch and pressure thresholds, and over the first three postnatal weeks they gradually withdraw from the superficial laminae to terminate in lamina III and below (Fitzgerald *et al.*, 1984; Beggs *et al.*, 2002). Their presence can be observed at EM level (Coggeshall *et al.*, 1996) and correlates with monosynaptic A beta input to lamina II cells observed in single-cell patching studies (see below). C fibres, on the other hand, grow specifically to laminae I and II (Fitzgerald, 1987*a*), and so for a considerable postnatal period these laminae are occupied by both A- and C-fibre terminals.

The laminar reorganization of primary afferent terminals does not occur following neonatal capsaicin treatment, suggesting that it is a process that involves an interaction between A and C fibres (Torsney *et al.*, 2000). Furthermore, it is an NMDA receptor-mediated, activity dependent process since chronic, local exposure of the dorsal horn of the lumbar spinal cord to the NMDA antagonist MK801 from birth prevents the normal functional and structural reorganization of A-fibre connections. The postnatal withdrawal of superficially projecting A-fibre primary afferents to deeper laminae does not occur in MK801-treated animals, although other aspects of dorsal horn development such as cell density and C-fibre afferent terminations are unaffected (Beggs *et al.*, 2002).

9.3.3 Development of nociceptor properties

The process of terminal elaboration of sensory nerves in the skin is a prolonged one, but all the main functional cutaneous afferent types found in the adult rat hindlimb can be found at birth, although the level of maturity depends on receptor type. C-fibre polymodal nociceptors are mature in their thresholds, pattern, and frequency of firing at birth, and are capable of showing sensitization to repeated heating from the embryonic period. High-threshold Aδ mechanoreceptors can also be distinguished at birth, but their peak firing frequencies are lower than in adults. Low-threshold Aβ mechanoreceptors are, relatively, the most immature at birth, with low frequencies of firing and amplitude of response. In addition, a group of less well-defined A-fibre 'pressure' receptors are observed in the newborn which decline in incidence with age. The absolute receptive field sizes of cutaneous receptors do not appear to change with age, despite the growth of body surface area (Fitzgerald, 1987*b*; Fitzgerald and Fulton, 1992; Koltzenburg and Lewin, 1997; Koltzenburg *et al.*, 1997; Woodbury and Koerber, 2003).

Nociceptors are characterized within the DRG by their chemical phenotype, but it appears that many of the functional markers used to identify them, such as receptors and neurotransmitters, are developmentally regulated. These changes no doubt reflect alterations in their function as sensory receptors over this period. The onset of nociceptor neuropeptide expression appears to be triggered by peripheral innervation (Jackman and Fitzgerald, 2000) and levels of expression increase with age (Marti *et al.*, 1987). The expression of trkA receptors is not restricted to the neuropeptide-expressing population in the newborn, but is developmentally downregulated (see Fig. 9.1 and Box 9.2). The expression of the vanilloid (capsaicin) receptor (TRV-1), which is activated by noxious heat and low pH (Caterina *et al.*, 1997), is also developmentally regulated in the DRG (Guo *et al.*, 2001). The voltage-gated, tetrodotoxin-resistant sodium channels, SNS 1 and 2, are expressed early in development (Benn *et al.*, 2001), but their onset and pattern of expression also varies postnatally (see Fig. 9.1). A functional consequence of this regulation is that neonatal nociceptors will be affected differently from adult nociceptors by any changes in activity or alterations in target properties that occur following tissue injury (e.g. the upregulation of growth factors during inflammation).

Another important group of receptors that are developmentally regulated over the postnatal period are the opioid receptors, and this may have important clinical implications. While opioid receptors are restricted to small, nociceptive afferents in the adult, μ- (MOR) and δ-opioid receptors (DOR) are also expressed in large primary sensory neurons in neonatal rats and are downregulated postnatally (Beland *et al.*, 2001). Calcium imaging studies show that these overexpressed MOR are functionally active and that morphine is more effective at depressing calcium entry in the neonatal compared to adult DRG neurons (Nandi *et al.*, 2003). This may be an explanation for the observed increased sensitivity to the analgesic epidural morphine in young animals (Marsh *et al.*, 1999*a,b*).

9.4 Development of dorsal horn cells and circuitry

9.4.1 Birth and maturation of dorsal horn neurons

The spinal cord develops in ventrodorsal gradient with deep dorsal horn neurones being born after motoneurones, and substantia gelatinosa (SG) neurons being the last to mature (Altman and Bayer, 1994). The homeobox gene, Lbx1, is expressed in and required for the correct specification of SG neurons and mice lacking Lbx1 lack these neurons and have disrupted sensory afferent innervation of the dorsal horn (Gross *et al.*, 2002). The late birth and postnatal axodendritic maturation of SG neurons is a key aspect of postnatal spinal sensory processing and is likely to be related to the slow synaptic maturation of C-fibre terminals mentioned above.

Studies in the spinal cord suggest that the period of neurogenesis is correlated with the projection target and its distance from the nerve cell body of origin. The neurogenesis of supraspinal projection neurons in laminae I and II proceeds along an axon-length gradient, such that neurons with the longest axons, projecting to rostral brain centres, complete neurogenesis before neurons with shorter axons, projecting only to the caudal brainstem. Furthermore, although the generation of both interneurons and supraspinal projection neurons in laminae I and II begins on embryonic day 13 (E13) and nearly equal numbers of neurons in each group are generated through E14, supraspinal projection neuron generation is complete by E14, two days before the completion of neurogenesis for interneurons (both local circuit neurons and propriospinal neurons) at E16 (Bice and Beal, 1997*a,b*).

9.4.2 Postsynaptic responses to primary afferent stimulation in the newborn spinal cord

Synaptogenesis in the rat dorsal horn is at its maximum in the first postnatal weeks. The maturation of cutaneous afferent input to the newborn dorsal horn has been analysed from extracellularly recorded spike activity evoked by electrical or natural stimulation of sensory afferents in individual cells in anesthetized rat pups (Fitzgerald and Jennings, 1999). It has also been studied using dorsal root stimulation or selective capsaicin stimulation in whole cell patch clamp recordings of dorsal horn cells in neonatal cord slices (Bardoni, 2001; Baccei *et al.*, 2003).

When neonatal cells are isolated for *in vivo* extracellular recording, they generally have no background activity. In whole cell patch recordings from lamina II neurons in slice preparations, spontaneous EPSCs can be observed from P3 but frequencies increase considerable with age. The frequency of neonatal spontaneous EPSCs in lamina II cells, unlike those in adults, are reduced by the addition of TTX, suggesting a strong influence of local circuit spike activity in this period (Baccei *et al.*, 2003).

9.4.2.1 A-fibre inputs

The widespread presence of A-fibre terminals in both SG and deeper laminae in the first weeks of life appears to influence the physiological responses of dorsal horn neurons. In slice preparations, a high incidence of Aβ-evoked monosynaptic responses has been observed in SG neurons in 3-week- old rats (Park *et al.*, 1999; Nakatsuka *et al.*, 2000). *In vivo*, low-intensity electrical skin stimulation, sufficient to recruit Aβ fibres, evokes spike activity in both superficial and deep laminae at latencies that progressively decrease with age (postnatal day (P) 3 mean, 33 ms; P21 mean, 7 ms). The variation in the A-fibre latencies within the population of recorded cells also decreases with age, so that the general pattern of cutaneous evoked activity in young animals is both variable and slow. In addition, repetitive A-fibre stimulation can produce sensitization in dorsal horn neurons in the neonate, which is not seen in adults (Jennings and Fitzgerald, 1999). This sensitization takes the form of a buildup of background activity in the cells during repetitive stimulation that outlasts the stimulation period and a prolonged afterdischarge of several minutes.

9.4.2.2 C-fibre inputs

In contrast to responses to A-fibre input, long-latency C-fibre-evoked spike responses are not evoked in dorsal horn neurons *in vivo* in the first postnatal week (Fitzgerald and Jennings, 1999; Torsney and Fitzgerald, 2002). At P10, only 13% of dorsal horn neurons appear to have a C-fibre input, while at P21 the value has risen to 32%. Repetitive peripheral stimulation at C-fibre strength also has no observable effects on spike responses recorded from dorsal horn neurons in the first week of life, but from P10, repetitive C-fibre stimulation produces a classical 'wind-up' in 18% of cells, increasing to 40% of cells by P21.

These results do not, of course, provide information about subthreshold C-fibre-evoked responses at this time. Indeed, whole cell patching of lamina II neurons shows that capsaicin activation of C-fibre nociceptor terminals in spinal cord slices increases glutamate mEPSC frequency from P3, although there is a marked enhancement of the effect between P5 and P10 (Baccei *et al.*, 2003). Capsaicin potently activates the noxious heat receptor TRPV1 or VR1 (Caterina *et al.*, 1997). TRPV1 is expressed on the central as well as peripheral terminals of some C and Aδ fibres and thus capsaicin may be used to selectively activate transmitter release from these afferents in the superficial dorsal horn. Menthol also significantly increased the mEPSC frequency, with a similar developmental pattern to capsaicin, without consistently affecting mEPSC amplitude (Baccei *et al.*, 2003). It therefore seems likely that C-fibre terminals are present and functional soon after arriving in the spinal cord, but that neurotransmitter release may be asynchronous and the synapses too immature to evoke spike activity *in vivo*.

9.4.2.3 Responses to natural skin stimulation

In vivo studies show that strong responses in dorsal horn neurons can be evoked by mechanical and thermal stimulation of the skin of the receptive field. Some neurons respond to both innocuous brushing and noxious pinching of the skin from birth, but the convergence of these two input modalities onto dorsal horn neurons changes over the postnatal period. The responses recorded from dorsal horn cells in younger animals are elicited mainly by low-threshold mechanoreceptors, and there are few cells with convergent input in the first week of life. This population gradually increases so that by P21 the percentage of neurones with convergent primary afferent input is similar to that seen in the adult (Fitzgerald and Jennings, 1999). The size of dorsal horn cell peripheral cutaneous mechanical receptive fields decreases with age (Fitzgerald and Jennings, 1999; Torsney and Fitzgerald, 2002). At P3, the mean (±SE) peripheral receptive field occupies $50 \pm 5.6\%$ of the plantar hindpaw. This value drops to $36 \pm 2.9\%$ at P6, $20 \pm 1.9\%$ at P10, and $15\% \pm 1.6$ at P21. The biggest change occurs in the first postnatal week. In the neonate, therefore, receptive fields overlap more than in the adult, increasing the chance of activation by peripheral skin stimulation.

9.4.3 **Descending and local inhibition**

One possible reason for large receptive fields of dorsal horn neurons and the enhanced cutaneous reflex sensitivity in young animals described in secion 9.2, is a lack of inhibitory processing in young animals. Gradual suppression or inhibition of neural connections is a feature of the developing somatosensory system. Not all segmental inhibition is absent in the newborn rat cord. Renshaw cell inhibition (Naka, 1984) and some contralateral inhibitory mechanisms (Fitzgerald, 1985) are well developed at birth. Nevertheless, as described above, the maturation of interneurons in SG, which appear to be particularly important for control of sensory processing, is largely postnatal. Furthermore, it may be that synapses destined to become inhibitory in the adult may be excitatory earlier in development (see below).

Descending inhibitory controls are immature at birth (Fitzgerald, 1991). Animals given a mid-thoracic spinal cord transection before P15 are markedly less affected than those transected at older ages (Weber and Stelzner, 1977). Descending inhibitory pathways travelling from the brainstem, via the dorsolateral funiculus of the spinal cord, to the dorsal horn grow down the spinal cord early in foetal life, but they do not extend collateral branches into the dorsal horn for some time. Furthermore, they do not begin to become functionally effective at inhibiting inputs to dorsal horn cells until postnatal day 10 in the rat, and are not fully functional for three postnatal weeks (Fitzgerald and Koltzenburg, 1986; Boucher *et al.*, 1998). This may in part be due to immaturity of neurotransmitter/receptor interactions (5-HT (serotonin) and noradrenaline) as well as delayed maturation of critical interneurones.

It has been suggested that the maturation of descending inhibition is dependent upon afferent C-fibre activity, because rats treated with capsaicin at birth have reduced inhibitory controls as adults (Cervero and Plenderleith, 1985). The lack of descending inhibition in the neonatal dorsal horn means that there is no endogenous analgesic system to 'dampen' noxious inputs as they enter the CNS, and their effects may therefore be more profound than in the adult. It also explains why stimulus-produced analgesia from the periacqueductal grey is not effective until P21 in rats (van Praag and Frenk, 1992).

9.4.4 Development of glutamatergic excitatory synapses in the dorsal horn

Most fast excitatory transmission in the spinal cord dorsal horn is mediated by the transmitter glutamate acting on postsynaptic ionotropic or channel-forming receptors. There are three types of ionotropic receptors sensitive to glutamate expressed postsynaptically including alpha-amino-3-hydroxy-5-methyl-4-isoxazolepropionic acid (AMPA), N-methyl-D-aspartate (NMDA), and kainate receptors. The best character-ized excitatory synapses in the dorsal horn are the primary afferent inputs onto laminae I and II neurons. In was in the late 1980s that glutamate was shown to function as the fast transmitter at these synapses in adult rodents (Schneider and Perl, 1988; Yoshimura and Jessell, 1990). Postsynaptic AMPA receptors are primary mediators of these responses. Postsynaptic NMDA receptors are often present as well but seem to contribute more potently to changing neuronal excitability when the synapses are activated repetitively. This is due to the activity dependent release of the Mg^{2+} block of NMDA channels that keeps them from passing ions at more negative membrane potentials (see Box 9.2).

Glutamatergic synaptic currents are clearly evident in the superficial dorsal horn around birth in rats (Bardoni et al., 1998), including those synapses due specifically to glutamate release from nociceptive primary afferent terminals (Baccei et al., 2003). As in the adult, both AMPA and NMDA receptors are expressed postsynaptically in the neonate and contribute to this activity. Overall, the synaptic currents observed at rest-ing membrane potentials are dominated by AMPA receptors and are fast but heteroge-neous in their kinetics. This is consistent with reports of regional differences in GluR subunit expression in postnatal dorsal horn, as well as changes in expression of overall levels of GluR subunits over the first three postnatal weeks (Jakowec et al., 1995). Kainate receptors are also expressed postsynaptically in neonates and appear to be primarily at high-threshold rather than low-threshold primary afferent synapses (Li et al., 1999).

AMPA receptors are tetrameric assemblies of different combinations of four subunits, GluR 1, 2, 3, and 4, each of which is expressed as at least two splice variants (Dingledine et al., 1999). Different combinations of subunits and their splice variants produce different channel properties such as kinetics and ion permeability. These properties in turn strongly influence synaptic characteristics. One particularly interest-ing property is Ca^{2+} permeability. NMDA receptors are the most Ca^{2+} permeable of the ionotropic glutamate receptors. The entry of Ca^{2+} into neurons through synaptic

Box 9.2 **NMDA receptors and silent synapses**

When a synapse morphologically exists but does not function, following stimulation of the presynaptic cell, it is often termed a silent synapse. An early report of silent synapses was based on studies of low-threshold mechanoreceptors projecting to the deep dorsal horn of the spinal cord (Wall, 1977). The inference of silent synapses was based in part on the observed mismatch between the extensive rostro-caudal projection of afferent sensory fibres and the restricted receptive fields of dorsal horn neurons. It was suggested that the synaptic inputs of each afferent to distant dermatomes are silent under normal conditions. A synapse may be silent because the presynaptic terminal fails to release transmitter or because the postsynaptic response is not detected due to inhibition or to the presence of post-synaptic receptors that do not produce significant changes in the resting membrane potential.

One well-studied form of silent synapses that become functional due to activity is when NMDA receptors are the only postsynaptic glutamate receptor at a gluta-matergic synapse. An important property of NMDA receptors is that they are blocked by extracellular Mg^{2+} at membrane potentials negative to ~-30 mV. The degree of block increases as the membrane potential becomes more negative. Therefore, at resting membrane potential, synaptic release of glutamate at synapses with only NMDA receptors will not be readily detectable and the synapse will appear silent. These kinds of silent synapses have been demonstrated to be present in the rat dorsal horn over the first two weeks after birth (Bardoni et al., 1998; Li and Zhuo, 1998; Baba et al., 2000). Because these synapses respond to activity by increases in expression of postsynaptic AMPA receptors, the synapses become no longer silent (Liao et al., 1995).

There are conflicting reports about whether silent synapses are no longer present in adults (Baba et al., 2000) or remain throughout life (Wang and Zhuo, 2002).

NMDA receptors has been shown to initiate long-lasting changes in synaptic strength. AMPA receptors are not usually permeable to Ca^{2+} due to incorporation of at least one GluR2 subunit in the receptor tetramer (Dinglendine et al., 1999), but Ca^{2+}-permeable AMPA receptors with no GluR2 subunit are expressed in neurons of laminae I and II_O and, to a lesser extent, II_I, in neonatal spinal cord. In lamina I, Ca^{2+}-permeable AMPA receptors are expressed by NK1-positive neurons (Engelman et al., 1999) believed to be projection neurons mediating some forms of hyperalgesia (Mantyh et al., 1997). Because Ca^{2+}-permeable AMPA receptors have been shown to mediate transient changes in synaptic strength (Gu et al., 1996), the receptors are potentially well situated to strongly influence projection neuron firing in the neonate.

Synaptic NMDA receptors are widely expressed in the developing dorsal horn, either together with AMPA receptors or alone. Even though little synaptic current flows through NMDA receptors at negative membrane potentials (see Box 9.2), the receptors bind synaptically released glutamate tightly and therefore remain activated longer than AMPA receptors in response to synaptically released glutamate. Thus, NMDA receptor-mediated synaptic currents can summate at lower input frequencies. This summation is coupled with an intrinsic positive feedback, because even the smallest depolarization will contribute to relief of Mg^{2+} block of the NMDA channel. Due to these properties, with repetitive activation, synapses with only NMDA receptors are not truly silent in the neonatal dorsal horn and are able to drive action potential firing even in the absence of AMPA receptor activation (Bardoni et al., 2000). In addition, NMDA receptors mediate long-term changes in mono- and polysynaptic synapse strength in young rat dorsal horn neurons following high-frequency dorsal root stimulation (Randic et al., 1993). In the developing dorsal horn, they thus contribute to fast synaptic transmission, influence the strength of synaptic connections, and impact on the presence of A-fibre connections.

Metabotropic glutamate receptors (mGluRs) also contribute to pain signalling in the spinal cord dorsal horn (Neugebauer, 2002). Little is known about how they contribute to signalling during development. It is known, however, that mRNA expression levels of the different mGluR proteins change over the first three postnatal weeks (Berthele et al., 1999). In general, mGluR 1, 5, and 3 are expressed at high levels by birth, and the levels decrease over the next three weeks. This expression pattern suggests both a role in pain signalling and possibly in development of relevant synaptic connections.

9.4.5 Development of other excitatory transmitters in the dorsal horn

There is a wide range of signalling molecules other than glutamate that have been identified but not well studied in the developing dorsal horn. ATP is released in a quantal manner onto postsynaptic P2X receptors in superficial dorsal horn neurons of young rat pups (Bardoni et al., 1997). P2X receptors are ionotropic receptors and are directly gated by ATP (Khakh, 2001). The frequency with which stimulation-evoked quantal ATP-gated currents occur in the developing dorsal horn, however, is very low, and it seems more likely that the major role for ATP P2X receptors is a presynaptic one where they regulate transmitter release at a wide variety of synapses.

Substance P is a neuromodulatory peptide released by a subset of nociceptive primary afferent neurons and a few dorsal horn neurons. It acts on the NK1 receptor, a G-protein-coupled receptor that stimulates phospholipase C, Ca^{2+} release, and protein kinase C activity. Substance P-positive afferent fibres terminate in laminae I and outer II, while NK1-expressing neurons are predominantly in laminae I and III (Todd, 2002). Substance P and its cognate receptor have a very early role to play in embryonic dorsal horn development and the directional growth of projection neurons (De Felipe et al., 1995) but their function in pain transmission is delayed until around birth when the substance P -expressing afferent fibres become synaptically connected to NK1 receptor-expressing neurons in the superficial dorsal horn.

Finally, serotonin is an important transmitter in the dorsal horn and can be either excitatory or inhibitory, depending on the receptor and cell type onto which it is released. The primary source of serotonin in the spinal cord is from descending fibres from nucleus raphe magnus. Little information is available about serotonin's role in dorsal horn development. However, it has been suggested that over the first few postnatal weeks in rat-developing spinal cord, serotonin is able to enhance synaptic transmission at low-threshold primary afferents to dorsal horn synapses when used at low doses, while it does not do so in adult dorsal horn (Wang and Zhuo, 2002).

9.4.6 Development of inhibitory synapses in the dorsal horn

The main, fast, inhibitory transmitters in the spinal cord are GABA and glycine. Receptors for both of these transmitters are heteropentameric configurations of subunits and both form anion channels (Moss and Smart, 2001). Early in development, neurons throughout the nervous system respond to GABA and glycine with a depolarization. This unexpected action of inhibitory transmitters is associated with developmental signalling and is also an early form of excitatory synaptic transmission (Ben–Ari, 2002). Some experiments suggest a similar fate for GABA and glycine receptors in the developing dorsal horn.

Embryonic dorsal horn neurons growing in culture show a developmental switch of GABA and glycine receptor function from a depolarizing to a hyperpolarizing effect on membrane potential (Wang *et al.*, 1994). Initially in culture, the depolarization is sufficiently strong to drive an increase in intracellular Ca^{2+} concentration. The developmental switch from depolarization to hyperpolarization has been shown, elsewhere in the nervous system, to be due primarily to an increase in expression of the $K^+ Cl^-$ coupled co-transporter, KCC2 (Ben–Ari, 2002). This pump moves Cl^- out of neurons, changing the Cl^- reversal potential from a value that is positive relative to resting potential to one that is negative. The Cl^- reversal potential is directly reflected in the sign of the response to GABA and glycine in developing dorsal horn neurons (Reichling *et al.*, 1994). The timing of the switch in response to GABA and glycine *in vivo* in the dorsal horn is soon after birth. The excitatory impact mediated by GABA and by P7 receptors on synaptic activity in lamina II is gone and has been replaced by an inhibitory effect (Baccei and Fitzgerald, 2004).

GABA and glycine are sometimes co-expressed in inhibitory dorsal horn neurons, although GABA is also expressed alone (Todd and Sullivan, 1990). In the adult rat, lamina I synapses are purely glycinergic, while in lamina II, the synapses are either GABAergic or glycinergic, even though both transmitters are often co-released. This was interpreted to mean that only one receptor family is postsynaptic, while the other may be in the peri-synaptic regions of the postsynaptic membrane (Chery and de Koninck, 1999). During postnatal development, as in the adult, GABA and glycine are often co-released from inhibitory synaptic terminals (Keller *et al.*, 2001). However, early in postnatal development, the postsynaptic receptor configuration is different than in the adult. In the neonate, GABA and glycine receptors may be mixed together

Box 9.3 **Pain behaviour in human infants**

Because human infants cannot report pain, we have to use indirect physiological and behavioural methods to assess its existence and severity. The debate on how best to measure pain in infants continues (Stevens and Franck, 2001) and it is clear that there is a lot of individuality of response even at very young ages (Morison *et al.*, 2001).

From 23 weeks gestational age, human foetuses mount a hormonal response when needles are inserted into the innervated intrahepatic vein (Giannakoulopoulos *et al.*, 1994). Noxious activation of nerve endings stimulates central pathways (most likely through the foetal hypothalamic-pituitary-adrenal axis) producing a biochemical 'stress' response. While the link between perceived pain and the hormonal stress response, even in adults, is unpredictable, noxious sensory stimulation clearly can produce a reaction from the nervous system at this young age. Hormonal responses are also used to measure pain in the youngest preterm infants (~24–26 weeks), along with many other physiological measures such as heart rate variability, crying and palmar sweating, and motor activity (Stevens and Franck, 2001). One well-validated method of pain assessment is facial expression or grimaces (Craig *et al.*, 2002).

Many of these measures can be applied to pain related to a particular noxious event, such as a needle prick, but are harder to use for persistent pain. Studies using cutaneous reflexes have been useful in that by focusing upon pain and sensitivity in and around an area of injury, prolonged cutaneous sensitization or hyperalgesia lasting days and weeks can be measured (Fitzgerald *et al.*, 1989; Andrews and Fitzgerald, 2002; Andrews *et al.*, 2002). These methods also have the advantage of direct parallels with laboratory studies (Fitzgerald and De Lima, 2001).

While providing important information as to human infant reactions to noxious stimulation and adequacy of analgesia, these physiological measures cannot be equated with true 'pain experience' which requires functional maturation of higher brain centres. Below 32 weeks, most pain responses, including facial expression, appear to be largely subcortical (Oberlander *et al.*, 2002). Stronger responses, therefore, do not necessarily mean more perceived pain but may be protective and beneficial to an organism that is unable (through cortical immaturity or malfunction) to perceive and organize a more directed response to the pain. They could reflect the absence of the normal inhibitory control or 'dampening' influences that higher brain structures normally exert at more mature stages.

in the postsynaptic membrane, making synaptic currents a complex of currents flowing through both GABA and glycine receptors. The subsequent restriction of postsynaptic receptors to GABA only, or glycine only, occurs over the next three to four postnatal weeks. GABA and glycine receptor kinetics differ from each other and both change with development. One possibility is that receptor kinetics are a key feature of synaptic function that require receptor segregation during development in order to mature.

9.4.7 Presynaptic receptors and regulation of transmitter release

There is a growing body of literature about presynaptic receptor expression near transmitter release sites at early developmental times. Presynaptic receptors are expressed throughout the superficial dorsal horn at neurotransmitter release sites for both inhibitory and excitatory transmitters, at both primary afferent and local interneuronal synapses. Some of these presynaptic receptors appear to perform a stable function throughout development, while others clearly change properties and thus, most likely, change their function over the first days and weeks after birth.

All of the glutamate receptors are expressed by at least some primary afferent terminals and all have been shown to regulate release there. Because all primary afferents release glutamate as their main transmitter, these receptors may be functioning as autoreceptors. Kainate receptors, best known for their ability to modulate release, depress transmitter release at the primary afferent synapses in neonatal spinal cord (Kerchner et al., 2001). Within the different populations of DRG neurons, kainate receptors are expressed almost exclusively by a subset of the non-peptidergic, IB4+ sensory neurons (Lee et al., 2001). Kainate receptors, like AMPA receptors, can be either Ca^{2+}-permeable or Ca^{2+}-impermeable, depending on the subunit configuration. Interestingly, kainate receptors expressed by the IB4+ sensory neurons are mostly permeable to Ca^{2+} before birth but become Ca^{2+}-impermeable over the first few postnatal days (Lee et al., 2001). It is tempting to speculate that kainate receptors may have a role in axon outgrowth or synapse formation between the C fibres on which they are expressed and their dorsal horn target neurons while still Ca^{2+}-permeable.

AMPA receptors are also expressed by a subpopulation of primary afferent neurons not positive for IB4, terminating in the superficial dorsal horn of neonatal rats (Lee et al., 2002) where they act to suppress glutamate release. While AMPA and kainate receptors both work to suppress transmitter release from sensory neurons terminating in the neonatal dorsal horn, they have different glutamate binding and channel properties and are expressed on different populations of fibres, suggesting they will contribute to regulation of synapse development and synaptic transmission in different ways.

NMDA receptors are also expressed at some primary afferent nerve terminals where they have been shown to drive release of substance P (Liu et al., 1997). This NMDA receptor-mediated release of substance P can be driven by dorsal root stimulation in young postnatal rats (Marvizon et al., 1997).

ATP activates P2X receptors on nerve terminals in the dorsal horn and can modulate release there. This is true on some sensory glutamatergic nerve terminals and on terminals releasing the inhibitory transmitters, GABA and glycine (Khakh, 2001). There is little developmental information about P2X receptor subunits and function in the spinal cord. However, pharmacology has been used to investigate developmental changes in P2X receptor properties that regulate glycine release onto dorsal horn neurons. The change in sensitivity to a subunit selective agonist, α,β-meATP, from none at P10 to nearly 50% at P28, while sensitivity to the pan agonist ATP remains steady across the same time period at around 60%, indicates a change in P2X receptor subunit composition (Jang et al., 2001). It is possible that this change in receptor subunit composition will be reflected by a change in receptor kinetics, that in turn is expected to change in impact of endogenous ATP on transmitter release.

Presynaptic kainate and AMPA receptors have also been demonstrated to regulate release of GABA and glycine from early postnatal neurons in the superficial dorsal horn (Kerchner et al., 2001; Engelman et al., in press). Regulation by AMPA receptors appears to remain constant for the first four postnatal weeks.

Opioid peptides and the opioid analgesics have an important role in the presynaptic regulation of glutamate release, but little is known about the developmental regulation of opioid receptor mechanisms. Opioid analgesia is widely used in young patients and is an effective analgesic in young animals (Marsh et al., 1998, 1999a,b). Opiate receptor expression and function in DRG cells is developmentally regulated as described above (Nandi et al., 2003). Opioid signalling is mediated by various effectors, including G protein-activated inwardly rectifying potassium (GIRK) channels, adenylyl cyclases, voltage-dependent calcium channels, phospholipase C beta (PLCbeta), and mitogen-activated protein kinases. All of these may alter during development, but as yet little is known about this.

9.5 Developmental mechanisms of persistent pain

In the adult, it is clear that persistent pain, both inflammatory and neuropathic, have very different underlying mechanisms from acute pain, and there is evidence for plasticity in both transmission and modulating systems in prolonged pain states. This is of great importance when considering persistent pain in infants and children, where this plasticity will be superimposed upon a nervous system that is immature and where sensory connections are still establishing themselves.

9.5.1 Inflammatory pain

Studies focusing upon pain and sensitivity in and around an area of inflammation have shown that even very young preterm babies are capable of showing a prolonged cutaneous sensitization or hyperalgesia lasting days and weeks (Fitzgerald et al., 1989). The area around an abdominal surgical wound shows a similar enhanced cutaneous sensitivity in the postoperative period (Andrews and Fitzgerald, 2002) and secondary hyperalgesia has also been observed in the contralateral limb following local ischaemic injury (Andrews and Fitzgerald, 1994). Pain reactions (grimace, and crying) to venipuncture on the forearm are also increased in full-term infants who have undergone repeated heel lances compared to normal infants (Taddio *et al.*, 2002).

Infant animal models of persistent inflammatory pain have also been established. Cutaneous mechanical thresholds fall in neonatal rat pups following local carrageenan injection (Marsh *et al.*, 1999b) and mustard oil application (Jiang and Gebhart, 1998), but the effect is less at P3 than at P21. This may partly reflect peripheral nociceptor terminal immaturity. C fibres are capable of peripheral sensitization from before birth (Koltzenburg and Lewin, 1997) but peripheral C-fibre terminals do not release sufficient substance P to produce neurogenic extravasation until P10 (Fitzgerald and Gibson, 1984), even though exogenously applied SP can produce extravasation before this age (Gonzales *et al.*, 1991). However, hyperalgesia and allodynia also result from central synaptic rather than peripheral receptor alterations.

Electrophysiological studies *in vivo* show that sensitization of dorsal horn cells can be observed 2–5 hours after carageenan inflammation of the hindpaw at all ages, although the exact pattern of effects is age- dependent. Increased spontaneous activity and response magnitude are observed from the earliest postnatal age examined (P3) but inflammation-induced expansion of mechanical receptive field size is not observed until at least the second postnatal week (Torsney and Fitzgerald, 2002), mainly because baseline receptive fields are already large at this age (Fitzgerald and Jennings, 1999). 'Wind-up' of C-fibre-evoked responses is not observed in dorsal horn cells *in vivo* until P10, but in slice preparations, NMDA- dependent C-fibre-evoked depolarization of spinal cord cells and wind-up of cells to repeated C-fibre stimulation has been demonstrated in the young (8–14 day) spinal cord (Sivilotti *et al.*, 1995). The development of glutamate/NMDA and substance P/NK1 interactions discussed above undoubtedly play an important role in these changing responses.

9.5.2 Neuropathic pain

The epidemiology of neuropathic pain in infants and children is not well established (Olsson and Berde, 1993). In contrast to the intense pain that occurs in adults, no chronic long-term pain follows brachial plexus avulsion at birth (Anand and Birch, 2002). While restoration of sensory function and localization occurs in avulsed spinal root dermatomes following surgical repair, a number of unusual sensations remain, and systematic testing of sensory receptive fields adjacent to the area of sensory loss would be interesting. Until recently, children were widely regarded not to experience phantom pain, but studies now show a 100% incidence of phantom sensations in children, with the majority also experiencing phantom pain (Krane and Heller, 1995). The phenomenon is highly associated with preoperative pain.

In animal models, peripheral nerve injury does not produce the allodynia observed following similar lesions in the adult (Howard *et al.*, 2005). This is consistent with the observation in rat pups that, despite profound alterations of plantar hindpaw innervation induced by early nerve transection, cutaneous nociceptive reflexes maintain an essentially normal spatial organization (Holmberg and Schouenborg, 1996). The cellular reactions to nerve injury, however, are far more dramatic. In the adult, axotomy induced DRG cell death does not begin until approximately three months after the lesion and is limited to the unmyelinated axons (Costigan et al., 1998). However, in the neonate, death occurs rapidly and involves all cell populations (Yip et al., 1984). Approximately 50% of neonatal motor and sensory neurones have died one week after peripheral nerve injury (Himes and Tessler, 1989). Application of exogenous NGF and GDNF and decreasing p75 expression with antisense oligos in axotomized sensory neurones can temporarily prevent the loss of DRG neurones occurring after neonatal axotomy (Cheema, 1996), and recently this cell loss has been linked with low levels of heat shock proteins, such as Hsp27 (Lewis et al., 1999; Benn et al., 2002), which are induced after stress in tissues, perhaps with a protective role.

The substantial cell loss following neonatal nerve injury leads to transganglionic degeneration and subsequent withdrawal of central terminals (Aldskogius and Risling, 1984; Bondok and Sansone, 1985). This is followed by sprouting of adjacent, intact axon collaterals into the denervated region (Fitzgerald, 1985; Fitzgerald et al., 1990; Shortland and Fitzgerald, 1994) disrupting the somatotopic organization of central terminals within the dorsal horn. Both intact A fibres and C fibres sprout and grow arbors outside of their normal central terminal field making functional synaptic connections within new areas of the cord (Shortland and Fitzgerald, 1991). The resulting rearrangement of connections in the developing rat nervous system are not confined to dorsal horn cells but are found in higher levels of the nervous system including the cortex (Kaas et al., 1983). Although in the short term this could be a useful compensatory device to restore sensory input from an area of the body surface in which it has been lost, the effects may be detrimental and trigger chronic pain.

The few surviving axotomized neurons also undergo a sprouting response (Shortland et al., 1994) similar to that seen in the adult, and could allow low-threshold inputs to excite nociceptive circuits and therefore contribute to allodynia. Sprouting may also partly explain the lack of neuropeptide depletion in the dorsal horn following nerve injury, that contrasts with the extensive depletion seen in the adult (Reynolds and Fitzgerald, 1992).

9.6 The role of experience in developing pain pathways

Studies in the wider field of developmental neurobiology have shown that CNS development over the postnatal period is dependent upon neural activity and that normal synaptic development requires defined patterns of afferent input (Ben–Ari, 2002; Debski and Kline, 2002; Fox, 2002). One possibility then is that abnormal or excessive activity related to pain and injury in early life may change the course of development and cause long-term changes in somatosensory and pain processing (Alvares et al., 2000; Anand, 2000). Clinical studies suggest that early pain related to surgical and

Box 9.4 **Does pain and injury in human infants lead to alterations in their perception of pain when they are adults?**

The plasticity of developing pain pathways has led scientists and clinicians to investigate the potential for tissue injury to cause prolonged changes in sensory responses lasting into childhood, adolescence, or adulthood. This is of particular importance for preterm infants who may undergo hundreds of painful procedures during their stay in intensive care (Stevens and Franck, 2001).

Boys who have been circumcised at birth show increased pain responses to vaccinations at 4–6 months compared to those who have not (Taddio *et al.*, 1995) and this is relieved by treatment with lidocaine-prilocaine cream (EMLA) during circumcision (Taddio *et al.*, 1997). This suggests that sensitization to one early painful procedure influences the reaction to a different one some time later. However, former preterm infants who have undergone multiple invasive procedures in intensive care show similar pain responses to finger lance blood collection at 4 months to term-born controls (Oberlander *et al.*, 2002).

An important study of 195 former preterm infants at 18 months, found that parents perceived the lowest birth weight groups to have the lowest pain responsiveness and that, unlike normal toddlers, there was no relationship between temperament and pain perception (Grunau *et al.*, 1994*a*). Also, at the older age of 4.5 years, somatization (the occurrence of numerous pains that cannot be accounted for medically) was significantly greater in the lowest birth weight children (Grunau *et al.*, 1994*b*). This was not observed at 8–10 years, but these children do rate pictures of painful events as more painful than their normal birth weight peers (Grunau and Whitfield, 1998). The complexity of such studies and the need for careful design and interpretation has been emphasized by Grunau (2000). For instance, learnt patterns of behaviour within families are a major determinant of perceived sensitivity to pain (MacGregor *et al.*, 1997).

procedural interventions during intensive care management of premature neonates can have long-term consequences upon pain behaviour and perception in later life (see Box 9.4) (Fitzgerald and Walker, 2003).

Exposure to repetitive paw needle prick four times a day in rat pups from postnatal (P) P0–P7 produces hyperalgesia, in the form of reduced hot-plate latencies, at P16, but this does not last into adulthood (Anand *et al.*, 1999). The neonatally injured animals do, however, show increased preference for alcohol and other behavioural changes as adults. On the other hand, a more severe injury of repeated 10% formalin injections into paws from P1–P7 leads to hypoalgesia in adulthood, in the form of increased hot-plate and tail-flick latency and decreased alcohol preference (Bhutta *et al.*, 2001). The differences in these results may be explained by the fact that formalin is a more damaging stimulus that may lead to some sensory neuron death (Tsujino *et al.*, 2000), whereas repeated needle prick will presumably produce a local inflammation only.

The long-term sensory effects of neonatal inflammation is a subject of some controversy and clearly depends upon the agent and dose used. Neonatal hindpaw carrageenan injection causing mechanical and heat hypoalgesia in adults, while increasing the hyperalgesia produced by an injection of complete Freund adjuvant (Lidow *et al.*, 2001; Ren *et al.*, 2004), but other, blinded studies report no changes in mechanical, heat, or inflammatory responses were observed in adults following neonatal carageenan injection (Alvares *et al.*, 2000; Walker *et al.*, 2003). Consistent with this is the finding that the acute response of neonatal dorsal horn cells to hindpaw carageenan injections (Torsney and Fitzgerald, 2002) does not last, so the dorsal horn cell properties at six weeks are no different from controls (Torsney and Fitzgerald, 2003).

A stronger inflammatory agent (50μl CFA) injected into hindpaw at birth also leaves adult baseline thermal withdrawal latencies unchanged but hyperalgesia, following a second challenge with CFA, increases, and the time course but not the magnitude of the formalin response is altered (Ruda *et al.*, 2000). CFA injections in the neonate also cause long-lasting changes in spinal circuitry that can be observed in the adult. These consist of expanded central C-fibre terminal fields and CGRP expression and increased fos-like immunoreactivity (Fos-LI) — a measure of neuronal activity in dorsal horn neurons (Ruda *et al.*, 2000; Tachibana *et al.*, 2001). These central changes must be viewed in the context of very severe tissue damage caused by large volumes of inflammatory agents that produce an inflammatory response that lasts into adulthood. The expansion of afferent terminals in lamina II following neonatal CFA inflammation is maintained into adulthood only if the inflammation is also maintained (Walker *et al.*, 2003). However, this effect of chronic inflammation is not seen in adult animals, emphasizing the plasticity of the system at this time.

Another type of injury that has been investigated is a full thickness skin wound in the hindpaw of the newborn rat pup. Despite rapid healing, such wounds cause a long-lasting hypersensitivity, in the form of lowered von Frey mechanical threshold, in the previously injured region (Reynolds and Fitzgerald, 1995; De Lima *et al.*, 1999). The effect is apparent after one week and lasts for at least six weeks (De Lima *et al.*, 1999) and only occurs if the wound is made in the postnatal period (Reynolds and Fitzgerald, 1995). Local sciatic nerve block with bupivicaine for the first 24 hours after wounding does not affect the onset or magnitude of mechanical hypersensitivity.

This hypersensitivity is likely to have a peripheral and central origin. In the skin, sensory nerve terminals in the wounded area show a profound sprouting response, which long outlasts the injury (at least 12 weeks in the rat) (Reynolds and Fitzgerald, 1995; De Lima *et al.*, 1999; Alvares *et al.*, 2000). The effect is most dramatic when wounds are performed at birth and decreases progressively with age at wounding. This is a sensory A- and C-fibre nerve response with no sympathetic involvement (Reynolds and Fitzgerald, 1995). In addition, this wounding triggers central changes in synaptic connections leading to a long-lasting expansion of dorsal horn cell receptive fields, which is clearly observed at six weeks (Torsney and Fitzgerald, 2003).

The mechanism by which early pain experience or inflammation might alter somatosensory processing is likely to involve activity dependent changes in the developing nervous system as has been reported in the rodent whisker barrel cortex, where the effects of sensory deprivation (selective whisker removal or repeated trimming) or sensory stimulation (repeated whisker stimulation) within critical time windows during development have striking effects upon the structural and functional development of cortical sensory maps (Fox, 2002). Some of these effects may be a result of structural plasticity in dendrites. Dendritic spines and filopodia are highly motile: spines and filopodia appear, disappear, or change shape over tens of minutes, and this motility is markedly influenced by sensory deprivation during a critical period around postnatal days (P)11–13 (Lendvai et al., 2000). Another mechanism whereby synaptic connections are strengthened is when both pre and postsynaptic activity is correlated, with those connections that are uncorrelated being weakened and eliminated. The molecular basis of this mechanism is thought to involve the induction of NMDA-dependent long-term potentiation and depression (LTP and LTD) (Cohen–Cory, 2002; Murphy, 2003).

Spinal cord dorsal horn somatosensory maps also undergo postnatal refinement over a critical postnatal period. Chronic, local exposure of the dorsal horn of the lumbar spinal cord to the NMDA antagonist, MK801, from birth prevents the normal functional and structural reorganization of A-fibre connections (Beggs et al., 2002). Dorsal horn cells in spinal MK801-treated animals, investigated at eight weeks of age by in vivo electrophysiological recording, have significantly larger cutaneous mechanoreceptive fields and greater A-fibre-evoked responses than vehicle controls. C-fibre-evoked responses are unaffected. Chronic MK801 also prevents the normal structural reorganization of A-fibre terminals in the spinal cord. The postnatal withdrawal of superficially projecting A-fibre primary afferents to deeper laminae does not occur in treated animals, although C-fibre afferent terminals and cell density in the dorsal horn are apparently unaffected. Spinal MK801-treated animals also have significantly reduced behavioural reflex thresholds to mechanical stimulation of the hindpaw compared to naïve and vehicle- treated animals, whereas noxious heat thresholds remain unaffected.

These results indicate that the normal postnatal structural and functional development of A-fibre sensory connectivity within the spinal cord is an activity dependent process requiring NMDA receptor activation (Beggs et al., 2002) and provides a cellular basis for potential effects of early pain experience upon synaptic development.

9.7 Conclusions

In this chapter we have highlighted the importance of the postnatal period in the development of primary afferent nociceptors and their synaptic connections within the dorsal horn, the development of dorsal horn circuitry, and the maturation of spinal sensory reflex responses to noxious stimulation. This postnatal period is time when pain transmission and modulation is becoming organized. As a result, responses to noxious stimulation, tissue damage, and to analgesic agents is under developmental control and is not easily predicted from adult data. Only by fully understanding this control can we aim to improve pain management for infants and children.

References

Albers KM, Wright DE, Davis BM (1994) Overexpression of nerve growth factor in epidermis of transgenic mice causes hypertrophy of the peripheral nervous system. *J Neurosci* **14**:1422–1432.

Aldskogius H, Risling M (1983) Preferential loss of unmyelinated L7 dorsal root axons following sciatic nerve resection in kittens. *Brain Res* **289**:358–361.

Altman J, Bayer SA (1984) The development of the rat spinal cord. *Adv Anat Embryol Cell Biol* **85**:1–164.

Alvares D, Fitzgerald M (1999) Building blocks of pain: the regulation of key molecules in spinal sensory neurones during development and following peripheral axotomy. *Pain* **Suppl 6**:S71–85.

Alvares D, Torsney C, Beland B, Reynolds M, Fitzgerald M (2000) Modelling the prolonged effects of neonatal pain. *Prog Brain Res* **129**:365–373.

Anand KJS (2000) Pain, plasticity and premature birth: a prescription for permanent suffering? *Nature Medicine* **6**:971–973 .

Anand KJS, Coskun V, Thrivikraman KV, Nemeroff CB, Plotsky PM (1999) Long-term behavioural effects of repetitive pain in neonatal rat pups. *Physiology & Behaviour* **66**:627–637.

Anand P, Birch R (2002) Restoration of sensory function and lack of long-term chronic pain syndromes after brachial plexus injury in human neonates. *Brain* **125**:113–122.

Anderson DJ (1999) Lineages and transcription factors in the specification of vertebrate primary sensory neurons. *Curr Opin Neurobiol* **9**:517–524.

Andrews K, Fitzgerald M (1994) The cutaneous withdrawal reflex in human neonates: sensitization, receptive fields and the effects of contralateral stimulation. *Pain* **56**:95–101.

Andrews K, Fitzgerald M (2002) Wound sensitivity as a measure of analgesic effects following surgery in human neonates and infants. *Pain* **99**:185–192.

Andrews KA, Desai D, Dhillon HK, Wilcox DT, Fitzgerald, M (2002) Abdominal sensitivity in the first year of life: comparison of infants with and without prenatally-diagnosed unilateral hydronephrosis. *Pain* **100**:35–46.

Baba H, Doubell TP, Moore KA, Woolf CJ (2000) Silent NMDA receptor-mediated synapses are developmentally regulated in the dorsal horn of the rat spinal cord. *J Neurophysiol* **83(2)**:955–962.

Baccei ML, Bardoni R, Fitzgerald M (2003) Development of nociceptive synaptic inputs to the neonatal rat dorsal horn: glutamate release by capsaicin and mentnol. *J Physiol* **549**:231–242.

Baccei ML, Fitzgerald M (2004) Development of GABAergic and glycinergic transmission in the neonatal dorsal horn. *J Neurosci* **24**:4749–4757.

Bardoni R (2001) Excitatory synaptic transmission in neonatal dorsal horn: NMDA and ATP receptors. *News Physiol Sci* **16**:95–100.

Bardoni R, Goldstein PA, Lee CJ, Gu JG, MacDermott AB (1997) ATP P2X receptors mediate fast synaptic transmission in the dorsal horn of the rat spinal cord. *J Neurosci* **17**:5297–5304.

Bardoni R, Magherini PC, MacDermott AB (1998) NMDA EPSCs at glutamatergic synapses in the spinal cord dorsal horn of the postnatal rat. *J Neurosci* **18**:6558–6567.

Bardoni R, Magherini PC, MacDermott AB (2000) Activation of NMDA receptors drives action potentials in superficial dorsal horn from neonatal rats. *Neuroreport* **11**:1721–1727.

Beggs S, Torsney C, Drew LJ, Fitzgerald M (2002) The postnatal reorganization of primary afferent input and dorsal horn cell receptive fields in the rat spinal cord is an activity-dependent process. *Eur J Neurosci* **16**:1249–1258.

Beland B, Fitzgerald M (2001) Mu- and delta-opioid receptors are down-regulated in the largest diameter primary sensory neurons during postnatal development in rats. *Pain* **90**:143–150.

Ben–Ari Y (2002) Excitatory actions of gaba during development: the nature of the nurture. *Nat Rev Neurosci* **3**:728–739.

Benn SC, Costigan M, Tate S, Fitzgerald M, Woolf CJ (2001) Developmental expression of the TTX-resistant voltage-gated sodium channels Nav1.8 (SNS) and Nav1.9 (SNS2) in primary sensory neurons. *J Neurosci* **21**:6077–6085.

Bennett DL, Averill S, Clary DO, Priestley JV, McMahon SB (1996) Postnatal changes in the expression of the trkA high-affinity NGF receptor in primary sensory neurons. *Eur J Neurosci* **8**:2204–2208.

Berthele A, Boxall SJ, Urban A, *et al.* (1999) Distribution and developmental changes in metabotropic glutamate receptor messenger RNA expression in the rat lumbar spinal cord. *Brain Res Dev Brain Res* **112**:39–53.

Bhutta AT, Rovnaghi C, Simpson PM, Gossett JM, Scalzo FM, Anand KJS (2001) Interactions of inflammatory pain and morphine in infant rats. Long term behavioural effects. *Physiology & Behaviour* **73**:51–58.

Bice TN, Beal JA (1997*a*) Quantitative and neurogenic analysis of the total population and subpopulations of neurons defined by axon projection in the superficial dorsal horn of the rat lumbar spinal cord. *J Comp Neurol* **388**:550–564.

Bice TA and Beal JA (1997*b*) Quantitative and neurogenic analysis of neurons with supraspinal projections in the superficial dorsal horn of the rat lumbar spinal cord. *J Comp Neurol* **388**:565–574.

Bicknell HRJ, Beal JA (1984) Axonal and dendritic development of substantia gelatinosa neurons in the lumbosacral spinal cord of the rat. *J Comp Neurol* **226**:508–522.

Bondok AA, Sansone FM (1984) Retrograde and transganglionic degeneration of sensory neurons after a peripheral nerve lesion at birth. *Exp Neurol* **86**:322–330.

Boucher T, Jennings E, Fitzgerald M (1998) The onset of diffuse noxious inhibitory controls (DNIC) in postnatal rat pups – a c-Fos study. *Neurosci Lett* **257**: 9–12.

Caterina MJ, Schumacher MA, Tominaga M, Rosen TA, Levine JD, Julius D (1997) The capsaicin receptor: a heat-activated ion channel in the pain pathway (see comments). *Nature* **389**:816–824.

Cervero F, Plenderleith MB (1985) C-fibre excitation and tonic descending inhibition of dorsal horn neurones in adult rats treated at birth with capsaicin. *J Physiol* **365**:223–237.

Cheema XX (1996) Reducing p75 nerve growth factor receptor levels using antisense oligoneucleotides prevents the loss of axotomized sensory neurons in the dorsal root ganglia of newborn rats. *J Neurosci Res* **46**:239–245.

Chery N, de Koninck Y (1999) Junctional versus extrajunctional glycine and GABA(A) receptor-mediated IPSCs in identified lamina I neurons of the adult rat spinal cord. *J Neurosci* **19**:7342–7355.

Chong MS, Fitzgerald M, Winter J, *et al.* (1992) GAP-43 mRNA in rat spinal cord and dorsal root ganglia neurons: developmental changes and re-expression following peripheral nerve injury. *Eur J Neurol* **4**:883–895.

Cohen–Cory S (2002) The developing synapse: construction and modulation of synaptic structures and circuits. *Science* **298(5594)**:770–776.

Coggeshall RE, Jennings EA, Fitzgerald M (1996) Evidence that large myelinated primary afferent fibers make synaptic contacts in lamina II of neonatal rats. *Brain Res Dev Brain Res* **92**:81–90.

Coggeshall RE, Pover CM, Fitzgerald M (1994) Dorsal root ganglion cell death and surviving cell numbers in relation to the development of sensory innervation in the rat hindlimb. *Brain Res Dev Brain Res* **82**:193–212.

Constantinou J, Reynolds ML, Woolf CJ, Safieh–Garabedian B, Fitzgerald M (1994) Nerve growth factor levels in developing rat skin: upregulation following skin wounding. *NeuroReport* **5**:2281–2284.

Costigan M, Mannion RJ, Kendall G, *et al.* (1998) Heat shock protein 27: developmental regulation and expression after peripheral nerve injury. *J Neurosci* **18**:5891–5900.

Craig KD, Korol CT, Pillai RR (2002) Challenges of judging pain in vulnerable infants. *Clin Perinatol* **29**(3):445–457.

Davies AM (2000) Neurotrophins: neurotrophic modulation of neurite growth. *Curr Biol* **10**:R198–200.

Davies AM, Bandtlow C, Heumann R, Korsching S, Rohrer, Theonen H (1987) Timing and site of nerve growth factor synthesis in developing skin in relation to innervation and expression of the receptor. *Nature* **326**:353–358.

Debski EA, Cline HT (2002) Activity-dependent mapping in the retinotectal projection. *Curr Opin Neurobiol* **12**:93–99.

De Felipe C, Pinnock RD, Hunt SP (1995) Modulation of chemotropism in the developing spinal cord by substance P. *Science* **267**:899–902.

De Lima J, Alvares D, Hatch DJ, Fitzgerald M (1999) Sensory hyperinnervation after neonatal skin wounding: effect of bupivacaine sciatic nerve block. *Br J Anaesth* **83**:662–664.

Dickson BJ (2002) Molecular mechanisms of axon guidance. *Science* **298**:1959–1964.

Dingledine R, Borges K, Bowie D, Traynelis SF (1999) The glutamate receptor ion channels. *Pharmacol Rev* **51**:7–61.

Ekholm J (1967) Postnatal changes in cutaneous reflexes and in the discharge pattern of cutaneous and articular sense organs. *Acta Physiologica Scandinavica* **Suppl. 297**:1–130.

ElShamy WM, Ernfors P (1996) A local action of neurotrophin-3 prevents the death of proliferating sensory neuron precursor cells. *Neuron* **16**:963–972.

Engelman HS, Allen TB, MacDermott AB (1999) The distribution of neurons expressing calcium-permeable AMPA receptors in the superficial laminae of the spinal cord dorsal horn. *J Neurosci* **19**:2081–2089.

Engelman HS, Anderson RL, MacDermott AB (submitted) AMPA receptors modulate release of inhibitory amino acids in the spinal cord dorsal horn.

Ernfors P, Henschen A, Olsen L, Persson H (1989) Expression of nerve growth factor mRNA is developmentally regulated and increased after axotomy in rat spinal cord neurons. *Neuron* **2**:1605–1612.

Ernfors P, Merlio J–P, Persson H (1992) Cells expressing mRNA for neurotrophins and their receptors during embryonic rat development. *Eur J Neurosci* **4**:1140–1158.

Falcon M, Guendellman D, Stolberg A, Frenk H, Urca G (1996) Development of thermal nociception in rats. *Pain* **67**:203–208.

Farinas I, Wilkinson GA, Backus C, Reichardt LF, Patapoutian A (1998) Characterization of neurotrophin and Trk receptor functions in developing sensory ganglia: direct NT-3 activation of TrkB neurons *in vivo*. *Neuron* **21**:325–334.

Felts PA, Yokoyama S, Dib–Hajj S, Black JA, Waxman SG (1997) Sodium channel subunit mRNAs I, II, III, NaG, Na6 and hNE (PN1): different expression patterns in developing rat nervous system. *Brain Res Mol Brain Res* **45**:71–82.

Fitzgerald M (1985) The sprouting of saphenous nerve terminals in the spinal cord following early postnatal sciatic nerve section in the rat. *J Comp Neurol* **240**:407–413.

Fitzgerald M (1987*a*) The prenatal growth of fine diameter afferents into the rat spinal cord — a transganglionic study. *J Comp Neurol* **261**:98–104.

Fitzgerald M (1987*b*) Cutaneous primary afferent properties in the hindlimb of the neonatal rat. *J Physiol* **383**:79–92.

Fitzgerald M (1987*c*) Spontaneous and evoked activity of foetal primary afferents 'in vivo'. *Nature* **326**:603–605.

Fitzgerald M (1991) The development of descending brainstem control of spinal cord sensory processing. In: *The Fetal and Neonatal Brainstem* (ed. Hanson MA). Cambridge University Press, pp. 127–136.

Fitzgerald M, De Lima J (2001) Hyperalgesia and allodynia in infants. In: *Acute Pain in Infants and Children: Progress in Pain Research and Management*, Vol 20 (eds. McGrath PJ, Finlay A). IASP Press, Seattle, pp. 1–12.

Fitzgerald M, Fulton BP (1992) The physiological properties of developing sensory neurons. In: *Sensory Neurons: Diversity, Development and Plasticity* (ed. Scott SA). Oxford University Press, Oxford, pp. 287–306.

Fitzgerald M, Gibson SJ (1984) The postnatal physiological and neurochemical development of peripheral sensory C fibres. *Neurosci* **13**:933–944.

Fitzgerald M, Jennings E (1999) The postnatal development of spinal sensory processing. *Proc Natl Acad Sci USA* **96**:7719–7722.

Fitzgerald M, Koltzenburg M (1986) The functional development of descending inhibitory pathways in the dorsolateral funiculus of the newborn rat spinal cord. *Dev Brain Res* **24**:261–270.

Fitzgerald M, Walker S (2003) The role of activity in developing pain pathways Fitzgerald M, Butcher T, Shortland P (1994) Developmental changes in the laminar termination of A fibre cutaneous sensory afferents in the rat spinal cord dorsal horn. *J Comp Neurol* **348**:225–233.

Fitzgerald M, Millard C, Macintosh N (1988a) Hyperalgesia in premature infants. *The Lancet* **8580 (1)**:292.

Fitzgerald M, Millard C, Macintosh N (1989) Cutaneous hypersensitivity following peripheral tissue damage in newborn infants and its reversal with topical anaesthesia. *Pain* **39**:31–36.

Fitzgerald M, Shaw A, McIntosh N (1988*b*) Postnatal development of the cutaneous flexor reflex: comparative study of preterm infants and newborn rat pups. *Developmental Medicine and Child Neurology* **30**:520–526.

Fitzgerald M, Woolf CJ, Shortland P (1990) Collateral sprouting of the central terminals of cutaneous primary afferent neurons in the rat spinal cord: pattern, morphology, and influence of targets. *J Comp Neurol* **300**:370–385.

Fox K (2002) Anatomical pathways and molecular mechanisms for plasticity in the barrel cortex. *Neuroscience* **111(4)**:799–814.

Giannakoulopoulos X, Sepulveda W, Kourtis P, Glover V, Fisk NM (1994) Fetal plasma cortisol and beta-endorphin response to intrauterine needling. *Lancet* **344(8915)**:77–81.

Gonzales R, Coderre TJ, Sherbourne CD, Levine JD (1991) Postnatal development of neurogenic inflammation in the rat. *Neurosci Lett* **127**:25–27.

Gross MK, Dottori M, Goulding M (2002) Lbx1 specifies somatosensory association interneurons in the dorsal spinal cord. *Neuron* **34**:535–549.

Grunau RE (2000) Long-term consequences of pain in human neonates. *Pain Res Clin Man* **10**:101–134.

Grunau RE, Whitfield MF (1998) Children's judgements about pain at age 8–10 years: do extremely low birthweight (<=1000 g) children differ from full birthweight peers? *J Child Psychology & Psychiatry & Allied Disciplines* **39**.

Grunau R, Whitfield MF, Petrie JH (1994*a*) Pain sensitivity and temperament in extremely lowbirth-weight premature toddlers and preterm and fullterm controls. *Pain* **58**:341–346.

Grunau RVE, Whitfield MF, Petrie JH, Fryer EL (1994*b*) Early pain experience, child and family factors, as precursors of somatization: a prospective study of extremely premature and fullterm children. *Pain* **56**:353–359.

Guo A, Simone DA, Stone LS, Fairbanks CA, Wang J, Elde R (2001) Developmental shift of vanilloid receptor 1 (VR1) terminals into deeper regions of the superficial dorsal horn: correlation with a shift from TrkA to Ret expression by dorsal root ganglion neurons. *Eur J Neurosci* **(2)**:293–304.

Guy ER, Abbott FV (1992) The behavioral response to formalin in preweaning rats. *Pain* **51**:81–90.

Helmeke C, Ovtscharoff W Jr, Poeggel G, Braun K (2001) Juvenile emotional experience alters synaptic inputs on pyramidal neurons in the anterior cingulate cortex. *Cereb Cortex* **11**:717–727.

Himes BT, Tessler A (1989) Death of some dorsal root ganglion neurons and plasticity of others following sciatic nerve section in adult and neonatal rats. *J Comp Neurol* **284**:215–230.

Indo Y, Tsuruta M, Hayashida Y, *et al.* (1996) Mutations in the TrkA/NGF receptor gene in patients with congenital insensitivity to pain with anhidrosis. *Nat Genet* **13**:485–488.

Isaac JT, Nicoll RA, Malenka RC (1999) Silent glutamatergic synapses in the mammalian brain. *Can J Physiol Pharmacol* **77**:735–737.

Issler H, Stephens JA (1983) The maturation of cutaneous reflexes studied in the upper limb in man. *J Physiol* **335**:643–654.

Jackman A, Fitzgerald M (2000) Development of peripheral hindlimb and central spinal cord innervation by subpopulations of dorsal root ganglion cells in the embryonic rat. *J Comp Neurol* **418**:281–298.

Jakowec MW, Fox AJ, Martin LJ, Kalb RG (1995) Quantitative and qualitative changes in AMPA receptor expression during spinal cord development. *Neuroscience* **67**:893–907.

Jang IS, Rhee JS, Kubota H, Akaike N, Akaike N (2001) Developmental changes in P2X purinoceptors on glycinergic presynaptic nerve terminals projecting to rat substantia gelatinosa neurones. *J Physiol* **536(Pt 2)**:505–519.

Jennings E, Fitzgerald M (1996) C-fos can be induced in the neonatal rat spinal cord by both noxious and innocuous peripheral stimulation. *Pain* **68**:301–306.

Jennings E, Fitzgerald M (1998) Postnatal changes in responses of rat dorsal horn cells to afferent stimulation: a fibre-induced sensitization. *J Physiol (Lond)* **509**:859–868.

Jiang MC, Gebhart GF (1998) Development of mustard oil-induced hyperalgesia in rats. *Pain* **77**: 305–313.

Kaas JH, Merzenich MM, Killackey HP (1983) The reorganization of somatosensory cortex following peripheral nerve damage in adult and developing mammals. *Annu Rev Neurosci* **6**:325–356.

Keller AF, Coull JA, Chery N, Poisbeau P, De Koninck Y (2001) Region-specific developmental specialization of GABA-glycine cosynapses in laminas I-II of the rat spinal dorsal horn. *J Neurosci* **21**:7871–7880.

Kerchner GA, Wang GD, Qiu CS, Huettner JE, Zhuo M (2001) Direct presynaptic regulation of GABA/glycine release by kainate receptors in the dorsal horn: an ionotropic mechanism. *Neuron* **32**:477–488.

Kerchner GA, Wilding TJ, Huettner JE, Zhuo M (2002) Kainate receptor subunits underlying presynaptic regulation of transmitter release in the dorsal horn. *J Neurosci* **22**:8010–8017.

Khakh BS (2001) Molecular physiology of P2X receptors and ATP signalling at synapses. *Nat Rev Neurosci* **2**:165–174.

Kirstein M, Farinas I (2002) Sensing life: regulation of sensory neuron survival by neurotrophins. *Cell Mol Life Sci* **59**:1787–1802.

Koltzenburg M (1999) The changing sensitivity in the life of the nociceptor. *Pain* **Suppl 6**:S93–S102.

Koltzenburg M, Lewin GR (1997) Receptive properties of embryonic chick sensory neurons innervating skin. *J Neurophysiol* **78**:2560–2568.

Koltzenburg M, Stucky CL, Lewin GR (1997) Receptive properties of mouse sensory neurons innervating hairy skin. *J Neurophysiol* **78**:1841–1850.

Krane EJ, Heller LB (1995) The prevalence of phantom sensations and phantom pain in pediatric amputees. *J Pain Symptom Management* **10**:21–29.

Lee CJ, Bardoni R, Tong CK, *et al.* (2002) Functional expression of AMPA receptors on central terminals of rat dorsal root ganglion neurons and presynaptic inhibition of glutamate release. *Neuron* **35**:135–146.

Lee CJ, Kong H, Manzini MC, Albuquerque C, Chao MV, MacDermott AB (2001) Kainate receptors expressed by a subpopulation of developing nociceptors rapidly switch from high to low Ca2+ permeability. *J Neurosci* **21**:4572–4581.

LeMaster AM, Krimm RF, Davis BM, *et al.* (1999) Overexpression of brain-derived neurotrophic factor enhances sensory innervation and selectively increases neuron number. *J Neurosci* **19**: 5919–5931.

Lendvai B, Stern EA, Chen B, Svoboda K (2000) Experience-dependent plasticity of dendritic spines in the developing rat barrel cortex in vivo. *Nature* **404**:876–881.

Lewis SE, Mannion RJ, White FA, *et al.* (1999) A role for HSP27 in sensory neuron survival. *J Neurosci* **19**:8945–8953.

Li P, Wilding TJ, Kim SJ, Calejesan AA, Huettner JE, Zhuo M (1999) Kainate-receptor-mediated sensory synaptic transmission in mammalian spinal cord. *Nature* **397**:161–164.

Li P, Zhuo M (1998) Silent glutamatergic synapses and nociception in mammalian spinal cord. *Nature* **393**:695–698.

Liao D, Hessler NA, Malinow R (1995) Activation of postsynaptically silent synapses during pairing-induced LTP in CA1 region of hippocampal slice. *Nature* **375**:400–404.

Lidow MS, Song Z–M, Ren K (2000) Long-term effects of short lasting early local inflammatory insult. *Neuroreport* **12**:399–403.

Liu H, Mantyh PW, Basbaum AI (1997) NMDA-receptor regulation of substance P release from primary afferent nociceptors. *Nature* **386**:721–724.

Mantyh PW, Rogers SD, Honore P, *et al.* (1997) Inhibition of hyperalgesia by ablation of lamina I spinal neurons expressing the substance P receptor (see comments). *Science* **278**:275–279.

Markus A, Patel TD, Snider WD (2002) Neurotrophic factors and axonal growth. *Curr Opin Neurobiol* **12**:523–531.

Marsh D, Dickenson A, Hatch D, Fitzgerald M (1999*a*) Epidural opioid analgesia in infant rats. I: mechanical and heat responses. *Pain* **82**:23–32.

Marsh D, Dickenson A, Hatch D, Fitzgerald M (1999*b*) Epidural opioid analgesia in infant rats II: responses to carrageenan and capsaicin. *Pain* **82**:33–38.

Marsh DF, Hatch, DJ, Fitzgerald M (1998) Opioid systems and the newborn. *Brit J Anaesth* **79**:787–795.

Marti E, Gibson SJ, Polak JM, *et al.* (1987) Ontogeny of peptide- and amine-containing neurones in motor, sensory and autonomic regions of rat and human spinal cord, dorsal root ganglia and rat skin. *J Comparative Neurol* **266**:332–359.

Marvizon JC, Martinez V, Grady EF, Bunnett NW, Mayer EA (1997) Neurokinin 1 receptor internalization in spinal cord slices induced by dorsal root stimulation is mediated by NMDA receptors. *J Neurosci* **17**:8129–8136.

McGregor AJ, Griffiths GO, Baker J, Spector TD (1997) Determinants of pressure pain threshold in adult twins: evidence that shared environmental influences predominate. *Pain* **73**:253–257.

Micheva KD, Beaulieu C (1997) Development and plasticity of the inhibitory neocortical circuitry with an emphasis on the rodent barrel field cortex: a review. *Can J Physiol Pharmacol* **75**:470–478.

Mirnics K, Koerber HR (1995*a*) Prenatal development of rat primary afferent fibers: I. Peripheral projections. *J Comp Neurol* **355**:589–600.

Mirnics K, Koerber HR. (1995*b*) Prenatal development of rat primary afferent fibers: II. Central projections. *J Comp Neurol* **355**:601–614.

Molliver DC, Snider WD (1997) Nerve growth factor receptor TrkA is down-regulated during postnatal development by a subset of dorsal root ganglion neurons. *J Comp Neurol* **381**:428–438.

Morison SJ, Grunau RE, Oberlander TF, Whitfield MF (2001) Relations between behavioral and cardiac autonomic reactivity to acute pain in preterm neonates. *Clin J Pain* **17**:350–358.

Moss SJ, Smart TG (2001) Constructing inhibitory synapses. *Nat Rev Neurosci* **2**:240–250.

Murphy TH (2003) Activity-dependent synapse development: changing the rules. *Nat Neurosci* **6(1)**:9–11.

Nandi R, Beacham D, Middleten J *et al.* (2004) The functional expression of mu opioid receptors on sensory neurons is developmentally regulated, morphine analgesia is less selective in the neonate. *Pain* **111**:38–50.

Narayanan CH, Fox MV, Hamburger V (1971) Prenatal development of spontaneous and evoked activity in the rat. *Behaviour* **40**:100–134.

Neugebauer V (2002) Metabotropic glutamate receptors — important modulators of nociception and pain behavior. *Pain* **98**:1–8.

Oberlander TF, Grunau RE, Whitfield MF, Fitzgerald C, Pitfield S, Saul, JP (2000) Biobehavioral pain responses in former extremely low birth weight infants at four months' corrected age. *Pediatrics* **105**:e6.

Oberlander TF, Grunau RE, Fitzgerald C, Whitfield MF (2002) Does parenchymal brain injury affect biobehavioral pain responses in very low birth weight infants at 32 weeks' postconceptional age? *Pediatrics* **110**:570–576.

Olsson G, Berde CB (1993) Neuropathic pain in children and adolsecents. In: *Pain in Infants, Children and Adolescents* (eds. Schecter N, Berde CB, Yaster M). Williams and Wilkins, Baltimore, pp. 473–494.

Park JS, Nakatsuka T, Nagata K, Higashi H, Yoshimura M (1999) Reorganization of the primary afferent termination in the rat spinal dorsal horn during post-natal development. *Brain Res Dev Brain Res* **113**:29–36.

Peters EM, Botchkarev VA, Muller–Rover S, Moll I, Rice FL, Paus R (2002) Developmental timing of hair follicle and dorsal skin innervation in mice. *J Comp Neurol* **448**:28–52.

Petralia RS, Esteban JA, Wang YX, *et al.* (1999) Selective acquisition of AMPA receptors over postnatal development suggests a molecular basis for silent synapses. *Nat Neurosci* **2**:31–36.

Phillips HS, Armanini MP (1996) Expression of the trk family of neurotrophin receptors in developing and adult dorsal root ganglion neurons. *Philos Trans R Soc Lond B Biol Sci* **351**:413–416.

Pignatelli D, Ribeiro–da–Silva A, Coimbra A (1989) Postnatal maturation of primary afferent terminations in the substantia gelatinosa of the rat spinal cord. An electron microscopic study. *Brain Res* **491**:33–44.

Pryce CR, Ruedi–Bettschen D, Dettling AC, Feldon J (2002) Early life stress: long-term physiological impact in rodents and primates. *News Physiol Sci* **17**:150–155.

Randic M, Jiang MC, Cerne R (1993) Long-term potentiation and long-term depression of primary afferent neurotransmission in the rat spinal cord. *J Neurosci* **13**:5228–5241.

Reichling DB, Kyrozis A, Wang J, MacDermott AB (1994) Mechanisms of GABA and glycine depolarization-induced calcium transients in rat dorsal horn neurons. *J Physiol (Lond)* **476**:411–421.

Ren K, Anseloni V, Zou SP *et al.* (2004) Characterization of basal and re-inflammation-associated long-term alteration in pain responsivity following short-lasting neonatal local inflammatory insult. *Pain* **110**:558–596.

Reynolds ML, Fitzgerald M (1992) Neonatal sciatic nerve section results in TMP but not SP or CGRP depletion from the terminal field in the dorsal horn of the rat: the role of collateral sprouting. *Neuroscience* **51**:191–202.

Reynolds M, Fitzgerald M (1995) Long term sensory hyperinnervation following neonatal skin wounds. *J Comp Neurol* **358**:487–498.

Reynolds ML, Fitzgerald M, Benowitz LI (1991) GAP-43 expression in developing cutaneous and muscle nerves in the rat hindlimb. *Neuroscience* **41**:201–211.

Rios M, Treede R, Lee J, Lenz FA (1999) Direct Evidence of nociceptive input to human anterior cingulate gyrus and parasylvian cortex. *Curr Rev Pain* **3(4)**:256–264.

Rohrer H, Heumann H, Theonen H (1998) The synthesis of nerve growth factor (NGF) in developing skin is independent of innervation. *Dev Biol* **128**:240–244.

Ruda MA, Ling Q–D, Hohmann AG, Peng YB, Tachibana T (2000) Altered nociceptive neuronal circuits after neonatal peripheral inflammation. *Science* **289**:628–630.

Ruit KG, Elliott JL, Osborne PA, Yan Q, Snider WD (1992) Selective dependence of mammalian dorsal root ganglion neurons on nerve growth factor during embryonic development. *Neuron* **8**:573–587.

Sanes JR, Yamagata M (1999) Formation of lamina-specific synaptic connections. *Curr Opin Neurobiol* **9**:79–87.

Schecterson LC, Bothwell M (1992) Novel roles for neurotrophins are suggested by BDNF and NT-3 mRNA expression in developing neurons. *Neuron* **9**:449–463.

Schneider SP, Perl ER (1988) Comparison of primary afferent and glutamate excitation of neurons in the mammalian spinal dorsal horn. *J Neurosci* **8**:2062–2073.

Sebert ME, Shooter EM (1993) Expression of mRNA for neurotrophic factors and their receptors in the rat dorsal root ganglion and sciatic nerve following nerve injury. *J Neurosci Res* **36**:357–367.

Shortland P, Fitzgerald M. (1991) Functional connections formed by saphenous nerve terminal sprouts in the dorsal horn following neonatal nerve section. *Eur J Neurosci*, **3**:383–396.

Shortland P, Fitzgerald M (1994) Neonatal sciatic nerve section results in a rearrangement of the central terminals of saphenous and axotomized sciatic nerve afferents in the dorsal horn of the spinal cord of the adult rat. *Eur J Neurosci* **6**:75–86.

Shortland P, Molander C, Woolf CJ, Fitzgerald M (1990) Neonatal capsaicin treatment induces invasion of the substantia gelatinosa by the terminal arborizations of hair follicle afferents in the rat dorsal horn. *J Comp Neurol* **296**:23–31.

Sivilotti LG, Gerber G, Rawat B, Woolf CJ (1995) Morphine selectively depresses the slowest, NMDA-independent component of C-fibre-evoked synaptic activity in the rat spinal cord in vitro. *Euro J Neurosci* **7**:12–18.

Snider WD (1994) Functions of neurotrophins during nervous system development: what the knockouts are teaching us. *Cell* **77**:627–638.

Stelzner DJ (1971)The normal postnatal development of synaptic end-feet in the lumbosacral spinal cord and of responses in the hindlimbs of the albino rat. *Experimental Neurology* **31**:337–357.

Stevens BJ, Franck LS (2001) Assessment and management of pain in neonates. *Paediatr Drugs* **3**:539–558.

Tachibana T, Ling QD, Ruda MA (2001) Increased fos induction in adult rats that experienced neonatal peripheral inflammation. *Neuroreport* **12**:925–927.

Taddio A, Goldbach M, Ipp M, Stevens B, Koren G (1995) Effect of neonatal circumcision on pain responses during vaccination in boys. *Lancet* **345(8945)**:291–292.

Taddio A, Katz J, Ilersich AL, Koren G (1997) Effect of neonatal circumcision on pain response during subsequent routine vaccination. *Lancet* **349(9052)**:599–603.

Teng CJ, Abbott FV (1998) The formalin test: a dose-response analysis at three developmental stages. *Pain* **76**:337–347.

Todd AJ (2002) Anatomy of primary afferents and projection neurones in the rat spinal dorsal horn with particular emphasis on substance P and the neurokinin 1 receptor. *Exp Physiol* **87**:245–249.

Todd AJ, Sullivan AC (1990) Light microscope study of the coexistence of GABA-like and glycine-like immunoreactivities in the spinal cord of the rat. *J Comp Neurol* **296**:496–505.

Torsney C, Fitzgerald M (2002) Age-dependent effects of peripheral inflammation on the electrophysiological properties of neonatal rat dorsal horn neurons. *J Neurophysiol* **87**:1311–1317.

Torsney C, Fitzgerald, M (2003) Spinal dorsal horn cell receptive field size is increased in adult rats following neonatal hindpaw skin injury. *J Physiol* **550**:255–261.

Torsney C, Meredith–Middleton J, Fitzgerald M (2000) Neonatal capsaicin treatment prevents the normal postnatal withdrawal of A fibres from lamina II without affecting Fos responses to innocuous peripheral stimulation. *Brain Res Dev Brain Res* **121**:55–65.

Tsujino H, Kondo E, Fukuoka T, *et al.* (2000) Activating transcription factor 3 (ATF3) induction by axotomy in sensory and motoneurons: a novel neuronal marker of nerve injury. *Mol Cell Neurosci* **15**:170–182.

van Praag H, Frenk H (1992) The effects of systemic morphine on behavior and EEG in newborn rats. *Brain Res* **67**:19–26.

Walker SM, Meredith–Middleton J, Cooke–Yarborough C, Fitzgerald M (in press) Neonatal inflammation and primary afferent terminal plasticity in the rat dorsal horn. *Pain*.

Wall PD (1977) The presence of ineffective synapses and the circumstances which unmask them. *Philos Trans R Soc Lond B Biol Sci* **278**:361–372.

Wang G, Scott SA (2000) The 'waiting period' of sensory and motor axons in early chick hindlimb: its role in axon pathfinding and neuronal maturation. *J Neurosci* **20**:5358–5366.

Wang G, Scott SA (2002) Development of 'normal' dermatomes and somatotopic maps by 'abnormal' populations of cutaneous neurons. *Dev Biol* **251**:424–433.

Wang GD, Zhuo M (2002) Synergistic enhancement of glutamate-mediated responses by serotonin and forskolin in adult mouse spinal dorsal horn neurons. *J Neurophysiol* **87**:732–739.

Wang J, Reichling DB, Kyrozis A, MacDermott AB (1994) Developmental loss of GABA- and glycine-induced depolarization and Ca2+ transients in embryonic rat dorsal horn neurons in culture. *Eur J Neurosci* **6**:1275–1280.

Weber ED, Stelzner DJ (1977) Behavioural effects of spinal cord transection in the developing rat. *Brain Res* **125**:241–255.

White FA, Behar O (2000) The development and subsequent elimination of aberrant peripheral axon projections in Semaphorin3A null mutant mice. *Dev Biol* **225**:79–86.

Woodbury CJ, Koerber HR (2003) Widespread projections from myelinated nociceptors throughout the substantia gelatinosa provide novel insights into neonatal hypersensitivity. *J Neurosci* **23**:601–610.

Woodbury CJ, Ritter AM, Koerber HR (2001) Central anatomy of individual rapidly adapting low-threshold mechanoreceptors innervating the 'hairy' skin of newborn mice: early maturation of hair follicle afferents. *J Comp Neurol* **436**:304–323.

Wright DE, Snider WD (1996) Focal expression of glial cell line-derived neurotrophic factor in developing mouse limb bud. *Cell Tissue Res* **286**:209–217.

Yip HK, Rich KM, Lampe PA, Johnson EMJ (1984) The effects of nerve growth factor and its antiserum on the postnatal development and survival after injury of sensory neurons in rat dorsal root ganglia. *J Neurosci* **4**:2986–2992.

Yoshimura M, Jessell T (1990) Amino acid-mediated EPSPs at primary afferent synapses with substantia gelatinosa neurones in the rat spinal cord. *J Physiol* **430**:315–335.

Zirlinger M, Lo L, McMahon J, McMahon AP, Anderson DJ (2002) Transient expression of the bHLH factor neurogenin-2 marks a subpopulation of neural crest cells biased for a sensory but not a neuronal fate. *Proc Natl Acad Sci USA* **99**:8084–8089.

Zwick M, Davis BM, Woodbury CJ, *et al.* (2002) Glial cell line-derived neurotrophic factor is a survival factor for isolectin B4-positive, but not vanilloid receptor 1-positive, neurons in the mouse. *J Neurosci* **22**:4057–4065.

Chapter 10

Visceral and deep somatic pain

Jennifer M.A. Laird and Hans-Georg Schaible

10.1 Introduction

Disease processes in the deep tissue such as the viscera, muscle, and joint are the most common cause of clinically relevant pain. Pain is also the major, or in some cases, the only sensation that originates from deep tissues. In contrast, the skin gives rise to a wide range of sensations that include touch, tickle, itch, warmth, coolness, and complex sensations like wetness or stickiness. Cutaneous pain serves primarily as a warning of external threats and is much more rarely a clinical concern, although lesions, burns, and some skin diseases produce pain. This chapter will outline the basic principles of nociception in the viscera, muscle, and joint, with a particular emphasis on the similarities and differences in the neurobiology of pain from deep structures compared to pain from the skin.

10.2 Pain sensation in the viscera and somatic deep tissue

10.2.1 Characteristics of visceral pain sensation

There are five main characteristics of visceral pain — the clinical features that make visceral pain unique. These are that visceral pain:

1. is not evoked from all viscera

2. is not linked to visceral injury

3. is referred to other locations

4. is diffuse and poorly localized

5. is accompanied by strong motor and autonomic reflexes (Cervero and Laird 1999).

The referral of visceral pain to other locations (usually the body wall), the diffuse nature of visceral pain, and the strong reflexes it evokes are due to the central organization of visceral nociceptive mechanisms. Particularly important are the lack of a separate visceral sensory pathway and the low proportion of visceral afferent fibres compared to those of somatic origin. The clinical observation that visceral pain cannot be evoked from all viscera and the lack of a direct relationship between visceral injury and pain initially suggested that some viscera lacked an afferent innervation. However, it is now clear that all internal organs are innervated and that these features of visceral pain are due to the functional properties of the sensory receptors that innervate different visceral organs (Cervero 1994, 1996). Receptors whose activation does not evoke conscious perception and that are not *sensory* receptors in the strict sense innervate many viscera. These are receptors concerned with the homeostatic regulation of the internal environment and mainly activated by signals that do not reach consciousness, such as the level of blood pressure or the pH of the stomach (Cervero 1994).

10.2.1.1 Visceral sensitization and hyperalgesia

In psychophysical terms, hyperalgesia is best described as the consequences of the left-ward shift that occurs, following a peripheral injury, in the curve that relates stimulus intensity to pain sensation. This shift causes the lower portion of the pain curve to fall in the innocuous stimulus intensity range whereas the upper portion shows an increased pain sensation to noxious stimuli (Cervero and Laird 1996).

The areas of hypersensitivity produced by an injury to the skin include a zone that incorporates the injury site and a much larger area of undamaged skin around the site of injury. These regions are known as areas of primary and secondary hyperalgesia respectively (Cervero and Laird 1996). An injury to visceral tissue also produces areas equivalent to primary and secondary hyperalgesia seen after cutaneous lesions. *Primary visceral hyperalgesia* occurs in the damaged area, as for the skin. The secondary hyperalgesia area, (i.e. undamaged tissue showing hypersensitivity as a result of a nearby lesion) similarly includes adjacent undamaged regions of the same viscus. However, visceral damage may also result in hypersensitivity in other, undamaged viscera, or in undamaged areas of the same viscus. This is known as *viscero-visceral hyperalgesia*. Furthermore, visceral lesions may also give rise to hyperalgesia in the area to which the visceral pain is referred, on the body wall. This is known as *referred hyperalgesia* (Giamberardino 1999).

10.2.1.2 Referred hyperalgesia

Hyperalgesia of the somatic area to which visceral pain is referred, or referred hyperalgesia, is a common clinical observation. It is particularly obvious in conditions where visceral pain occurs intermittently (e.g. dysmenorrhoea or ureteric colic), since the referred hyperalgesia often continues during the pain-free periods. Patients report experiencing 'tenderness' in the referral zone. Referred hyperalgesia has been quantified in patients with a variety of different visceral pain states and has also been measured in animal models of visceral pain (e.g. Giamberardino *et al.* 1997, 2002; Laird *et al.* 2001*a*, 2002; Al–Chaer and Traub 2002). Referred hyperalgesia is more pronounced in subcutaneous tissues than in the skin and is directly related to the duration and intensity of visceral pain episodes (Giamberardino *et al.* 1997). The referral zone may also present trophic changes in visceral pain patients. For example, increases in the thickness of the subcutis and a reduction in muscle volume have been quantified ipsilateral to painful ureteric colics (Giamberardino 1999).

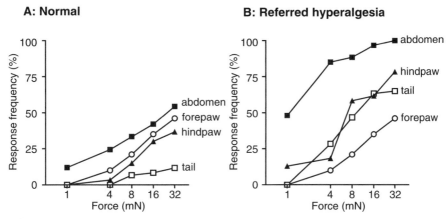

Fig. 10.1 Development of visceral hyperalgesia referred to the abdomen, hindpaw, and tail after colon inflammation in the mouse. Normal mice and mice with an experimental inflammation of the colon were tested for sensitivity of various body areas to mechanical stimuli by measuring the frequency of withdrawal responses evoked by a stimulus of a given force, applied using a von Frey probe. In normal animals, the abdomen was the most sensitive region tested and the tail the least sensitive **(A)**. After colon inflammation, the sensitivity of the abdomen, hindpaw, and tail all increased significantly, whereas the responses to stimulation of the forepaw did not change **(B)**. The shift to the left of the stimulus–response curve, or referred visceral hyperalgesia, occurs in body areas where the somatic afferents terminate in the spinal segments which also receive afferents innervating the affected viscus, the colon. (Data from Laird *et al.* 2001 and unpublished data.)

10.2.1.3 Viscero-visceral hyperalgesia

Painful events in one viscus may affect the responses to noxious stimuli of another viscus with partially overlapping innervation. For example, fertile women with repeated ureteric colics have been shown to be more likely to suffer a colic attack at a specific point in their monthly cycle. The effect of the cycle on the timing of colics was especially pronounced in those women with dysmenorrhoea (Giamberardino *et al.* 2001).

10.2.2 Characteristics of pain in deep somatic tissue

As for viscera, the major sensation that originates from deep tissue such as joint and muscle is pain (Schaible and Grubb 1993; Mense 1996). Sensory afferent inflow from muscle and joint is continuously regulating the activity of the motor system, but we are usually not aware of it. However, it can reach consciousness as 'position sense' (i.e. our ability to estimate the position of a limb quite accurately in the absence of visual control). Furthermore, non-painful pressure sensations can be elicited by mechanical stimulation of ligaments, joint capsule, and muscle bellies. Thus, most afferent fibres innervating the deep somatic tissues may elicit sensations in the appropriate context.

While innocuous stimulation of proprioceptive receptors may escape awareness, noxious stimulation usually evokes conscious pain. In humans, pain sensations from the joint can be experimentally elicited when noxious mechanical, thermal, and chemical stimuli are applied to the fibrous structures such as ligaments and fibrous cartilage. By contrast, stimulation of the synovial layer rarely evokes pain, and stimulation of the cartilage does not evoke any sensation (Schaible and Grubb 1993). This is surprising because degenerative diseases of cartilage (osteoarthritis) are considered quite painful. Squeezing of a tendon, ischaemia in a contracting muscle, or injection of algogenic compounds such as hypertonic saline into a muscle are very painful stimuli (Mense 1996; Mense *et al.* 1997). A very strong pain can be elicited when the tibial bone (or the overlying periosteum) is hit. Thus pain is usually elicited by noxious stimuli and, in contrast to the viscera, the relationship between the application of noxious stimuli and the experience of pain is much tighter than when noxious stimuli are applied to visceral organs.

As in the viscera or the skin, injury or inflammation of deep somatic tissues evokes hyperalgesia. When a joint or a muscle is inflamed, normal movements in the working range hurt, and palpation may elicit pain. This pain usually becomes worse when the limb is used, and so one attempts to limit movements (Schaible and Grubb 1993;

Box 10.1 Clinical characteristics of pain syndromes in deep somatic tissue

Acute arthritis (acute inflammation, rheumatoid fever, etc.)

♦ Pain during movements in the working range, local pain during light or modest pressure applied to the joint, spontaneous pain (in absence of movements).

♦ Joint is swollen and warm due to the acute inflammation.

Chronic arthritis (e.g. rheumatoid arthritis)

♦ Stiffness in the morning, pain during movements in the working range, local pain during light or modest pressure to the joint, spontaneous pain; weakness of muscle contraction (grip strength, etc.).

♦ Swelling of the joint, warm skin over joint; at later stages, joint destruction and deformation.

Osteoarthritis (degenerative joint destruction)

♦ Pain during walking in the morning, gets better during the day but gets worse with increasing load, pressure pain, sometimes spontaneous pain during the day and at night.

♦ At later stages, deformation of joints; intermittent swelling of the joint.

Mense *et al.* 1997). Another source of pain in deep tissue are degenerative diseases such as osteoarthritis. In this case pain may also occur at night or at rest, and in many cases the pain may go away when the joint is being moved. A clinically very impressive pain is caused by bone cancer or metastasis (Honore *et al.* 2000). In the final stage of cancer many patients suffer from dramatic pain that can only be treated with strong opioids.

Pain in the deep tissue may be relatively precisely localized (e.g. pain can be elicited by palpation of an injured meniscus), but pain is often also dull and poorly localized. In some cases the contralateral side is painful during a unilateral disease process that may be taken as secondary hyperalgesia. However, pain originating in deep tissue can also be referred to skin and other deep tissues (i.e. it is felt at a site remote from the site of origin/stimulation) (Arendt–Nielsen *et al.* 2000).

10.3 **Models of visceral and deep somatic pain**

10.3.1 **Visceral pain models**

The principal challenge of modelling visceral pain in animals is the relative inaccessibility of the target tissue compared to more superficial structures like the skin. The smaller the species chosen, the greater the problem. Mice are used increasingly in pain research because of the availability of transgenic and mutant strains, but visceral pain models in mice are essentially restricted to the larger organs like the colon and bladder (e.g. Laird *et al.* 2001*b*, 2002).

Intraperitoneal injection of algogens (the abdominal constriction or writhing test) is also widely used as a 'visceral' pain model in mice, although it is really a mixed viscerosomatic test since the peritoneum, partly innervated by somatic afferents, is also involved. There is a clear difference in behavioural profile between the writhing test and viscero-specific abdominal pain models in rodents. This difference correlates well with the differing clinical presentation of peritonitis and inflammation of visceral mucosa (e.g. cystitis, colitis) in human patients.

Another important consideration in developing visceral pain models is the use of an *adequate* stimulus (Ness and Gebhart 1990; Al–Chaer and Traub 2002). In viscera, the relationship between damage and pain is not as clear as in somatic tissues. In the early twentieth century, abdominal surgery was routinely performed with only local anaesthesia of the incision site. Surgeons noted that stretch of mesenteries and distension of hollow viscera produced much more pain than cauterization or cutting (Mackenzie 1909). Damage to the parenchyma of solid viscera like the liver or kidney does not produce pain at all. So the selection of a nociceptive rather than damaging stimulus is required.

However, in some respects, the behaviour in visceral pain models is easier to interpret than in models of cutaneous pain. Pain is the only sensation experienced from some internal organs (e.g. the ureter, the uterus, the gall bladder, and the pancreas). This means that in the study of basic mechanisms, behavioural responses evoked by noxious stimulation of these viscera can more reliably be interpreted in terms of their contribution to pain processing than equivalent responses evoked from the skin, where a number of alternative interpretations must be considered.

There are a number of visceral pain models that model specific disease states (e.g. ureteric calculosis, pancreatitis, endometriosis, irritable bowel syndrome) (Al–Chaer and Traub 2002; Giamberardino *et al.* 2002; Vera–Portocarrero *et al.* 2003). Using such models, complex mechanisms underlying chronic pain behaviour and hyperalgesia can be studied. However, these models are quite technically demanding and so simpler, acute noxious stimuli like distension and/or inflammation of hollow viscera are also widely used (Ness and Gebhart 1990; Al–Chaer and Traub 2002).

10.3.2 Deep somatic pain models

Inflammation and degenerative processes in joint and muscle are an important cause of chronic painful human disease. Rheumatoid arthritis, for example, is an inflammatory painful disease of joints that lasts decades because no disease-modifying treatment is available. Cancer pain, caused by the primary disease but especially by bone metastases, is also a clinically important pain problem. In animals, pain from deep somatic tissues has been most extensively modelled using inflammatory stimuli, but models are also being developed for joint degenerative diseases and bone cancer to address the clear need both to understand these conditions and to develop novel therapies.

Inflammation in the joint can be induced by the intra-articular injections of crystals such as urate and kaolin or of carrageenan. These injections produce an oedema and granulocytic infiltration within 1–3 hours, with a plateau after 4–6 hours. Awake animals show enhanced sensitivity to pressure onto the joint and limping. During this period the development of peripheral and spinal sensitization can be directly observed in long-term recordings from primary afferent neurones supplying the joint and spinal cord neurones with joint input (see below) (Schaible and Grubb 1993). This inflammatory process may also become more chronic. The muscle can also be inflamed by injections of carrageenan into the muscle belly (Mense 1996; Mense *et al.* 1997).

However, for chronic inflammation other models are usually used. The injection of Freund's complete adjuvant (FCA) into one joint produces monoarthritis. Usually the lesion is restricted to the injected joint, and the animals show no gross physical impairment except at the inflamed site. Signs of hyperalgesia (limping or guarding of the leg, enhanced sensitivity to pressure onto the joint) develop within a day, reach a peak within 3 days, but are maintained to some degree up to several weeks. When FCA is injected at a high dose in the footpad tail base or lymph node, a polyarthritis develops, with two stages. In the first stage an acute inflammation develops at the site of inoculation, that subsides after 3–5 hours. During the second, a diffuse inflammatory reaction develops in the distal joints of the animals and in other parts of the body such as the eyes, ears, tail, genitalia. The polyarthritis subsides after 4 weeks but may reoccur (Schaible and Grubb 1993).

Another form of chronic inflammation is the antigen-induced arthritis. Rats or mice are first immunized and, in the second step, the antigen (m-BSA) is injected into the knee joint. A unilateral inflammation develops that shows an acute phase with granu-locytic infiltration. At later stages, parameters of chronic inflammation such as fibrosis are more dominant. The rats show signs of hyperalgesia such as limping and increased pressure sensitivity, particularly in the first weeks, but signs of inflammatory hyperalgesia may be present for up to 5 or 6 weeks (Segond von Banchet *et al.* 2000).

Cutting joint ligaments such as the anterior cruciate ligament of the knee joint can induce degenerative osteoarthritis. This will lead to a morphologically degenerative joint, but the pain behaviour has not been rigorously tested so far.

Recently, a model of cancer pain has been introduced. Osteolytic sarcoma cells are injected into the femoral intramedullary space, and the injected mice develop a sarcoma with bone destruction. Mice with bone cancer exhibit painful behaviour in the form of guarding the limb, hyperalgesia, and a loss of grip strength that are correlated to the extent of bone destruction (Honore *et al.* 2000).

10.4 Nociceptive primary afferent neurones supplying the viscera and deep somatic tissue

10.4.1 Spinal projections of visceral, articular, and muscular afferents

Visceral afferent fibres with somata in the dorsal root ganglia convey visceral informa-tion to the spinal cord. Visceral spinal afferents terminate in the outermost layer of the spinal grey matter (lamina I), the neck of the dorsal horn (lamina V), and around the central canal (lamina X) (Cervero *et al.* 1984; Sugiura *et al.* 1993). Afferent fibres with somata in the nodose ganglion and running in the vagus nerve also provide the CNS with information about visceral events, but are probably not directly involved in mediating visceral pain sensation (Cervero 1994).

The spinal projection of joint and muscle afferents into the spinal cord shows similarities. Studies using HRP as a tracer have shown that nerves supplying the knee joint or the gastrocnemius-soleus muscle of the cat project to lamina I and to deeper laminae (V–VII). At least in the cat, usually no projections are found into laminae II–IV (Schaible and Grubb 1993; Mense 1996).

10.4.2 Response properties of visceral, articular, and muscular afferents

In addition to visceral homeostatic receptors mentioned above, there are other groups of sensory receptors in the viscera concerned with the encoding of noxious events and whose activation presumably accounts for the perception of visceral pain. Likewise, joint and muscle nerves contain a large proportion of fibres that are nociceptive and presumably account for pain in the deep somatic tissue. Traditionally, receptors are classified according to their responses to mechanical stimulation, although clearly a variety of chemical stimuli (including changes in pH, ischaemia, and release of chemical mediators like bradykinin) are also important in the physiology and pathophysiology

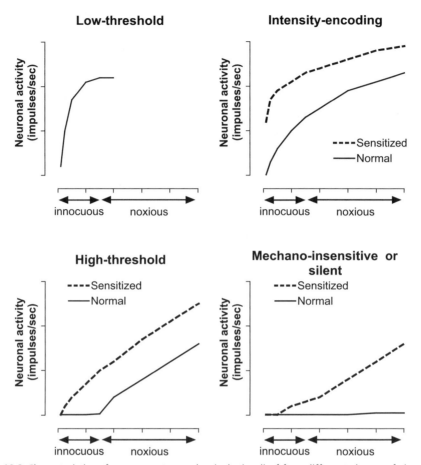

Fig. 10.2 Characteristics of responses to mechanical stimuli of four different classes of visceral and deep somatic afferents. The **low-threshold class** effectively encodes mechanical stimuli in the non-noxious range, but not in the noxious range. In viscera this class includes fibres responding to stimuli such as peristalsis and stroking of the mucosa. They are likely to be involved in homeostatic regulation of the viscera and to include most vagal afferents. In muscle and joints, this group of afferents are probably those involved in fine motor control and that give rise to position sense. The intensity-encoding class encodes mechanical stimuli effectively in the innocuous range and, therefore, potentially may be involved in regulation like the low-threshold class. However, this class encodes well into the noxious range and, therefore, may also contribute to pain sensations. After sensitization by inflammation or tissue damage, the responses of the intensity-encoding class increases significantly, such that the stimulus–response curve for these afferents shifts to the left. The **high-threshold class** consists of afferents that only encode effectively noxious intensities of mechanical stimulation. These afferents fulfil the criteria for nociceptors and are well suited to contribute to pain sensation produced by noxious mechanical stimuli. Sensitization of these afferents also shifts the stimulus–response curve for these afferents to the left, so that they are now excited by innocuous stimuli. The **mechano-insensitive or silent class** of afferents responds poorly, or not at all, to mechanical stimuli under normal conditions and, therefore, presumably does not contribute to mechanically evoked pain sensations under normal conditions but may function as chemoreceptors. However, after sensitization these afferents acquire novel responses to mechanical stimuli and thus contribute to mechanically evoked pain.

of sensation. Electrophysiological studies in experimental animals have revealed three distinct classes of receptor innervating internal organs and deep somatic structures that could contribute to conscious sensation from viscera, joint, muscle, etc. — intensity-encoding mechanoreceptors, high-threshold mechanoreceptors, and mechanically insensitive receptors.

10.4.2.1 Intensity-encoding mechanoreceptors

A number of reports have described sensory receptors in *internal organs* with a low threshold to mechanical stimulation but that encode both innocuous and noxious intensities. They may also respond to chemical and even thermal stimuli. These receptors have been described mainly in the gastrointestinal tract and the urinary bladder (Cervero 1994; Coutinho *et al.* 2000; Sengupta 2000). These receptors could be responsible for those visceral sensations that start as non-painful but that evolve towards pain as the stimulus intensity or duration increase (fullness, urge to void). This would explain their presence in viscera from which non-painful and well as painful sensations are experienced (Cervero 1994, 1996).

Low-threshold receptors in the *joint nerve* with thick myelinated axons may show higher discharge rate when a movement such as supination or pronation is continued from the innocuous working range into the painful range. However, when the responses of these fibres to all kinds of mechanical stimuli (e.g. different types of movements) are monitored, the discharge rate often does not properly discriminate innocuous from noxious mechanical stimuli. Furthermore, these fibres do not respond to bradykinin and other inflammatory mediators, and thus is unlikely that they play a major role in nociception. Other low-threshold fibres (mainly those with thinly myelinated and unmyelinated fibres) encode innocuous and noxious intensity of mechanical stimuli, and most of them also respond to bradykinin and some other inflammatory mediators (Schaible and Schmidt 1996).

10.4.2.2 High-threshold mechanoreceptors

These are sensory receptors with a high threshold to mechanical stimuli (around the threshold for pain in man) and an encoding function contained entirely within the noxious range of stimulation. *Visceral* high-threshold receptors have been described in the heart, veins, lungs and airways, oesophagus, biliary system, small intestine, colon, ureter, urinary bladder, and uterus (Cervero 1994; Foreman 1999; Coutinho *et al.* 2000; Sengupta 2000). Their functional properties mean that these sensory receptors will be activated by intensities of mechanical stimulation perceived as painful. A large proportion of these receptors are also excited by chemical stimuli such as bradykinin or brief ischaemia and reperfusion. In addition, these receptors can be sensitized by prolonged and intense stimuli so that their threshold decreases and their excitability increases in the presence of tissue injury and inflammation.

Joint nerves contain numerous thinly myelinated and unmyelinated fibres that respond only to high-intensity mechanical stimulation such as firm painful pressure and movements carried out with torque against the resistance of the tissue (Schaible and Schmidt 1996). In the *muscle nerve* high-threshold receptors respond to strong compression of the muscle belly but not to light pressure and contractions in the physiological range. These high-threshold receptors encode mechanical stimuli only in the noxious range (Mense 1996). Many of these units are also chemosensitive and respond to bradykinin, prostaglandin E2 or prostaglandin I2, serotonin, histamine, substance P, or several of these and possibly other compounds (see below).

10.4.2.3 Mechanically insensitive receptors

Mechanically insensitive receptors were first described in joints (Schmidt *et al.* 1994). This prompted the search for a similar population in *viscera*. Experiments searching for receptors using chemical or electrical stimuli or brief episodes of ischaemia revealed a chemosensitive component of the afferent innervation of internal organs that respond poorly or only at rather high thresholds to mechanical stimuli under normal conditions (e.g. Longhurst and Dittman 1987; Habler *et al.* 1990; Pan and Longhurst 1996; Pan and Chen 2002). Like the high-threshold population, they can be sensitized by prolonged and intense stimuli or inflammation and then may become sensitive to low- intensity mechanical stimuli. Because of their lack of mechanosensitivity and ability to be sensitized and respond to mechanical stimuli after inflammation, it has been suggested that these afferents only contribute to chronic visceral pain sensation resulting from tissue injury or inflammation. However, as mentioned above, chemical stimuli would also be expected to be important in generating acute visceral pain sensation, and many mechanically insensitive receptors respond briskly to chemical stimuli, suggesting they may function as chemonociceptors.

A proportion of primary afferent neurones in the *joint nerve*, most of them with unmyelinated axons, are not activated even by noxious mechanical stimuli under normal conditions. These units respond to a bolus injection of KCl into the joint artery, and inflammatory compounds also activate many of them. In the first instance they were named silent nociceptors because they become mechanosensitive under inflammatory conditions but a proportion of them could also function as chemonociceptors (Schmidt *et al.* 1994). Muscle afferents probably also include a proportion of mechanically insensitive or silent nociceptors, because not all units seem to be initially mechanosensitive. However, this has been less extensively investigated (Mense 1996).

In summary, noxious events may cause afferent fibres innervating deep tissues encoding the intensity of mechanical stimuli to fire at maximal rates. Whether this intensity-dependent input, and in particular the high discharge rates, actually produce pain, is difficult to say. While it has been possible to study fibre activities in single human skin nerve fibres in parallel with the exploration of pain sensation, such information is not available for visceral and deep somatic afferents, with the exception of a few studies in muscle nerves (Simone *et al.* 1994). Clearly, however, noxious stimuli activate a large number of high-threshold afferents that fulfil the criteria for nociceptors, and it is reasonable to assume that this nociceptive-specific input will result in a specific pain sensation. In deep somatic tissue, pain is elicited by high-intensity stimuli that activate specific high-threshold nociceptors. Furthermore, it is reasonable to assume that the recruitment of mechanically insensitive or silent nociceptors during chemical stimulation and/or inflammation will contribute to pain sensations. Again, however, no information is available whether, for example, the electrical stimulation of a silent joint nociceptor is sufficient to elicit a pain sensation in a joint.

10.4.3 Sensitization of visceral, articular, and muscular nociceptors

Tissue injury induces a process of nociceptor sensitization whereby the excitability of the nociceptors is increased and their thresholds lowered. It is generally thought that sensitization is an important neuronal mechanism underlying primary hyperalgesia at the site of injury or inflammation.

10.4.3.1 Sensitization of visceral nociceptors

The decrease in threshold to stimulation of injured or inflamed tissue (primary visceral hyperalgesia) can be demonstrated in patients and in animals, for example by distension of the gut with an intraluminal balloon (Coutinho *et al.* 2000; Mayer *et al.* 2001). However, the viscera are normally inaccessible to external stimuli. So is primary visceral hyperalgesia really of any relevance to visceral pain sensation?

Visceral nociceptors innervate motile, secretory tissue. Thus sensitization of these nociceptors to chemical or mechanical stimuli may result in their activation by the normal physiological activity of the viscus. Furthermore, this effect may be potentiated by increases in motility or secretion induced by the lesion, either directly, or by activation of reflex arcs. So, sensitization of visceral nociceptors will lead to visceral pain by a dual mechanism — as a result of any spontaneous activity induced, and also by ongoing excitation produced either by the normal physiological activity of the viscus and further enhanced by pathological changes in motility or secretion induced by the initiating injury (Cervero and Laird 1999).

10.4.3.2 Sensitization of deep tissue nociceptors

Typically, high-threshold units become more sensitive under inflammatory conditions. Whereas it often seems to be difficult to show sensitization for mechanical stimuli in single cutaneous afferent units (hence mostly thermal sensitization is measured in single-fibre studies), mechanical sensitization is a robust phenomenon in deep tissue afferents. High-threshold afferents start to respond to mechanical stimuli within the physiological range (such as movements in the working range in the case of joint nociceptors). In addition, a proportion of the initially mechanoinsensitive neurones is rendered sensitive for mechanical stimuli, thus providing a recruitment of fibres that contribute to the inflow into the spinal cord during inflammation. However, also some low-threshold neurones show enhanced responses, and therefore the input into the spinal cord is dramatically increased during inflammation by the contribution of all types of fibres (Schaible and Grubb 1993; Schmidt *et al.* 1994).

Mechanisms of sensitization in deep tissue afferents have been investigated in nerve recordings in intact animals. It was shown that the application of inflammatory mediators (either topical application or intra-arterial injection) could increase the responses of joint and muscle afferents to mechanical stimuli. The effects of bradykinin and prostaglandins have been studied most extensively. Bradykinin activates a large proportion of joint and muscle afferents. After a short-lived activation, a reduction of threshold was noted outlasting the period of activation. Prostaglandins, in particular PGE_2 and PGI_2, can also sensitize joint afferents. In general, such chemical effects are observed in thinly myelinated and unmyelinated afferents, but there is no strict correlation between original mechanical threshold and sensitization (Schaible, 2004). These mediators can sensitize a proportion of low-threshold as well as high-threshold and initially unresponsive units. Sensitization of some joint afferents has also been observed after application of other inflammatory mediators like serotonin or substance P.

The molecular mechanisms of sensitization are most often studied in isolated dorsal root ganglion neurones, and usually no attempt is made to define whether the cell body corresponds to a cutaneous, deep somatic, or visceral afferent fibre. Furthermore, changes of mechanosensitivity have not been the focus of molecular studies of sensitization.

From work on chronic inflammatory models it appears that in the long term, sensitization may be supported by enhanced receptor expression in the primary afferent neurones. For example, a significantly higher proportion of dorsal root ganglion neurones in rats with acute and chronic antigen-induced arthritis express the bradykinin B2 receptor (Segond von Banchet *et al.* 2000).

10.5 Central processing of visceral and deep somatic pain

Spinal neurones are the first point of processing and integration of pain-related information within the CNS. Spinal neurones are usually classified by their thresholds to external stimulation, their receptive fields, and the convergence pattern of their inputs.

10.5.1 Spinal neurones processing visceral pain

The major feature of spinal processing of visceral information is the convergence of visceral and somatic afferents onto the same population of spinal neurones. There is no evidence for a population of spinal neurones receiving purely visceral information that would provide a 'private pathway' for the signalling of visceral sensation. The viscero-somatic afferent convergence in the spinal cord underlies the referral of visceral pain to somatic tissue in the same segments. Electrophysiological recordings from single neurones in the spinal cord of animals have found that neurones excited by stimulation of a particular viscus are also activated by stimulation of somatic tissues in the appropriate dermatomes. For example, neurones with an excitatory input from the ureter are also activated by stimulation of the flanks of the animal (Roza *et al.* 1998).

The somatic input to viscero-somatic neurons is predominately from deep tissues, which may help to explain the dull, diffuse nature of referred visceral pain.

The area of somatic tissue whose stimulation affects the activity of the neurones, known as the somatic receptive field of the neurone, is larger in spinal neurones with both visceral and somatic input (viscerosomatic neurones) than in neighbouring neurones with a purely somatic input (e.g. Olivar *et al.* 2000). Many viscerosomatic neurones, even those excited by one side of a bilateral viscus, such as the ureter, have bilateral somatic receptive fields (e.g. Laird *et al.* 1996). These observations help to explain the poorly localized nature of visceral pain sensations.

Visceral sensation depends on a relatively small population of afferent fibres compared to the numbers innervating somatic targets. Even in the mid-thoracic segments, where visceral innervation is at its greatest and somatic innervation density is low, there are approximately 10-fold more somatic than visceral afferent fibres

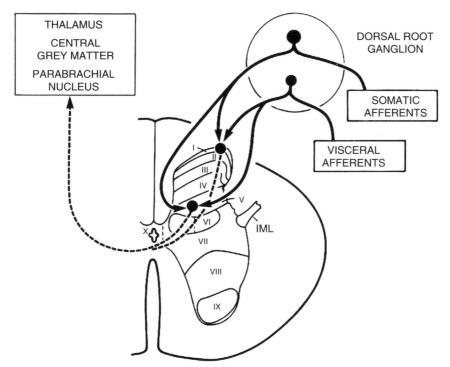

Fig. 10.3 Spinal circuitry underlying referral of visceral sensation to somatic areas. Separate groups of spinal afferents with cell bodies in the dorsal root ganglia innervate visceral and somatic structures ('somatic afferents' and 'visceral afferents'). However, visceral afferents synapse with spinal neurones that also receive synapses from somatic afferents, known as viscerosomatic neurones. Thus, mixed viscerosomatic information is transmitted to higher centres in the brain. (Reproduced from Cervero and Foreman 1990.)

(Cervero *et al.* 1984). Visceral afferent fibres nonetheless branch extensively within the spinal cord and excite many spinal neurones (Sugiura *et al.* 1993). This diffuse termination pattern within the spinal cord further contributes to the poor localization of visceral pain sensations. The extensive branching also serves to amplify the visceral nociceptive input at the level of the spinal cord, and may contribute to the very strong autonomic and skeletal muscle reflex responses evoked by visceral noxious stimulation.

Some spinal neuronal populations receive excitatory inputs from more than one viscus. This viscero-visceral convergence likely explains the similarities of the sensations evoked by stimulation of certain viscera. For example, afferents from the oesophagus and the heart converge onto a population of thoracic spinal neurones (Garrison *et al.* 1992). This convergence may underlie the phenomenon of non-cardiac chest pain, where patients present with symptoms typical of angina, yet on exploration have normal heart function (Foreman 1999). In many cases, such patients have been shown to suffer from oesophageal disease.

The characteristics of visceral stimuli that excite spinal neurones reflect the response properties of visceral afferents and, in turn, underlie the characteristics of sensation from the organ in question. For example, neurones excited by distension of the colon show a range of thresholds from very low to above the normal pain threshold. Almost all encode in the noxious range with the exception of a very small number of neurones that have low thresholds and do not encode in the noxious range (Olivar *et al.* 2000). The afferent innervation of the colon includes a large population of intensity-encoding afferents, and a smaller proportion of fibres that have high thresholds (Sengupta and Gebhart 1994). Both non-painful and painful sensations can be experienced from distension of the colon. In contrast, stimulation of organs such as the ureter or gallbladder exclusively evokes the sensation of pain. Spinal neurones excited by distension of the ureter or gallbladder recorded in animals have relatively high thresholds (Cervero 1983; Laird *et al.* 1996), similar to the thresholds of pain sensation in man, and the afferents innervating these organs include a large proportion of high-threshold fibres (Cervero 1982; Cervero and Sann 1989).

10.5.1.1 Referred hyperalgesia

Referred hyperalgesia can be explained by an extension of the viscero-somatic convergence that underlies referred pain. A continuous low level of activity in nociceptors innervating an area of visceral damage may not produce sufficient spinal activation to evoke pain. However, if the somatic area of referral is stimulated, the somatic input summates with the ongoing visceral activity and the threshold to evoke pain sensations is reached more quickly. Referred hyperalgesia is correlated with the intensity and duration of visceral pain, suggesting that this reflects the level of activity in visceral nociceptors (Giamberardino 1999). However, noxious inputs can also change the way that subsequent inputs are processed, usually resulting in an enhanced response. Thus, referred hyperalgesia also reflects these 'memory traces' or changes in spinal processing.

10.5.1.2 Viscero-visceral hyperalgesia

There is evidence for single visceral afferent fibres that innervate more than one viscus and a good deal of evidence for viscero-visceral convergence onto neurones of the spinal cord. These findings could provide the anatomical substrate for viscero-visceral hyperalgesia. The underlying spinal mechanism is probably similar to that of referred hyperalgesia. However, in addition to the pain sensation *per se*, an additional factor in viscero-visceral hyperalgesia may be the activation of reflex pathways by disease in one viscus that initiate or exacerbate problems in another organ. Since reflexes are segmentally organized, the greatest effects are likely to occur in viscera innervated by the same or adjacent spinal segments (Giamberardino 1999).

10.5.2 **Spinal neurones processing deep somatic pain**

Nociceptive inputs from joint and muscle are either processed in dorsal horn neurones that respond solely to mechanical stimulation of deep tissue, or in neurones that respond to mechanical stimulation of both deep tissue and the skin (Schaible and Grubb 1993; Mense 1996). Thus, there is a 'private pathway' of neurones that only process deep inputs. However, more neurones show convergent inputs from deep tissue and skin. Whether neurones with input from deep tissue have also inputs from viscera has never been explored systematically, although the converse has often been observed, as described above. This may depend on the segment. While heart disease may cause pain in the arm (possibly involving neurones with visceral, cutaneous, and deep somatic inputs), visceral diseases do not usually cause pain in the knees or lower legs.

The receptive field of neurones with deep somatic inputs may be large including, for example, convergent inputs from muscles of the thigh and lower limb, knee, and ankle joints. The size of receptive fields of neurones with deep input from distal parts of the limbs such as small joints in the foot has not been explored because it is extremely difficult to differentiate receptive fields in skin and underlying deep tissue. Given the larger representation of inputs from distal parts of the limbs in cortical areas, it may be expected that neurones with inputs from distal parts of the limbs have, in general, smaller receptive fields.

Whereas visceral sensation is thought to depend on a relatively small population of afferent fibres, the deep tissue seems to be densely innervated. For example, the nerves to the gastrocnemius soleus muscle or other big muscles are relatively thick nerve branches. Although muscle nerves contain numerous motoneurones and thick myelinated afferent fibres such as Ia and Ib fibres supplying muscle spindles and tendon organs, the majority of the fibres are thinly myelinated or unmyelinated (Mense 1996). Joints also seem to be densely innervated. Three nerves that altogether contain ~2000 fibres supply the knee joint of the cat (Schaible and Grubb 1993).

Usually neurones can easily be identified by pressure applied to deep tissue, showing that mechanical stimuli are in general adequate to activate spinal neurones processing input from joints. From their mechanical thresholds, neurones appear either nociceptive-specific and respond only to intense pressure or painful twisting of the leg, or are wide dynamic range cells and respond to both innocuous pressure and noxious pressure, encoding stimulus intensity in a graded fashion. By and large, nociceptive specific neurones have smaller receptive fields and receive specific deep inputs with no receptive field on the skin (Schaible and Grubb 1993).

10.5.3 Spinal pathways of visceral and deep somatic pain

Several pathways originating in the spinal grey matter and terminating in the brain have been identified as carrying information related to visceral pain. Of these, the spinothalamic tract is thought to be the most important for sensory-discriminative functions (i.e. the localization and quality of pain sensation). Recent evidence suggests that the postsynaptic dorsal column pathway, classically considered as a pathway responsible for cutaneous tactile discrimination, also has an important role in transmission of signals related to visceral nociceptive processing (Willis and Westlund 2001). This discovery explains descriptions of pain relief produced by surgical spinal lesions of midline white matter in patients with terminal cancer affecting abdominal viscera. Other pathways, which carry axons of viscerosomatic spinal neurones (e.g. the spinohypothalamic or spino-parabrachial-amygdaloid pathways), are obvious candidates for carrying signals related to the affective components of the sensation of visceral pain. Spinal viscerosomatic neurones also project rostrally in the spinosolitary and spinoreticular tracts.

Spinal neurones with nociceptive input from muscle and joint project rostrally in the ventrolateral quadrant suggesting that the information is carried in the spinothalamic and spinoreticular tracts. In particular many neurones in the spinoreticular tract seem to be excited by deep inputs and not by cutaneous inputs (Fields *et al.* 1977).

10.6 Central sensitization of dorsal horn neurones with visceral or deep somatic input

A cardinal feature of nociceptive dorsal horn neurones is that they can be rendered more responsive to external stimuli by intense noxious stimulation or inflammation of the periphery. This central hyperexcitability is known as 'central sensitization' and is characterized by:

1. increased responses to external stimuli
2. decreased thresholds
3. enlargement of receptive fields
4. increase of background activity in some cases.

Central sensitization is not just a reflection of increased input from sensitized peripheral nociceptors, even though it is driven by input from the periphery. It is thought that central sensitization, in addition to peripheral sensitization, is an important neural mechanism underlying pain during visceral disease and deep somatic pain.

10.6.1 **Sensitization of neurones with visceral input**

Spinal neurones with visceral input show the characteristic signs of central sensitization after inflammation or injury. These changes are due to central events, rather than just a reflection of the sensitization of visceral afferents, since electrical stimulation of visceral afferents (bypassing the sensitized peripheral terminals) also produces an enhanced effect after visceral inflammation (Olivar *et al.* 2000).

In contrast to somatic tissues, acute stimulation of the viscera at noxious intensities may produce signs of central sensitization. For example, a single 20-second noxious distension of the colon or ureter produces a marked increase in the somatic receptive field size and other signs of hyperexcitability in spinal neurones in experimental animals (Laird *et al.* 1996; Olivar *et al.* 2000). A psychophysical correlate of the increased somatic receptive field can be observed in normal human subjects. In volunteers, the area to which the pain of bladder distension is referred is larger on the second or third of a series of brief, moderately painful distensions (Ness *et al.* 1998).

These observations suggest that central sensitization is more easily induced after visceral stimulation. However, viscero-somatic neurones in the spinal cord with visceral input show frequency-dependent facilitation (wind-up) to stimulation of their somatic inputs, but do not show a similar facilitation to electrical stimulation of visceral afferent fibres (Herrero *et al.* 2000). Overall, there seem to be fundamental differences in the central consequences of somatic versus visceral nociceptive input, which may contribute to the differences in the sensations of visceral and somatic pain.

10.6.2 **Sensitization of neurones with deep somatic input**

Central sensitisation of neurones with deep input is an important consequence of inflammation in joint and muscle. The particular effectiveness of deep inputs to induce central sensitization has been demonstrated with electrical nerve stimulation. The electrical stimulation of muscular afferents caused a more pronounced facilitation of synaptic transmission than the electrical stimulation of cutaneous nerves (Woolf and Wall 1986). During development of an acute inflammation in the knee joint, neurones with knee joint input show enhanced responses to innocuous and noxious mechanical stimulation of the inflamed knee joint, and nociceptive-specific neurones often exhibit a lowering of threshold such that innocuous mechanical stimulation of the knee joint is sufficient to drive the neurone. In addition, responses to mechanical stimulation of adjacent and remote non-inflamed tissue (ankle, paw) also increase substantially, and the receptive field often shows an expansion, towards ankle and paw. Similar phenomena are observed in nociceptive neurones with input from the muscle. The responses of the neurones to electrical nerve stimulation are increased simultaneously, showing that some of the spinal changes take place in the spinal cord. Collectively, these changes show that a state of hyperexcitability is generated by inflammation (Schaible and Grubb 1993).

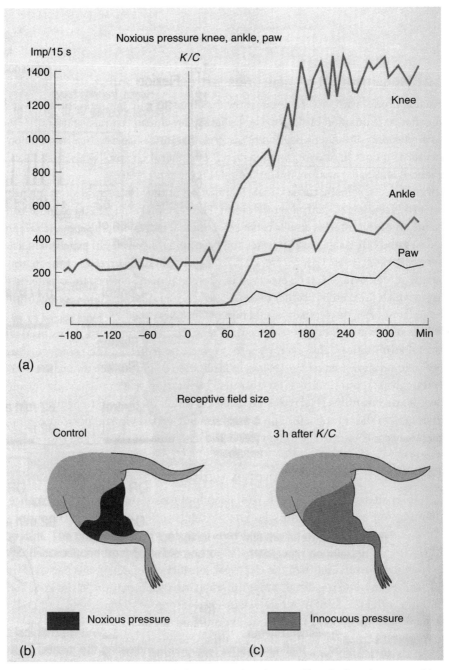

Fig. 10.4 Development of hyperexcitability in a nociceptive-specific spinal cord neuron with knee input after inflammation of the knee. The neuron was recorded at a depth of 1052 μm. Before inflammation it had a high-threshold receptive field in the knee joint and the deep structures adjacent to the knee **(b)**. **(a)** Responses to noxious pressure applied to the knee joint, the ankle region, and the paw before and during development of inflammation, post injections of kaolin and carrageenan into the knee joint. **(c)** Receptive field of the neuron 3 hours after injections of kaolin and carrageenan (K/C) into the knee joint. The time-scale was set to 0 at the injection of kaolin. (Data from Neugebauer *et al.* 1993.)

While it is possible to show the generation of hyperexcitability directly in long-term recordings from neurones lasting several hours, it is more difficult to know whether central sensitization is maintained during prolonged or chronic inflammation. From the comparison of samples of neurones in normal and arthritic rats (monoarthritis and polyarthritis) it appears that the state of sensitization may last for several weeks. On average, neurones with input from inflamed areas have larger receptive fields, and in the polyarthritic model in particular, neurones may exhibit periods of bursting spontaneous discharges (Menetréy and Besson 1982; Grubb *et al.* 1993). Thus, there is some evidence that central sensitization may last for weeks.

It is unknown whether central sensitization resolves during healing of the joint, when peripheral sensitisation disappears. When patients are operated for joint replacement (e.g. in the course of degenerative osteoarthritis), pain may disappear completely, even for many years. On the other hand, pain may persist during arthritis even when the inflammatory process seems to be under control. The understanding of the neuronal processes of chronic pain in deep tissue is still quite limited.

10.7 Mechanisms of central sensitization during deep tissue and visceral inflammation

The mechanisms of inflammation-evoked central sensitization have been identified to some extent. Because peripheral nociceptors are sensitized, they release more transmitter during stimulation of inflamed tissue (for transmitters, see section 10.8). The enhanced transmitter release may thus constitute a tonic *presynaptic component* of central sensitization. On the other hand, as a *postsynaptic component* of central sensitization, the gain of spinal cord neurones is increased by changes of receptor activation. Most important is the activation of NMDA receptors for glutamate. Central sensitization by inflammation can be completely blocked by spinal application of antagonists at NMDA receptors. Furthermore, when inflammation and inflammation-evoked hyperexcitability are established, NMDA receptor antagonists can reduce or even reverse enhanced responses to stimulation (even after several weeks). Thus, NMDA receptors in the nociceptive spinal cord neurones with deep input are important for the generation as well as for the maintenance of central sensitization. Other glutamate receptors (metabotropic receptors) are also involved.

In addition to glutamate, substance P can facilitate spinal processing of deep input. The application of substance P to the spinal cord can cause an enlargement of receptive fields and stronger responses (see Fig. 10.5). On the other hand, central sensitization is not abolished but is significantly attenuated when antagonists at either tachykinin NK1, NK2, or CGRP receptors are applied to the spinal cord during development of inflammation, showing that substance P, neurokinin A, and CGRP contribute to the full development of central sensitization (Schaible 1996: Schaible *et al.* 2002). An attenuation of central sensitization is also found when the prostaglandin synthesis inhibitor, indomethacin, is applied topically to the spinal cord before inflammation, suggesting that spinal prostanoids play a role in this process. Indeed, topical application of PGE2 to the spinal cord produces a response pattern in nociceptive spinal cord neurones with knee joint input that is similar to that induced by knee joint inflammation (Vasquez *et al.* 2001).

Responses of spinal cord neurones and changes of response properties during joint inflammation are under the control of ***descending influences***. Most descending inputs are inhibitory, but some facilitate spinal nociceptive processing. When descending influences are eliminated (either by transection of the spinal cord or by cooling of descending tracts), the development of inflammation-evoked spinal hyperexcitability is more pronounced. Furthermore, the effects of descending influences increase when an inflammation develops. Thus, descending pathways, at least in the acute stages of inflammation, control spinal hyperexcitability (Danziger *et al.* 2001). The possible long-term changes in descending inputs are not known.

Descending control of spinal viscero-somatic neurons, even under normal conditions, includes a substantial component of descending facilitation. This may be part of the central amplification of the visceral signal required, because the number of afferent neurones carrying visceral information from the periphery is so small.

10.8 **Transmitters involved in visceral and deep somatic pain**

10.8.1 **Transmitters in visceral afferents**

There are two distinct biochemical classes of fine-calibre primary afferents — those that contain peptide neurotransmitters such as the tachykinins (substance P, neurokinin A and B) and calcitonin gene-related peptide (CGRP), and those that do not. There is also a range of other receptors that are expressed by one group and not the other, and the two groups seem to have different trophic requirements to maintain their normal phenotypes. Somatic fine afferent fibres include both biochemical classes, and the functional role of the two classes in somatic pain is still not clear. However, almost all visceral afferent fibres contain peptides, and they do not express the carbohydrate membrane markers that are characteristic of the non-peptide class (Lawson 1996). Furthermore, the peptide-containing afferents terminate in the most superficial layers of the dorsal horn (laminae I and IIa), lamina V, and around the central canal (lamina X), matching the distinctive termination patterns in laminae I, V, and X of the spinal cord of visceral afferent fibres (Cervero 1996). The biochemical identification of visceral afferents as part of the peptide-containing class suggests that peptides are particularly important in the transmission of information from viscera.

Pharmacological evidence also supports a greater role for peptides in visceral rather than cutaneous pain transmission. Recent studies with specific antagonists for tachykinin receptors and with transgenic mice with a disruption of the gene for the substance P (tachykinin NK1) receptor have suggested peripheral NK2 receptors and central NK1 receptors are involved in visceral pain (Laird *et al.* 2001*b,c*). CGRP has been proposed as a marker for pathways throughout the neuraxis carrying visceral

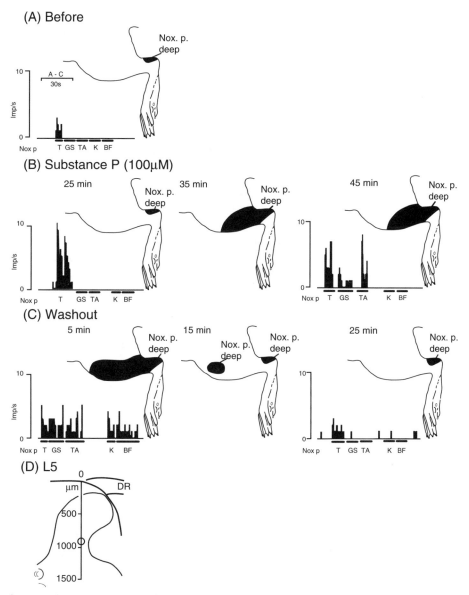

Fig. 10.5 Changes in receptive field (RF) size of a nociceptive spinal cord neuron with input from deep somatic structures during spinal (SP) superfusion with substance P (100 μM). The recording site is indicated in D (CC, central canal; DR, dorsal root). Size and location of the RF (black area) on the hind limb are shown before SP superfusion **(A)**, during superfusion **(B)**, and during washout with CSF **(C)**. The histograms underneath the outlines of the hind limb show the neurone's responses to noxious deep pressure stimulation (Nox.p.deep) of the calcaneal tendon (T), gastrocnemius-soleus muscle (GS), tibialis anterior muscle (TA), knee joint (K), and biceps femoris muscle (BF). Before SP superfusion, the neurone was only excited by activation of nociceptors in the calcaneal tendon **(A)**. During SP superfusion **(B)** (35 and 45 min after the start of the SP superfusion) and in the early phase of the washout period **(C)** (5 min), the RF expanded. At the time of greatest RF expansion, noxious pressure stimulation of gastrocnemius-soleus muscle, tibialis anterior muscle, knee joint, and biceps femoris muscle excited the neurone. The effect was reversible after a washout period of 25 min **(C: far right)**. (Reproduced from Mense et al. 1996.)

information, since it is found in more than 98% of primary afferents innervating viscera (Lawson 1996) and also in brain nuclei (e.g. the parabrachial nucleus and visceral sensory cortex) associated with processing visceral information in general, not just pain-related information.

10.8.2 Transmitters in deep somatic afferents

Probably most deep somatic afferents use glutamate as their principal transmitter. This derives from the observation that the application of antagonists at glutamate receptors (AMPA and NMDA receptors) to spinal cord neurones reduces their responses to mechanical stimulation of the joint. Proportions of primary afferents contain neuropeptides, but the percentage is not as high as for visceral afferents. Substance P is found in around 20–30% of joint afferents, and CGRP in about 50% (Lawson 1996). Other peptides have also been identified in deep somatic afferents. The neuropeptides are either transported to the periphery where they produce neurogenic inflammation, or to the spinal cord where they support central sensitization (see above). As already mentioned, peripheral sensitization not only facilitates excitation of the nociceptors but also increases intraspinal release of mediators such as substance P, neurokinin A, and CGRP (Schaible and Grubb 1993; Schaible *et al.* 2002).

10.9 Representation of visceral and deep somatic pain in higher centres

Information on the processing of *visceral pain* in higher centres has come from animal experiments and, increasingly in recent years, from studies in man, including imaging studies and microstimulation during intracranial surgery in conscious patients. Studies in animals have demonstrated a viscerotopic representation of the viscera in the thalamus and somatosensory cortex. Imaging experiments in normal subjects comparing non-painful somatic and visceral stimuli suggest that visceral sensations are represented in the secondary rather than in primary somatosensory cortex. When visceral pain is experienced, the hypothalamus and periaqueductal grey, the thalamus, and various limbic cortical regions (anterior cingulate cortex, lateral prefrontal cortex) are activated (Aziz *et al.* 2000; Strigo *et al.* 2003). This pattern of activation is consistent with the strong affective component of visceral pain and also the poor localization of the pain sensation.

Microstimulation of the thalamus in patients undergoing intracranial surgery can evoke visceral pain experiences, such as angina or labour pain, sometimes many years after the original episode. These observations suggest the existence of long-term neural mechanisms capable of storing the results of a previous pain experience. The pain memories evoked in these studies are of pain with a strong affective component, almost all of visceral pain experiences, presumably because they are very frequent in the general population and relatively intense (Cervero and Laird 1999).

Irritable bowel syndrome (IBS) accounts for half of all GI referrals in the US and is a chronic disorder characterized by abdominal pain and changes in motility in the absence of structural or biochemical abnormalities. Imaging and psychophysical studies reveal two coexisting disorders underlying IBS: visceral hypersensitivity (perhaps due to sensitization of nociceptors or alterations in spinal processing) and cortical hypervigilance to visceral events (Mayer *et al.* 2001). Patients with IBS show increased activation in the anterior cingulate cortex during painful colorectal distension and abnormal patterns of cortical activation when they anticipate a painful visceral stimulus. IBS is a good example of visceral pain as a disease *per se*, where pain (or hyperalgesia) is the problem, and highlights the contribution of cortical processing to clinically relevant pain.

In general, the supraspinal processing of **deep somatic pain** has not been as extensively studied as the processing of cutaneous pain. Recordings from thalamic and cortical areas in the cat and rat have shown that proportions of the nociceptive neurons are activated by nociceptive deep input from muscle and joint. In the cat thalamus, neurons were located at the ventral and dorsolateral periphery of the ventroposterolateral nucleus that received input from group III and group IV muscle afferents in addition to cutaneous inputs. In the cat cortical area 3a, some neurons were identified to process nociceptive input from the muscle. In the ventrobasal complex of rat thalamus, nociceptive neurons seem to be intermingled with neurons that receive, exclusively, input from low-threshold fibres. Possibly the localization of nociceptive neurons in the thalamus and cortex is species-dependent (Guilbaud 1988).

In polyarthritic rats, dramatic changes of the responses of thalamic neurons have been observed. A large proportion of neurons in the thalamic ventrobasal complex respond to gentle pressure onto inflamed joints and movements, whereas only few neurons respond to this stimulus in normal rats, and often long-lasting afterdischarges were noted. Some neurons also displayed paroxsymal discharges. Similar alterations were noted in the somatosensory cortex (Guilbaud 1988). Thus, sensitization of neurons is observed at all levels of the neuraxis. Whether the discharge pattern in supraspinal neurons reflects entirely the discharge pattern of spinal cord neurons, or whether additional supraspinal components come into play, is difficult to say.

Studies on supraspinal nociceptive processing of deep somatic pain in humans have just begun. Comparisons are being made of which cortical areas are activated by cutaneous stimulation and stimulation of the muscle. However, firm conclusions seem to be premature at the moment.

10.10 **Concluding remarks**

Although there are some common principles of nociception for skin, somatic deep tissue, and viscera, available data suggest that there are also fundamental differences in the processing of nociceptive information from skin, deep tissue and viscera. Thus, the different character of cutaneous, deep tissue, and visceral pain does not only reflect

Box 10.2 Release of mediators in the CNS (spinal cord)

1. **Indirect methods** measure effects which are produced or induced by mediators that are released.

Examples using electrophysiology:

♦ **Recording of EPSPs or IPSPs:** Electrical stimulation of a presynaptic ending will produce an EPSP or an IPSP in the postsynaptic neuron. From the occurrence, amplitude and frequency of EPSPs or IPSPs conclusions are made on the release of the synaptic transmitter. When several mediators are released, the contribution of a transmitter can be estimated by using receptor-specific antagonists.

♦ **Recording spikes from neurons:** Assessment of the responses of a neuron to peripheral stimulation before and during administration of a receptor-specific antagonist to the neuron will reveal whether a transmitter or mediator is released and contributes to the response.

Examples using immunohistochemistry:

♦ **Visualization of depletion**: After extensive stimulation immunohistochemical staining of a compound may be reduced.

♦ **Visualization of receptor internalization**: Some receptors are internalized when a ligand has bound. The internalization can be visualized using confocal microscopy.

2. **Direct methods** detect release by measuring the compound of interest.

In vitro experiments:

♦ **Superfusion of a slice:** Mediators can be measured in the superfusate. One can measure basal release and release of compounds after stimulation (e.g. after electrical stimulation of attached dorsal roots or after administration of drugs to the bath). Particularly suitable for pharmacological studies.

In vivo experiments:

♦ **Superfusion of CNS region:** A region is superfused and compounds are measured in the superfusate. Only compounds can be measured that diffuse to the surface.

♦ **Push–pull cannula:** A cannula is inserted into the grey matter to a defined depth. Through an opening at the tip, solutions can be applied locally and fluid can be collected to measure compounds. *Advantage*: measurement of mediators within the grey matter. *Disadvantage*: big size of cannula may cause tissue damage.

♦ **Microdialysis:** A small tube is inserted in the grey matter (e.g. in a transverse direction). The part of the tube in the grey matter consists of a permeable membrane that allows fluid exchange from tube to tissue and from tissue to tube.

Box 10.2 **Release of mediators in the CNS (spinal cord)** *(continued)*

The dialysis tube is continuously perfused. Suitable for sample collection and local application of drugs. *Disadvantages*: tissue damage, low recovery rate for some compounds.

♦ **Antibody microprobes:** Glass capillaries are coated with antibodies and are then inserted to defined depths in the grey matter, where ligands bind to the microprobe at the site of release. *Advantages*: show spatial distribution of compounds in the grey matter (e.g. in the ventral, deep, and superficial dorsal horn), minor tissue damage. *Disadvantages*: only suitable for compounds that can be measured with antibodies, only one compound can be measured per probe, semi-quantitative.

differences in the disease processes that might affect these tissues but may also depend to a large extent on the neuronal organization of the particular nociceptive system. Considerable progress in the understanding of pain syndromes in different tissue should be made as basic and clinical pain research continues to define the differences in nociceptive processing of different types of tissue.

References

Al–Chaer ED, Traub RJ (2002) Biological basis of visceral pain: recent developments. *Pain*, **96**, 221–225.

Arendt–Nielsen L, Laursen RJ, Drewes AM (2000) Referred pain as an indicator for neural plasticity. In (eds. Sandkühler J, Bromm B, Gebhart GF) *Nervous System Plasticity and Chronic Pain*, pp. 343–356. Elsevier, Amsterdam.

Aziz Q, Schnitzler A, Enck P (2000) Functional neuroimaging of visceral sensation. *Journal of Clinical Neurophysiology*, **17**, 604–612.

Cervero F (1982) Afferent activity evoked by natural stimulation of the biliary system in the ferret. *Pain*, **13**, 137–151.

Cervero F (1983) Somatic and visceral inputs to the thoracic spinal cord of the cat: effects of noxious stimulation of the biliary system. *Journal of Physiology*, **337**, 51–67.

Cervero F (1994) Sensory innervation of the viscera: peripheral basis of visceral pain *Physiological Reviews*, **74**, 95–138.

Cervero F (1996) Visceral nociceptors. In (eds. Belmonte C, Cervero F) *Neurobiology of Nociceptors*, pp. 220–240. Oxford University Press, Oxford.

Cervero F, Foreman DD (1990) Sensory innervation of the viscera. In (eds. Loewy AD, Spyer KM) *Central Regulation of Autonomic Functions*, pp. 104–125. Oxford University Press, New York.

Cervero F, Laird JM (1996) Mechanisms of touch-evoked pain (allodynia): a new model. *Pain*, **68**, 13–23.

Cervero F, Laird JMA (1999) Visceral pain. *Lancet*, **353**, 2145–2148.

Cervero F, Sann H (1989) Mechanically evoked responses of afferent fibres innervating the guinea-pig's ureter: an in vitro study. *Journal of Physiology*, **412**, 245–266.

Cervero F, Connell LA, Lawson SN (1984) Somatic and visceral primary afferents in the lower thoracic dorsal root ganglia of the cat. *Journal of Comparative Neurology*, **228**, 422–431.

Coutinho SV, Su X, Sengupta JN, Gebhart GF (2000) Role of sensitized pelvic nerve afferents from the inflamed rat colon in the maintenance of visceral hyperalgesia. *Progress in Brain Research*, **129**, 375–387.

Danziger N, Weil–Fugazza J, LeBars D, Bouhassira D (2001) Stage-dependent changes in the modulation of nociceptive neuronal activity during the course of inflammation. *European Journal of Neuroscience*, **13**, 230–240.

Fields HL, Clanton CH, Anderson SD (1977) Somatosensory properties of spinoreticular neurons in the cat. *Brain Research*, **120**, 49–66.

Foreman RD (1999) Mechanisms of cardiac pain. *Annual Review of Physiology*, **61**, 143–167.

Garrison DW, Chandler MJ, Foreman RD (1992) Viscerosomatic convergence onto feline spinal neurons from esophagus, heart and somatic fields: effects of inflammation. *Pain*, **49** 373–382.

Giamberardino MA (1999) Recent and forgotten aspects of visceral pain *European Journal of Pain*, **3**, 77–92.

Giamberardino MA, Berkley KJ, Affaitati G, *et al.* (2002) Influence of endometriosis on pain behaviors and muscle hyperalgesia induced by a ureteral calculosis in female rats. *Pain*, **95**, 247–257.

Giamberardino MA, Berkley KJ, Iezzi S, de Bigontina P, Vecchiet L (1997) Pain threshold variations in somatic wall tissues as a function of menstrual cycle, segmental site and tissue depth in non-dysmenorrheic women, dysmenorrheic women and men. *Pain*, **71**, 187–197.

Giamberardino MA, De Laurentis S, Affaitati G, Lerza R, Lapenna D, Vecchiet L (2001) Modulation of pain and hyperalgesia from the urinary tract by algogenic conditions of the reproductive organs in women. *Neuroscience Letters*, **304**, 61–64.

Grubb BD, Stiller RU, Schaible H–G (1993) Dynamic changes in the receptive field properties of spinal cord neurons with ankle input in rats with unilateral adjuvant-induced inflammation in the ankle region. *Experimental Brain Research*, **92**, 441–452.

Guilbaud G (1988) Peripheral and central electrophysiological mechanisms of joint and muscle pain. In (eds. Dubner R, Gebhart GF, Bond MR) *Proceedings of the Vth World Congress on Pain*, pp. 210–215. Elsevier, Amsterdam.

Habler HJ, Janig W, Koltzenburg M (1990) Activation of unmyelinated afferent fibres by mechanical stimuli and inflammation of the urinary bladder in the cat. *Journal of Physiology*, **425**, 545–562.

Herrero JF, Laird JM, Lopez–Garcia JA (2000) Wind-up of spinal cord neurones and pain sensation: much ado about something? *Progress in Neurobiology*, **61**, 169–203.

Honore P, Schwei MJ, Rogers SD, *et al.* (2000) Cellular and neurochemical remodeling of the spinal cord in bone and cancer pain. In (eds. Sandkühler J, Bromm B, Gebhart GF) *Nervous System Plasticity and Chronic Pain*, pp. 389–397. Elsevier, Amsterdam.

Laird JMA, Martinez–Caro L, Garcia–Nicas E, Cervero F (2001) A new model of visceral pain and referred hyperalgesia in the mouse. *Pain*, **92**, 335–342.

Laird JMA, Olivar T, Lopez–Garcia JA, Maggi CA, Cervero F. (2001) Responses of rat spinal neurons to distension of inflamed colon: role of tachykinin NK2 receptors. *Neuropharmacology*, **40**, 696–701.

Laird JM, Roza C, Cervero F (1996) Spinal dorsal horn neurons responding to noxious distension of the ureter in anesthetized rats. *Journal of Neurophysiology*, **76**, 3239–3248.

Laird JMA, Roza C, de Felipe C, Hunt SP, Cervero F (2001) Role of central and peripheral tachykinin NK1 receptors in capsaicin-induced pain and hyperalgesia in mice. *Pain*, **90**, 97–103.

Laird JMA, Souslova V, Wood JN, Cervero F (2002) Deficits in visceral pain and referred hyperalgesia in Nav1.8 (SNS/PN3) null mice. *Journal of Neuroscience*, **22**, 8352–8356.

Lawson, S (1996) Neurochemistry of cutaneous afferents In (eds. Belmonte C, Cervero F) *Neurobiology of Nociceptors*, pp. 72–91. Oxford University Press, Oxford.

Longhurst JC, Dittman LE (1987) Hypoxia, bradykinin, and prostaglandins stimulate ischemically sensitive visceral afferents. *American Journal of Physiology*, **253**, H556–H567.

MacKenzie J (1909) *Symptoms and Their Interpretation*, pp. 1–297. Shaw and Sons, London.

Mayer EA, Naliboff BD, Chang L (2001) Basic pathophysiologic mechanisms in irritable bowel syndrome. *Digestive Diseases*, **19**, 212–218.

Menetréy D, Besson J–M (1982) Electrophysiological characteristics of dorsal horn cells in rats with cutaneous inflammation. *Pain*, **13**, 343–364.

Mense S (1996) Nociceptors in skeletal muscle and their reaction to pathological tissue changes. In (eds. Belmonte C, Cervero F) *Neurobiology of Nociceptors*, pp. 184–201. Oxford University Press, Oxford.

Mense S, Hoheisel U, Reinert A (1996) The possible role of substance P in eliciting and modulating deep somatic pain. In (eds. Carli G, Zimmermann M) *Progress in Brain Research, Towards the Neurobiology of Chronic Pain*, Vol 110, pp. 125–135. Elsevier, Amsterdam.

Mense S, Hoheisel U, Kaske A, Reinert A (1997) Muscle pain: basic mechanisms and clinical correlates. In (eds. Jensen TS, Turner JA, Wiesenfeld–Hallin Z) *Proceedings of the 8th World Congress on Pain*, pp. 479–496. IASP Press, Seattle.

Ness TJ, Gebhart GF (1990) Visceral pain: a review of experimental studies. *Pain*, **41**, 167–234.

Ness TJ, Richter HE, Varner RE, Fillingim RB (1998) A psychophysical study of discomfort produced by repeated filling of the urinary bladder. *Pain*, **76**, 61–69.

Neugebauer, Luecke T, Schaible H–G (1993) N-methyl-D-aspartate (NMDA) and non-NMDA receptor antagonists block the hyperexcitability of dorsal horn neurons during development of acute arthritis in rat's knee joint. *Jounal of Neurophysiology*, **70**, 1365–1377.

Olivar T, Cervero F, Laird JM (2000) Responses of rat spinal neurones to natural and electrical stimulation of colonic afferents: effect of inflammation. *Brain Research*, **866**, 168–177.

Pan HL, Chen SR (2002) Myocardial ischemia recruits mechanically insensitive cardiac sympathetic afferents in cats. *Journal of Neurophysiology*, **87**, 660–668.

Pan HL, Longhurst JC (1996) Ischaemia-sensitive sympathetic afferents innervating the gastrointestinal tract function as nociceptors in cats. *Journal of Physiology*, **492**, 841–850.

Roza C, Laird JM, Cervero F (1998) Spinal mechanisms underlying persistent pain and referred hyperalgesia in rats with an experimental ureteric stone. *Journal of Neurophysiology*, **79**, 1603–1612.

Schaible H–G (1996) On the role of tachykinins and calcitonin gene-related peptide in the spinal mechanisms of nociception and in the induction and maintenance of inflammation-evoked hyperexcitability in spinal cord neurons (with special reference to nociception in joints). In (eds. Kumazawa T, Kruger L, Mizumura K) *The Polymodal Receptor: A Gateway to Pathological Pain*, pp. 423–441. Elsevier, Amsterdam.

Schaible H–G (2004) The neurophysiology of pain. In (eds. Maddison PJ, Isenberg DA, Woo P, Glass DN) *The Oxford Textbook of Rheumatology*. Oxford University Press, Oxford.

Schaible H–G, Grubb BD (1993) Afferent and spinal mechanisms of joint pain. *Pain*, **55**, 5–54.

Schaible H–G, Schmidt RF (1996) Neurobiology of articular nociceptors. In (eds. Belmonte C, Cervero F) *Neurobiology of Nociceptors*, pp. 202–219 Oxford University Press, Oxford.

Schaible H–G, Ebersberger A, Segond von Banchet G (2002) Mechanisms of pain in arthritis. *Annuals of the New York Academy of Science*, **966**, 343–354.

Schmidt RF, Schaible H–G, Messlinger K, Heppelmann B, Hanesch U, Pawlak M (1994) Silent and active nociceptors: structure, functions, and clinical implications. In (eds. Gebhart GF, Hammon DL, Jensen TS). *Proceedings of the 7th World Congress on Pain*, pp. 213–250. IASP Press, Seattle.

Segond von Banchet G, Petrow PK, Bräuer R, Schaible H–G (2000) Monoarticular antigen-induced arthritis leads to pronounced bilateral upregulation of the expression of neurokinin 1 and bradykinin 2 receptors in dorsal root ganglion neurons of rats. *Arthritis Research*, 2, 424–427.

Sengupta JN (2000) An overview of esophageal sensory receptors. *American Journal of Medicine*, 108, 87S–89S.

Sengupta JN, Gebhart GF (1994) Characterization of mechanosensitive pelvic nerve afferent fibers innervating the colon of the rat. *Journal of Neurophysiology*, 71, 2046–2060.

Simone DA, Marchettini P, Caputi G, Ochoa JL (1994) Identification of muscle afferents subserving sensation of deep pain in humans. *Journal of Neurophysiology*, 72, 883–889.

Strigo IA, Duncan GH, Boivin M, Bushnell MC (2003) Differentiation of visceral and cutaneous pain in the human brain. *Journal of Neurophysiology*, 89, 3294–3303.

Sugiura Y, Terui N, Hosoya Y, Tonosaki Y, Nishiyama K, Honda T. (1993) Quantitative analysis of central terminal projections of visceral and somatic unmyelinated (C) primary afferent fibers in the guinea pig. *Journal of Comparative Neurology*, 332, 315–325.

Vasquez E, Bär K–J, Ebersberger A, Klein B, Vanegas H, Schaible H–G (2001) Spinal prostaglandins are involved in the development but not the maintenance of inflammation-induced spinal hyperexcitability. *Journal of Neuroscience*, 21, 9001–9008.

Vera–Portocarrero LP, Lu Y, Westlund KN (2003) Nociception in persistent pancreatitis in rats: effects of morphine and neuropeptide alterations. *Anesthesiology*, 98, 474–484.

Willis WD Jr, Westlund KN (2001) The role of the dorsal column pathway in visceral nociception. *Current Pain and Headache Reports*, 5, 20–26.

Woolf CJ, Wall PD (1986) Relative effectiveness of C primary afferent fibres of different origins in evoking a prolonged facilitation of the flexor reflex in the rat. *Journal of Neuroscience*, 6, 1433–1442.

Chapter 11

The organization of the midbrain periaqueductal grey and the integration of pain behaviours

Thelma Lovick and Richard Bandler

11.1 The periaqueductal grey matter and endogenous analgesia

The perception of pain is a highly individual experience. Whilst the anatomical location of individual nociceptors and their mode of activation by the algogenic stimulus undoubtedly determine the basic sensation, many other factors contribute to the complex sensory and emotional experience which makes up the pain state. Environmental factors and the emotional states which they invoke play an important role in modulating activity at all levels of the neuronal circuitry which transmits signals from nociceptor afferents to the higher levels of the CNS. The influence of the environment and its intimate link with emotional status was first dramatically put on scientific record in the middle of the last century by Beecher (1946), who reported the absence of pain in soldiers during the acute period after being wounded in battle. Whilst Beecher attributed the analgesia as a response to the 'relief' of being wounded and the prospect of being removed from the battlefield, a more contemporary view is to consider such analgesia as an adaptive response which optimizes the chances of survival in a life-threatening environment. Thus, under extreme conditions, pain may be subjugated temporarily in favour of emergency fight-or-flight behaviour.

Identifying such 'endogenous' analgesia-producing systems and harnessing them to therapeutic advantage became the primary goal for many researchers in the pain field. Indeed, more than 30 years ago, the description of surgical analgesia following activation of the periaqueductal grey matter (PAG) and adjacent midbrain regions of the rat (Reynolds, 1969) provided the impetus for an explosion of interest in these structures of the brainstem, which continues to the present time. It has now been established beyond doubt that electrical or chemical stimulation within the periaqueductal region in conscious animals can produce a significant reduction in the overall responsiveness to stimulation of nociceptors. The PAG is the source of a number of descending pathways that exert powerful modulatory influences on the transmission of afferent impluses from nociceptors to the dorsal horn and the spinal trigeminal nucleus (for reviews see Besson and Chaouch, 1987; Willis, 1982). The hypoalgesia which results from activation of the midbrain is, however, only one single component of a far more complex and highly integrated pattern of activity involving behavioural, somatomotor, and autonomic changes. Moreover, the properties of the hypoalgesia, and even the emotional and autonomic changes that accompany it, differ considerably according to the precise site of stimulation within the PAG itself.

11.2 **Stimulation-produced analgesia in man**

The early reports of stimulation-produced analgesia in animals led to a rush of enthusiasm to adapt the technique for use in man as a new method of pain relief. Initially, studies were carried out on patients with persistent intractable pain which had previously proved resistant to conventional analgesic therapy. Stimulating electrodes were implanted stereotactically into both periventricular and periaqueductal sites, and high levels of success were claimed in several studies (Hosobuchi *et al.*, 1977; Young and Brechner, 1986). Others, however, were more circumspect (Nashold *et al.*, 1969), and several investigators emphasized the importance of patient selection and the precise location of the stimulating electrode (Kumar *et al.*, 1997; Young, 1989).

The best results, where stimulation produced a relatively 'pure' pain relief, were obtained following electrode placements at rostrally- and ventrally-located periventricular sites (Hosobuchi *et al.*, 1977; Kumar *et al.*, 1997). Indeed, following stimulation at such optimal sites patients reported 'warmth and relaxing pleasurable sensation' (Kumar *et al.*, 1997) or 'warmth, floating, or generalised well-being' (Young, 1989), as well as relief from their pain. Stimulation at more rostral sites, presumably those that encroached the hypothalamic area, produced adverse responses that included sensations of fear and anxiety, smothering, vertigo, and nausea (Kumar *et al.*, 1997). Stimulation further caudally in the PAG proper also evoked side-effects which the patients found intolerable, despite obtaining some relief from their pain (Nashold *et al.*, 1969). Following similar reports of highly aversive side-effects (Kumar *et al.*, 1997), the procedure became more controversial and its popularity has declined in recent years. Indeed, the procedure is no longer licenced in the USA, although it is continued elsewhere.

11.3 **Functional organization of the PAG — two forms of analgesia**

The PAG is a longitudinally orientated tubular structure surrounding the aqueduct. It tapers towards its rostral end and expands towards its caudal end as the aqueduct opens into the fourth ventricle. It is organized functionally into at least four longitudinal neuronal columns of unequal dimensions, which lie in the dorsomedial, dorsolateral, lateral, and ventrolateral sectors of the PAG on either side of the aqueduct (Bandler and Shipley, 1994; Keay and Bandler, 2002*a*) (Fig. 11.1). In its caudal half, the area ventromedial to the PAG is occupied by the dorsal raphe nucleus, whilst the motoneurones of the trochlear and oculomotor nuclei are embedded in its ventral aspect at more rostral levels.

In terms of analgesia, the PAG can be divided into a dorsal zone which corresponds approximately to the dorsolateral and lateral columns (dl/lPAG), and a ventral zone which encompasses the ventrolateral column of the PAG (vlPAG). Although stimulation

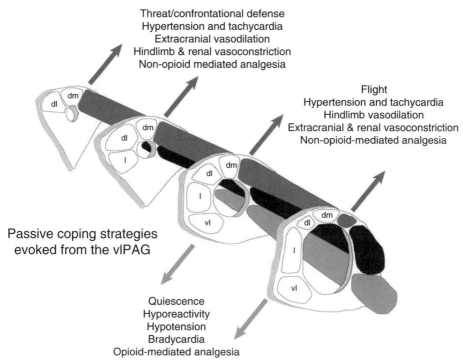

Active coping strategies evoked from the lPAG and the dlPAG

Threat/confrontational defense
Hypertension and tachycardia
Extracranial vasodilation
Hindlimb & renal vasoconstriction
Non-opioid mediated analgesia

Flight
Hypertension and tachycardia
Hindlimb vasodilation
Extracranial & renal vasoconstriction
Non-opioid-mediated analgesia

Passive coping strategies evoked from the vlPAG

Quiescence
Hyporeactivity
Hypotension
Bradycardia
Opioid-mediated analgesia

Fig. 11.1 A series of schematic sections of the PAG illustrating the four main longitudinal neuronal columns: dorsomedial (dm), dorsolateral (dl), lateral (l), and ventrolateral (vl) (rostral is to the left, caudal is to the right). Note that microinjections of excitatory amino acids (EAA) made within the dlPAG/lPAG (dark shadings) versus vlPAG (light shading) evoke distinct emotional coping strategies. EAA microinjections made within the rostral half of the dl/lPAG evoke a confrontational/ defensive reaction, tachycardia, and hypertension (associated with decreased blood flow to viscera and limbs and increased blood flow to extracranial vascular beds). EAA microinjections within the caudal half of the dl/lPAG evoke flight, tachycardia, and hypertension (associated with decreased blood flow to viscera and extracranial vascular beds and increased blood flow to limbs). In contrast, EAA microinjections made within the vlPAG evoke a cessation of all spontaneous movements (quiescence), a decreased responsiveness to the environment (hyporeactivity), hypotension, and bradycardia. Note also that non-opioid-mediated analgesia versus opioid-mediated analgesia are evoked from dl/lPAG versus vlPAG. (Modified from Fig, 1, Bandler et al., 2000.)

in either zone reduces the responsiveness to stimulation of nociceptors, the characteristics of the analgesia evoked from the dorsal versus the ventral site are quite distinct (see Fig. 11.1). Analgesia elicited from stimulation at dorsal sites (i.e within the dl/lPAG sectors) is typically short-lasting and non-opioid- mediated. On the other hand, stimulation at ventrolateral sites elicits analgesia that may outlast the initial period of stimulation and can be blocked by opiate antagonists (see Besson *et al.*, 1991; Lovick, 1991*b*; Morgan, 1991 for more extensive discussions). Moreover analgesia can be evoked by microinjection of opiates into the vlPAG but not at more dorsally located sites (Yaksh *et al.*, 1976).

There is some evidence that dorsal PAG-evoked analgesia may be due to selective attenuation of inputs arising from C-fibre nociceptors, whilst the ventrolateral system produces a more generalized decrease in sensory responsiveness to both A- and C-fibre inputs (Duggan and Morton, 1983). Others, however, have challenged this view (Waters and Lumb, 1997). Nevertheless, it is clear that the analgesia evoked from dorsal and ventral sites is mediated by anatomically distinct but partially overlapping pathways, which originate from neurones situated in the lateral and ventrolateral columns of the PAG respectively. Descending pathways to the spinal dorsal horn and spinal trigeminal nucleus from the lateral column of the PAG relay predominantly via ventrolateral medullary sites (Lovick, 1985), whilst analgesia from the vlPAG relays via ventromedial medullary sites (Besson and Chaouch, 1987). In addition, the vlPAG- mediated analgesia involves activation of ascending circuitry (Morgan *et al.*, 1989).

The dorsolateral column of the PAG does not fit easily into this scheme. Maps of effective analgesia-producing sites clearly show positive sites in the dlPAG suggesting that, functionally, the dorsolateral and lateral columns act as one. Yet based on anatomical and neurochemical criteria, the dlPAG column is an anatomically distinct entity which, unlike the neighbouring lateral column, does not send significant direct projections to medullary antinociceptive nuclei (for a recent review see Keay and Bandler, 2002*a*). In the rat (the species in which most studies of analgesia have been carried out), the dlPAG column occupies a relatively small area of tissue and it is likely that unless very low intensities of stimulation are used to activate this region, the stimulus would spread to activate neurones in the lateral column. The dlPAG appears to consist principally of interneurones with intrinsic connections within the PAG itself (Jansen *et al.*, 1998). More recent studies (see below) suggest that it is a functionally distinct region within the PAG which may have an important role in processing the cognitive aspects of the pain experience and may also be involved in setting the gain of output neurones from the other columns.

11.4 Functional significance of antinociceptive circuitry in the PAG

The presence of two descending antinociceptive systems which evoke qualitiatively different forms of analgesia is initially puzzling. However, the situation becomes clearer if the analgesia evoked from dorsolateral/lateral versus ventrolateral sites is considered in the context of the accompanying behavioural and autonomic sequalae.

11.4.1 Dorsolateral/lateral PAG (dl/lPAG)

Behavioural studies designed to investigate the affective nature of the response evoked from the dl/lPAG in animals have shown it to be highly aversive (see Besson *et al.*, 1991 for a discussion). It is remarkable, given the extensive literature that already existed, that so many of the early studies of stimulation-produced analgesia overlooked the 'secondary' behavioural effects. Rats will readily learn to carry out simple tasks that lead to a reduction in the intensity of a stimulus to the dl/lPAG (switch-off behaviour) or even to avoid it completely (Kiser *et al.*, 1978; Schmitt *et al.*, 1974). Indeed, in later studies, as more workers recognized the behavioural side-effects, the dorsal half of the PAG was delineated an 'aversive' zone (Besson *et al.*, 1991; Prado and Roberts, 1985), a concept which appeared to support the clinical reports of intolerable aversive sensations evoked by stimulation at dorsal periventricular and periaqueductal sites in man (Nashold *et al.*, 1969; Young, 1989).

In most of the early animal studies, electrical current was used to activate neurones in the PAG and it was these studies which emphasized the 'explosive' nature of the behavioural reaction that was evoked from stimulation at sites in the dorsal half of the PAG. However, when graded low-intensity electrical stimulation was employed or if microinjections of excitatory amino acids were used to activate neurones, a more natural and recognizable pattern of behaviour ensued. In the rat or cat, an initially quiet animal could be transformed into one that reacted as if challenged by a threatening stimulus, initially showing alerting, then freezing, and culminating often in escape behaviour (Bandler and Carrive, 1988; Depaulis *et al.*, 1992; Krieger and Graeff, 1985; Vianna *et al.*, 2001) (for a historical review see Bandler, 1988). Moreover, the exact pattern of response which was evoked appeared to be related to the rostrocaudal location of the stimulus. As indicated in Fig. 11.1, stimulation within the rostral half of the dl/lPAG evokes a confrontational defensive-type behaviour as if the animal were facing and ready to actively engage with the threat or stressor. In contrast, stimulation at more caudal levels initiates a stereotypic escape or flight response that is consistent with fleeing from, rather than confronting, the stressor (Bandler and Depaulis, 1991; Bandler *et al.*, 2000; Keay and Bandler, 2002*a*).

These behavioural changes, which are integrated by neurones in the dorsal half of the PAG, are invariably accompanied by pronounced autonomic changes. Typically, blood pressure rises and the pressor response is accompanied by tachycardia and constriction in the renal and mesenteric vascular beds with either a constriction (stimulation sites in the rostral dl/lPAG) or dilatation (stimulation sites in the caudal dl/lPAG) in skeletal muscle (Carrive *et al.*, 1989; Carrive and Bandler, 1991*a*; Lovick, 1985; Nakai and Maeda, 1994*a*; Schenberg and Lovick, 1995). Respiration also increases and there are other signs of autonomic arousal such as pupillodilatation with exophthalmus (rats) or retraction of the nictitating membrane and piloerection (cats) (Duggan and Morton, 1983; Lovick, 1985). This neurally-mediated response, termed the 'defence reaction' in early studies (Abrahams *et al.*, 1960; Hunsperger, 1956), is reinforced at the level of the effector organs by catecholamines released from the adrenal medulla (Yardley and Hilton, 1987).

11.4.2 Ventrolateral PAG (vlPAG)

The behavioural response which is evoked by stimulation in the vlPAG column is almost the antithesis of its dorsally-located counterpart. In the rat or cat, microinjections of an excitatory amino acid into sites in the vlPAG produced a state of 'hyporeactive immobility' characterized by quiescence and a lack of responsiveness to tactile or visual stimuli (e.g. social approaches by another rat) (Bandler and Depaulis, 1991; Depaulis *et al.*, 1994; Morgan and Carrive, 2001; Zhang *et al.*, 1990). Stimulation in ventrolateral parts of the PAG also produces characteristic changes in cardiovascular function. In anaesthetized rats and unanaesthetized decerebrate cats, blood pressure and heart rate fell and dilatation was seen in certain peripheral vascular beds (Carrive and Bandler, 1991*b*; Lovick, 1991*a*; Morgan and Carrive, 2001; Waters and Lumb, 1997). However, in a recent study in conscious, freely moving rats, only bradycardia was present (Morgan and Carrive, 2001). The hypotension seen so readily under anaesthesia or in a decerebrate animal is perhaps exaggerated in a preparation in which the cardiovascular control system may be somewhat depressed compared to the intact, conscious, freely moving animal.

11.4.3 Peripheral sensory stimuli which activate the PAG

When considered in the context of the accompanying bodily changes, the analgesia which is evoked by stimulation at sites within the PAG appears as a relatively small but nonetheless important component part of one of two highly integrated behavioural responses. The functional role of these responses becomes more apparent when considered in the context of stimuli which activate neurones in the different columns of the PAG.

In terms of peripheral sensory inputs to the dorsal half of the PAG, the lateral, but not the dorsolateral, column receives a dense afferent input from spinomesencephalic tract neurones and neurones in the laminar portion of the trigeminal nucleus, both of which relay information from peripheral nociceptors (Blomqvist and Craig, 1991; Keay *et al.*, 1997). Studies utilizing expression of the immediate early gene, c-fos, as a marker of neuronal activation, have been particularly effective in revealing the precise nature of the nociceptive inputs to the PAG. The lateral column has been shown to be activated preferentially following cutaneous nociceptive stimuli such as intermittent radiant heat or pinch (Keay and Bandler, 1993; Parry *et al.*, 2002), compared to deep noxious, deep somatic, or visceral stimuli (Clement *et al.*, 1996; Keay *et al.*, 2000; Snowball *et al.*, 2000). Interestingly, mice which received repeated bites from an aggressive conspecific, developed a non-opioid PAG-mediated analgesia — a finding which is consistent with activation of the lPAG descending system by intermittent stimulation of cutaneous nociceptors (Canto–de–Souza *et al.*, 1997, 1998).

In addition to these direct spinal inputs, the dorsal half of the PAG also receives sensory information which is relayed indirectly via the medial hypothalamus. The input from these diencephalic sites appears to relate more to the type of afferent fibre which is stimulated (cutaneous or visceral), rather than its anatomical location. Thus, preferential activation of Aδ but not C-fibre inputs originating from the same somatic source (the rat hindpaw) preferentially activated only those hypothalamic neurones with projections to the dorsolateral/lateral columns of the PAG (Lumb *et al.*, 2002). However, bearing in mind the mixed nature of cutaneous afferents compared to the predominantly C-fibre composition of visceral afferents, the data would suggest that the lateral PAG system is concerned primarily with processing information from cutaneous nociceptors.

In contrast to the dorsal half of the PAG, the neurones in the vlPAG appear to be activated preferentially by stimulation of nociceptive afferents from deep somatic structures (muscles and joints) or thoracic and abdominal viscera (Clement *et al.*, 1996; Keay *et al.*, 2000). Interestingly, PET scans in humans have shown activation of the PAG during angina attacks, confirming the suggestion from the animal work that cardiac nociceptors project to the PAG (Rosen *et al.*, 1994). However, in these studies the resolution of the imaging technique was not sufficient to determine whether activity was restricted to the ventrolateral column of the PAG.

The differential targeting of the lateral and ventrolateral columns of the PAG by cutaneous and deep nociceptors respectively, may provide the basis for the long-recognized dichotomy between the affective responses evoked by deep pain arising from joints, muscles, and viscera and that evoked by cutaneous pain. As first described by Lewis (1942), the response to deep pain is typified by quiescence, decreased reactivity, hypotension, and bradycadia (the same pattern of response evoked by activation of the vlPAG), whilst cutaneous pain triggers an active response characterized by increased vigilance, hyper-reactivity, hypertension, and tachycardia (the characteristic pattern of response evoked from the lPAG). Usually however, superficial (cutaneous) pain is escapable, whereas pain of deep somatic or visceral origin is inescapable, raising the question of whether the escapability/inescapability of a noxious stimulus, rather than its tissue origin, is another important factor which is represented in the PAG. In particular, cutaneous pain does not always trigger active coping.

Clinically, when cutaneous pain persists (e.g. burns, even moderate sunburn) it evokes a passive rather than an active emotional response. Similarly in rodents, a persistent noxious cutaneous stimulus (a clip applied to the skin of the nape of the neck) has been found to evoke both a passive emotional coping response (Fleischmann and Urca, 1988, 1993) and a selective neural activation of the vlPAG as revealed by expression of the immediate early gene, *c-fos* (Keay *et al.*, 2001; Keay and Bandler, 2002*b*). Such data suggest that pain representation in supraspinal regions such as the PAG likely reflects a quality akin to behavioural significance (i.e. escapability or inescapability) rather than simply the tissue of origin (see also Lumb, 2002).

It should be noted that, under normal conditions, the descending control systems from the PAG appear not to be active. Responses to an acute noxious visceral stimulus did not change following microinjections of GABA into the PAG to suppress any ongoing activity (Monhemius *et al.*, 2001). On the other hand, when the same experiment was performed in a neuropathic pain model, responsiveness to acute visceral pain was found to be reduced (Monhemius *et al.*, 2001). Thus, the presence of persistent and inescapable sensory input from nociceptors appears to engage descending control from the PAG.

11.5 **Activation of muscle afferents and acupuncture activate the ventrolateral PAG**

Whilst it is clear that activation of deep nociceptors can activate the vlPAG, non-nociceptive stimuli which originate from deep structures may also be effective. Acupuncture stimulation has been widely used for relief of pain in Eastern cultures for centuries and, in recent decades, has become increasingly popular in Western society. The classical view of acupuncture, which was developed without the benefit of present-day anatomical and physiological insight, is that needling releases the flow of blocked energy or 'Qi', which somehow normalizes the underlying disturbance of bodily function giving rise to the pain. The recent application of modern scientific investigative techniques to the phenomenon now indicates that this age-old method for pain relief may actually represent one of man's first successful attempts to engage one of the endogenous pain control systems in the PAG.

It is well-established now that acupuncture analgesia is opioid-mediated (see Han and Terenius, 1982 for a review). By mapping expression of the immediate early gene, c-fos, effective acupuncture stimulation in the rat has been shown to activate a descending pathway from the hypothalamic arcuate nucleus to the vlPAG (the PAG site for opioid-mediated analgesia) and engages the descending inhibitory system to the spinal cord (Lee and Beitz, 1993; Takeshige *et al.*, 1992). Interestingly, PET scans in humans also revealed activation in the hypothalamus and PAG following stimulation at the analgesia point, Ho Ku (Li4) (Hsieh *et al.*, 2001).

Traditional acupuncture (e.g. needling or low-frequency electroacupuncture) at point Zu San Li (St36) first activates predominantly group II and III skeletal muscle afferents in the deep peroneal nerve, and then evokes analgesia (Lovick *et al.*, 1995; Lu *et al.*, 1981). For maximimal effectiveness, the acupuncture stimulus is typically sustained for some 10–20 minutes. Interestingly, a similar prolonged stimulation of afferent nerves supplying muscles and joints occurs during intense exercise. Prolonged intense exercise is typically followed by a period of recuperation which is characterized by quiescence, hyporeactivity, endorphin-mediated analgesia (Shyu *et al.*, 1982), and a feeling of well-being (the 'jogger's high'). This pattern of response bears a close resemblance to the quiescence, hyporeactivity, and opioid-mediated analgesia evoked by stimulating the vlPAG in animals (see above). Increased sensory input from muscles and joints during prolonged exercise may constitute yet another example of deep somatic stimuli which, in order to trigger a period of passive coping following severe physical exertion, activate and engage descending systems from the vlPAG (see below).

11.6 **Functional significance of PAG activation — active and passive emotional coping**

Initially, a cutaneous noxious event is an alerting or alarm stimulus. The manner in which the individual responds depends on the context in which the information is perceived. Under emergency conditions which pose a threat to physical survival (e.g. soldiers in battle or confrontation by an aggressor), the engagement of the descending control systems which emanate from the dorsal half of the PAG evoke a type of 'stress-induced analgesia' in which the perception of pain associated with acute physical injury is temporarily suppressed. By mobilizing the cardio-respiratory systems and redistributing a raised cardiac output to vascular beds of potentially highest metabolic need, the body becomes primed for physical activity. At the same time, the subjugation of responses to acute pain enables fight-or-flight behaviour to proceed in the face of physical injury which would otherwise provide a distraction (Bandler and Shipley, 1994; Lovick, 1993). In other words, the responses may be viewed as active coping strategies which favour survival of self in response to classes of threat that are perceived as escapable (Bandler *et al.*, 2000; Keay and Bandler, 2002*a*).

This complex pattern of autonomic and behavioural responses, which occurs when the lateral column of the PAG is mobilized, has considerable adaptive value in an emergency. However, in less extreme circumstances, where the noxious stimulus is of a moderate intensity and not received in the context of an overtly life-threatening situation, such a response is clearly inappropriate. With increasing encephalization, primates, and especially man, have developed sophisticated strategies to deal with pain according to context. Indeed, recent studies indicate that on a minute-to-minute basis, attention levels may be sufficient to activate descending control systems from the PAG in a graded manner. Magnetic resonance imaging studies in humans have shown a significant correlation between the increase in signal intensity in the PAG and decreased perception of the intensity of a noxious cutaneous stimulus when subjects were distracted from their pain (Tracey *et al.*, 2002).

For the individual suffering from persistent pain (e.g. pain arising from inflamed viscera and joints, or from burns), the active coping strategies outlined above are inappropriate. The characteristic reaction to persistent pain is a disengagement from the environment. Such a passive coping strategy accompanied by a long-term, opioid-mediated analgesia may be viewed as a functionally adaptive response designed to promote recovery and healing. A similar passive emotional coping or 'conservation- withdrawal' response (Henry and Stephens, 1977) is observed also in animals following repeated defeats in social encounters or in situations in which organisms repeatedly encounter an inescapable stressor (e.g. Blanchard *et al.*, 1994). Experimentally, such situations are well modelled by learnt helplessness paradigms (e.g. swim stress, conditioned fear). Under such conditions, the environmental cues, often in the absence of a physical stressor, become sufficient to trigger an appropriate emotional coping response.

In the context of emotional reactions triggered by psychological, rather than physical stressors, it is important to note that:

1. there is a dramatic expansion of cortex in higher mammals, particularly prefrontal cortex (PFC)

2. PFC damage in humans dramatically alters the capacity to cope emotionally with perceived as well as real threats (see, for example, Bechara *et al.*, 1994; Price *et al.*, 1996).

The anatomy of PFC projections to the specific PAG columns has been studied recently in both the macaque and the rat (An *et al.*, 1998; Floyd *et al.*, 2000). Retrograde tracing studies first revealed that projections to the PAG arose predominantly from the medial PFC wall and a few select orbital/anterior insular PFC regions. Anterograde tracers were then injected into each PAG-projecting PFC region of the primate in order to obtain information about the precise patterns of termination. Distinct columnar patterns of PAG termination were revealed (Fig. 11.2). The most striking finding was the extent of the projection from the medial PFC wall (areas 10, 25, and 32) to the dlPAG. This raises the possibility that the dlPAG column, which receives no direct somatic or

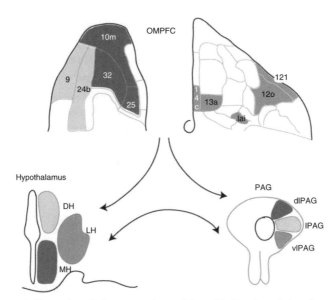

Fig. 11.2 Schematic illustration of the connections of the orbital and medial prefrontal cortex (OMPFC), hypothalamus, and PAG of the macaque. Three distinct OMPFC networks can be distinguished by their preferred projections to distinct PAG columns and different hypothalamic fields. Orbito-insular PFC areas (12l, 12o, Iai, 13a, 14c) project preferentially to the vlPAG and the lateral hypothalamus (LH). Medial wall PFC areas (10m, 32, and 25) project preferentially to the dlPAG and medial hypothalamus (MH). Dorsomedial PFC areas (9 and 24b) project preferentially to the lPAG and dorsal hypothalamus. Note also the interconnections of specific PAG columns and specific hypothalamic fields projected upon by the same OMPFC areas (dlPAG — MH; lPAG — DH; vlPAG — LH). (Modified from Fig. 6, Bandler *et al.*, 2000.)

visceral inputs (see above), is driven predominantly by information related to the cognitive aspects of stress/pain. In contrast, the vlPAG column received an exclusive input from orbital and anterior insular PFC areas (12o, 12l, 13a, 14c, Iai), as well as a weaker input from medial and dorsomedial PFC. Input to the lPAG column arose mainly from the dorsomedial PFC convexity (areas 9 and 24).

The projections from select PFC regions to specific PAG columns (described above) demonstrate the presence of anatomical pathways via which 'psychological' (cortical) stimuli could activate the PAG. In particular, the density of medial PFC projections to the dlPAG suggests that this column could be activated selectively by social stressors of the type likely to trigger active coping (e.g. presence of a potential predator). In support of this idea, innate 'psychological' stimuli known to induce active coping (i.e. flight mixed with immobility), such as the exposure of a rat to a cat (but without any physical contact), have been shown to preferentially activate neurones within the dlPAG (Canteras and Goto, 1999; Chiavegatto et al., 1998; see also Keay and Bandler, 2002a). In contrast, projections to the vlPAG from select orbital PFC areas appear to provide a structural basis for 'psychological" stressors (e.g. learnt helplessness paradigms) to trigger passive coping. 'Psychological' stimuli which rely upon conditioning (e.g. exposure of a rat to an environment in which it previously received a foot shock) trigger *only* immobility and serve as a powerful activator of the vlPAG (Carrive et al., 1997).

As illustrated in Fig. 11.2, the same OMPFC regions which project to different PAG columns, also project selectively to medial versus lateral hypothalamic regions (Floyd et al., 2001; Öngür et al., 1998). Specific regions of the amygdala and parabrachial complex have been found also to participate in these circuits (Bernard and Bandler, 1998). Thus, the distinct PAG columns which mediate active and passive emotional coping lie embedded within parallel, but anatomically distinct, OMPFC-hypothalamic-PAG-amygdaloid-parabrachial circuits. Indeed, it has been shown that the integrity of the vlPAG and of afferent inputs to it from the amygdala are criticial to the manifestation of immobility triggered by conditioned fear paradigms (prior exposure to foot shock) in rats (Carrive et al., 2000; De Oca et al., 1998; Fanselow et al., 1995; Kim et al., 1993; Vianna et al., 2001).

In summary, both the stressful/noxious qualities of a stimulus and the environmental context in which it is received are important determinants of PAG activation. PAG columns which trigger reactions of engagement with the environment (i.e. active emotional coping) appear to be differentially activated by 'escapable' physical (lPAG-activating) or 'escapable' psychological (dlPAG-activating) stressors such as acute superficial pain, confrontion by an attacker/predator, and a threat of mortal injury (Bandler and Shipley, 1994; Keay and Bandler, 2002a,b; Lovick, 1993) (see Fig. 11.3). In contrast, 'inescapable' stressors (e.g. severe traumatic injury, persistent pain, strong physical exertion, or learnt helplessness paradigms) selectively active the vlPAG and trigger a reaction of passive emotional coping or disengagement from the environment (Bandler et al., 2000; Clement et al., 1996; Keay and Bandler, 2002a,b) (see Fig. 11.3).

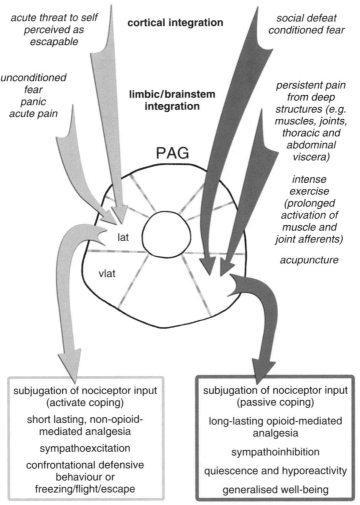

Fig. 11.3 Schematic illustration summarizing the functional characteristics of the analgesia-producing systems which orginate from different regions of the PAG, and their role in mediating behavioural responses of the whole animal to different types of physical and psychological challenge.

11.7 Disturbance of PAG function and generation of pain states

11.7.1 Migraine

Although it is generally accepted that activation of the PAG produces a reduced responsiveness to stimulation of nociceptors, under certain conditions, activation of the PAG may initiate rather than suppress pain. Ironically, one of the earliest indications that the PAG may be able to initiate pain arose from attempts to relieve pain in humans. Headache resembling migraine was reported in patients in whom stimulating electrodes had been implanted into the PAG for relief of intractable pain (Raskin *et al.*, 1987). Severe headache was also reported in a patient with a discrete sclerotic lesion of the PAG (Hass *et al.*, 1993). Similarly, in patients experiencing a migraine attack, PET scans revealed an area of increased neuronal activity in the dorsal and rostral brainstem in the region of the aqueduct (Bahra *et al.*, 2001; Weiller *et al.*, 1995).

High-resolution MRI has localized the disturbed neuronal function to the PAG in patients with episodic migraine or chronic daily headache (Welch *et al.*, 2001). Interestingly, the central disturbance did not appear to be secondary to the presence of pain, since the brainstem activation persisted after complete relief from the headache using sumatriptan (Bahra *et al.*, 2001; Weiller *et al.*, 1995). In recent animal studies, activation of the PAG has also been found to evoke changes in cerebral blood flow, suggesting that the PAG may be able to influence the cerebral vasculature directly (Nakai and Maeda 1994*b*, 1996*a,b*). Thus it has been suggested that a primary cause of the pain of migraine leading to stimulation of trigeminal nociceptors may be a 'dysfunctional' control of the trigemino-vascular nociceptive system rather than a peripheral pathology (Welch *et al.*, 2001).

11.7.2 **Non-cardiac chest pain**

In addition to migraine, involvement of the PAG has been implicated in other painful conditions including non-cardiac chest pain (NCCP). Often, no pathological cause for the pain can be found and patients appear to have an illness without organic disease — a situation which presents a particularly difficult challenge for the physician. These types of pain are surprisingly common. For example, some 50% of patients who present with chest pain have been reported to have no detectable cardiac abnormality (Mayou, 1999). These patients pose a significant clinical problem. With their pain unresolved, they become frequent users of the health services and represent a considerable drain on resources (Thurston *et al.*, 2001).

Not unexpectedly, patients in pain worry about the long-term outcome for their pain, their long-term health prospects, the effects on their family, their job, etc. Pain is often associated with high levels of anxiety. Paradoxically, it appears that in some cases anxiety itself may lead to the development of pain states. Mild anxiety or fear is commonly associated with autonomic disturbances such as sweating, palpitations, 'butterflies' in the stomach. In clinical anxiety states such as panic, these autonomic disturbances may become so severe that in some patients, the symptoms appear to indicate a recognized pathological condition.

Co-morbidity of NCCP and panic disorder is surprisingly common. Some 30% of patients with NCCP have been diagnosed as suffering from panic disorder (Fleet *et al.*, 1996; Katon *et al.*, 1988; Mayou, 1999). Interestingly, the symptoms of a panic attack closely resemble the extreme form of the response evoked by electrical stimulation in the dl/lPAG in conscious animals and in humans (Lovick, 2000). Indeed, the concept of panic attacks as a complex pyschophysiological response, with elements of freezing behaviour, which can rapidly transform into fight/flight reactions (Bystrisky *et al.*, 2000), corresponds almost exactly with the sequence of functional responses evoked by graded stimulation of the dl/lPAG (discussed above). The dl/lPAG therefore appears to contain a locus for panic behaviour.

During a panic attack, the period of irrational fear and intense autonomic disturbance is often accompanied by angina-like chest pain (DSM–IV). Recent studies in animals have shown that within a population of outbred Wistar rats, a significant proportion of animals responded to electrical stimulation in the dl/lPAG with electrocardiographic signs of ischaemia and a significant increase in coronary resistance (Fig. 11.4) (Lovick *et al.*, in preparation). This subgroup of rats appeared to show an abnormal or inappropriate response to dl/lPAG stimulation, and in this respect they resemble the 30% of patients with NCCP who have angiographically normal hearts but who suffer from panic disorder. Other studies in rats have shown that in susceptible individuals, intense sympathoactivation can produce coronary spasm and transient myocardial damage (Gutstein *et al.*, 1987).

The chest pain of panic attacks and the pain of patients with NCCP may therefore represent a dysfunctional response of the coronary vascular bed which triggers ischaemic pain from the myocardium when the dl/lPAG is activated. In these patients a paradoxical situation may arise whereby engagement of active coping mechanisms

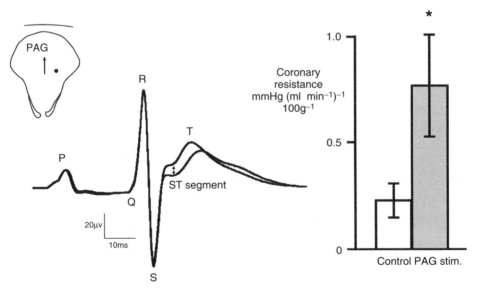

Fig. 11.4 Electrical stimulation in the PAG evoked signs of myocardial ischaemia in a subpopulation of anaesthetized rats. A brief (60 μA, 1ms, 80Hz for 10s) period of stimulation within the lateral column of the PAG (solid dot on drawing of histological section) produced depression of ST segment and prolongation of the T-wave of the ECG. Histogram shows mean data from 15 rats in which the PAG-evoked change in the ECG was accompanied by an increase in coronary vascular resistance.

(dl/lPAG) associated usually with analgesia and sympathoactivation, actually gives rise to pain as a consequence of an aberrant response of the coronary vasculature to increased sympathetic drive. Indeed, during a panic attack, the patient's perception that his/her chest pain indicates a heart attack may exacerbate the situation by leading to a further fear-induced activation of the PAG and an increase in the severity of the pain.

11.7.3 Irritable bowel syndrome (IBS)

In contrast to the increased activity in the PAG during migraine and attacks of NCCP, the pain of IBS is associated with reduced activity in this region of the midbrain. Imaging studies in normal human subjects have reported that distension of the sygmoid colon was associated with activation in the PAG (Mayer, 2000). Patients with IBS reported the procedure to be more painful than normal subjects, but in patients, the level of activation of the PAG was lower than in the normal controls, both in response to actual distension and in the anticipatory phase prior to application of the stimulus (i.e. where there was no sensory input from the colon). One possible interpretation of these data is that for patients with IBS, a reduced (dysfunctional) descending antinociceptive control from the PAG may underlie the visceral hyperalgesic state (Mayer, 2000).

The clinical data outlined above are highly suggestive of a link between activity of the PAG and non-organic pain states such as migraine, NCCP, and IBS. One of the problems associated with data obtained from imaging studies using PET or MRI in humans is that current techniques are unable to resolve the area of activation much beyond the central core of the midbrain. This leads to problems of interpretation and, at present, it is impossible to determine whether the signal originates from a particular column within the PAG, or even whether neighbouring structures might be involved. Nevertheless, the available evidence does suggest that the control systems of the PAG are altered in painful conditions such as migraine, NCCP, and IBS. A 'disturbance' of PAG function may give rise to:

1. an abnormal vascular smooth muscle response that leads to activation of nociceptors in the mycocardium or trigeminal vasculature, or

2. colonic hyperalgesia conseqent to decreased descending antinociceptive control of inputs from abdominal viscera.

11.8 Summary

The data reviewed in this chapter suggest that analgesia evoked from the PAG is best viewed as a component of one or more complex adaptive emotional coping responses. The PAG is organized functionally into four longitudinal columns of neurons. Two distinct forms of analgesia arise from activation specifically of the dorsolateral/lateral PAG columns or the ventrolateral PAG column. A long-acting, opioid-mediated analgesia is a component of a vlPAG-mediated passive coping or conservation-withdrawal reaction which promotes recovery and healing, typically as a response to extreme, inescapable physical stress, including traumatic injury. In contrast, a short-acting, non-opioid-mediated analgesia represents a component of a dlPAG- or lPAG-mediated active coping or defensive reaction to an escapable threat or stress, including acute pain.

Anatomical data indicate that each PAG column lies embedded within a distinct forebrain circuit that includes select medial and orbital PFC, hypothalamic and amygdaloid areas. These circuits provide a basis whereby psychological (as well as physical) stressors can influence neural activity in the PAG in a graded and distinct columnar manner.

Finally, activation of the PAG is invariably accompanied by pronounced changes in autonomic function. In humans, an involvement of the PAG has been implicated in several 'visceral' pain states (e.g. migraine, NCCP, IBS). We argue that in such cases, pain may arise as a consequence of abnormal activity in the PAG which generates pain as a result of 'dysfunctional' ischaemic changes or spasm in regional smooth muscle and/or alterations in descending antinociceptive control.

References

Abrahams, V.C., Hilton, S.M., and Zbrozyna, A.W. (1960) Active muscle vasodilatation produced by stimulation of the brainstem: its significance for the defence reaction. *J Physiol* **154**, 491–513.

An, X., Bandler, R., Ongur, D., and Price, J.L. (1998) Prefrontal cortical projections to longitudinal columns in the midbrain periaqueductal gray in macaque monkeys. *J Comp Neurol* **401**, 455–479.

Bahra, A., Matharu, M.S., Buchnel, C., Frackowiak, R.S.J., and Goadsby, P.J. (2001) Brainstem activation specific to migraine headache. *Lancet* **357**, 1017.

Bandler, R. (1988) Brain mechanisms of aggression as revealed by electrical and chemical stimulation: suggestion of a central role for the midbrain periaqueductal gray. *Prog Psychobiol Physiol Psychol* **13**, 67–154.

Bandler, R. and Carrive, P. (1988) Integrated defense reaction elicited by excitatory amino acid microinjection in the midbrain periaqueductal gray of the unrestrained cat. *Brain Res* **439**, 95–106.

Bandler, R. and Depaulis, A. (1991) Midbrain periaqueductal gray control of defensive behavior in the cat and the rat. In: (Depaulis, A. and Bandler, R.) *The Midbrain Periaqueductal Grey Matter*. Plenum Press, New York, pp. 175–198.

Bandler, R. and Shipley, M.T. (1994) Columnar organisation in the midbrain periaqueductal gray: modules for emotional expression? *Trends in Neurosci* **17**, 379–389.

Bandler, R., Keay, K., Floyd, N., and Price, J. (2000) Central circuits mediating patterned autonomic activity during active vs. passive emotional coping. *Brain Res Bull* **53**, 95–104.

Bechara, A., Damasio, A.R., Damasio, H., and Anderson, S.W. (1994) Insensitivity to future consequences following damage to human prefrontal cortex. *Cognition* **50**, 7–15.

Beecher, H.K. (1946) Pain in men wounded in battle. *Ann Surg* **123**, 96–105.

Bernard, J–F. and Bandler, R. (1998) Commentary: parallel circuits for emotional coping behavior: new pieces in the puzzle. *J Comp Neurol* **401**, 429–436.

Besson, J.M. and Chaouch, A. (1987) Peripheral and spinal mechanisms of pain. *Physiol Rev* **67**, 67–186.

Besson, J.M., Fardin, V., and Olivéras. J.L. (1991) Analgesia produced by stimulation of the periaqueductal gray matter: true antinociceptive versus stress effects. In: (Depaulis, A. and Bandler, R.) *The Midbrain Periaqueductal Grey Matter*. Plenum Press, New York, pp. 121–138.

Blanchard, D.C., Sakai, R.R., McEwen, B., Weiss, S.M., and Blanchard, R.J. (1993) Subordination stress: behavioural brain and neuroendocrine correlates. *Behav Brain Res* 58, 113–121.

Blomqvist, A. and Craig, A.D. (1991) Organisation of spinal and trigeminal input to the PAG. In: (Depaulis, A. and Bandler, R.) *The Midbrain Periaqueductal Grey Matter*. Plenum Press, New York, pp. 345–364.

Bystristky, A., Craske, M., Maidenburg, E., Vapnik, T., and Shapiro, D. (2000) Autonomic reactivity of panic patients during CO_2 inhalation procedure. *Depression and Anxiety* 11, 15–26.

Canteras, N.S. and Goto, M. (1999) Fos-like immunoreactivity in the periaqueductal gray of rats exposed to a natural predator. *NeuroReport* 10, 413–418.

Canto–de–Souza, A., Nunes de Souza, R.L., Pela, I.R., and Graeff, F.G. (1997) High intensity social conflict in the Swiss albino mouse induces analgesia modulated by $5-HT_{1A}$ receptors. *Pharmacol Biochem Behav* 56, 481–486.

Canto–de–Souza, A., Nunes de Souza, R.L., Pela, I.R., and Graeff, F.G. (1998) Involvement of the midbrain periaqueductal gray $5-HT_{1A}$ receptors in social conflict induced analgesia in mice. *Europ J Pharmacol* 345, 253–256.

Carrive, P. and Bandler, R. (1991*a*) Control of extracranial and hindlimb blood flow by the midbrain periaqueductal gray of the cat. *Exp Brain Res* 84, 599–606.

Carrive, P. and Bandler, R. (1991*b*) Viscerotopic organization of neurons subserving hypotensive reactions within the midbrain periaqueductal grey: a correlative functional and anatomical study. *Brain Res* 541, 206–215.

Carrive, P., Bandler, R., and Dampney, R.A. (1989) Somatic and autonomic integration in the midbrain of the unanaesthetised decerebrate cat: a distinctive pattern evoked by excitation of neurons in the subtentorial portion of the midbrain periaqueductal gray. *Brain Res* 483, 251–258.

Carrive, P., Lee, J., and Su, A. (2000) Lidocaine blockade of amygdala ouptut in fear-conditioned rats reduces fos expression in the ventrolateral periaqueductal gray. *Neuroscience* 95, 1071–1080.

Carrive, P., Leung, P., Harris, J., and Paxinos, G. (1997) Conditioned fear to context is associated with increased fos expression in the caudal ventrolateral region of the midbrain periaqueductal gray. *Neuroscience* 78, 165–177.

Chiavegatto, S., Scavone, C., and Canteras, N.S. (1998) Nitric oxide synthase in the dorsal periaqueductal gray of rats expressing innate fear responses. *NeuroReport* 9, 571–576.

Clement, C.I., Keay, K.A., Owler, B.K., and Bandler, R. (1996) Common patterns of increased and decreased Fos expression in midbrain and pons evoked by noxious deep somatic and noxious visceral manipulations in the rat. *J Comp Neurol* 366, 495–575.

De Oca, B.M., DeCola, J.P., Maren, S., and Fanselow, M.S. (1998) Distinct regions of the periaqueductal gray are involved in the acquisition and expression of defensive responses. *J Neurosci* 18, 3426–3432.

Depaulis, A., Keay, K.A., and Bandler, R. (1992) Longitudinal neuronal organisation of defensive reactions in the midbrain periaqueductal gray of the rat. *Exp Brain Res* 90, 307–320.

Depaulis, A., Keay, K.A., and Bandler, R. (1994) Quiescence and hyporeactivity evoked by activation of cell bodies in the ventrolateral midbrain periaqueductal gray of the rat. *Exp Brain Res* 99, 75–83.

DSM–IV (1994) *Diagnostic and Statistical Manual for Mental Disorders, 4th Ed*. Washington DC, American Psychological Press.

Duggan, A.W. and Morton, C.R. (1983) Periaqueductal grey stimulation: an association between selective inhibition of dorsal horn neurones and changes in peripheral circulation. *Pain* 15, 237–248.

Fanselow, M.S., De Cola, J.P., and De Oca, B.M. (1995) Ventral and dorsolateral regions of midbrain periaqueductal gray (PAG) control different stages of defensive behavior — dorsolateral PAG lesions enhance defensive freezing produced by massed and immediate shock. *Aggres Behav* **21**, 63–77.

Fleet, R.O.P., Dupuis, G., Marchand, A., Burelle, D., Arsenault, A., and Beitman, B.D. (1996) Panic disorder in emergency department chest pain patients: prevalence, comorbidity, suicidal ideation, and physician cognition. *Am J Med* **101**, 3371–3380.

Fleischmann, A. and Urca, G. (1988) Clip induced analgesia and immobility in the mouse: activation by different sensory modalities. *Physiol Behav* **44**, 39–45.

Fleischmann, A. and Urca, G. (1993) Tail-pinch induced analgesia and immobility: altered responses to noxious tail-pinch by prior pinch of the neck. *Brain Res* **601**, 28–33.

Floyd, N.S., Price, J.L., Ferry, A., Keay, K.A., and Bandler, R. (2000) Orbitomedial prefrontal cortical projections to distinct longitudinal column of the periaqueductal gray in the rat. *J Comp Neurol* **422**, 556–578.

Floyd, N.S., Price, J.L., Ferry, A., Keay, K.A., and Bandler, R. (2001) Orbitomedial prefrontal cortical projections to hypothalamus in the rat. *J Comp Neurol* **432**, 307–328.

Gutstein, W.H., Anversa, P., and Guideri, G. (1987) Spasm of small coronary arteries and ischemic myocardial injury induced by hypothalamic stimulation in the rat. *Am J Path* **129**, 287–294.

Haas, D.C., Kent, P.F., and Friedman, D.I. (1993) Headache caused by a single lesion of multiple sclerosis in the periaqueductal gray area. *Headache* **33**, 452–455.

Han, J.S. and Terenius, L. (1982) Neurochemical basis of acupuncture analgesia. *Ann Rev Pharmacol Toxicol* **22**, 193–220.

Henry, J.P. and Stephens, P.M. (1977) *Stress, health and social environment: a sociobiological approach to medicine.* New York, Springer.

Hosobuchi, Y., Adamas, J.E., and Linchitz, K. (1977) Pain relief by electrical stimulation of the central gray in humans and its reversal by naloxone. *Science* **197**, 183–186.

Hsieh, J.C., Tu, C.H., Chen, F.P., *et al.* (2001) Activation of the hypothalamus characterizes the acupuncture stimulation at the analgesic point in human: a positron emission tomography study. *Neurosci Lett* **307**, 105–108.

Hunsperger, R.W. (1956) Affektreaktionen auf elektrische Reizung im Hirnstamm der Katze. *Helv Physiol Pharmacol Acta* **14**, 70–92.

Jansen, A.S.P., Farkas, E., Sams, J.M., and Loewy, A.D. (1998) Local connections between columns of the periaqueductal grey matter: a case for intrinsic modulation. *Brain Res* **784**, 329–336.

Katon, W., Hall, M.L., Russo, J., *et al.* (1988) Chest pain: relationship of psychiatric illness to coronary arteriographic results. *Am J Med* **84**, 1–9.

Keay, K.A. and Bandler, R. (1993) Deep and superficial noxious stimulation increases Fos-like immunoreactivity in different regions of the midbrain periaqueductal gray. *Neurosci Lett* **154**, 23–26.

Keay, K.A. and Bandler, R. (2002*a*) Parallel circuits mediating distinct emotional coping reactions to different types of stress. *Neurosci Biobehav Rev* **25**, 669–678.

Keay, K. and Bandler, R. (2002*b*) Distinct central representations of inescapable and escapable pain: observations and speculation. *Exp Physiol* **87**, 275–279.

Keay, K.A., Clement, C., and Bandler, R. (2000) The neuroanatomy of cardiac nociceptive pathways: differential representation of 'deep' and 'superficial' pain. In: (ed. Ter Horst, G.J.) *The Nervous System and the Heart.* Humana Press, New Jersey, pp. 303–342.

Keay, K.A., Clement, C.I., Depaulis, A., and Bandler R. (2001) Different representations of inescapable noxious stimuli in the periaqueductal grey and upper cervical spinal cord of freely moving rats. *Neurosci Lett* **313**, 17–20.

Keay, K.A., Feil, K., Gordon, B.D., Herbert, H., and Bandler, R. (1997) Spinal afferents to functionally distinct periaqueductal gray columns in the rat. An anterograde and retrograde tracing study. *J Comp Neurol* **385**, 207–229.

Kim, J.J., Rison, R.A., and Fanselow, M.S. (1993) Effects of amygdala, hippocampus, and periaqueductal gray lesions on short-term and long-term contextual fear. *Behav Neurosci* **107**, 1093–1098.

Kiser, R., German, D.C., and Lebowitz, R.M. (1978) Serotonergic modulation of dorsal central gray area stimulation-produced aversion. *Pharmacol Biochem Behav* **8**, 27–31.

Krieger, J.E. and Graeff, F.G. (1985) Defensive behaviour and hypertension induced by glutamate in the midbrain central gray of the rat. *Braz J Med Biol Res* **18**, 61–67.

Kumar, K., Toth, C., and Nath, R.K. (1997) Deep brain stimulation for intractable pain: a 15 year experience. *Neurosurgery* **40**, 736–746.

Lee, J.H. and Beitz, A.J. (1993) The distribution of brain-stem and spinal cord nuclei associated with different frequencies of electroacupuncture analgesia. *Pain* **52**, 11–28.

Lewis, T. (1942) *Pain.* McMillan, London.

Lovick, T.A. (1985) Ventrolateral medullary lesions block the antinociceptive and cardiovascular responses elicited by stimulating in the dorsal periaqueductal grey matter in rats. *Pain* **21**, 241–252.

Lovick, T.A. (1991*a*) Central nervous system integration of pain control and autonomic function. *News in Physiol Sci* **6**, 82–86.

Lovick, T.A. (1991*b*) Interactions between descending pathways from the dorsal and ventrolateral periaqueductal grey matter in the rat. In: (eds. Depaulis, A., and Bandler, R.) *The Midbrain Periaqueductal Gray Matter.* Plenum Press, New York, pp. 101–120.

Lovick, T.A. (1993) Midbrain and medullary regulation of defensive cardiovascular functions. *Prog Brain Res* **107**, 301–314.

Lovick, T.A. (2000) Panic disorder — a malfunction of multiple transmitter control systems in the midbrain periaqueductal grey matter? *The Neuroscientist* **6**, 48–59.

Lovick, T.A., Li, P., and Schenberg, L.C. (1995) Modulation of the cardiovascular defence response by low frequency stimulation of a deep somatic nerve in rats. *J Auton Nerv Sys* **50**, 347–354.

Lu, G.W., Xie, J.Q., Yang, Y.N., and Wang, Q.L. (1981) Afferent nerve fibre composition at point zusanli in relation to acupuncture analgesia: a morphological investigation. *Chin Med J* **95**, 255–263.

Lumb, B.M. (2002) Inescapable and escapable pain is represented in distinct hypothalamic-midbrain circuits: specific roles for A-delta and C-nociceptors. *Exp Physiol* **13**, 281–286.

Lumb, B.M., Parry, D.M., Semenenko, F.M., McMullan, S., and Simpson, D.A.A. (2002) C-nociceptor activation of hypothalamic neurones and the columnar organisation of their projections to the periaqueductal grey in the rat. *Exp Physiol* **87**, 123–128.

Mayer, E.A. (2000) Spinal and supraspinal modulation of visceral sensation. *Gut* **47**(**Suppl IV**), 69–72.

Mayou, R. (1998) Chest pain, palpitations and panic. *J Psychosom Res* **44**, 53–70.

Monhemius, R., Green, D.L., Roberts, M.H.T., and Azami, J. (2001) Periaqueductal grey mediated inhibition of responses to noxious stimulation is dynamically activated in a rat model of neuropathic pain. *Neurosci Lett* **298**, 70–74.

Morgan, M.M. (1991) Differences in antinociception evoked from dorsal and ventral regions of the caudal periaqueductal grey matter. In: (eds. Depaulis, A and Bandler, R.) *The Midbrain Periaqueductal Gray Matter.* Plenum Press, New York, pp. 139–150.

Morgan, M.M. and Carrive, P. (2001) Activation of the ventrolateral periaqueductal grey reduces locomotion but not mean arterial pressure in awake, freely moving rats. *Neuroscience* **102**, 905–910.

Morgan, M.M., Sohn, J.H., and Liebeskind, J.C. (1989) Stimulation of the periaqueductal gray matter inhibits nociception at the supraspinal as well as the spinal level. *Brain Res* **502**, 61–66.

Nakai, M. and Maeda, M. (1994*a*) Systemic and regional hameodynamic responses elicited by microinjection of N-methyl-D-aspartate into the lateral periaqueductal gray matter in anaesthetised rats. *Neuroscience* **58**, 777–783.

Nakai, M. and Maeda, M. (1994*b*) Cerebrovasodilatation of metabolic and non-metabolic origin elicited by chemical stimulation of the lateral periaqeuductal gray matter in anaesthetised rats. *Neuroscience* **58**, 785–791.

Nakai, M. and Maeda, M. (1996*a*) Vasodilatation and enhanced oxidative metabolism of the cerebral cortex provided by the periaqueductal gray mater in anesthetised rats. *Neuroscience* **72**, 1133–1140.

Nakai, M. and Maeda, M. (1996*b*) Nitrergic cerebral vasodilatation provoked by the periaqueductal gray. *NeuroReport* **7**, 2571–2574.

Nashold, B.S., Wilson, W.P., and Slaughter, D.G. (1969) Sensations evoked by stimulation in the midbrain in man. *J Neurosurg* **30**, 14–24.

Öngür, D.F., An, X., and Price, J. (1998) Prefrontal cortical projections to the hypothalamus in macaque monkeys. *J Comp Neurol* **401**, 480–505.

Parry, D.M., Semenenko, F.M., Conley, R.K., and Lumb, B.M. (2002) Noxious inputs to hypothalamic-midbrain projection neurones: a comparison of the columnar organisation of somatic and visceral inputs to the periaqueductal grey in the rat. *Exp Physiol* **87**, 117–122.

Prado, W.A. and Roberts, M.H.T. (1985) An assessment of the antinociceptive and aversive effects of identified stimulation sites in the rat brain. *Brain Res* **340**, 219–228.

Price, J.L., Carmichael, S.T., and Devrets, W.C. (1996) Networks related to the orbital and prefrontal cortex, a substrate for emotional behavior? *Prog Brain Res* **107**, 523–536.

Raskin, N.Y., Hosobuchi, Y., and Lamb, S. (1987) Headache may arise from peturbation of brain. *Headache* **27**, 416–420.

Rosen, S.D., Paulescu, E., Frith, C.D., *et al.* (1994) Central nervous pathways mediating angina-pectoris. *Lancet* **344**, 147–150.

Reynolds, D.V. (1969) Surgery in the rat during electrical analgesia induced by focal brain stimulation. *Science* **164**, 444–445.

Schenberg, L.C. and Lovick, T.A. (1995) Attenuation of the midbrain-evoked defence reaction by selective stimulation of medullary raphe neurones in rats. *Am J Physiol* **261**, R1378–R1389.

Schmitt, P., Eclancher, F., and Karli, P. (1974) Etudes des systèmes de renforcement negatif et de renforcement positif au niveau de la substance grise centrale chez le rat. *Physiol Behav* **12**, 271–279.

Shyu, B.C., Andersson, S.A., and Thoren, P. (1982) Enkephalin mediated increase in pain threshold induced by long-lasting exercize in rats. *Life Sci* **30**, 833–840.

Snowball, R.K., Semenenko, F.M., and Lumb, B.M. (2000) Visceral inputs to neurones in the anterior hypothalamus including those that project to the periaqueductal grey: a functional and anatomical study. *Neuroscience* **99**, 351–361.

Takeshige, C., Sato, T., Mera, T., Hisamitsu, T., and Fang, J.Q. (1992) Descending pain inhibitory system involved in acupuncture analgesia. *Brain Res Bull* **29**, 617–634.

Thurston, R.C., Keefe, F.J., Bradley, L., Ranga, K., Krishnan, R., and Caldwell, D.S. (2001) Chest pain in the absence of coronary artery disease: a biopsychosocial perspective. *Pain* **93**, 95–100.

Tracey, I., Ploghaus, A., Gati, J.S., *et al.* (2002) Imaging attentional modulation of pain in the periaqueductal gray in humans. *J Neurosci* **22**, 2748–2752.

Vianna, D.M.L., Landeira–Fernandez, J., and Brandao, M.L. (2001) Dorsolateral and ventral regions of the periaqueductal gray matter are involved in distinct types of fear. *Neurosci Biobehav Rev* **25**, 711–719.

Waters, A.J. and Lumb, B.M. (1997) Inhibitory effects evoked from both the lateral and ventrolateral periaqueductal grey are selective for the nociceptive responses of rat dorsal horn neurones. *Brain Res* **752**, 239–249.

Weiller, C., May, A., Limmroth, V., Jüptner, M., Kaube, H., Schayck, R.V., Coenen, H.H., and Dlener, H.C. *et al.* (1995) Brain stem activation in spontaneous human migraine. *Nature Medicine* **1**, 658–660.

Welch, K.M.A., Nagesh, V., Aurora, S.J., and Gemman, N. (2001) Periaqueductal gray matter dysfunction in migraine: cause or burden of illness? *Headache* **41**, 629–637.

Willis, W.D. (1982) Control of nociceptive transmission in the spinal cord. In: (eds. Autrum, H., Ottson, D., Perl, E.R., and Schmidt, R.F.) *Progress in Sensory Physiology: 3*. Springer–Verlag, Berlin.

Yaksh, T.L., Yeung, J.C., and Rudy, T.A. (1976) Systematic examination of brain sites sensitive to direct application of morphine: observation of differential effects within the periaqueductal grey. *Brain Res* **114**, 83–103.

Yardley, C.P. and Hilton, S.M. (1987) Vasodilatation in hind-limb muscle evoked as part of the defence reaction in the rat. *J Auton Nerv Sys* **19**, 127–136.

Young, R.F. (1989) Brain and spinal stimulation: how and to whom? *Clin Neurosurg* **35**, 429–447.

Young, R.D. and Brechner, T. (1986) Electrical stimulation of the brain for relief of intractable pain due to cancer. *Cancer* **57**, 1266–1272.

Zhang, S.P., Bandler, R., and Carrive, P. (1990) Flight and immobility evoked by excitatory amino acid miroinjection within distinct parts of the subtentorial midbrain periaqueductal gray of the cat. *Brain Res* **520**, 73–82.

Chapter 12

Descending control of pain processing

G.F. Gebhart and H.K. Proudfit

12.1 Perspective

Interest in supraspinal modulation of spinal cord excitability dates back at least to Sherrington, who had long studied reflexes and showed that a flexion reflex was increased after spinal cord transection (Sherrington and Sowton 1915), thus revealing the presence of tonic inhibitory influences descending from the brainstem. Others subsequently investigated descending modulation of flexion reflexes evoked by activation of 'flexion reflex afferents', which included myelinated cutaneous afferent fibers and some small, unmyelinated muscle and joint afferent fibers (see review by Lundberg 1964), and nociceptive withdrawal reflexes (see review by Willis 1982). In the 1960s, primary interest turned to nociceptive transmission in the spinal cord. Wall (1967) used a cold block of the thoracic spinal cord to demonstrate that lumbar spinal dorsal horn neurons were subject to tonic descending inhibitory influences; peripheral receptive field size expanded and neuron excitability increased when descending influences from the brainstem were blocked.

It was a report by Reynolds (1969), however, that generated widespread interest in descending control of spinal pain processing. He demonstrated that during, and for some time after, electrical stimulation in the rat midbrain periaqueductal gray (PAG), abdominal surgery in the absence of an anesthetic could be carried out. The stimulation-produced effects were subsequently confirmed and extended to humans (Hosobuchi *et al.* 1977, Richardson and Akil 1977), which established the relationship between stimulation-produced antinociception in animals and stimulation-produced analgesia in humans. Further study revealed that opioids given directly into the same area of the PAG produced antinociception. Opioid receptors and endogenous opioid peptides were subsequently shown to be present in these and other areas in the brainstem that have since been implicated in nociception or modulation of nociception.

An obvious implication of these findings was the existence of an endogenous pain control system that included endogenous opioids. This concept provided a rational mechanism to explain the analgesia produced by exogenous opioids. This concept galvanized investigators, who undertook anatomical, behavioral, electrophysiological, and neurochemical experiments to reveal the neuronal pathways and mechanisms that contribute to the descending inhibition of pain processing.

12.2 **Anatomical organization of descending pain modulation**

Early studies rapidly established the central importance of the ventrolateral PAG (vlPAG) in descending pain modulation. Selective activation of neurons in the vlPAG by excitatory amino acids or opioid analgesics such as morphine injected into the vlPAG was shown to inhibit spinal nociceptive reflexes (Yaksh and Rudy 1978, Jensen and Yaksh 1984) and spinal nociceptive transmission (Jones and Gebhart 1988). It was soon realised, however, that descending effects from the vlPAG were indirect and acted through relays in the brainstem region known as the rostral ventromedial medulla (RVM). This region includes a large number of serotonin-containing neurons in the nucleus raphe magnus (NRM) (Steinbusch 1981) that project to the spinal cord dorsal horn (Bowker *et al.* 1982), and the RVM became a primary focus of study.

The contribution of spinally projecting RVM serotonin neurons to the antinociception produced by activation of neurons in the vlPAG was demonstrated by numerous studies (Yaksh 1979, Yaksh and Tyce 1979, Jensen and Yaksh 1984, Aimone *et al.* 1987, Fang and Proudfit 1996). It was soon established that direct activation of spinally projecting neurons in the RVM produced antinociception, using the same agents that were antinociceptive when applied in the vlPAG (electrical stimulation, glutamate, or morphine). As was found in studies of the midbrain (Gebhart 1986), however, inhibition of spinal nociceptive reflexes and dorsal horn neurons from the medulla was produced from relatively widespread sites and not restricted to the midline NRM (Gebhart 1986) (Fig. 12.1). Moreover, descending inhibitory effects produced by stimulation in the vlPAG were not blocked fully by disruption of synaptic transmission through the midline NRM. Rather, sites in the RVM both medial (i.e. NRM) and lateral to the NRM had to be blocked to significantly reduce PAG-produced inhibition of either spinal nociceptive reflexes or dorsal horn neurons (Gebhart *et al.* 1983, Sandkühler and Gebhart 1984, Aimone and Gebhart 1986).

Other work implicated additional brainstem areas as important to descending inhibition of spinal nociception. For example, it was learnt that blockage of both serotonin and noradrenergic spinal receptors, by intrathecal administration of receptor-selective antagonists, was required to prevent the antinociception produced by stimulation of neurons in either the vlPAG or the RVM. These findings stimulated investigations that ultimately revealed the role of the dorsolateral pontine tegmentum (DLPT), which is the principal source of noradrenergic innervation of the spinal dorsal horn, in the modulation of pain processing at the level of the spinal cord (Gebhart 1986, Proudfit 1988, Jones 1992). The DLPT also receives projections from the PAG (Bajic and Proudfit 1999, Bajic *et al.* 2001), and like the RVM, sends axons to the spinal cord (Clark and Proudfit 1991*b*) which, when activated electrically (Yeomans *et al.* 1992) or pharmacologically (Yeomans and Proudfit 1992), similarly modulates spinal pain processing. Importantly, the RVM and DLPT are anatomically interconnected (Holden and Proudfit 1998, Clark and Proudfit 1991*c*) and apparently act in concert to modulate nociceptive processing in the spinal cord.

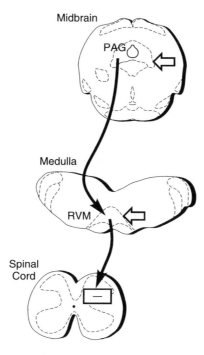

Fig. 12.1 Summary of the pain modulation pathways in the brainstem and spinal cord that reflects the state of understanding circa 1980. Neurons in the vlPAG were thought to activate inhibitory neurons in the RVM that project to the spinal cord dorsal horn. The arrows indicate brainstem sites where electrical stimulation or microinjection of morphine or glutamate were shown to produce antinociceptive effects. Abbreviations: PAG, periaqueductal gray; RVM, rostral ventromedial medulla; [–], inhibition.

It should be noted that in some rat stocks, noradrenergic neurons in the locus coeruleus innervate the spinal dorsal horn (Fritschy and Grzanna 1990, Clark and Proudfit 1991*a*, Grzanna and Fritschy 1991, Proudfit and Clark 1991) and modulate nociception (Gebhart 1986, Jones 1992, West *et al.* 1993). These findings imply the existence of genetic differences in ponto-spinal noradrenergic neurons that innervate the spinal cord dorsal horn and modulate nociception.

Figure 12.2 summarizes the interconnections among the principal cell groups in the brainstem that reflect current thinking about the organization of endogenous pain modulating systems. In addition to understanding how these systems are organized, we now appreciate that the descending modulation of spinal nociceptive processing can be either inhibitory or facilitatory (pronociceptive) and that hyperalgesic or chronic pain states may be sustained or opposed by descending influences from the brainstem.

12.3 **Functional aspects of descending systems**

12.3.1 **Descending inhibition**

Advances since the initial report of Reynolds (1969) have been remarkable and frequent (see reviews: Fields and Basbaum 1978, Sandkühler 1996, Millan 2002). We now know that inhibition of spinal nociceptive transmission can be produced by stimulation in the sensory cortex, ventrobasal thalamus, hypothalamus, and widespread areas in the midbrain, pons, and medulla (see Gebhart 1986, Hammond 1986, Jones 1992).

Many of these sites rostral to the midbrain have direct projections to the lumbar spinal cord, but they also project to areas of the caudal midbrain, pons, and medulla (and are not illustrated in Fig. 12.2). Descending influences from these rostral sites contribute to inhibition of spinal nociceptive transmission indirectly by multi-neuronal relays in the brainstem, where they modulate the excitability of neurons that send projections to all levels of the spinal cord. As indicated above, descending inhibition from the PAG or RVM is mediated by both serotonergic and noradrenergic receptors in the spinal cord. In addition, it was shown that electrical stimulation in RVM increased the spinal release of both noradrenaline and serotonin (Hammond et al. 1985).

The location of noradrenergic neurons in the brainstem activated by stimulation of neurons in the NRM was not obvious, and included several candidates: the A5, A6 (locus coeruleus), and A7 cell groups in the pons, and the A1 cell group located in the lateral reticular nucleus in the caudal ventrolateral medulla. The A designation indicates cell groups in the brainstem that contain noradrenergic neurons (Dahlström and Fuxe 1964). It had been established that activation of these cell groups produced descending inhibition that is antagonized predominantly, if not exclusively, by a_2-adrenoceptor antagonists given into the lumbar intrathecal space, confirming the release of noradrenaline in the spinal cord. Many studies, summarized in reviews by Jones (1991) and Proudfit (1992), documented that potent behavioral antinociception and inhibition of spinal nociceptive transmission can be produced by activation of these noradrenaline-containing cell groups in the brainstem. It was subsequently shown that noradrenergic neurons in the A7 cell group are activated by stimulation of neurons in the RVM (Brodie and Proudfit 1986, Nuseir et al. 1999), and the prominent projections from the vlPAG to noradrenergic A7 neurons (Bajic and Proudfit 1999, Bajic et al. 2001) provide the noradrenergic component of descending modulation engaged by stimulation in the vlPAG.

The importance of spinal noradrenergic receptors in the control of nociceptive transmission has been confirmed by numerous reports which demonstrate that intrathecal or epidural administration of a_2-adrenoceptor agonists (e.g. clonidine and dexmedetomidine) produces antinociception in animals (Reddy et al. 1980, Takano and Yaksh 1992) and analgesia in humans (Coombs et al. 1985, Gordh 1988, Eisenach 1989, Bonnet et al. 1990), respectively.

Activation of cells in the NRM also increases the spinal release of serotonin (Hammond et al. 1985), and intrathecal administration of serotonin is antinociceptive (Yaksh and Wilson 1979). Serotonin, however, is involved in multiple non-nociceptive spinal functions, such as motor control (White and Neuman 1980, White and Fung 1989) and vasomotor regulation (Solomon and Gebhart 1988), and identification of the spinal serotonergic receptor(s) that participates in nociceptive transmission and its modulation has been challenging. The principal serotonergic receptors present in spinal cord are 5-HT_1 (Pazos and Palacios 1985), 5-HT_2 (Pazos et al. 1985), and 5-HT_3 (Hamon et al. 1989), and several of these have multiple subtypes (e.g. 5-$HT_{1a,b,c}$). In addition, 5-HT4 receptors are found on primary sensory neurons (Chen et al. 1998a).

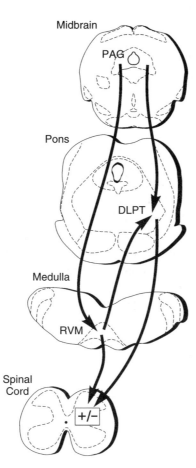

Fig. 12.2 Summary of brainstem pain modulation pathways that reflects the current state of understanding. Neurons in the vlPAG modulate the activity of neurons in both the RVM and the DLPT that constitute parallel descending pathways to the spinal cord dorsal horn. These descending pathways can both inhibit and facilitate nociceptive processing in the dorsal horn, and the relative activity of these opposing actions controls the output of second order nociceptive neurons that project to more rostral brain sites that relay nociceptive information to somatosensory cortical and other brain regions where pain is perceived and interpreted. Abbreviations: DLPT, dorsolateral pontine tegmentum; PAG, periaqueductal gray; RVM, rostral ventromedial medulla; +/−, excitatory/inhibitory.

The 5-HT$_3$ receptor, a ligand-gated ion channel, is present on nociceptor terminals and other locations in the spinal dorsal horn (Hamon *et al.* 1989) and 5-HT$_3$ receptor-selective antagonists dose-dependently block serotonin-produced nociceptive behaviors (Bardin *et al.* 2000).

The roles of the other serotonin receptors in spinal cord, all of which are G protein-coupled receptors, are less clear. Intrathecal administration of receptor selective agonists or antagonists in different experiments provide data suggesting that one or another of these receptors is antinociceptive, pronociceptive, or without effect (Fasmer *et al.* 1986, Solomon and Gebhart 1988, Glaum *et al.* 1990, Crisp *et al.* 1991). These conflicting results likely reflect the absence of specificity of the drugs tested, the nature of the noxious stimulus employed (thermal, mechanical), the nociceptive test, whether inflammation is present, and the multiple functions of serotonin in the spinal cord. Although the spinal serotonergic receptors that mediate the descending effects of serotonin have not been clearly defined, the importance of serotonin to descending control of pain processing remains undiminished.

Although the primary focus of study has been on noradrenergic and serotonergic modulation of nociception in the spinal cord, it should be appreciated that other neurotransmitters descending from the brainstem also contribute to modulation of spinal nociceptive transmission. The RVM is the principal source of spinal serotonin, but this region also contains a large proportion of non-serotonergic cells, including those that contain GABA (Jones *et al.* 1991), enkephalin (Bowker *et al.* 1988), glutamate (Minson *et al.* 1991), somatostatin (Millhorn *et al.* 1987), substance P (Bowker *et al.* 1983), and cholecystokinin (Mantyh and Hunt 1984) that project to the spinal cord. RVM neurons that contain substance P (Yeomans and Proudfit 1990), GABA (Nuseir and Proudfit 1999), and enkephalin (Holden and Proudfit 1998) also project to the DLPT (Fig. 12.3). Thus, stimulating electrically or injecting an excitatory neurotransmitter like glutamate into the RVM activates multiple, chemically heterogeneous cells that contribute, in incompletely understood ways, to spinal cord modulation of pain processing.

These descending axons do not all terminate in the spinal dorsal horn, the site of termination of nociceptor input, but there is evidence to support a role for most of these substances in nociceptive processing (Duggan and Weihe 1991). For example, intrathecal administration of naloxone, the opioid receptor antagonist, has been reported by some (Zorman *et al.* 1982), but not others (Aimone *et al.* 1987), to antagonize RVM stimulation-produced spinal inhibition, suggesting a role for endogenous opioids in spinal nociceptive modulation. Similarly, intrathecal injection of the GABA$_A$ receptor antagonist, bicuculline, reduces the antinociception produced by chemical stimulation of RVM neurons (McGowan and Hammond 1993). In contrast, activation of cholecystokinin cells in RVM, produced by microinjection of neurotensin, enhances responses to noxious stimuli (Urban *et al.* 1996, Friedrich and Gebhart 2003), and thus may be important to descending facilitatory influences that can be activated in the RVM (see below).

The existence of an endogenous pain modulation system implies a physiological function that can be engaged or activated by appropriate stimuli. The stimuli that activate this modulatory system have been studied and several classes of such stimuli identified. Certainly, opioids given systemically for control of pain produce receptor-mediated actions in the PAG and RVM, and thus functionally activate the endogenous pain inhibitory system (e.g. see Fig. 12.1). Although opioids like morphine generally inhibit neurons, they appear to indirectly activate descending inhibitory neurons by inhibition of local GABAergic interneurons that disinhibit (activate) the descending neurons. For example, in the PAG it has been shown that morphine inhibits a GABAergic interneuron that disinhibits descending excitatory influences on neurons in the RVM (Moreau and Fields 1986).

In the RVM, similar indirect effects of opioids (i.e. disinhibition of GABAergic interneurons) are believed to activate cells with axons that descend the spinal cord and inhibit spinal nociceptive transmission in the dorsal horn (Drower and Hammond 1988, Heinricher and Kaplan 1991). Opioids like morphine, of course, have actions at

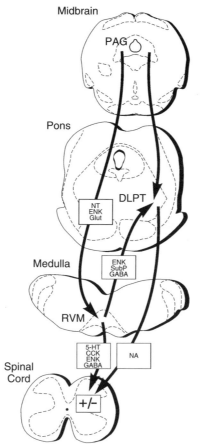

Fig. 12.3 Summary of the neurotransmitters involved in brainstem pain modulation pathways. Neurons in the vlPAG that contain neurotensin, enkephalin, and glutamate project to the RVM and modulate the activity of spinally projecting neurons. Activation of enkephalin and gluta-mate neurons in the PAG directly or indirectly activates descending inhibitory RVM neurons, while activation of neurotensin neurons produces a bi-directional effect. Descending RVM neurons that contain serotonin, enkephalin, and GABA inhibit nociceptive processing in the spinal cord, while those that contain cholecystokinin facilitate nociception. PAG neurons also project to the DLPT and activate ponto-spinal noradrenergic neurons. Several types of neurons in the RVM, including enkephalin-, substance P-, and GABA-containing, also project to the DLPT. Substance P neurons directly activate, GABA neurons directly inhibit, and enkephalin neurons indirectly activate ponto-spinal DLPT neurons. Abbreviations: 5-HT, serotonin; CCK, cholecystokinin; DLPT, dorsolateral pontine tegmentum; ENK, enkephalin; GABA, gamma aminobutyric acid; Glut, glutamic acid; NT, neurotensin; NA, noradrenaline; PAG, periaque-ductal gray; RVM, rostral ventromedial medulla; SubP, substance P; +/−, excitatory/inhibitory.

other sites in the CNS, including at opioid receptors in the spinal dorsal horn (Duggan and North 1984, Zieglgänsberger 1984) and in the periphery (Herz 1995, Arguelles *et al.* 2002, Martinez *et al.* 2002, Shannon and Lutz 2002). However, the antinociception produced by morphine given systemically is significantly reduced when opioid receptors are blocked in either supraspinal (Yaksh and Rudy 1978, Dickenson *et al.* 1979) or spinal sites (Yaksh and Rudy 1977), revealing that endogenous inhibitory systems are extensively distributed and the parts act in concert to reduce nociception.

Natural stimuli that have also been shown to engage the endogenous pain control system include stress (stress-induced analgesia), fear and anxiety, intense exercise (e.g. running a marathon), and sexual activity (Watkins and Mayer 1982, Bodnar 1986). Some forms of acupuncture may also access this system (Chen *et al.* 1998*b*). Disease states also certainly engage the endogenous modulatory system. For example, cardiopulmonary input (Randich and Maixner 1984, 1986, Randich and Gebhart 1992) and experimentally-induced illness (Watkins and Maier 2000) both alter nociceptive response thresholds by accessing the modulatory system. Experimentally increasing blood pressure in normotensive individuals increases response thresholds to experimentally applied noxious stimuli (see Maixner and Randich 1984), whereas illness behavior typically leads to increased sensitivity to stimuli, or hyperalgesia (see Watkins and Maier 2000).

Interestingly, both cardiopulmonary and illness-induced changes in nociceptive responding are conveyed to the brainstem *via* the vagus nerve, which previously has been established as contributing to spinal pain modulation (see Randich and Gebhart 1992). The intracranial pathways for vagal-produced modulation of spinal nociception have been studied and clearly integrate with the brainstem organization described above; that is, the RVM appears to function as a final common pathway for descending modulation of spinal nociceptive processing. The relevance of this information is supported by evidence that vagal afferent stimulation reduces experimental pain in humans (Kirchner *et al.* 2000).

12.3.2 Descending facilitation

It has been appreciated for some time that stimulation in the brainstem, and particularly the RVM, could excite spinal neurons or enhance their responses to nociceptive input (McCreery *et al.* 1979, Light *et al.* 1986, McMahon and Wall 1988). This descending facilitation of nociception produced by RVM stimulation was initially shown to be partly mediated by descending noradrenergic neurons acting at spinal cord alpha$_1$-adrenoceptors (Brodie and Proudfit 1986). These observations, however, were not systematically investigated until Ren noted that low-intensity stimulation of vagal afferent fibers significantly reduced the latency of the nociceptive tail-flick reflex in the rat (Ren *et al.* 1988). In subsequent studies of descending modulation from RVM, additional spinal pathways of descending inhibition and facilitation, and the spinal receptors involved were determined by Zhuo (see Millan 2002 for review). Consequently, the notion that descending systems could be pronociceptive gained wider acceptance.

The scope of this work has expanded to include modulation of visceral nociceptive transmission (Zhuo *et al.* 2002), spinal nociceptive and non-nociceptive mechanical transmission (Zhuo and Gebhart 2002), and also includes the caudal medullary dorsal reticular nucleus (Lima and Almeida 2002), the vlPAG (Fang and Proudfit 1998), and the A7 catecholamine cell group in the DLPT (Holden and Proudfit 1999, Nuseir and Proudfit 2000).

It has been documented for several sites in the brainstem (e.g. NRM, n. gigantocellularis, gigantocellularis pars a, dorsal reticular nucleus, A7 cell group, and vlPAG) that either inhibition or facilitation of spinal nociceptive transmission can be produced, depending on the intensity of stimulation or the concentration of microinjected agonist drugs. In general, facilitation is produced by low intensities of electrical stimulation, whereas inhibition is produced by greater intensities of stimulation (Zhuo and Gebhart 1991), explaining why early investigations of descending modulation from the brainstem failed to note facilitatory effects. Importantly, both the inhibitory and facilitatory effects of electrical stimulation are replicated by agonist drugs such as cholinergic agonists (Brodie and Proudfit 1986, Iwamoto and Marion 1993), the GABA receptor agonist, baclofen (Thomas *et al.* 1995), glutamate (Zhuo and Gebhart 1990), opioid agonists (Fang and Proudfit 1998, Holden and Proudfit 1999), or neurotensin (Urban and Smith 1993, Urban *et al.* 1996, Smith *et al.* 1997) injected into brainstem sites, including the RVM, vlPAG, and A7 cell group. These effects have been shown to be receptor-mediated, which confirms the role of neurons in these brainstem areas to the descending effects produced. These investigations also confirmed that descending inhibitory influences are prepotent (and often tonically active).

12.3.3 Interactions among brainstem pain modulation neurons

There are significant interactions among the major cell groups in the brainstem that modulate nociception. For example, activation of the DLPT exerts both facilitatory and inhibitory influences on spinal nociceptive transmission that are mediated by adrenoceptors in the spinal cord (Holden and Proudfit 1999, Nuseir *et al.* 1999). More specifically, local injection of morphine (Holden and Proudfit 1999) or the GABA receptor antagonist, bicuculline, (Nuseir and Proudfit 2000) into the A7 cell group can bi-directionally modulate spinal nociceptive reflexes by disinhibiting different populations of spinally projecting DLPT neurons. One population produces facilitation of nociception that is mediated by alpha$_1$-adrenoceptors and another produces inhibition of nociception that is mediated by alpha$_2$-adrenoceptors. Furthermore, the bi-directional effects of stimulating neurons in the RVM (Brodie and Proudfit 1986, Iwamoto and Marion 1993) or the vlPAG (Fang and Proudfit 1996, Fang and Proudfit 1998) are mediated in part by activation of ponto-spinal noradrenergic neurons located in the DLPT. These conclusions are supported by anatomical evidence that demonstrates that significant populations of neurons in both the RVM (Clark and Proudfit 1991*c*, Holden and Proudfit 1998) and vlPAG (Bajic and Proudfit 1999, Bajic *et al.* 2001) project to noradrenergic A7 neurons.

Neurons in the vlPAG form synapses with both noradrenergic and non-noradrenergic neurons in the DLPT (Bajic *et al.* 2001). Several populations of RVM neurons that project to the DLPT have been identified, including enkephalin (Holden and Proudfit 1998), substance P (Yeomans and Proudfit 1990), and GABA (Nuseir and Proudfit 1999). Although the function of these neurons has not been systematically determined, RVM GABAergic neurons appear to tonically inhibit ponto-spinal A7 neurons (Nuseir and Proudfit 2000), and RVM enkephalinergic neurons appear to inhibit DLPT GABA neurons that also tonically inhibit ponto-spinal A7 neurons (Holden and Proudfit 1999). Together, the RVM, vlPAG, and A7 cell group constitute a highly integrated system of neurons that modulates nociceptive transmission in the spinal cord by both active inhibition and active facilitation.

Recent evidence indicates that cortical areas such as the rostral agranular insular cortex also interact with brainstem neurons and appear to bi-directionally modulate nociception (Jasmin *et al.* 2003). It is notable that neurons that modulate nociceptive processing are widely distributed and are present in all major divisions of the CNS: the cortex, thalamus, midbrain, pons, medulla, and spinal cord.

12.3.4 Interactions among RVM cells

In 1983, Fields described physiologic classes of putative nociceptive modulatory cells in RVM (Fields *et al.* 1983). These cells were characterized in the lightly anesthetized rat during tail withdrawal from noxious heat. *Off* cells displayed an abrupt pause in ongoing activity immediately before the withdrawal reflex and were proposed to contribute the inhibitory influence on spinal nociceptive processing that descended from RVM. *On* cells gave a burst of activity immediately before the withdrawal reflex and were proposed to contribute to facilitatory influences on spinal nociceptive processing. A third group of cells, *neutral* cells, was unresponsive in this preparation, showing no changes in activity related to noxious thermal stimulation. Subsequent work established that the latency of nociceptive responsiveness correlated with on and off cell activity and that cells of the same class (on or off) tended to discharge at the same time (Fields and Heinricher 1989).

This work led to the proposition that on and off cells mediated spinal nociceptive facilitation and inhibition, respectively. Given the extensive and compelling evidence for the involvement of 5-HT in the modulation of spinal nociceptive processing (Millan 1997), it was surprising that neither on nor off cells were serotonin-containing. More recently, serotonergic cells in RVM have been suggested to be a fourth class of cells with different physiological and functional characteristics (see Mason 2001 for overview). Thus, a class of cells distinct from on and off cells, that likely includes some neutral cells and contains a transmitter long associated with descending inhibition of spinal nociceptive processing and opioid-produced antinociception, also contributes to descending modulation of spinal pain transmission.

The model proposed by Fields and colleagues is supported by studies of the opioid analgesic morphine, which tonically activates off cells and inhibits on cells (Fields *et al.* 1991), suggesting that each class of RVM cell functions as a unit that exerts non-topographical descending modulation of spinal nociceptive transmission. Heinricher *et al.* (1992) documented that morphine directly inhibits on cells (which thus must express a μ-opioid receptor), but had no direct effect on off or neutral cells in RVM. The activation of off cells by morphine was proposed to arise indirectly by inhibition of tonically active GABAergic inhibitory interneurons (i.e. by disinhibition) (Heinricher and Kaplan 1991). In addition to electrophysiologic evidence for the expression of μ-opioid receptors by on cells, there is anatomic evidence that both bulbospinal serotonergic and non-serotonergic RVM cells contain μ- (and δ-) opioid receptor mRNA or protein and that some bulbospinal RVM cells that express μ-opioid receptors also express GABA (Kalyuzhny and Wessendorf 1998).

The heuristic value of the on and off cell model has been enormously important. However, aspects of this model have been challenged by contradictory and inconsistent findings. For example, innocuous auditory and somatic stimuli excite and inhibit on and off cells, respectively (Oliveras *et al.* 1989, 1990, Leung and Mason 1999), and responses to these innocuous stimuli are as great as are responses to noxious stimuli. In addition, neutral cells, which are unresponsive to noxious thermal stimulation, have been reported to be on or off in response to mechanical stimuli (Ellrich *et al.* 2000, Schnell *et al.* 2002), which led to speculation that there were on and off cell subtypes responsive to a different stimulus modality. More recently, on, off, and neutral cells were characterized as described above and then studied for responses to noxious colon distension, a mechanical visceral stimulus (Brink and Mason 2003). It was found that most on cells were not excited and most off cells were not inhibited by the noxious visceral stimulus, whereas most neutral cells were excited or inhibited by the stimulus. These and other considerations related to state-dependence of RVM neuron activity and convergent afferent input led Mason (2001) to propose a broader role for RVM neurons associated with behavioral states and not restricted only to modulation of nociception. Although the functions of on, off, neutral, serotonergic, and other RVM cells in the modulation of nociception require much more study, it is clear that cells in RVM play an important modulatory role and should remain a focus of investigation.

An important approach to understanding the function of RVM neurons is the characterization of neurotransmitter actions on the various RVM cell types. Cells in RVM also have been characterized *in vitro*, initially using sharp electrodes, and later using whole cell patch clamp methods. In an early *in vitro* study, μ-opioid receptor agonists — (Met[5]) enkephalin, DAMGO — were found to directly hyperpolarize a subset of RVM neurons (termed secondary cells) by increasing a K^+ channel conductance (Pan *et al.* 1990). In the same study, μ-opioid receptor agonists reduced a GABAergic inhibitory postsynaptic potential on a different subset of RVM neurons (termed primary cells). Primary cells most closely correspond to the population of RVM cells whose activation results in antinociception (i.e. off cell-like). Secondary cells were suggested to tonically inhibit primary cells and to contain GABA; they were further distinguished from primary cells by insensitivity to the κ-opioid receptor agonist, U69,593.

Several recent reports, however, suggest that the division of RVM cells into primary or secondary, based on how they respond to a μ-opioid receptor agonist, is an oversimplification. For example, it has been shown that some cells in RVM respond to both μ- *and* κ-opioid receptor agonists as well as to deltorphin II, a δ-opioid receptor agonist (Marinelli *et al.* 2002), confirming that the present characterization of cells in RVM is incomplete.

These different means of classifying cells in the RVM, which are considered to mediate the descending influences exerted on spinal nociceptive processing, are not wholly consonant. The on-cell, off-cell, and neutral-cell classification, which is based on responses to noxious thermal stimulation, does not accommodate responses to either somatic mechanical or visceral mechanical stimuli (see Brink and Mason 2003). The primary and secondary cell classification developed *in vitro* appears to be an oversimplification, and the number of cell types and their interactions is more complex than originally advanced (see Marinelli *et al.* 2002).

There are advantages and limitations associated with both means of RVM cell classification. In the intact animal, the relation of cell responses to relevant stimuli is emphasized. Typically, however, only one modality of stimulation is tested and it has only been recently that stimuli other than thermal have been studied. The principal limitation of these studies is the inability to study cellular mechanisms, which is the principal attraction of the *in vitro* slice approach. *In vitro*, direct and indirect synaptic effects of drugs can be tested, ion currents isolated, and intracellular signaling cascades studied. The principal limitation of the *in vitro* approach is that immature animals are typically used (8–15 days old), when peripheral afferent inputs and descending systems are still in development. Behavioral reactions to noxious stimuli are non-specific in rats until at least postnatal day 10 (Fitzgerald and Jennings 1999) and the typical biphasic response to intraplantar injection of formalin is not apparent until postnatal day 15 (Guy and Abbott 1992). Secondary hyperalgesia, which is dependent on central (spinal and likely supraspinal) mechanisms, is not adult-like until day 21 (Jiang and Gebhart 1998). Furthermore, descending control mechanisms are immature at birth and stimulation-produced antinociception from the midbrain does not develop until postnatal day 21 (van Praag and Frenk 1991). These developmental issues are a significant limitation of using neonatal animals to study the responses of modulatory neurons in the RVM to neurotransmitter agonists.

Another significant limitation of using neonatal slice preparations to study the functional significance of RVM cells has been a lack of suitable methods to identify recorded neurons. This limitation has recently been overcome to some extent (Marinelli *et al.* 2002). Our understanding of the functional interactions among RVM neurons that modulate nociception will remain rudimentary until these limitations are overcome.

The importance of understanding the role of RVM cells in pain processing is underscored by compelling evidence demonstrating their contribution to the maintenance of altered states of pain processing such as allodynia and hyperalgesia. It is now clear that cells in the RVM undergo significant plasticity in response to persistent pain.

That is, peripheral tissue injury activates spino-bulbospinal circuitry that contributes to the development of central sensitization, an increase in the excitability of spinal neurons, and to secondary hyperalgesia (see reviews by Urban and Gebhart 1999, Pertovaara 2000, Porreca *et al.* 2002, Ren and Dubner 2002). For example, Hurley and Hammond (2000, 2001) showed that the antihyperalgesic and antinociceptive potency of μ- and δ-opioid receptor agonists given directly into the RVM was significantly increased for up to two weeks after hindpaw inflammation in the rat. Interestingly, changes in potency for both μ- and δ-agonists was apparent for the inflamed as well as the contralateral, uninflamed hindpaw, suggesting a general change in descending modulation. Hindpaw inflammation also increases NMDA subunit NR1, NR2A, and NR2B receptor mRNAs for a week (Miki *et al.* 2002). In addition, neutral-like cells in RVM were initially unresponsive to thermal stimulation of the hindpaw, but most became off-like or on-like during the development of hindpaw inflammation.

Indirect evidence that on cells contribute to the development of neuropathic pain was reported by Porreca and colleagues (2001) who selectively destroyed RVM cells containing μ-opioid receptors by injecting a μ-opioid receptor agonist conjugated to saporin; the complex is internalized when the agonist binds to the μ-opioid receptor. The saporin then dissociates and kills the cell. The loss of RVM neurons that express μ-opioid receptors either prevented the development of, or reversed, the neuropathic pain behaviors in rats, depending upon when the conjugate was injected into the RVM. They postulated that a presumed loss of on cells eliminated descending facilitation required for the expression of nerve-injury produced tactile and thermal hypersensitivity. This complex and growing literature suggests that descending facilitatory influences engaged in the RVM contribute to the development and maintenance of secondary hyperalgesia. In contrast, descending inhibitory influences from RVM are enhanced when tested at the site of peripheral insult (i.e. primary hyperalgesia), illustrating the bi-directional nature of descending modulation of spinal pain transmission.

Although research efforts to date have greatly expanded our understanding of the functions of RVM neurons under acute pain conditions (e.g. Mason 2001), they have also revealed the highly complex and altered nature of the interactions among brainstem neurons that occurs during persistent and chronic pain states.

12.4 **Summary**

Since the seminal observation by Reynolds (1969), significant progress has been made in understanding the circuitry and function of brainstem neurons that modulate nociception. There is now compelling evidence that neurons in the vlPAG control the activity of neurons in both the RVM and the DLPT which constitute a parallel descending pathway to the spinal cord dorsal horn (see Fig. 12.2). These descending pathways can both inhibit and facilitate nociceptive processing in the dorsal horn, and the relative activity of these opposing actions controls the output of second order nociceptive neurons that project to more rostral brain sites that relay pain signals to somatosensory cortical and other brain regions where pain is perceived and interpreted. The function of descending control systems is significantly altered by the presence of persistent or chronic pain, which appears to be at least partially responsible for the initiation and maintenance of these pain states.

Although the function of these systems has been primarily studied in rodents, a similar system of neurons appears to control pain perception in humans with, of course, added layers of complexity contributed by cognitive and other influences. Thus, electrical stimulation of neurons in the midbrain PAG/periventricular gray produces potent relief of pain in humans, and the importance of descending noradrenergic neurons in human pain modulation is supported by the clinical efficacy of epidural administration of the adrenoceptor agonist, clonidine. These observations support the relevance of investigating mechanisms of pain and pain modulation in non-human animals.

12.5 **Future directions**

Although significant advances have been made in delineating the location, neurotransmitter content, and interconnections among neurons in the brainstem and spinal cord that modulate nociception, there are still significant deficiencies in our understanding of the specific connections among these many neurons. For example, a large number of neurons have been immunochemically identified in the RVM, PAG, DLPT, and spinal cord, but information related to the specific interconnections among these neurons is very rudimentary and based largely on the results of anterograde and retrograde tracing studies that provide relatively gross descriptions of connections among neurons in different nuclei or cell groups. Furthermore, relatively little is known about specific neuronal interconnections in local circuits within a given nucleus or cell group. Finally, there is also relatively little information related to specific synaptic connections among immunochemically identified neurons in the brainstem and spinal cord. These deficiencies in our understanding of the specific anatomical interconnections among neurons that modulate nociception is a significant obstacle to the unequivocal interpretation of behavioral, pharmacological, and electrophysiological studies designed to determine the function of these neuronal systems.

Another deficiency is our incomplete understanding of the signal transduction mechanisms that operate in the various neurons that comprise the brainstem modulatory systems. Some transmitters are coupled to G-proteins and others to ligand-gated ion channels. The interactions among signaling pathways activated by different receptors on the same neurons are not well understood, but are likely to have important functional ramifications. The complexity of these signaling pathways and their alteration during persistent inflammatory or neuropathic pain states presents an especially difficult challenge, but one that needs to be overcome as evidence of plasticity in these systems accumulates. For example, there are numerous chronic pain conditions that are characterized as 'functional', meaning that we do not understand their cause. Many such pain states exist in the absence of apparent pathology, and it is intriguing to speculate that they may persist as a consequence of an alteration in the normal balance between descending inhibitory and facilitatory influences on spinal transmission, including interpretation of non-noxious input as painful. Accordingly, an important future direction is anatomical identification of neurons that produce these opposing actions and characterization of the signaling and electrophysiological mechanisms that control the activity of these neurons.

References

Aimone LD and Gebhart GF (1986). Stimulation-produced spinal inhibition from the midbrain in the rat is mediated by an excitatory amino acid neurotransmitter in the medial medulla. *J. Neurosci.*, **6**, 1803–13.

Aimone LD, Jones SL, and Gebhart GF (1987). Stimulation-produced descending inhibition from the periaqueductal gray and nucleus raphe magnus in the rat: mediation by spinal monoamines but not opioids. *Pain*, **31**, 123–36.

Arguelles CF, Torres–Lopez JE and Granados–Soto V (2002). Peripheral antinociceptive action of morphine and the synergistic interaction with lamotrigine. *Anesthesiology*, **96**, 921–5.

Bajic D and Proudfit HK (1999). Projections of neurons in the periaqueductal gray to pontine and medullary catecholamine cell groups involved in the modulation of nociception. *J. Comp. Neurol.*, **405**, 359–79.

Bajic D, Van Bockstaele EJ, and Proudfit HK (2001). Ultrastructural analysis of ventrolateral periaqueductal gray projections to the A7 catecholamine cell group. *Neuroscience*, **104**, 181–97.

Bardin L, Lavarenne J, and Eschalier A (2000). Serotonin receptor subtypes involved in the spinal antinociceptive effect of 5-HT in rats. *Pain*, **86**, 11–18.

Bodnar RJ (1986). Neuropharmacological and neuroendocrine substrates of stress-induced analgesia. *Ann. New York Acad. Sci.*, **467**, 345–60.

Bonnet F, Boico O, Rostaing S, Loriferne JF, and Saada M (1990). Clonidine-induced analgesia in postoperative patients: epidural versus intramuscular administration. *Anesthesiology*, **72**, 423.

Bowker RM, Abbott LC, and Dilts RP (1988). Peptidergic neurons in the nucleus raphe magnus and nucleus gigantocellularis: their distributions, interrelationships and projections to the spinal cord. *Prog. Brain Res.*, **88**, 95–128.

Bowker RM, Westlund KN, and Coulter JD (1982). Organization of descending serotonergic projections to the spinal cord. *Prog. Brain Res*, **57**, 239–65.

Bowker RM, Westlund KN, Sullivan MC, Wilber JF, and Coulter JD (1983). Descending serotonergic, peptidergic and cholinergic pathways from the raphe nuclei: a multiple transmitter complex. *Brain Res.*, **288**, 33–48.

Brink TS and Mason P (2003). Raphe magnus neurons respond to noxious colorectal distension. *J. Neurophysiol.*, **89**, 2506–15.

Brodie MS and Proudfit HK (1986). Antinociception induced by local injection of carbachol into the nucleus raphe magnus: Alteration by intrathecal injection of noradrenergic antagonists. *Brain Res.*, **371**, 70–9.

Chen JJ, Vasko MR, Wu X, *et al.* (1998*a*). Multiple subtypes of serotonin receptors are expressed in rat sensory neurons in culture. *J. Pharmacol. Exp. Ther.*, **287**, 1119–27.

Chen XH, Geller EB, and Adler MW (1998*b*). CCK(B) receptors in the periaqueductal grey are involved in electroacupuncture antinociception in the rat cold water tail-flick test. *Neuropharmacology*, **37**, 751–7.

Clark FM and Proudfit HK (1991*a*). The projection of locus coeruleus neurons to the spinal cord in the rat determined by anterograde tracing combined with immunocytochemistry. *Brain Res.*, **538**, 231–45.

Clark FM and Proudfit HK (1991*b*). The projection of noradrenergic neurons in the A7 catecholamine cell group to the spinal cord in the rat demonstrated by anterograde tracing combined with immunocytochemistry. *Brain Res.*, **547**, 279–88.

Clark FM and Proudfit HK (1991*c*). Projections of neurons in the ventromedial medulla to pontine catecholamine cell groups involved in the modulation of nociception. *Brain Res.*, **540**, 105–15.

Coombs DW, Saunders RL, Lachance D, Savage S, Ragnarsson T, and Jensen LE (1985). Intrathecal morphine tolerance: use of intrathecal clonidine, DADLE, and intraventricular morphine. *Anesthesiology*, **62**, 358–63.

Crisp T, Stafinsky JL, Spanos LJ, Uram M, Perni VC, and Donepudi HB (1991). Analgesic effects of serotonin and receptor-selective serotonin agonists in the rat spinal cord. *Gen. Pharmacol.*, **22**, 247–51.

Dahlström A and Fuxe K (1964). Evidence for the existence of monoamine neurons in the central nervous system. I. Demonstration of monoamines in the cell bodies of brain stem neurons. *Acta Physiol. Scand.*, **Suppl 232, 62**, 1–55.

Dickenson AH, Oliveras JL, and Besson JM (1979). Role of the nucleus raphe magnus in opiate analgesia as studied by the microinjection technique in the rat. *Brain Res.*, **170**, 95–111.

Drower EJ and Hammond DL (1988). GABAergic modulation of nociceptive threshold: effects of THIP and bicuculline microinjected into the ventral medulla of the rat. *Brain Res.*, **450**, 316–24.

Duggan AW and North RA (1984). Electrophysiology of opioids. *Pharmacol. Rev.*, **35**, 219–81.

Duggan AW and Weihe E (1991). Central transmission of impulses in nociceptors: events in the superficial dorsal horn. In (eds. AI Basbaum and J–M Besson) *Towards a New Pharmacology of Pain*, pp. 35–67. John Wiley & Sons, New York.

Eisenach JC (1989) Epidural clonidine analgesia following surgery: phase 1. *Anesthesiology*, **71**, 640–46.

Ellrich J, Ulucan C, and Schnell C (2000). Are 'neutral cells' in the rostral ventro-medial medulla subtypes of on- and off-cells? *Neurosci. Res.*, **38**, 419–23.

Fang F and Proudfit HK (1996). Spinal cholinergic and monoamine receptors mediate the antinociceptive effect of morphine microinjected in the periaqueductal gray on the rat tail, but not the feet. *Brain Res.*, **722**, 95–108.

Fang F and Proudfit HK (1998). Antinociception produced by microinjection of morphine in the periaqueductal gray is enhanced in the rat foot, but not the tail, by intrathecal injection of alpha1-adrenoceptor antagonists. *Brain Res.*, **790**, 14–24.

Fasmer OB, Berge O–G, Post C, and Hole K (1986). Effects of the putative 5-HT1A receptor agonist 8-OH-2-(di-n-propylamino)tetraline on nociceptive sensitivity in mice. *Pharmacol. Biochem. Behav.*, **25**, 883–88.

Fields HL and Basbaum AI (1978). Brainstem control of spinal pain transmission neurons. *Ann. Rev. Physiol.*, **40**, 217–48.

Fields HL and Heinricher MM (1989). Brainstem modulation of nociceptor-driven withdrawal reflexes. *Ann. NY Acad. Sci.*, **563**, 34–44.

Fields HL, Bry J, Hentall I, and Zorman G (1983). The activity of neurons in the rostral medulla of the rat during withdrawal from noxious heat. *J. Neurosci.*, **3**, 2545–52.

Fields HL, Heinricher MM, and Mason P (1991). Neurotransmitters in nociceptive modulatory circuits. *Ann. Rev. Neurosci.*, **14**, 219–45.

Fitzgerald M and Jennings E (1999). The postnatal development of spinal sensory processing. *Proc. Natl. Acad. Sci. USA*, **96**, 7719–22.

Friedrich AE and Gebhart GF (2003). Modulation of visceral hyperalgesia by morphine and cholecystokinin from the rat rostroventral medial medulla. *Pain*, **104**, 93–101.

Fritschy JM and Grzanna R (1990). Demonstration of two separate descending noradrenergic pathways to the rat spinal cord: evidence for an intragriseal trajectory of locus coeruleus axons in the superficial layers of the dorsal horn. *J. Comp. Neurol.*, **291**, 553–82.

Gebhart GF (1986). Modulatory effects of descending systems on spinal dorsal horn neurons. In (ed. TL Yaksh) *Spinal Afferent Processing*, pp. 391–416. Plenum, New York.

Gebhart GF, Sandkühler J, Thalhammer JG, and Zimmerman M (1983). Inhibition of spinal nociceptive information by stimulation in midbrain of the cat is blocked by lidocaine microinjections in nucleus raphe magnus and medullary reticular formation. *J. Neurophysiol.*, **50**, 1446–59.

Glaum SR, Proudfit HK, and Anderson EG (1990). 5-HT$_3$ receptors modulate spinal nociceptive reflexes. *Brain Res.*, **510**, 12–16.

Gordh T (1988). Epidural clonidine for treatment of post-operative pain after thoracotomy. A double- blind placebo-controlled study. *Acta Anaesthesiol. Scand.*, **32**, 702–9.

Grzanna R and Fritschy J–M (1991). Efferent projections of different subpopulations of central noradrenaline neurons. *Prog. Brain Res.*, **88**, 89–101.

Guy ER and Abbott FV (1992). The behavioral response to formalin in preweanling rats. *Pain*, **51**, 81–90.

Hammond DL (1986). Control systems for nociceptive afferent processing: the descending inhibitory pathways. In (ed. TL Yaksh) *Spinal Afferent Processing*, pp. 363–90. Plenum Press, New York.

Hammond DL, Tyce GM, and Yaksh TL (1985). Efflux of 5-hydroxytryptamine and noradrenaline into spinal cord superfusates during stimulation of the rat medulla. *J. Physiol.*, **359**, 151–62.

Hamon M, Gallissot MC, Menard F, Gozlan H, Bourgoin S, and Verge D (1989). 5-HT3 receptor binding sites are on capsaicin-sensitive fibres in the rat spinal cord. *Eur. J. Pharmacol.*, **164**, 315–22.

Heinricher MM and Kaplan HJ (1991). GABA-mediated inhibition in rostral ventromedial medulla: role in nociceptive modulation in the lightly anesthetized rat. *Pain*, **47**, 105–13.

Heinricher MM, Morgan MM, and Fields HL (1992). Direct and indirect actions of morphine on medullary neurons that modulate nociception. *Neuroscience*, **48**, 533–43.

Herz A (1995). Opioid peptides, opioid receptors and peripheral analgesia. In (ed. LF Tseng) *The Pharmacology of Opioid Peptides*, pp. 287–301. Harwood, New York.

Holden JE and Proudfit HK (1998). Enkephalin neurons that project to the A7 catecholamine cell group are located in brainstem nuclei that modulate nociception: ventromedial medulla. *Neuroscience*, **83**, 929–47.

Holden JE and Proudfit HK (1999). Microinjection of morphine in the A7 catecholamine cell group produces opposing effects on nociception that are mediated by alpha1- and alpha2-adrenoceptors. *Neuroscience*, **91**, 979–90.

Hosobuchi Y, Adams JE, and Linchitz R (1977). Pain relief by electrical stimulation of the central gray matter in humans and its reversal by naloxone. *Science*, **197**, 183–86.

Hurley RW and Hammond DL (2000). The analgesic effects of supraspinal mu and delta opioid receptor agonists are potentiated during persistent inflammation. *J Neurosci*, **20**, 1249–59.

Hurley RW and Hammond DL (2001). Contribution of endogenous enkephalins to the enhanced analgesic effects of supraspinal mu opioid receptor agonists after inflammatory injury. *J. Neurosci.*, **21**, 2536–45.

Iwamoto ET and Marion L (1993). Adrenergic, serotonergic and cholinergic components of nicotinic antinociception in rats. *J. Pharmacol. Exp. Ther.*, **265**, 777–89.

Jasmin L, Rabkin SD, Granato A, Boudah A, and Ohara PT (2003). Analgesia and hyperalgesia from GABA-mediated modulation of the cerebral cortex. *Nature, 424,* 316–20.

Jensen TS and Yaksh TL (1984). Spinal monoamine and opiate systems partly mediate the antinociceptive effects produced by glutamate at brainstem sites. *Brain Res., 321,* 287–97.

Jiang MC and Gebhart GF (1998). Development of mustard oil-induced hyperalgesia in rats. *Pain, 77,* 305–13.

Jones BE, Holmes CJ, Rodriguez–Veiga E, and Mainville L (1991). GABA-synthesizing neurons in the medulla: their relationship to serotonin-containing and spinally projecting neurons in the rat. *J. Comp. Neurol., 313,* 349–67.

Jones SL (1991). Descending noradrenergic influences on pain. *Prog. Brain Res., 88,* 381–94.

Jones SL (1992). Descending control of nociception. In (ed. AR Light) *The Initial Processing of Pain and its Descending Control: Spinal and Trigeminal Systems,* Vol. 12, pp. 203–95. Karger, New York.

Jones SL and Gebhart GF (1988). Inhibition of spinal nociceptive transmission from the midbrain pons and medulla in the rat: activation of descending inhibition by morphine, glutamate and electrical stimulation. *Brain Res., 460,* 281–96.

Kalyuzhny AE and Wessendorf MW (1998). Relationship of mu- and delta-opioid receptors to GABAergic neurons in the central nervous system, including antinociceptive brainstem circuits. *J. Comp. Neurol., 392,* 528–47.

Kirchner A, Birklein F, Stefan H, and Handwerker HO (2000). Left vagus nerve stimulation suppresses experimentally induced pain. *Neurology, 55,* 1167–71.

Leung CG and Mason P (1999). Physiological properties of raphe magnus neurons during sleep and waking. *J. Neurophysiol., 81,* 584–95.

Light AR, Casale EJ, and Menétrey DM (1986). The effects of focal stimulation in nucleus raphe magnus and periaqueductal grey on intracellularly recorded neurons in spinal laminae I and II. *J. Neurophysiol., 56,* 555–71.

Lima D and Almeida A (2002). The medullary dorsal reticular nucleus as a pronociceptive centre of the pain control system. *Prog. Neurobiol., 66,* 81–108.

Lundberg A (1964). Supraspinal control of transmission in reflex paths to motoneurons and primary afferents. In (eds. JC Eccles and JP Schade) *Physiology of Spinal Neurons,* pp. 197–221. Elsevier, Amsterdam.

Maixner W and Randich A (1984). Role of the right vagal nerve trunk in antinociception. *Brain Res., 298,* 374–77.

Mantyh PW and Hunt SP (1984). Evidence for cholecystokinin-like immunoreactive neurons in the rat medulla oblongata which project to the spinal cord. *Brain Res., 291,* 49–54.

Marinelli S, Vaughan CW, Schnell SA, Wessendorf MW, and Christie MJ (2002). Rostral ventromedial medulla neurons that project to the spinal cord express multiple opioid receptor phenotypes. *J. Neurosci., 22,* 10847–55.

Martinez V, Christensen D, and Kayser V (2002). The glycine/NMDA receptor antagonist (+)-HA966 enhances the peripheral effect of morphine in neuropathic rats. *Pain, 99,* 537–45.

Mason P (2001). Contributions of the medullary raphe and ventromedial reticular region to pain modulation and other homeostatic functions. *Annu. Rev. Neurosci., 24,* 737–77.

McCreery DB, Bloedel JR, and Hames EA (1979). Effects of stimulating in raphe nuclei and in reticular formation on responses of spinothalamic neurons to mechanical stimuli. *J. Neurophysiol., 42,* 166–82.

McGowan MK and Hammond DL (1993). Antinociception produced by microinjection of L-glutamate into the ventromedial medulla of the rat: mediation by spinal GABA$_A$ receptors. *Brain Res., 620,* 86–96.

McMahon SB and Wall PD (1988). Descending excitation and inhibition of spinal cord lamina I projection neurons. *J. Neurophysiol., 59,* 1204–19.

Miki K, Zhou QQ, Guo W, *et al.* (2002). Changes in gene expression and neuronal phenotype in brain stem pain modulatory circuitry after inflammation. *J. Neurophysiol.,* **87,** 750–60.

Millan MJ (1997). The role of descending noradrenergic and serotoninergic pathways in the modulation of nociception: focus on receptor multiplicity. In (eds. A Dickenson and J–M Besson) *The Pharmacology of Pain,* Vol. 130, pp. 385–446. Springer–Verlag, Berlin.

Millan MJ (2002). Descending control of pain. *Progress in Neurobiology,* **66,** 355–474.

Millhorn DE, Seroogy K, Hökfelt T, *et al.* (1987). Neurons of the ventral medulla oblongata that contain both somatostatin and enkephalin immunoreactivities project to nucleus tractus solitarii and spinal cord. *Brain Res.,* **424,** 99–108.

Minson J, Pilowsky P, Llewellyn–Smith I, Kaneko T, Kapoor V, and Chalmers J (1991). Glutamate in spinally projecting neurons of the rostral ventral medulla. *Brain Res.,* **555,** 326–31.

Moreau JL and Fields HL (1986). Evidence for GABA involvement in midbrain control of medullary neurons that modulate nociceptive transmission. *Brain Res.,* **397,** 37–46.

Nuseir K and Proudfit HK (1999). Modulation of nociception by GABA neurons that tonically inhibit noradrenergic neurons in the A7 cell group. *Soc. Neurosci. Abstr.,* **25,** 1675.

Nuseir K and Proudfit HK (2000). Bidirectional modulation of nociception by GABA neurons in the dorsolateral pontine tegmentum that tonically inhibit spinally-projecting noradrenergic A7 neurons. *Neuroscience,* **96,** 773–83.

Nuseir K, Heidenreich BA, and Proudfit HK (1999). The antinociception produced by microinjection of a cholinergic agonist in the ventromedial medulla is mediated by noradrenergic neurons in the A7 catecholamine cell group. *Brain Res.,* **822,** 1–7.

Oliveras JL, Martin G, Montagne J, and Vos B (1990). Single unit activity at ventromedial medulla level in the awake, freely moving rat: effects of noxious heat and light tactile stimuli onto convergent neurons. *Brain Res.,* **506,** 19–30.

Oliveras JL, Vos B, Martin G, and Montagne J (1989). Electrophysiological properties of ventromedial medulla neurons in response to noxious and non-noxious stimuli in the awake, freely moving rat: a single-unit study. *Brain Res.,* **486,** 1–14.

Pan ZZ, Williams JT, and Osborne PB (1990). Opioid actions on single nucleus raphe magnus neurons from rat and guinea-pig in vitro. *J. Physiol. (Lond.),* **427,** 519–32.

Pazos A and Palacios JM (1985). Quantitative autoradiographic mapping of serotonin receptors in the rat brain. I: serotonin-1 receptors. *Brain Res.,* **346,** 205–30.

Pazos A, Cortes M, and Palacios JM (1985). Quantitative autoradiographic mapping of serotonin receptors in the rat brain. II: serotonin-2 receptors. *Brain Res.,* **346,** 231–45.

Pertovaara A (2000). Plasticity in descending pain modulatory systems. *Prog. Brain Res.,* **129,** 231–42.

Porreca F, Burgess SE, Gardell LR, *et al.* (2001). Inhibition of neuropathic pain by selective ablation of brainstem medullary cells expressing the μ-opioid receptor. *J. Neurosci.,* **21,** 5281–88.

Porreca F, Ossipov MH, and Gebhart GF (2002). Chronic pain and medullary descending facilitation. *Trends Neurosci.,* **25,** 319–25.

Proudfit HK (1988). Pharmacologic evidence for the modulation of nociception by noradrenergic neurons. *Prog. Brain Res.,* **88,** 359–72.

Proudfit HK (1992). The behavioural pharmacology of the noradrenergic descending system. In (ed. J–M Besson) *Toward the Use of Noradrenergic Agonists for the Treatment of Pain,* pp. 119–36. Elsevier, Amsterdam.

Proudfit HK and Clark FM (1991). The projections of locus coeruleus neurons to the spinal cord. *Prog. Brain Res.,* **88,** 123–41.

Randich A and Gebhart GF (1992). Vagal afferent modulation of nociception. *Brain Res. Rev.,* **17,** 77–99.

Randich A and Maixner W (1984). Interactions between cardiovascular and pain regulatory systems. *Neurosci. Biobehav. Rev.,* **8,** 343–67.

Randich A and Maixner W (1986). The role of sinoaortic and cardiopulmonary baroreceptor reflex arcs in nociception and stress-induced analgesia. *Ann. N Y Acad. Sci.*, **467**, 385–401.

Reddy SVR, Maderdrut JL, and Yaksh TL (1980). Spinal cord pharmacology of adrenergic agonist-mediated antinociception. *J. Pharmacol. Exp. Ther.*, **213**, 525–33.

Ren K and Dubner R (2002). Descending modulation in persistent pain: an update. *Pain*, **100**, 1–6.

Ren K, Randich A, and Gebhart GF (1988). Vagal afferent modulation of a nociceptive reflex in rats: involvement of spinal opioid and monoamine receptors. *Brain Res.*, **446**, 285–94.

Reynolds DV (1969). Surgery in the rat during electrical analgesia induced by focal brain stimulation. *Science*, **164**, 444–45.

Richardson DE and Akil H (1977). Pain reduction by electrical brain stimulation in man. Part II: chronic self administration in the periaqueductal gray matter. *J. Neurosurg*, **47**, 184–94.

Sandkühler J (1996). The organization and function of endogenous antinociceptive systems. *Prog. Neurobiol.*, **50**, 49–81.

Sandkühler J and Gebhart GF (1984). Relative contributions of the nucleus raphe magnus and adjacent medullary reticular formation to the inhibition by stimulation in the periaqueductal gray of a spinal nociceptive reflex in the pentobarbital-anesthetized rat. *Brain Res.*, **305**, 77–87.

Schnell C, Ulucan C, and Ellrich J (2002). Atypical on-, off- and neutral cells in the rostral ventromedial medulla oblongata in rat. *Exp. Brain Res.*, **145**, 64–75.

Shannon HE and Lutz EA (2002). Comparison of the peripheral and central effects of the opioid agonists loperamide and morphine in the formalin test in rats. *Neuropharmacology*, **42**, 253–61.

Sherrington CS and Sowton SCM (1915). Observations on reflex responses to single break shocks. *J. Physiol. (Lond.)*, **49**, 331–48.

Smith DJ, Hawranko AA, Monroe PJ, *et al.* (1997). Dose-dependent pain-facilitatory and -inhibitory actions of neurotensin are revealed by SR 48692, a nonpeptide neurotensin antagonist: influence on the antinociceptive effect of morphine. *J. Pharmacol. Exp. Ther.*, **282**, 899–908.

Solomon RE and Gebhart GF (1988). Mechanisms of effects of intrathecal serotonin on nociception and blood pressure in rats. *J. Pharmacol. Exp. Ther.*, **245**, 905–12.

Steinbusch HWM (1981). Distribution of serotonin-immunoreactivity in the central nervous system of the rat. Cell bodies and terminals. *Neuroscience*, **6**, 557–618.

Takano Y and Yaksh TL (1992). Characterization of the pharmacology of intrathecally administered alpha-2 agonists and antagonists in rats. *J. Pharmacol. Exp. Ther.*, **261**, 764–72.

Thomas DA, McGowan MK, and Hammond DL (1995). Microinjection of baclofen in the ventromedial medulla of rats: antinociception at low doses and hyperalgesia at high doses. *J. Pharmacol. Exp. Ther.*, **275**, 274–84.

Urban MO and Gebhart GF (1999). Supraspinal contributions to hyperalgesia. *Proc. Natl. Acad. Sci. USA*, **96**, 7687–92.

Urban MO and Smith DJ (1993). Role of neurotensin in the nucleus raphe magnus in opioid-induced antinociception from the periaqueductal gray. *J. Pharmacol. Exp. Ther.*, **265**, 580–86.

Urban MO, Smith DJ, and Gebhart GF (1996). Involvement of spinal cholecystokinin, receptors in mediating neurotensin hyperalgesia from the medullary nucleus raphe magnus in the rat. *J. Pharmacol. Exp. Ther.*, **278**, 90–96.

van Praag H and Frenk H (1991). The development of stimulation-produced analgesia (SPA) in the rat. *Brain Res. Dev. Brain Res.*, **64**, 71–6.

Wall PD (1967). The laminar organization of dorsal horn and effects of descending impulses. *J. Physiol.*, **188**, 403–23.

Watkins LR and Maier SF (2000). The pain of being sick: implications of immune-to-brain communication for understanding pain. *Annu. Rev. Psychol.*, **51**, 29–57.

Watkins LR and Mayer DJ (1982). Organization of endogenous opiate and nonopiate pain control systems. *Science,* **216,** 1185–92.

West WL, Yeomans DC, and Proudfit HK (1993). The function of noradrenergic neurons in mediating antinociception induced by electrical stimulation of the locus coeruleus in two different sources of Sprague–Dawley rats. *Brain Res.,* **626,** 127–35.

White SR and Fung SJ (1989). Serotonin depolarizes cat spinal motoneurons in situ and decreases motoneuron afterhyperpolarizing potentials. *Brain Res.,* **502,** 205–13.

White SR and Neuman RS (1980). Facilitation of spinal motoneurone excitability by 5-hydroxytryptamine and noradrenaline. *Brain Res.,* **188,** 119–27.

Willis WD (1982). Control of nociceptive transmission in the spinal cord. In (ed. D Ottoson) *Progress in Sensory Physiology,* Vol. 3, pp. 159. Springer–Verlag, New York.

Yaksh TL (1979). Direct evidence that spinal serotonin and noradrenaline terminals mediate the spinal antinociceptive effects of morphine in the periaqueductal gray. *Brain Res.,* **160,** 180–85.

Yaksh TL and Rudy TA (1977). Studies on the direct spinal action of narcotics in the production of analgesia in the rat. *J. Pharmacol. Exp. Ther.,* **202,** 411–28.

Yaksh TL and Rudy TA (1978). Narcotic analgetics: CNS sites and mechanisms of action as revealed by intracerebral injection techniques. *Pain,* **4,** 299–359.

Yaksh TL and Tyce GM (1979). Microinjection of morphine into the periaqueductal gray evokes the release of serotonin from spinal cord. *Brain Res.,* **171,** 176–81.

Yaksh TL and Wilson PR (1979). Spinal serotonin terminal system mediates antinociception. *J. Pharmacol. Exp. Ther.,* **208,** 446–53.

Yeomans DC and Proudfit HK (1990). Projections of substance P-immunoreactive neurons located in the ventromedial medulla to the A7 noradrenergic nucleus of the rat demonstrated using retrograde tracing combined with immunocytochemistry. *Brain Res.,* **532,** 329–32.

Yeomans DC and Proudfit HK (1992). Antinociception induced by microinjection of substance P into the A7 catecholamine cell group in the rat. *Neuroscience,* **49,** 681–91.

Yeomans DC, Clark FM, Paice JA, and Proudfit HK (1992). Antinociception induced by electrical stimulation of spinally-projecting noradrenergic neurons in the A7 catecholamine cell group of the rat. *Pain,* **48,** 449–61.

Zhuo M and Gebhart GF (1990). Characterization of descending inhibition and facilitation from the nucleus reticularis gigantocellularis and gigantocellularis pars alpha in the rat. *Pain,* **42,** 337–50.

Zhuo M and Gebhart GF (1991). Spinal serotonin receptors mediate descending facilitation of a nociceptive reflex from the nuclei reticularis gigantocellularis and gigantocellularis pars alpha in the rat. *Brain Res.,* **550,** 35–48.

Zhuo M and Gebhart GF (2002). Modulation of noxious and non-noxious spinal mechanical transmission from the rostral medial medulla in the rat. *J. Neurophysiol.,* **88,** 2928–41.

Zhuo M, Sengupta JN, and Gebhart GF (2002). Biphasic modulation of spinal visceral nociceptive transmission from the rostroventral medial medulla in the rat. *J. Neurophysiol.,* **87,** 2225–36.

Zieglgänsberger W (1984). Opioid action on mammalian spinal neurons. *Int. Rev. Neurobiol.,* **25,** 243–75.

Zorman G, Belcher G, Adams JE, and Fields HL (1982). Lumbar intrathecal naloxone blocks analgesia produced by microstimulation of the ventromedial medulla in the rat. *Brain Res.,* **236,** 77–84.

Chapter 13

Central imaging of pain

Herta Flor and M. Catherine Bushnell

13.1 Introduction

This chapter concentrates on the representation of pain in the human brain, covering relevant work from neuroelectric and neuromagnetic source imaging (ESI and MSI), functional magnetic resonance imaging (fMRI), magnetic resonance spectroscopy (MRS), positron emission (PET), and single photon emission computed tomography (SPECT) performed in healthy humans during acute pain, as well as studies performed in chronic pain sufferers. The focus is on the central imaging of pain in humans, although animal studies will be included when necessary. Rather than being exhaustive, this chapter will discuss persistent research questions and methodological developments related to imaging the central representation of pain in humans. Comprehensive reviews on this topic can, for example, be found in Treede *et al.* (1999), Casey and Bushnell (2000), Peyron *et al.* (2000), Chen (2001), Jones *et al.* (2002), Petrovic and Ingvar (2002), and Rainville (2002).

13.2 Multidimensionality of the acute pain experience and its neural correlates

Numerous studies have been performed that used various imaging methods to detect the brain regions that are active during acute painful stimulation (e.g. by laser, heat or cold, electric shock, capasicin, or pressure). There is great convergence in these data. In most studies, independent of the imaging method, the insular (IC), secondary somatosensory (SII), and anterior cingulate (ACC) cortices (Brodman areas (BA) 24 and 32) were active, usually bilaterally (e.g. Jones *et al.* 1991; Talbot *et al.* 1991; Kunde and Treede 1993; Coghill *et al.* 1994; 1999; Casey *et al.* 1996; Davis *et al.* 1998, 2002). In many studies, additional areas of activation included primary somatosensory cortex (SI) contralateral to the stimulation, the thalamus, the prefrontal cortex (BA 10, 45, 46, 47), the supplementary motor area, the cerebellum, the basal ganglia (striatum), the peraqueductal gray, the amygdala, the hippocampus, and the posterior parietal cortex (BA 40) (e.g. Jones *et al.* 1991; Coghill *et al.* 1994, 1999; Casey *et al.* 1996; Tölle *et al.* 1999; Bingel *et al.* 2002).

Melzack and Casey (1968) noted that pain has a sensory-discriminative, a motivational-affective, and a cognitive-evaluative component. These components have been separated by imaging studies. Activation in SI has been associated with the sensory-discriminative aspect of pain (Bushnell *et al.* 1999; Hofbauer *et al.* 2001). SI receives inputs from several thalamic nuclei, including ventroposterior lateral (VPL), medial (VPM), and inferior (VPI) nuclei, and has neurons that are responsive to nociceptive stimuli (Kenshalo *et al.* 1988). It is not only active during tactile stimulation but also shows differential activation to increasing intensities of painful stimulation, as a recent fMRI study that used contact-free laser stimuli showed (Bornhövd *et al.* 2002). Activation in SI is linearly related to the intensity of painful stimuli (Coghill *et al.* 1999; Timmermann *et al.* 2001; Bornhövd *et al.* 2002). However, the function of SI in pain processing may be complicated and also involve inhibitory mechanisms (Apkarian *et al.* 1992; Tommerdahl *et al.* 1996). The imaging data are in accordance with primate data showing that firing rates of wide dynamic range neurons in SI are positively correlated with the intensity of the physical stimulus (Kenshalo *et al.* 1988).

SI activation is observed only in about one half of the imaging studies (Bushnell *et al.* 1999; Peyron *et al.* 2000). Based on a meta-analysis, Peyron *et al.* (2000) have suggested that the amount of spatial summation may be a crucial variable for SI activation and that temporal summation may also be important. Moreover, since nociceptive and non-nociceptive neurons are in close proximity, activation of non-nociceptive neurons in the control condition may mask the nociceptive activation (Rainville *et al.* 2000). Also, attentional factors may modulate activity in SI (Bushnell *et al.* 1999).

SII seems to be activated via a direct pathway from the thalamus (Ploner *et al.* 1999*b*) when painful stimulation is used and also has a role in the sensory component of pain. It also receives projections via SI and from non-nociceptive thalamic nuclei. It seems to code the 'painfulness' of the stimulation (e.g. Coghill *et al.* 1999; Treede *et al.* 2000) and is also involved in the temporal coding of the pain experience (Chen *et al.* 2002).

Insular cortex is involved in memory functions, emotional responses, and visceral sensory and motor integration, and is unlikely to be a structure specific to the processing of painful stimulation. It has, however, been consistently activated in imaging studies of pain (see Treede *et al.* 2000) and seems to have a complicated role in pain processing. In primates there is a direct projection from nociceptive regions of the thalamus to the insular cortex (Dostrovsky and Craig 1996), and nociceptive activity has been recorded in humans (Frot and Mauguiere 2003). Coghill *et al.* (1999) observed a systematic relationship between the intensity of painful heat stimuli and IC activation, and Craig *et al.* (2000) observed a similar correlation between IC activity and intensity of cold stimuli, suggesting that IC may be involved in coding of noxious and innocuous temperature. Nevertheless, other data indicate that IC activity may be important in pain affect. Insular lesions are sometimes characterized by the condition of pain asymbolia, in which pain sensations appear to be normal but behaviorial and physiological responses to the offending stimulus are inappropriate (Berthier *et al.* 1988). Both animal and human studies implicate IC in autonomic control (Oppenheimer *et al.* 1996;

Verberne and Owens 1998), and Craig (2002) has suggested that pain-related responses in this region are related to homeostasis and maintaining the sense of self.

The anterior cingulate cortex (ACC) has sensory, affective, and cognitive subdivisions (Devinsky *et al.* 1995) and has been associated with both affective and cognitive aspects of the pain experience. Specifically, a midcingulate caudal 'cognitive' part with projections to the lateral prefrontal and motor areas and a ventral perigenual cingulate 'emotional' part have been identified. The midcingulate region is activated in most pain imaging studies (Peyron *et al.* 2000), and nociceptive neurons have been identified there in patients undergoing neurosurgical procedures (Hutchison *et al.* 1999). An adjacent region of ACC appears to be involved in attentional processes and may interact with ACC pain processing (Davis *et al.* 1997, 2000; Kwan *et al.* 2000). Activation in the rostral part may be associated with anticipation of pain (Ploghaus *et al.* 1999) and the emotional evaluation of the pain experience, since cingulotomy preferentially reduces the emotional component of pain.

Single unit studies in rabbits show that ACC nociceptive neurons have large, usually bilateral receptive fields, further indicating that this region is unlikely to code pain location (Sikes and Vogt 1992). In a study on the 'thermal grill illusion', where alternating warm and cold bars create the experience of pain without peripheral nociceptive input, ACC activation was only found when pain was experienced (Craig *et al.* 1996). The aversiveness of pain is positively correlated with activation in the mid- or posterior ACC (Rainville *et al.* 1997; Tölle *et al.* 1999; Büchel *et al.* 2002). However, attentional effects also increase activation in the mid-ACC, thus confirming the view that the ACC is a multi-integrative structure (Peyron *et al.* 2000).

Rainville *et al.* (1997) used hypnotic instructions to vary the level of unpleasantness of a painful thermal stimulus, and PET to record cerebral activations. They found a highly significant correlation between the level of unpleasantness and activation of the ACC, whereas the activation level of SI was unaffected by the affective variation of pain. In a complementary study, Hofbauer *et al.* (2001) used hypnotic instructions to increase or decrease perceived pain intensity and found significant changes in SI using PET. These studies suggest that the sensory-discriminative component of pain is preferentially coded in the somatosensory cortex, whereas affective processing of pain is associated more with activity in ACC (Fig. 13.1). These imaging data were confirmed by a case report in which a patient had sustained a lesion in the postcentral gyrus and parietal operculum (SI and SII) due to stroke. This patient could no longer discriminate pain location or intensity but had preserved pain affect (Ploner *et al.* 1999a).

Several studies have shown that psychological factors such as attention, anticipation, or anxiety can influence pain perception as well as the central representation of pain. These variables may be viewed as the correlate of the central control or cognitive-evaluative dimension of pain originally proposed by Melzack and Casey (1968). The effects of attention on pain have been known for a long time and have been used in cognitive-behavioral pain treatment programs (Turk 1983). Imaging studies confirm that attentional demands alter activity in pain pathways. For example, Bushnell *et al.* (1999)

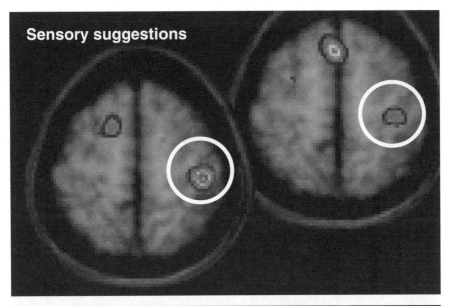

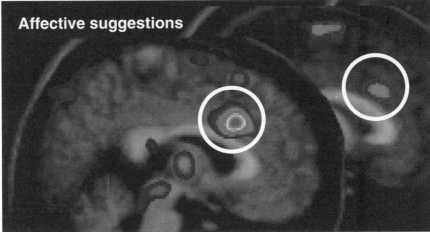

Fig. 13.1 Pain-evoked activation in SI and ACC during equally intense noxious heat stimuli applied to the hand. **(Top)** SI activation during hypnotic suggestions of high pain intensity (left) and low pain intensity (right). Despite the equally intense physical stimulus, SI was significantly more activated when subjects perceived it as more intense (from Hofbauer *et al.* 2001). **(Bottom)** ACC activation during hypnotic suggestions of high pain unpleasantness (left) and low pain unpleasantness (right). The suggestions for pain unpleasantness, but not those for pain intensity, produced a significant modulation of pain-evoked ACC activation (from Rainville *et al.* 1997).

showed, using PET, that pain-evoked activation in SI cortex was greater when subjects were required to attend to the pain than when they were required to attend to the simultaneously presented auditory stimulus. Similarly, Bantick *et al.* (2002) used fMRI to examine how attention to versus distraction from pain affects its central processing. Subjects either had to attend to the intensity of the painful stimulus or were distracted by a cognitively demanding counting Stroop task. Cognitive distraction reduced activation in a number of areas such as the thalamus, the insula, and the cognitive division of the ACC. Increased activation was found in the affective division of the ACC and orbito-frontal regions. The authors concluded that these activation patterns were due to a synergistic effect of pain and distraction. Davis *et al.* (1997) found that pain and attention activate non-overlapping separate portions of the posterior and anterior ACC, respectively. Finally, Tracey *et al.* (2002) showed that the periaqueductal gray, an area important for opioid analgesia, is also involved in attentional control and, thus, cognitive functions related to pain.

Anticipation of pain is another variable that may greatly influence the subsequent processing of noxious stimulation. Sawamoto *et al.* (2000) found that the expectation of pain enhanced the response to non-painful stimuli in ACC and SII. Further, Porro *et al.* (2002), examining the anticipation of pain related to a subcutaneous injection of ascorbic acid, found a significant positive relationship between later pain ratings and anticipatory activation in the SI, ACC, IC, and medial prefrontal cortex. Less pain was associated with bilateral activation in the anteroventral and perigenual cingulate cortices. Interestingly, anticipation of pain led to a somatotopic activation of SI cortex. Ploghaus *et al.* (1999) and Ploghaus and Tracey (2001) observed that the anticipation of pain activated very similar brain regions as the experience of pain itself, although the foci of activation were adjacent. The regions involved in pain experience were the caudal ACC, the mid-insula, and the anterior cerebellum, whereas anticipation of pain activated the anterior medial frontal cortex, the anterior insula, and the posterior cerebellum.

Activation in the dorsolateral prefrontal cortex and the intraparietal sulcus may be related to attention and working memory (Coghill *et al.* 1999; Peyron *et al.* 1999; Bornhövd *et al.* 2002; Strigo *et al.* in press), irrespective of painful or non-painful stimulation. Amygdala activation has been found to be associated with the expectation of pain and may be related to fear of pain (e.g. Ploghaus *et al.* 1999; Bornhövd *et al.* 2002). The hippocampus may also have a role in pain processing, particularly in relation to attentional and emotional factors in the anticipation of pain (Ploghaus and Tracey 2001; Bantick *et al.* 2002).

Activation in the cerebellum, the red nucleus, and the putamen has been related to the production of motor withdrawal responses (or their inhibition), and seem to be mainly lateralized to the side contralateral to the stimulation (Bingel *et al.* 2002). However, Becerra *et al.* (2001) showed that several brain regions such as the basal forebrain, the ventral tegmentum/periaqueductal gray, the ventral striatum, and the nucleus accumbens were differentially activated to painful stimulation, suggesting that neural circuitries involved in punishment/reward are also active during painful stimulation.

The medial thalamic nuclei are also activated by painful stimulation in many studies (e.g. Tracey *et al.* 2000) and may reflect not only a sensory response but also an arousal reaction to pain, since attentional processes can enhance medial thalamic activation (Bushnell and Duncan 1989).

Finally, there is fMRI evidence that the orbito-frontal cortex is involved in the emotional processing of pain (Rolls *et al.* 2003). Activation in this area is generally difficult to detect in fMRI studies due to susceptibility artifacts in this region, and thus has not been studied extensively.

13.3 **The central representation of chronic pain**

One difficulty in assessing chronic pain in imaging studies is the lack of controllability. Several methods have been introduced to analyze the processing of pain in chronic pain patients. Apkarian *et al.* (2001) used two strategies to study changes in event-related fMRI in patients with chronic pain. In one experiment finger-span scaling was used to record spontaneous fluctuations of chronic pain. In another experiment pain intensity was modulated by a straight leg-raising procedure in patients suffering from chronic back pain. Other studies have induced acute pain and observed to what extent the processing of these stimuli differs between chronic pain patients and healthy controls (e.g. Derbyshire *et al.* 2002; Gracely *et al.* 2002).

Di Piero *et al.* (1991) used PET to determine pain-related activation patterns in patients with cancer pain and found, as the most prominent characteristic, decreased rCBF in the thalamus. In a subsequent study, patients who underwent cordotomy, with substantial pain relief, were tested and reversal of this activation pattern was observed. The reduced activation in the thalamus in states of chronic pain and its increase related to effective treatment was confirmed in several other studies of neuropathic pain conditions (e.g. Hsieh *et al.* 1995; Iadarola *et al.* 1995; Duncan *et al.* 1998).

Several studies have examined central activation patterns in fibromyalgia syndrome (FMS). Mountz *et al.* (1999) reviewed PET and SPECT studies in FMS and came to the conclusion that the most prominent finding in chronic patients is a reduced activation in the thalamus. In addition, FMS patients showed reduced blood flow in the region of the caudate nucleus. The authors related these reduced activations to hypersensitivity of spinal cord neurons. Using fMRI, Gracely *et al.* (2002) reported a marked hyperreactivity to painful stimulation in a number of brain regions including SI cortex in fibromyalgia patients (Fig. 13.2). These data are in accordance with previous EEG studies that examined laser-related evoked responses and found enhanced activity of the long-latency components in FMS patients (Gibson *et al.* 1994; Lorenz *et al.* 1996).

Silvermann *et al.* (1997) found that painful colorectal distention in irritable bowel syndrome patients did not activate the ACC as in healthy controls, but activation was found in the left prefrontal cortex (BA10), suggesting that chronic pain might activate other brain regions than does experimental pain. Grachev *et al.* (2000) used proton magnetic resonance spectroscopy to determine to what extent abnormal brain chemistry is

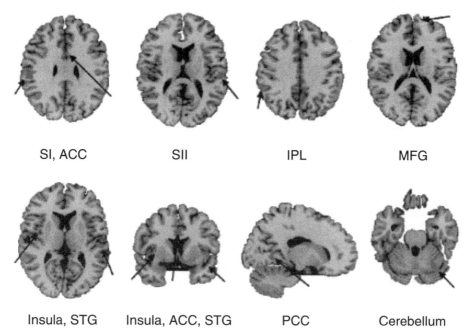

| SI, ACC | SII | IPL | MFG |

| Insula, STG | Insula, ACC, STG | PCC | Cerebellum |

Fig. 13.2 Comparison of the effects of similar stimulus pressures in patients and controls. Results of unpaired *t*-tests of the mean difference in signal (arrows) between pain pressure and innocuous touch for each group are shown in standard space superimposed on an anatomic image of a standard brain. Images are shown in radiologic view, with the right brain shown on the left. Regions in which the response in patients was significantly greater than the response in controls are shown in red; regions in which the response in controls was significantly greater than that in patients are shown in green. The level of significance was adjusted for multiple comparisons at $P < 0.05$. Patients showed significant activations that were markedly different from those in the healthy controls in the primary somatosensory cortex (SI), inferior parietal lobe (IPL), insula, posterior cingulate cortex (PCC), secondary somatosensory cortex (SII), superior temporal gyrus (STG), and cerebellum. The peak of the significant difference in anterior cingulate cortex (ACC) is in the right hemisphere, although the activation is near the midline and spreads into both hemispheres. Significant increases in the contralateral STG and in a second region of ipsilateral cerebellum are not shown. In contrast to these regions of greater signal differences in patients, similar stimulus pressures resulted in one region of significantly increased stimulus intensity in control subjects, located in the medial frontal gyrus (MFG). (From Gracely *et al.* 2002, with permission.) See plate section, Plate 4 (centre of book) for a colour version.

present in the anterior cingulate, the thalamus, or the prefrontal cortex. They observed reduced levels of N-acetyl aspartate and glucose in the dorsolateral prefrontal cortex in patients with chronic low back pain.

A number of studies have examined the central correlates of headache. Weiller *et al.* (1995) found activation of the cingulate cortex, the auditory and visual association cortices, as well as an area in the dorsal midbrain that included the periaqueductal gray and dorsolateral pontine tegmentum, including the nucleus ceruleus, related to migraine attacks without aura. These activations seem to be specific for migraine headaches (e.g. May *et al.* 2000). In cluster headache, by contrast, the posterior hypothalamus may play a special role (e.g. May and Goadsby 2001).

The neural correlates of allodynia have been examined in patients with neuropathic pain and in normal subjects, using capsaicin-provoked allodynia. Some data suggest that allodynia, whether related to neuropathic pain or capsaicin application, is processed differently in the cerebral cortex than is nociceptive pain. Witting *et al.* (2001), using a capsaicin-evoked tactile allodynia, found an allodynia-specific activation in parietal association cortex (BA5/7). Lorenz *et al.* (2002), comparing heat pain and thermal allodynia in a PET study, found allodynia-specific activations in the medial thalamus, putamen, and prefrontal cortex. Further, whereas the ACC is almost always activated in PET or fMRI studies of nociceptive pain, Peyron *et al.* (1998, 2000) failed to find ACC activation during allodynia in central pain patients. Similarly, Baron *et al.* (1999) also did not observe ACC activation when examining dynamic tactile allodynia during a capsaicin model in normal subjects and suggested that Aβ-mediated pain has a unique cortical presentation. Nevertheless, other data do not support this interpretation, but rather suggest that pain arising from aberrant or normal processes ultimately activates the same cortical structures. For example, Iadarola *et al.* (1998) reported ACC activation during dynamic tactile allodynia after capsaicin injection in normal subjects. Similarly, Petrovic *et al.* (1999) showed ACC activation related to dynamic tactile allodynia in a neuropathic pain patient.

13.4 **Cortical plasticity and chronic pain**

In the last two decades, our understanding of the modifiability of the primary sensory and motor areas of the brain has greatly changed. Whereas it was previously assumed that plastic changes in these cortical areas are limited to an early period in development, it is now accepted that substantial plastic changes of the primary cortical areas occur throughout life.

Cortical reorganization has been observed as a consequence of both injury and stimulation (for review see Kaas 2000; Recanzone 2000). For example, in the owl monkey, the amputation of a digit leads to a 'take-over' of the cortical representation zone of this digit by neuronal input from adjacent digits (Merzenich *et al.* 1984). This 'shift' of neighboring areas into the amputation zone develops over the course of several weeks and might be due to the unmasking of normally inhibited connections as well as the sprouting of new axonal connections (Florence *et al.* 1998). An even larger cortical reorganization was observed by Pons *et al.* (1991) in the macaque monkey subsequent to longstanding dorsal rhizotomies. Here, the representation of the face 'invaded' the representation of the deafferented arm and hand — a shift that was in the range of several centimeters and that is probably related to altered thalamocortical projections (Jones and Pons 1998).

Cortical representation zones are not only altered by injury but also by behaviorally relevant stimulation and training. For example, Jenkins *et al.* (1990) observed that sensory discrimination training of individual fingers led to an expansion of the cortical representation zone of the trained fingers. This change occurred only if the training was behaviorally relevant and was not observed after passive stimulation.

13.4.1 Chronic pain and cortical reorganization

Animal models have shown that long-lasting and/or intense states of pain (e.g. when an inflammation is present) lead to the sensitization of spinal cord neurons (e.g. Woolf and Salter 2000) as well as an altered representation of the painful area in the thalamus (Vos *et al.* 2000) and the cortex (Benoist *et al.* 1999). In chronic pain patients, hyperreactivity to tactile or noxious stimuli was also observed (e.g. Lorenz *et al.* 1996; Kleinböhl *et al.* 1999). Although peripheral as well as spinal and thalamic mechanisms have been implicated in some of these changes in nociception, cortical changes might also play a role in these alterations in nociceptive sensitivity.

Flor *et al.* (1997) reported elevated responses to painful and non-painful tactile stimulation as assessed by magnetencephalography in chronic back pain patients. Stimulation at the affected site of the back, but not at the finger, led to a significantly higher magnetic field in the time window less than 100 msec, whereas both types of stimulation caused higher fields in the later time windows in patients compared to controls. This hyperreactivity of the somatosensory system increased with chronicity. When the source of this early activity was localized, it was shown to originate from SI. Whereas the localization of the fingers was not significantly different between patients and controls, the localization of the back was more inferior and medial in the patients, indicating a shift and expansion toward the cortical representation of the leg. These data suggest that chronic pain leads to an expansion of the cortical representation zone related to nociceptive input, much like the expansions of cortical representations that have been documented to occur with other types of behaviorally relevant stimulation. Nociceptive input is of high relevance for the organism, and it might be useful to enhance the representation of this type of stimulation to prepare the organism for the adequate response. The amount of expansion of the back region was positively correlated with chronicity suggesting that this pain-related cortical reorganization develops over time.

This type of cortical alteration may correspond to what Katz and Melzack (1990) have termed a 'somatosensory pain memory' in phantom limb pain patients. Although they referred mainly to explicit memories (i.e. the patients' recollection that the phantom pain was similar to previously experienced pains), somatosensory memories can also be implicit. Implicit pain memories are based on changes in the brain that are not open to conscious awareness but lead to behavioral and perceptual changes of which the patient is not aware, such as hyperalgesia and allodynia. It is therefore impossible for the patient to counteract these pain memories. This type of memory trace may lead to pain perception in the absence of peripheral stimulation, since an expansion of a representational zone is related to higher acuity in the perception of tactile input.

Similar alterations in the cortical processing of sensory information were recently reported in patients with complex regional pain syndrome (Juottonen *et al.* 2002).

These reorganizational processes are also modifiable by cognitive and affective processes. For example, Buchner *et al.* (1999) showed that attention modifies the somatotopic map in SI cortex. Flor *et al.* (2002) reported that verbal reinforcement of increased or decreased pain ratings leads to a persistence of elevated pain ratings in chronic pain patients that are accompanied by an elevated electrocortical response originating in SII cortex. It would be interesting to further explore these learning-related changes in the central representation of pain, because they might play an important role in the maintenance of these problems.

13.4.2 Phantom limb pain and cortical reorganization

As noted above, not only enduring nociceptive input but also the loss of input (e.g. subsequent to amputation or nerve injury) can alter the cortical map. Several studies examined cortical reorganization after amputation in humans. These studies were inspired by the report of Ramachandran *et al.* (1992) that phantom sensation could be elicited in upper extremity amputees when they were stimulated on the face. There was a point-to-point correspondence between stimulation sites on the face and the localization of sensation in the phantom. Moreover, the sensations in the phantom matched the modality of the stimulation (e.g. warmth was perceived as a warm phantom sensation, painful touch was perceived as pain). The authors assumed that this phenomenon might be the perceptual correlate of the type of reorganization previously described in animal experiments. The invasion of the cortical hand or arm area by the mouth representation might lead to activity in the cortical amputation zone that would be projected into the no longer present limb. Subsequently, Elbert *et al.* (1994) used a combination of magnetoencephalographic recordings and structural MRI to test this hypothesis. They observed a significant shift of the mouth representation into the zone that formerly represented the now amputated hand or arm; however, this shift occurred in patients with and without phantom sensation referred from the mouth.

Flor *et al.* (1995) showed that phantom limb pain rather than referred sensation was the perceptual correlate of these cortical reorganizational changes. Patients with phantom limb pain displayed a significant shift of the mouth into the hand representation, whereas this was not the case in patients without phantom limb pain. The intensity of phantom limb pain was significantly positively correlated with the amount of displacement of the mouth representation. It was later shown that referred sensations, such as those described by Ramachandran *et al.* (1992), can also be elicited from areas far removed from the amputated limb (e.g. from the foot in arm amputees). It was concluded that alterations in the organization of S1 — where arm and foot are represented far apart — are most likely not the neuronal substrate of referred phantom sensations (Flor *et al.* 2000; Grüsser *et al.* in press).

Similar results were obtained when the motor cortex was investigated. For example, an fMRI study where upper extremity amputees had to perform pursing lip movements showed that the representation of the lip in primary motor cortex had also shifted into the area that formerly occupied the amputated hand (Lotze *et al.* 1999, 2001) (see Fig. 13.3). The magnitude of this shift was also highly significantly correlated with the amount of phantom limb pain experienced by the patients, thus suggesting parallel processes in the somatosensory and motor system. A high concordance of changes in the somatosensory and the motor system was reported by Karl *et al.* (2001), who used transcranial magnetic stimulation to map the motor cortex and neuroelectric source imaging (that combines the determination of cortical sources by evoked potential recordings with structural MRI) to map the somatosensory cortex. This close interconnection of changes in the somatosensory and motor system suggests that rehabilitative efforts directed at one modality may also affect the other.

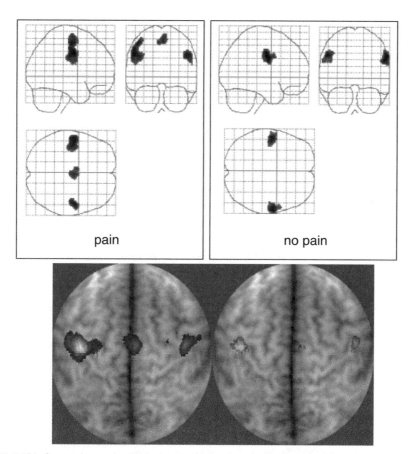

Fig. 13.3 This figure shows the SPM glass brain **(top)** and superimposed functional and structural imaging data of groups of phantom limb pain patients **(left)** and amputees without pain **(right)** during lip pursing. Note that the lip movement not only activates the cortical representation zone of the lip but also that of the hand in the patients with pain, but not in the pain-free amputees.

The close association between cortical alterations and phantom limb pain was further underscored by Birbaumer *et al.* (1997). In upper limb amputees, anesthesia of the brachial plexus led to the elimination of phantom limb pain in about 50% of the amputees, whereas phantom limb pain remained unchanged in the other half. Neuroelectric source imaging revealed that cortical reorganization was also reversed in those amputees who showed a reduction of phantom limb pain. Patients who continued to have phantom limb pain during the elimination of sensory input from the residual limb had an even more reorganized mouth representation. These data suggest that in some patients peripheral factors might be important in the maintenance of phantom limb pain, whereas in others, pain and reorganizational processes might have become independent of peripheral input.

As Devor (1997) and others have pointed out, it is, to date, not clear on which level of the neuraxis the cortical changes that have been observed in imaging studies originate. In addition to intracortical changes, alterations might be present in the dorsal root ganglion, the dorsal horn, the brainstem, or the thalamus. Recent imaging studies (e.g. Willoch *et al.* 2000) have also shown that not only SI, SII, and posterior parietal cortex, but also regions such as IC and ACC, are involved in the processing of phantom phenomena. In animal studies, additional reorganizational changes have also been observed in ACC (Wei and Zhuo 2001).

Based on these findings, Flor (2002) has suggested that phantom limb pain might be related to the establishment of central traces of ongoing nociceptive input that become activated when the deafferentation and the subsequent reorganization occur. Huse *et al.* (in press) found that chronic pain before the amputation significantly predicted phantom limb pain one year after the surgery. Interventions aimed at reducing cortical reorganization by providing behaviorally relevant input to the reorganized cortical representation zone have subsequently been found efficacious (Lotze *et al.* 1999; Flor *et al.* 2001). Likewise, the prevention of phantom limb pain seems to be possible when an NMDA receptor antagonist which prevents reorganizational change is given early in the postoperative phase (Wiech *et al.* 2001).

To summarize, somatosensory pain represented by alterations in the topographic map of SI cortex may underlie the development of phantom limb pain. Longstanding states of chronic pain prior to the amputation may be instrumental in the formation of these pain memories by inducing representational and excitability changes. Deafferentation does not alter the original assignment of cortical representation zones to peripheral input zones, and leads to double coding. Peripheral factors such as loss of C-fiber activity, spontaneous activity from neuroma, or psychophysiological activation may also influence the cortical representational changes.

13.5 Central imaging of the therapeutic modulation of pain

Both pharmacological and non-pharmacological interventions have been studied in their effects on the central processing of pain. Casey *et al.* (2000) used PET imaging to study the changes in rCBF related to the administration of the opioid, fentanyl.

Fentanyl reduced the subjective intensity of pain related to cold water and reduced, simultaneously, activation in all cortical and thalamic areas. Increased activation was, however, found in the perigenual region of the ACC, suggesting that it may mediate opioid analgesia. Vibratory stimuli and their cortical activation patterns were unaffected by fentanyl.

Recently, Petrovic *et al.* (2002) used remifentanyl versus placebo to induce opioid and placebo analgesia in a PET study and found involvement of the rostral ACC in both types of pain reduction. In addition, a close interaction was found between activation in the ACC and the brainstem, and some activation was observed in the lateral orbito-frontal cortex. Altered occupation of mu-opioid receptors was examined using carfentanil in a PET study with healthy volunteers during acute muscle pain (Zubieta *et al.* 2001). Activation of mu-opioid receptors was found in a number of brain regions including the dorsal ACC, IC, lateral prefrontal cortex, thalamus, hypothalamus, and amygdala. The highest correlations between reduced pain ratings and opiod receptor activation were found in the nucleus accumbens, the thalamus, and the amygdala.

Other studies examined the effects of thalamic stimulation on rCBF (e.g. Duncan *et al.* 1998; Davis *et al.* 2000). Duncan *et al.* (1998) found increased activation in SI and anterior IC, a region activated by thermal stimulation (Craig *et al.* 2000). Davis *et al.* (2000) observed activation in ACC during thalamic stimulation. Activation of thermal pathways is possibly involved in analgesia produced by thalamic stimulation — an idea supported by the report of both tingling paresthesias and thermal sensation induced by thalamic stimulation in some patients and a vast literature suggesting that activation of thermal pathways modulates pain (e.g. Strigo *et al.* 2000). The emotional or attentional modulation of pain might, however, be an additional factor, since such factors modulate nociceptive input into cortical pain regions (Bushnell *et al.* 1999; Bushnell and Villemure 2002). Studies on motor cortex stimulation found increased activation of several thalamic nuclei and limbic regions, suggesting that activation of non-nociceptive pathways might inhibit nociceptive neurons (Peyron *et al.* 1995; Garcia–Larrea *et al.* 1997, 1999).

Hsieh *et al.* (2001) used PET to examine the central effect of acupuncture and reported specifically increased activation in the hypothalamus as well as the ACC, midbrain, IC, and cerebellum, with the best correlation between hypothalamic activity and acupuncture sensation. Another study (Biella *et al.* 2001) found activation in several areas related to pain processing, but not the hypothalamus.

13.6 **Summary and conclusions**

The current literature on the imaging of acute pain shows that sensory, affective, and cognitive components of pain are represented by different but interacting networks in the brain. Many of the inconsistencies in the imaging literature may be related to insufficient attention to procedural variations between studies that may differentially engage these networks. For example, anticipation of pain and its emotional processing

---

Box 13.1 **Inducing and measuring pain in humans**

Pain induction methods

Studies that focus on acute pain in humans use a variety of stimulation methods to induce pain perception. One of the most frequently used methods is the induction of heat or cold pain via a *contact thermode*. The disadvantage of this method is that it also stimulates Aβ fibers. This disadvantage can be overcome by the use of CO_2 laser stimuli that can selectively activate Aδ and C fibers.

Experimental pain assessment in humans

The most commonly used instruments in pain assessment are visual analogue or numeric rating scales. In order to separately assess affective and sensory components of pain, the short form of the McGill Pain Questionnaire or separate scales for the unpleasantness and the intensity of pain are used.

Quantitative sensory testing

This refers to psychophysical evaluations of altered pain sensation in patients as compared to healthy controls. Most commonly, perception thresholds (when is a stimulus first perceived?), pain thresholds (when is it first perceived as painful?), and (in some cases) pain tolerance (when is a stimulus unbearably painful?) are assessed for mechanical and thermal stimuli. Additional assessments may involve two-point discrimination as a measure of receptive field size and measurements of sensitization (where a series of stimuli is given and the slope of the increase in pain intensity ratings is determined). In patients, determination of allodynia and hyperalgesia can be performed using mechanical and thermal stimulation.

---

may vary depending on the temporal and spatial distribution of the painful stimulation, instructions, and concurrent tasks, as well as the amount of control a subject has over the painful stimulation. One important task in future pain-imaging studies will be to precisely delineate these modulating factors and their underlying neural correlates. Pain not only involves affective, sensory, and cognitive components, but also a motor component that initiates pain-related action. This important pain-related response has so far not been examined sufficiently.

Although hampered by insufficient control over the underlying stimulus, imaging studies of chronic pain have shown that it seems to lead to distinct alterations in the cerebral pain-related networks, most notably, reduced activation in the thalamus and additional engagement of frontal cortical areas. There is also evidence that chronic pain leads to enhanced activation as well as somatotopic reorganization in SI cortex as well as other brain regions. These pain-related somatosensory memories may be instrumental in maintaining and exacerbating chronic pain. In phantom limb pain, pre-existing pain experiences and their central correlates may be a major

Box 13.2 **Imaging pain in humans**

Imaging methods in humans can be differentiated by the underlying physiological process they measure. **Electroencephalographic (EEG)** and **magnetoencephalographic (MEG)** recordings measure the neuronal activity related to painful stimulation. They thus reflect, directly, excitatory and inhibitory neuronal processes. They also have the advantage that they have a very high time resolution (in the msec range) and can thus adequately capture the dynamics of the central processing of pain. When multi-channel EEG or MEG recordings are combined with source analysis methods that often involve the co-registration of structural magnetic resonance images, the terms **neuroelectric (ESI)** or **neuromagnetic (MSI)** source imaging are used. They can be used to localize the brain regions that are active during nociceptive processing. However, they show much lower spatial resolution than the methods that are based on hemodynamic responses. They are also limited to processes readily recordable from the surface of the scalp. They do, however, have a high temporal resolution and can thus trace the method of information processing. Positron emission tomography (PET), single photon emission computed tomography (SPECT), and functional magnetic resonance imaging (fMRI) are methods that make use of the fact that neuronal changes are coupled with alteration in blood flow in the respective region. PET and SPECT involve the measurement of radioactively labeled molecules that are injected or inhaled. They measure regional blood flow. The most commonly used tracer in PET studies is ^{15}O-water with a relatively short half-life of 124 seconds that permits multiple scans. The advantage of PET is that the relationship of the signal and the physiological mechanism is known. Disadvantages are the relatively low temporal resolution and the need for group data, as well as the need to use a radioactive tracer. Compared to PET, SPECT uses technetium radiotracers with a long half-life that make it impossible to use repeat scans on the same day. It also has lower sensitivity and spatial resolution. fMRI uses changes based on blood oxygenation. The signal contrast used has thus been termed the BOLD (blood oxygen level dependent) contrast. fMRI assessments have a better temporal resolution (in the range of seconds) than the PET assessments and they can be repeated many times. In addition, individual analyses can be performed: group data are not absolutely necessary to draw conclusions. However, the relationship of the BOLD signal and neuronal activity is still under investigation.

pain-generating mechanism. Learning processes may further alter and enhance these pain-related memory traces.

Major knowledge about the processing of pain and the mechanisms of algesia and analgesia are now coming from studies that examine the effects of pharmacological, surgical, and other therapeutic procedures on activation of pain-related networks.

Acknowledgement

Supported by grants from the Deutsche Forschungsgemeinschaft and the Max Planck Research Award for International Cooperation to H.F., and Canadian Institutes of Health Research and the US National Institutes of Health to M.C.B.

References

Apkarian AV, Krauss BR, Fredrickson BE, and Szeverenyi MM (2001). Imaging the pain of low back pain: functional magnetic resonance imaging in combination with monitoring subjective pain perception allows the study of clinical pain states. *Neuroscience Letters*, **299**, 57–60.

Apkarian AV, Stea RA, Manglos SH, Szeverenyi NM, King RB, and Thomas FD (1992). Persistent pain inhibits contralateral somatosensory cortical activity in humans. *Neuroscience Letters*, **140**, 141–147.

Bantick SJ, Wise RG, Ploghaus A, Clare S, Smith SM, and Tracey I (2002). Imaging: how attention modulates pain in humans using functional MRI. *Brain*, **125**, 310–319.

Baron R, Baron Y, Disbrow E, and Roberts TP (1999). Brain processing of capsaicin-induced secondary hyperalgesia: a functional MRI study. *Neurology*, **53**, 548–557.

Becerra L, Breiter HC, Wise R, Gonzales RG, and Borsook D (2001). Reward circuitry activation by noxiuos thermal stimuli. *Neuron*, **32**, 927–946.

Benoist JM, Gautron M, and Guilbaud G (1999). Experimental model of trigeminal pain in the rat by constriction of one infraorbital nerve: changes in neuronal activities in the somatosensory cortices corresponding to the infraorbital nerve. *Experimental Brain Research*, **126**, 383–398.

Berthier M, Starkstein S, Leiguarda R (1988). Asymbolia for pain; a sensory-limbic disconnection syndrome. *Annals of Neurology*, **24**, 41–49.

Biella G, Sotgiu ML, Pellegata G, Paulesu E, Castiglioni I, and Fazio F (2001). Acupuncture produces central activations in pain regions. *Neuroimage*, **14**, 60–66.

Bingel U, Quante Q, Knab R, Bromm B, Weiller C, and Büchel C (2002). Subcortical structures involved in pain processing: evidence from single-trial fMRI. *Pain*, **99**, 313–321.

Birbaumer N, Lutzenberger W, Montoya P, *et al.* (1997). Effects of regional anesthesia on phantom limb pain are mirrored in changes in cortical reorganization. *Journal of Neuroscience*, **17**, 5503–5508.

Bornhövd K, Quante M, Glauche V, Bromm B, Weiller C, and Büchel C (2002). Painful stimuli evoke different stimulus–response functions in the amygdala, prefrontal, insula and somatosensory cortex: a single trial fMRI study. *Brain*, **125**, 1326–1336.

Büchel C, Bornhövd K, Quante M, Glauche V, Bromm B, and Weiller C (2002). Dissociable neural response related to pain intensity, stimulus intensity and stimulus awareness within the anterioir cingulate cortex: a parametric single trial laser functional magnetic resonance imaging study. *Journal of Neuroscience*, **22**, 970–976.

Buchner H, Reinhartz U, Waberski TD, Gobbele R, Noppeney U, and Scherg M (1999). Sustained attention modulates the immediate effect of deafferentation on the cortical representation of the digits: source localization of somatosensory evoked potentials in humans. *Neuroscience Letters*, **260**, 57–60.

Bushnell MC and Duncan GH (1989). Sensory and affective aspects of pain perception: is medial thalamus restricted to emotional issues? *Experimental Brain Research*, **78**, 415–418.

Bushnell MC and Villemure C (2002). Cognitive modulation of pain: how do attention and emotion influence pain processing? *Pain*, **95**, 195–199.

Bushnell MC, Duncan GH, Hofbauer RK, Ha B, Chen JL, and Carrier B (1999). Pain perception: is there a role for primary somatosensory cortex? *Proceedings of the National Academy of Sciences USA*, **96**, 7705–7709.

Casey KL and Bushnell MC (2000). *Pain imaging.* IASP Press, Seattle.

Casey KL, Minoshima S, Morrow TJ, and Koeppe RA (1996). Comparison of human cerebral activation patterns during cutaneous warmth, heat pain, and deep cold pain. *Journal of Neurophysiology,* **76**, 571–581.

Casey KL, Svensson P, Morrow TJ, Raz J, Jone C, Minoshima S (2000). Selective opiate modulation of nociceptive processing in the human brain. *Journal of Neurophysiology*, **84**, 525–533.

Chen AC (2001). New perspectives in EEG/MEG brain mapping and PET/fMRI neuroimaging of human pain. *International Journal of Psychophysiology*, **42**, 147–159.

Chen JI, Ha B, Bushnell MC, Pike B, Duncan GH (2002). Differentiating noxious- and innocuous-related activation of human somatosensory cortices using temporal analysis of fMRI. *Journal of Neurophysiology*, **10**, 464–474.

Coghill RC, Sang CN, Maisong JM, and Iadarola MJ (1999). Pain intensity processing within the human brain: a bilateral, distributed mechanism. *Journal of Neurophysiology*, **82**,1934–1943.

Coghill RC, Talbot JD, Evans AC, *et al.* (1994). Distributed processing of pain and vibration by the human brain. *Journal of Neuroscience*, **14**, 4095–4108.

Craig AD (2002). How do you feel? interoception: the sense of physiological condition of the body. *Nature Review Neuroscience*, **3**, 655–666.

Craig AD, Chen L, Brandy D, and Reiman EM (2000). Thermosensory activation of insular cortex. *Nature Neuroscience*, **3**, 184–190.

Craig AD, Reimann EM, Evans A, and Bushnell MC (1996). Functional imaging of an illusion of pain. *Nature*, **384**, 258–260.

Davis KD, Kwan CL, Crawley AP, and Mikulis DJ (1998). Functional MRI study of thalamic and cortical activations evoked by cutaneous heat, cold, and tactile stimuli. *Journal of Neurophysiology*, **80**, 1533–1546.

Davis KD, Pope GE, Crawley AP, and Mikulis DJ (2002). Neural correlates of prickle sensation: a percept-related fMRI study. *Nature Neuroscience*, **5**, 1121–1122.

Davis KD, Taub E, Duffner F, *et al.* (2000). Activation of the anterior cingulate cortex by thalamic stimulation in patients with chronic pain: a positron emission tomography study. *Journal of Neurosurgery*, **92**, 64–69.

Davis KD, Taylor SJ, Crawley AP, Wood ML, and Mikulis DJ (1997). Functional MRI of pain- and attention-related activations in the human cingulate cortex. *Journal of Neurophysiology*, **77**, 3370–3380.

Derbyshire SW, Jones AK, Creed F, *et al.* (2002). Cerebral responses to noxious thermal stimulation in chronic low back pain patients and normal controls. *Neuroimage*, **16**, 158–168.

Devinsky O, Morell MJ, and Vogt BA (1995). Contributions of anterior cingulate to behaviour. *Brain*, **118**, 279–306.

Devor M (1997). Phantom pain as an expression of referred and neuropathic pain. In (ed. RA Sherman) *Phantom Pain*, pp. 33–57. Plenum Press, New York.

Di Piero V, Jones AKP, Iannotti F, *et al.* (1991). Chronic pain: a PET study of the central effects of percutaneous high cervical cordotomy. *Pain*, **46**, 9–12.

Dostrovsky JO and Craig AD (1996). Nociceptive neurons in primate insular cortex. *Society of Neuroscience Abstracts*, **22**, 111.

Duncan GH, Kupers RC, Marchand S, Villemure JG, Gybels JM, and Bushnell M. (1998). Stimulation of human thalamus for pain relief: possible emodulatory circuits revealed by positron emission tomography. *Journal of Neurophysiology*, **80**, 3326–3330.

Elbert T, Flor H, Birbaumer N, *et al.* (1994). Extensive reorganization of the somatosensory cortex in adult humans after nervous system injury. *Neuroreport*, **5**, 2593–2597.

Flor H (2002). Phantom-limb pain: characteristics, causes and treatment. *Lancet*, **1**, 182–189.

Flor H, Braun C, Elbert T, and Birbaumer N (1997). Extensive reorganization of primary somatosensory cortex in chronic back pain patients. *Neuroscience Letters*, **224**, 5–8.

Flor H, Denke C, Schaefer M, and Grüsser M (2001). Sensory discrimination training alters both cortical reorganization and phantom limb pain. *Lancet,* **357**, 1763–1764.

Flor H, Elbert T, Knecht S, *et al.* (1995). Phantom-limb pain as a perceptual correlate of cortical reorganization following arm amputation. *Nature*, **375**, 482–484.

Flor H, Knost B, and Birbaumer N (2002). The role of operant conditioning in chronic pain: an experimental investigation. *Pain,* **95**, 111–118.

Flor H, Muhlnickel W, Karl A, *et al.* (2000). A neural substrate for nonpainful phantom limb phenomena. *Neuroreport*, **11**, 1407–1411.

Florence SL, Taub HB, and Kaas JH (1998). Large-scale sprouting of cortical connections after peripheral injury in adult macaque monkeys. *Science*, **282**, 1117–1121.

Frot M and Mauguiere F (2003) Dual representation of pain in the operculo-insular cortex in humans. *Brain*, **126**, 438–450.

Garcia–Larrea L, Peyron R, Mertens P, *et al.* (1997). Positron emission tomography during motor cortex stimulation for pain control. *Stereotactic and Functional Neurosurgery*, **68**, 141–148.

Garcia–Larrea L, Peyron R, Mertens P, *et al.* (1999). Electrical stimulation of motor cortex for pain control: a combined PET- scan and electrophysiological study. *Pain*, **83**, 259–273.

Gibson SJ, Littlejohn GO, Gorman MM, Helme RD, and Granges G (1994). Altered heat pain thresholds and cerebral event-related potentials following painful CO_2 laser stimulation in subjects with fibromyalgia syndrome. *Pain*, **58**, 185–193.

Gracely RH, Petzke F, Wolf JM, and Clauw DJ (2002). Functional magnetic resonance imaging evidence of augmented pain processing in fibromyalgia. *Arthritis and Rheumatism*, **46**, 1333–1343

Grachev ID, Fredrickson BE, and Apkarian AV (2000). Abnormal brain chemistry in chronic back pain : an in vivo proton magnetic resonance spectroscopic study. *Pain*, **89**, 7–18.

Grüsser SM, Mühlnickel W, Schaefer M, *et al.* (in press). Remote activation of referred phantom sensation and cortical reorganization in human upper extremity amputees.

Hofbauer RK, Rainville P, Duncan GH, and Bushnell MC (2001). Cortical representation of the sensory dimension of pain. *Journal of Neurophysiology*, **86**, 402–411.

Hsieh JC, Belfrage M, Stone–Elander S, Hansson P, and Ingvar M (1995). Central representation of chronic ongoing neuropathic pain studied by positron emission tomography. *Pain*, **63**, 225–236.

Hsieh JC, Tu CH, Chen FP, *et al.* (2001). Activation of the hypothalamus characterizes the acupuncture stimulation at the analgesic point in human: a positron emission tomography study. *Neuroscience Letters*, **307**, 105–108.

Huse E, Larbig W, Gerstein J, *et al.* (in press). Pain-related and psychological predictors of phantom limb and residual limb pain and non-painful phantom phenomena.

Hutchison WD, Davis KD, Lozano AM, Tasker RR, and Dostrovsky JO (1999). Pain-related neurons in the human cingulate cortex. *Nature Neuroscience*, **2**, 403–405.

Iadarola MJ, Berman KF, Zeffiro TA, *et al.* (1998). Neural activation during acute capsaicin-evoked pain and allodynia assessed with PET. *Brain*, **121**, 931–947.

Iadarola MJ, Max MB, Berman KF, *et al.* (1995). Unilateral decrease in thalamic activity observed with positron emission tomography in patients with chronic neuropathic pain. *Pain*, **63**, 55–64.

Jenkins WM, Merzenich MM, Ochs MT, Allard T, and Guic–Robles E (1990). Functional reorganization of primary somatosensory cortex in adult owl monkeys after behaviorally controlled tactile stimulation. *Journal of Neurophysiology*, **63**, 82–104.

Jones AKP, Brown WD, Friston KJ, Qi LY, and Frackowiak RS (1991). Cortical and subcortical localization of response to pain in man using positron emission tomography. *Proceedings of the Royal Society of London. Series B. Biological Sciences*, **244**, 39–44.

Jones AKP, Kulkarni B, and Stuart WG (2002). Functional imaging of pain perception. *Current Rheumatology Reports*, **4**, 329–333.

Jones EG and Pons TP (1998). Thalamic and brainstem contributions to large-scale plasticity of primate somatosensory cortex. *Science*, **6**, 1121–1125.

Juottonen K, Gockel M, Silen T, Hurri H, Hari R, and Forss N (2002). Altered central sensorimotor processing in patients with complex regional pain syndrome. *Pain*, **98**, 315–323.

Kaas JH (2000). The reorganization of sensory and motor maps after injury in adult mammals. In (ed. Gazzaniga MS) *The New Cognitive Neurosciences*, pp. 223–236. The MIT Press, Cambridge, London.

Karl A, Birbaumer N, Lutzenberger W, Cohen L, and Flor H (2001). Reorganization of motor and somatosensory cortex in upper extremity amputees with phantom limb pain. *Journal of Neuroscience*, **21**, 3609–3618.

Katz J and Melzack R (1990). Pain 'memories' in phantom limbs: review and clinical observations. *Pain*, **43**, 319–336.

Kenshalo DR Jr, Chudler EH, Anton F, and Dubner R (1988). SI nociceptive neurons participate in the encoding process by which monkeys perceive the intensity of noxious thermal stimulation. *Brain Research*, **454**, 378–382.

Kleinböhl D, Hölzl R, Möltner A, Rommel C, Weber C, and Osswald PM (1999). Psychophysical measures of sensitization to tonic heat discriminate chronic pain patients. *Pain*, **81**, 35–43.

Kunde V and Treede RD (1993) Topography of middle latency somatosensory evoked potentials following painful laser stimuli and non-painful electric electrical stimuli. *Encephalography and Clinical Neurophysiology*, **88**, 280–289.

Kwan CL, Crawley AP, Mikulis DJ, and Davis KD (2000). An fMRI study of the anterior cingulate cortex and surrounding medial wall activations evoked by noxious cutaneous heat and cold stimuli. *Pain*, **85**, 359–374.

Lorenz J, Cross D, Minoshima S, Morrow T, Paulson P, and Casey K (2002). A unique representation of heat allodynia in the human brain. *Neuron*, **35**, 383–393.

Lorenz J, Grasedyck K, and Bromm B (1996) Middle and long latency somatosensory evoked potentials after painful laser stimulation in patients with fibromyalgia syndrome. *Electroencephalography and Clinical Neurophysiology*, **100**, 165–168.

Lotze M, Flor H, Grodd W, Larbig W, and Birbaumer N (2001). Phantom movements and pain. An fMRI study in upper limb amputees. *Brain*, **124**, 2268–2277.

Lotze M, Grodd W, Birbaumer N, Erb M, Huse E, and Flor H (1999). Does use of a myo-electric prosthesis reduce cortical reorganization and phantom limb pain? *Nature Neuroscience*, **2**, 501–502.

May A and Goadsby PJ (2001). Hypothalamic involvement and activation in cluster headache. *Current Pain Headache Report*, **5**, 60–66.

May A, Bahra A, Buchel C, Frackowiak RS, and Goadsby PJ (2000). PET and MRA findings in cluster headache and MRA in experimental pain. *Neurology*, **55**, 1328–1335.

Melzack R and Casey KL (1968). Sensory, motivational and central control determinants of pain: a new conceptual model. In (ed. Kenshalo DR) *The Skin Senses*, pp. 423–443. IL, Thomas, Springfield.

Merzenich MM, Nelson RJ, Stryker MP, Cynader MA, Schoppmann A, and Zook JM (1984). Somatosensory cortical map changes following digit amputation in adult monkeys. *The Journal of Comparative Neurology*, **224**, 591–605.

Mountz JM, Bradley LA, and Alarcon GS (1999). Abnormal functional activity of the central nervous system in fibromyalgia syndrome. *American Journal of the Medical Sciences*, **315**, 385–396.

Petrovic P and Ingvar M (2002). Imaging cognitive modulation of pain processing. *Pain*, **95**, 1–5.

Petrovic P, Ingvar M, Stone–Elander S, Petersson KM, and Hansson P. (1999) A PET activation study of dynamic mechanical allodynia in patients with mononeuropathy. *Pain*, **83**, 459–470.

Petrovic P, Kalso E, Petersson KM, and Ingvar M (2002). Placebo and opioid analgesia — imaging a shared neuronal network. *Science*, **295**, 1737–1740.

Peyron R, Garcia–Larrea L, Deiber MP, *et al.* (1995). Electrical stimulation of precentral cortical area in the treatment of central pain: electrophysiological and PET study. *Pain*, **62**, 275–286.

Peyron R, Garcia–Larrea L, Gregoire MC, *et al.* (1998). Allodynia after lateral-medullary (Wallenberg) infarct. A positron emission tomography (PET) study. *Brain*, **121**, 345–356.

Peyron R, Garcia–Larrea L, Gregoire MC, *et al.* (1999). Haemodynamic brain responses to acute pain in humans: sensory and attentional networks. *Brain*, **122**, 1765–1779.

Peyron R, Laurent B, and Garcia–Larrea L (2000). Functional imaging of brain responses to pain. A review and meta-analysis. *Neurophysiologie Clinique*, **30**, 263–288.

Ploghaus A and Tracey I (2001). Exacerbation of pain by anxiety is associated with activity in a hippocampal network. *Journal of Neuroscience*, **21**, 9896–9903.

Ploghaus A, Tracey I, Gati JS, Clare S, Menon RS, Matthews PM, and Rawlins JN (1999). Dissociating pain from its anticipation in the human brain. *Science*, **284**, 1979–1981.

Ploner M, Freund HJ, and Schnitzler A (1999*a*). Pain affect without pain sensation in a patient with a postcentral lesion. *Pain*, **81**, 211–214.

Ploner M, Schmitz F, Freund HJ, and Schnitzler A (1999*b*). Parallel activation of primary and secondary somatosensory cortices in human pain processing. *Journal of Neurophysiology*, **81**, 3100–3104.

Pons TP, Garraghty PE, Ommaya AK, Kaas JH, Taub E, and Mishkin M (1991). Massive cortical reorganization after sensory deafferentation in adult macaques. *Science*, **252**, 1857–1860.

Porro CA, Baraldi P, Pagnoni G, *et al.* (2002). Does anticipation of pain affect cortical nociceptive systems? *Journal of Neuroscience*, **22**, 3206–3214.

Rainville P (2002). Brain mechanisms of pain affect and pain modulation. *Current Opinion Neurobiology*, **12**, 195–204.

Rainville P, Bushnell MC, and Duncan GH (2000). PET studies of the subjective experience of pain. In (eds. Casey K and Bushnell MC) *Pain Imaging*, pp. 123–156. IASP Press, Seattle.

Rainville P, Duncan GH, Price DD, Carrier B, and Bushnell MC (1997). Pain affect encoded in human anterior cingulate but not somatosensory cortex. *Science*, **277**, 968–971.

Ramachandran VS, Steward M, and Rogers–Ramachandran D (1992). Perceptual correlates of massive cortical reorganization. *Neuroreport*, **3**, 583–586.

Recanzone GH (2000). Cerebral cortical plasticity: perception and skill acquisition. In (ed. Gazzaniga MS) *The New Cognitive Neuroscience* (2nd edn), pp.237–247. MIT Press, Boston, MA.

Rolls ET, O'Doherty J, Kringelbach ML, Francis S, Bowtell R, and McGlone F (2003). Representations of pleasant and painful touch in the human orbitofrontal and cingulate cortices. *Cerebel Cortex*, **13**, 308–317.

Sawamoto N, Honda M, Okada T, *et al.* (2000). Expectation of pain enhances responses to nonpainful somatosensory stimulation in the anterior cingulate cortex and parietal operculum/posterior insula: an event-related functional magnetic resonance imaging study. *Journal of Neuroscience*, **20**, 7438–7445.

Sikes RW and Vogt BA (1992). Nociceptive neurons in area 24 of rabbit cingulate cortex. *Journal of Neurophysiology*, **68**, 1720–1732.

Silverman DH, Munakata JA, Ennes H, Mandelkern MA, Hoh CK, and Mayer EA(1997). Regional cerebral activity in normal and pathological perception of visceral pain. *Gastroenterology*, **112**, 64–72.

Strigo IA, Carli F, Bushnell MC (2000). Effect of ambient temperature on human pain and temperature perception. *Anesthesiology*, **92**, 699–707.

Strigo IA, Duncan GH, Boivin M, and Bushnell, MC (in press) Differentiation of visceral and cutaneous pain in human cerebral cortex. *Journal of Neurophysiology*

Talbot JD, Marrett S, Evans AC, Meyer E, Bushnell MC, and Duncan GH (1991). Multiple representations of pain in the human cerebral cortex. *Science*, **251**, 1355–1361.

Timmermann L, Ploner M, Haucke K, Schmitz F, Baltissen R, and Schnitzler A (2001). Differential coding of pain intensity in the human primary and secondary cortex. *Journal of Neurophysiology*, **86**, 1499–1503.

Tölle TR, Kaufmann T, Siessmeier T, *et al.* (1999). Region-specific encoding of sensory and affective components of pain in the human brain: a positron emission tomography correlation analysis. *Annals of Neurology*, **45**, 40–47.

Tommerdahl M, Delemos KA, Vierck CJ Jr, Favorov AV, and Whitsel BL (1996). Anterior parietal cortex response to tactile and skin-heating stimuli applied to the same skin site. *Journal of Neurophysiology*, **75**, 2662–2670.

Tracey I, Becerra L, Chang I, *et al.* (2000). Noxious heat and cold stimulation produce common patterns of brain activation in humans: a functional magnetic resonance imaging study. *Neuroscience Letters*, **288**, 159–162.

Tracey I, Ploghaus A, Gati JS, *et al.* (2002). Imaging attentional modulation of pain in the periaqueductal gray in humans. *Journal of Neurophysiology*, **22**, 2748–2752.

Treede RD, Apkarian AV, Bromm B, Greenspan JD, and Lenz FA (2000). Cortical representation of pain: functional characterization of nociceptive areas near the lateral sulcus. *Pain*, **87**, 113–119.

Treede RD, Kenshalo DR, Gracely RH, and Jones AKP (1999). The cortical representation of pain. *Pain*, **79**, 105–111.

Turk DC, Meichenbaum D, and Genest M (1983). *Pain and Behavioral Medicine*. The Guilford Press, New York, London.

Verberne AJ and Owens NC (1998). Cortical modulation of the cardiovascular system. *Progress in Neurobiology*. **54**, 748–754.

Vos BP, Benoist JM, Gautron M, and Guilbaud G (2000). Changes in neuronal activities in the two ventral posterior medial thalamic nuclei in an experimental model of trigeminal pain in the rat by constriction of one infraorbital nerve. *Somatosensorsory and Motor Research*, **17**, 109–122.

Wei F and Zhuo M (2001). Potentiation of sensory responses in the anterior cingulate cortex following digit amputation in the anaesthetised rat. *Journal of Physiology*, **532**, 823–833.

Weiller C, May A, Limmroth V, *et al.* (1995). Brain stem activation in spontaneous human migraine attacks. *Nature Medicine*, **1**, 658–660.

Wiech K, Preissl H, Kiefer T, *et al.* (2001). Prevention of phantom limb pain and cortical reorganization in the early phase after amputation in humans. *Society of Neuroscience Abstracts*, **28**, 163.9.

Willoch F, Rosen G, Tölle TR, *et al.* (2000). Phantom limb pain in the human brain: unraveling neural circuitries of phantom limb sensations using positron emission tomography. *Annals of Neurology*, **48**, 842–849.

Witting N, Kupers RC, Svensson P, Arendt–Nielsen L, Gjedde A, and Jensen TS (2001). Experimental brush-evoked allodynia activates posterior parietal cortex. *Neurology*, **57**, 1817–1824.

Woolf CJ and Salter MW (2000). Neuronal plasticity: increasing the gain in pain. *Science*, **288**, 1765–1769.

Zubieta JK, Smith YR, Bueller JA, *et al.* (2001). Regional mu opioid receptor regulation of sensory and affective dimensions of pain. *Science*, **293**, 311–315.

Chapter 14

Headache

Peter J. Goadsby and Michel D. Ferrari

14.1 Introduction

Headache is among the most fascinating and most common of medical problems (Rasmussen *et al.*, 1991). It can be a manifestation of a disease process in its own right, without a clearly defined other cause (primary headaches such as migraine, tension-type headache, or cluster headache), or headache can be due to a defined other disease process, such as that associated with infection, brain tumour, or head trauma (secondary headaches) (Table 14.1). The International Headache Society recognizes 96 pages' worth of headache types (Headache Classification Committee of The International Headache Society, 1988), and no doubt as the system is now under revision (Olesen, 2001), there will be more.

For this chapter we will set out the common biology of pain processing for headache, since it is likely to be shared to some extent by most forms of headache. We will then present the unique biology that underlies migraine as a form of primary headache that exemplifies some of the basic principles of headache biology. The clinical features of the various headache types and their management are dealt with in recent books (Lance˙and Goadsby, 1998; Olesen and Goadsby, 1999; Olesen *et al.*, 2000; Silberstein *et al.*, 2002) and are beyond the scope of this chapter.

It is appropriate to emphasize at the outset that, while secondary headaches can easily adopt most principles of pain, primary headaches, particularly the neurovascular syndromes such as migraine and cluster headache, are much more complex than simple pain syndromes.

14.2 Pain mechanisms underlying particularly primary headaches

There are many pain-producing structures in the head, such as the teeth and paranasal sinuses. However, when activated these are generally considered forms of facial pain and not headache, at least in clinical parlance. Headache is generally used to express a sensation of pain experienced in, or referred to, the first (ophthalmic) division of the trigeminal nerve, and this innervation is referred to as the trigeminovascular system (Fig. 14.1). We will use this clinical meaning when considering the anatomy and physiology of headache.

Table 14.1 Common causes of headache*

Primary headache		Secondary headache	
Type	Lifetime prevalence (%)	Type	Lifetime prevalence (%)
Migraine	16	Systemic infection	63
Tension-type	69	Head injury	4
Cluster headache	0.1	Sub-arachnoid haemorrhage	<1
Idiopathic stabbing	2	Vascular disorders	1
Exertional	1	Brain tumour	0.1

* Data from Rassmussen (1995)

14.2.1 Anatomy of the innervation of the intracranial contents

The brain itself is largely insensate. It is surrounded by a protective covering, the meninges, that produces pain in humans when directly stimulated (Wolff, 1948). Pain-producing components of the meninges include the large cerebral vessels, pial vessels, large venous sinuses, and dura mater. These are surrounded by a plexus of largely unmyelinated fibres arising from the ophthalmic division of the trigeminal ganglion

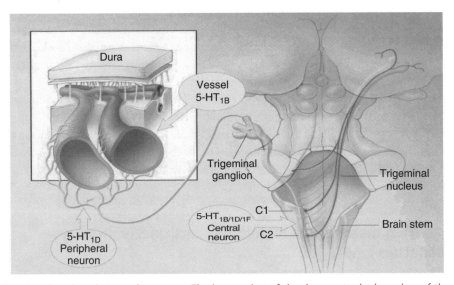

Fig.14.1 The trigeminovascular system. The innervation of the dura mater by branches of the first (ophthalmic) division of the trigeminal nerve. Vessels contain serotonin 5-HT$_{1B}$ receptors, while the peripheral nerves contain 5-HT$_{1D}$ receptors. Afferent fibres synapse in the trigeminocervical complex that extends from the trigeminal nucleus caudalis to the dorsal horns of C$_1$ and C$_2$ and contains 5-HT$_{1B/1D/1F}$ receptors. Second order neurons project to more rostral brain areas such as periaqueductal grey and thalamus (Goadsby et al., 2002b).

(McNaughton, 1938, 1966; Penfield and McNaughton, 1940) and, in the posterior fossa, from the upper cervical dorsal roots (Arbab *et al.*, 1986, 1988; Kerr, 1961; Kerr and Olafson, 1961). Stimulation of the cranial vessels, such as the superior sagittal sinus (SSS), is certainly painful in humans (Feindel *et al.*, 1960). Indeed, it has been shown that after trigeminal root section the dura mater is itself insensate (Cushing, 1904).

Trigeminal fibres innervating cerebral vessels arise from neurons in the trigeminal ganglion that contain substance P (Liu–Chen *et al.*, 1983*a,b*, 1984) and calcitonin gene-related peptide (CGRP) (Uddman *et al.*, 1985), both of which can be released when the trigeminal ganglion is stimulated either in humans or the cat (Goadsby *et al.*, 1988). Other potentially important neurotransmitters or receptors identified in the trigeminal ganglion include nitric oxide (identified in histological sections by its synthezing enzyme as nitric oxide synthase; NOS) (Edvinsson *et al.*, 1998), vanilloid 1 (TRPV1) receptors (Hou *et al.*, 2002), and nociceptin (Hou *et al.*, 2001*b*). Substance P, CGRP, and NOS are co-localized in the cell bodies in the trigeminal ganglion with serotonin 5-$HT_{1B/1D}$ receptors (Hou *et al.*, 2001*a*); agents stimulating these receptors are recognized effective and specific treatments of migraine and cluster headache (Goadsby, 2000).

14.2.2 Physiology of innervation of the intracranial contents — peripheral

14.2.2.1 Plasma protein extravasation (PPE)

Neurogenic plasma protein extravasation can be seen during electrical stimulation of the trigeminal ganglion in the rat (Markowitz *et al.*, 1987), and it has been suggested to play a role in the generation of pain in migraine and cluster headache. PPE can be blocked by ergot alkaloids (Markowitz *et al.*, 1988), indomethacin, acetylsalicylic acid (Buzzi *et al.*, 1989), and sumatriptan and other serotonin 5-$HT_{1B/1D}$ agonists (triptans) (Moskowitz and Cutrer, 1993). In addition, trigeminal ganglion stimulation may cause other structural changes in the dura mater, such as mast cell degranulation (Dimitriadou *et al.*, 1991) and changes in post-capillary venules including platelet aggregation (Dimitriadou *et al.*, 1992).

While it is generally thought that such changes, and particularly the initiation of a sterile inflammatory response, can contribute to pain (Burstein *et al.*, 1998; Strassman *et al.*, 1996), it is not clear whether this is sufficient of itself or requires other stimulators or promoters. Clearly, blockade of neurogenic PPE is not completely predictive of anti-migraine efficacy in humans, as evidenced by the failure of providing pain relief in clinical trials of substance P, neurokinin-1 antagonists (Connor *et al.*, 1998; Diener and The RPR100893 Study Group, 2003; Goldstein *et al.*, 1997; Norman *et al.*, 1998); specific PPE blockers, CP122,288 (Roon *et al.*, 2000) and 4991w93 (Earl *et al.*, 1999); an endothelin antagonist, bosentan (May *et al.*, 1996); and a neurosteriod, ganaxolone (Data *et al.*, 1998). Moreover, although PPE in the retina, which is blocked by sumatriptan, is seen after trigeminal ganglion stimulation in the rat, no such changes are seen with retinal angiography during acute attacks of migraine or cluster headache (May *et al.*, 1998*c*).

Despite these negative studies, the possible effect of any retrograde activation of the trigeminovascular system during migraine or cluster headache remains an interesting issue. Local release of pro-inflammatory substances in the dura mater is likely to sensitize trigeminal neurons (Strassman *et al.*, 1996), which enhances trigeminal transmission of other non-noxious facial inputs (Burstein *et al.*, 1998). Certainly, allodynia occurs in migraine (Burstein *et al.*, 2000*a,b*; Selby and Lance, 1960). It has recently been suggested, based on an open label study, that treatment with triptans prior to the onset of headache predicts a successful outcome (Burstein *et al.*, 2003). This would be an important clinical observation if it can be repeated. It would support new studies showing that treatment of migraine when the pain is mild can be a successful strategy (Klapper *et al.*, 2002; Lipton and Goadsby, 2001; Winner *et al.*, 2002), and suggests that future acute studies need to have consideration of these advances in understanding the biology of the condition.

14.2.2.2 Neuropeptide studies

Monitoring neuropeptides released from trigeminal nerves that innervate pain-producing intracranial structures may offer insights into the populations of neurons activated in primary headache syndromes, and guide development of new therapies. Electrical stimulation of the trigeminal ganglion in both humans and the cat leads to increases in cerebral (Tran–Dinh *et al.*, 1992) and extracerebral blood flow (Drummond *et al.*, 1983) and local release of both calcitonin gene-related peptide (CGRP) and substance P (SP) (Goadsby *et al.*, 1988). In the cat, trigeminal ganglion stimulation also increases cerebral blood flow by a pathway traversing the greater superficial petrosal branch of the facial nerve (Goadsby and Duckworth, 1987) releasing a powerful vasodilator peptide, vasoactive intestinal polypeptide (VIP) (Goadsby *et al.*, 1984). Stimulation of the more specifically vascular pain-producing superior sagittal sinus increases cerebral blood flow (Lambert *et al.*, 1988) and jugular vein CGRP levels (Zagami *et al.*, 1990) as well as resulting in more restricted changes in cranial blood flow (Goadsby *et al.*, 1997).

Human evidence that CGRP is elevated in the headache phase of migraine (Gallai *et al.*, 1995; Goadsby *et al.*, 1990), cluster headache (Fanciullacci *et al.*, 1995; Goadsby and Edvinsson, 1994), and chronic paroxysmal hemicrania (Goadsby and Edvinsson, 1996) supports the view that the trigeminovascular system may be activated in a protective role in these conditions. Furthermore, CGRP infusion will trigger headache, some clearly migrainous, in humans (Lassen *et al.*, 2002). It is of interest in this regard that compounds which have *not* shown activity in human migraine, notably the conformationally restricted analogue of sumatriptan, CP122,288 (Knight *et al.*, 1999), and the conformationally restricted analogue of zolmitriptan, 4991w93 (Knight *et al.*, 2001), were both also ineffective inhibitors of CGRP release after superior sagittal sinus in the cat. In contrast, the highly specific and potent analgesic CGRP antagonist,

BIBN 4096 (Palmer and Dalton, 2000), was recently shown to be effective in the acute treatment of migraine attacks.

14.2.3 Physiology of innervation of the intracranial contents — central nervous system

14.2.3.1 The trigeminocervical complex

Using Fos immunohistochemistry (a method for anatomically defining activated neurons in the CNS), stimulation of the superior sagittal sinus induces Fos-like immunoreactivity in the trigeminal nucleus caudalis and in the dorsal horn at the C_1 and C_2 levels in the cat (Kaube *et al.*, 1993*c*) and monkey (Goadsby and Hoskin, 1997). Using 2-deoxyglucose measurements after superior sagittal sinus stimulation it has also been shown that neuronal activity is increased in the trigeminal nucleus caudalis and in the dorsal horn at the C_1 and C_2 levels (Goadsby and Zagami, 1991). By recording from neurons in the C_2 dorsal horn that are activated by stimulation of both anterior dural and greater occipital nerves, it can be seen that there is a population of neurons that could subserve referred pain from these structures (Bartsch and Goadsby, 2002). Taken together, it is likely that the trigeminal nucleus extends beyond the traditional nucleus caudalis to the dorsal horn of the high cervical region in a functional continuum that could be regarded as a *trigeminocervical complex*. This structure provides second order neurons for the entire set of intracranial pain-producing structures. This arrangement explains why patients with primary headache complain of pain in the head that does not respect the cutaneous distribution of either the trigeminal or cervical nerves. Moreover, stimulation of a lateralized structure, the middle meningeal artery, produces Fos expression bilaterally in both the cat and monkey brain (Hoskin *et al.*, 1999) — a finding that is consistent with the fact that at least one-third of patients complain of bilateral pain or pain switching from one side to the other during attacks.

Experimental pharmacological evidence suggests that some abortive anti-migraine drugs, such as dihydroergotamine (Hoskin *et al.*, 1996), acetylsalicylic acid (Kaube *et al.*, 1993*a*), sumatriptan — but only after blood-brain barrier disruption (Kaube *et al.*, 1993*b*; Shepheard *et al.*, 1993), eletriptan (Goadsby and Hoskin, 1999), naratriptan (Cumberbatch *et al.*, 1998; Goadsby and Knight, 1997*b*), rizatriptan (Cumberbatch *et al.*, 1997), and zolmitriptan (Goadsby and Hoskin, 1996) can have actions at these second order neurons. It is clear from iontophoretic studies that 5-HT$_{1B/1D}$ agonists can block trigeminovascular nociceptive transmission locally (Storer *et al.*, 2001*a*; Storer and Goadsby, 1997). It has further been shown that triptans will antagonize the excitatory effect of local L-glutamate iontophoresis in the trigeminocervical complex (Goadsby *et al.*, 2001). This predicts the existence of postsynaptic triptan-sensitive 5-HT receptors on second order trigeminal neurons.

Novel targets for therapy in the trigeminocervical complex
Serotonin receptors   Since some of the triptans also activate the 5-HT$_{1F}$ receptor, the above data raise the question as to whether there is a 5-HT$_{1F}$ neuronal inhibitory

receptor (Adham *et al.*, 1993) that may be a possible target for an anti-migraine drug (Branchek and Archa, 1997). The potent specific 5HT$_{1F}$ agonist, LY334,370, has been developed (Phebus *et al.*, 1997) and shown to block PPE (Johnson *et al.*, 1997), consistent with early molecular studies (Wainscott *et al.*, 1998). Activation of 5-HT$_{1F}$ receptors does not seem to have vascular constrictive effects (Cohen and Schenck, 1999; Razzaque *et al.*, 1999). LY334,370 has been reported to be effective in acute migraine, albeit at relatively high doses with some central nervous system side-effects (Goldstein *et al.*, 2001). No cardiovascular problems were seen in these studies (Goldstein *et al.*, 1999), but unfortunately development has stopped because of a toxicity problem in the dog. There are 5HT$_{1F}$ receptors in the trigeminal nucleus (Castro *et al.*, 1997; Fugelli *et al.*, 1997; Pascual *et al.*, 1996; Waeber and Moskowitz, 1995) and trigeminal ganglion (Bouchelet *et al.*, 1996). Moreover, 5-HT$_{1F}$ agonism is inhibitory in the trigeminal nucleus in the rat (Mitsikostas *et al.*, 1999; Shepheard *et al.*, 1999).

It must be borne in mind that sumatriptan and a number of other *triptans* — notably eletriptan, naratriptan, and zolmitriptan — are also agonists at the 5HT$_{1F}$ site. However, alniditan, which is certainly active in migraine (Diener *et al.*, 2001), but is no longer being clinically developed, is relatively inactive at the 5HT$_{1F}$ receptor (Leysen *et al.*, 1996). On pre-clinical grounds, the 5-HT$_{1F}$ receptor seems to represent a second target that does not displace the 5HT$_{1B/1D}$ receptors but adds to our understanding of this pivotal synapse.

Adenosine receptors   It has recently been shown that the adenosine A$_1$ receptor may provide a target for therapeutic development. There is a considerable literature to suggest that the purine, adenosine, may have some role in nociception (Sawynok, 1998, 1999). It was originally observed that methylxanthine adenosine antagonists decreased nociceptive thresholds in rats (Paalzow and Paalzow, 1973). Based on studies comparing the rank order of potency of adenosine analogues (Sawynok *et al.*, 1986), or on the use of selective adenosine agonists and antagonists (Sjolund *et al.*, 1996), it is likely that the anti-nociceptive effects of adenosine are mediated via the A$_1$ receptor (Sawynok *et al.*, 1986). A$_1$ receptors are located in the trigeminal nucleus (Schindler *et al.*, 2001). A$_1$ receptor agonists inhibit PPE (Honey *et al.*, 2000). The potent A$_1$ receptor agonist, GR79236, blocks transmission in the trigeminocervical complex, at least as potently as triptans, in the rat (Bland–Ward *et al.*, 2000) and cat. It also blocks cranial release of CGRP in the cat (Goadsby *et al.*, 2002*a*) probably by inhibition of protein kinase A induced CGRP release (Carruthers *et al.*, 2001). It can be shown in humans that this compound inhibits the nociceptive-specific blink reflex (Giffin *et al.*, 2003), and it is therefore a candidate for acute treatment of migraine and cluster headache.

Other targets   Other possible targets for inhibition of the trigeminocervical complex would include GABA$_A$ receptor agonists (Storer *et al.*, 2001*b*), receptors from the transient receptor potential (TRP) family (Gunthorpe *et al.*, 2002; Montell *et al.*, 2002) such as vanilloid receptor TRPV1 (Akerman *et al.*, 2002), ORL-1 (NOP$_1$) (nociception) receptor agonists (Bartsch *et al.*, 2002), and μ-opiate receptor agonists (Storer *et al.*, 2001*c*; Williamson *et al.*, 2001).

14.2.4 **Higher order processing of trigeminal afferents**

Following transmission in the caudal brain stem and high cervical spinal cord, information is relayed in a group of fibres (the quintothalamic tract) to the thalamus. Processing of vascular pain in experimental animals in the thalamus occurs in the ventroposteromedial thalamus, medial nucleus of the posterior complex, and in the intralaminar thalamus (Zagami and Goadsby, 1991). Zagami has shown, by application of capsaicin to the superior sagittal sinus, that trigeminal projections with a high degree of nociceptive input are processed in neurons particularly in the ventroposteromedial thalamus and in its ventral periphery (Zagami and Lambert, 1991). Human imaging studies have confirmed activation of the thalamus contralateral to pain in acute migraine (Bahra *et al.*, 2001), cluster headache (May *et al.*, 1998*a*), and in SUNCT (short-lasting unilateral neuralgiform headache with conjunctival injection and tearing) (May *et al.*, 1999*a*). The properties and further higher-centre connections of these neurons are the subject of ongoing studies that will allow us to build up a more complete picture of the trigeminovascular pain pathways (Table 14.2).

14.2.5 **Primary neurovascular headache and the role of the cranial vessels**

Given the anatomy and physiology of the trigeminovascular system that is described above, it might be assumed that the vessels and dura mater are the source of pain in all forms of headache. This issue is far from clear and will be explored before some of the main forms of headache are discussed in more detail. These issues apply to both

Table 14.2 Neuroanatomical processing of vascular head pain

Target innervation	Structure	Comments
Cranial vessels	Ophthalmic branch of trigeminal nerve	
Dura mater		
1st	Trigeminal ganglion	Middle cranial fossa
2nd	Trigeminal nucleus (*quintothalamic tract*)	Trigeminal n. caudalis & C_1/C_2 dorsal horns
3rd	Thalamus	Ventrobasal complex
		Medial n. of posterior group
		Intralaminar complex
Final	Cortex	Insulae
		Frontal cortex
		Anterior cingulate cortex
		Basal ganglia

migraine and the trigeminal autonomic cephalgias, such as cluster headache (Goadsby and Lipton, 1997).

In a study of experimental head pain in which capsaicin was injected into the forehead of volunteers without headache (May *et al.*, 1998*b*) there was a bilateral activation pattern in midline structures over several planes, slightly lateralized to the left, anterior to the brainstem, and posterior to the chiasmatic region. Superimposed on a MRI template, the location of the activation covers intracranial arteries, as well as the region of the cavernous sinus. It is bilateral, but more marked on the side of the injection. Similarly, in the cluster headache study, there is a strong activation observed in the same region, the cavernous sinus, during acute attacks of pain (May *et al.*, 1998*a*). This change might be interpreted as an increased venous inflow from the superior ophthalmic vein draining the ophthalmic artery (Waldenlind *et al.*, 1993), or a longer transit time for the tracer in this region possibly due to impeded venous drainage. Another possibility is that the observed increase in activation might be due to a bilateral dilation of the internal carotid artery, since such a change would suggest a vasodilatation mediated by the ophthalmic division of the trigeminovascular system, a neurally driven vasodilatation.

To further address this question, magnetic resonance angiography (MRA) was performed using the same study design as in the PET study (May *et al.*, 1998*a*). Using an image calculation tool, the angiographies were subtracted from each other and it was demonstrated that after inhalation of the NO-donor nitroglycerine (NTG), there was bilateral dilatation of the internal carotid arteries compared to the rest state, even before the headache started (May *et al.*, 1999*b*). These vessels stayed dilated during the acute NTG-induced cluster headache that did not develop for a further 20–30 minutes. Given that we have observed vasodilatation in large vessels in cluster headache using MRA, and increased signal in the region of the cavernous sinus after capsaicin injection to the forehead, again in a PET study (May *et al.*, 1998*b*), it seems clear that the vascular changes occur whatever the trigger to the pain. The vascular change is therefore likely to be an epiphenomenon of activation of the trigeminovascular system (Goadsby and Duckworth, 1987). We have seen the very same change in this region in acute migraine studied with PET (Bahra *et al.*, 2001).

In a study of volunteers who had injections of capsaicin into the forehead, chin, and leg, on separate days in random order, MRA measurements of internal carotid diameter demonstrated that only the forehead (ophthalmic division of trigeminal innervated skin) produced dilation (May *et al.*, 2001). These findings are consistent with the preferential somatopically activated dilation seen in experimental animals during trigeminal ganglion or superior sagittal sinus stimulation (Goadsby *et al.*, 1997). It seems that dilation of the large cerebral vessels is non-specific to the headache syndrome and only dependent on activation of ophthalmic, first, division of trigeminal afferents.

14.3 **Migraine**

14.3.1 **Clinical features and epidemiology**

Migraine is a chronic disorder typically characterized by recurrent attacks (1–3 days each) of disabling headaches associated with nausea, vomiting, and sensitivity to light, sound, and movement (migraine without aura; MO). In one-third of patients, attacks are accompanied by transient focal neurological aura symptoms (migraine with aura; MA). More than 12% (two-thirds female) of the general population have regular migraine attacks; the median attack frequency is 18 per year and 10% of migraineurs have weekly attacks. Overuse of acute headache drugs may increase the attack frequency leading to daily or nearly daily headaches (chronified migraine) (Ferrari, 1998; Goadsby *et al.*, 2002*b*; Menken *et al.*, 2000; Stewart *et al.*, 1992). The associated symptoms described above distinguish migraine from tension-type headache, the latter being, in essence, featureless headache.

14.3.2 **Pathogenesis**

The essential aspects to be considered in understanding migraine as a whole, as opposed to its pain manifestations, are:

- Brainstem and diencephalic modulatory systems that modulate sensory processing and are dysfunctional during an attack.
- Hyperresponsiveness of the cerebral cortex and the role of cortical spreading depression (CSD) in causing the migraine aura and, potentially, in activating the trigeminovascular system.
- The genetic and molecular basis for migraine.

In essence, primary neurovascular headaches, such as migraine and cluster headache, entrain or engage the trigeminovascular system in some way for pain expression, but are primarily driven, in terms of pathogenesis, from the brain.

14.3.3 **Central modulation sensory input**

Activation of the rostral brainstem has been seen using PET during acute migraine without aura (Bahra *et al.*, 2001; Weiller *et al.*, 1995). The brainstem areas were active during headache and immediately after successful treatment of the headache, but not active interictally. In contrast, cingulate cortex and visual and auditory association cortex were only active during headache and not after treatment. This differentiation suggests that the brainstem activation represented some fundamental part of the disorder, not simply a response to pain. The activation corresponds with the brain region that Raskin and colleagues (1987) initially reported, and Veloso and colleagues (1998) confirmed, to cause migraine-like headache when stimulated in patients with electrodes implanted for pain control. Moreover, Welch and colleagues (2001) have shown abnormal iron homeostasis in these regions in both episodic and chronic migraine. Chronic migraine has the same brainstem areas of activation that are independent of the perception of pain (Matharu *et al.*, 2003). Moreover, lesions involving the rostral brainstem, such those seen in multiple sclerosis (Haas *et al.*, 1993), a bleed into an arteriovenous malformation in the midbrain (Goadsby, 2002), or a cavernous angioma involving the midbrain (Afridi and Goadsby, 2003), can be accompanied by typical migraine.

14.3.4 Some neurobiology of central dysfunction in migraine

It has been shown in the experimental animal that stimulation of a discrete nucleus in the brainstem, nucleus locus coeruleus (the main central noradrenergic nucleus), reduces cerebral blood flow in a frequency-dependent manner (Goadsby *et al.*, 1982) through an a$_2$-adrenoceptor-linked mechanism (Goadsby *et al.*, 1985). This reduction is maximal in the occipital cortex (Goadsby and Duckworth, 1989). While a 25% overall reduction in cerebral blood flow is seen, extracerebral vasodilatation occurs in parallel (Goadsby *et al.*, 1982). In addition, the main serotonin-containing nucleus in the brainstem, the midbrain dorsal raphe nucleus, can increase cerebral blood flow when activated (Goadsby *et al.*, 1991). It has been shown that stimulation of this ventrolateral periaqueductal grey region will inhibit sagittal sinus evoked trigeminal neuronal activity in the cat (Knight and Goadsby, 2001), and that with activation of pain-producing intracranial trigeminal afferents, ventrolateral PAG neurons are activated (Hoskin *et al.*, 2001).

These data suggest a reflex loop designed to minimize nociceptive signals at a subcortical level. Moreover, given the finding that one form of migraine, familial hemiplegic migraine (see below) involves missense mutations of the P/Q voltage-gated calcium channel gene, it is remarkable that injection of the P/Q channel toxin agatoxin-IVA into the ventrolateral PAG has a pronociceptive effect on trigeminovascular afferent traffic (Knight *et al.*, 2002). It is also remarkable, given the clinical problem of medication overuse, that this region of the brain has opiate (Fields and Basbaum, 1994), ergot (Goadsby and Gundlach, 1991), and triptan receptors (Goadsby and Knight, 1997*a*). Taken together, it seems entirely plausible to consider that rostral brainstem areas play a pivotal, if not defining, role in migraine.

14.3.5 Cortical spreading depression (CSD) and cortical responsiveness

Neuroimaging findings strongly suggest that migraine aura is due to CSD (Lauritzen, 1994). In animals, CSD is characterized by a slowly propagating wave of sustained strong neuronal depolarization (Bures *et al.*, 1974). This triggers a transient intense spike activity as it progresses along the cortex, followed by long-lasting neuronal suppression (Kraig and Nicholson, 1978). The neuronal changes drive secondary changes in regional cerebral blood flow (Goadsby *et al.*, 1992; Lauritzen, 1984).

There is some controversy in the literature as to whether CSD can activate neurons of the trigeminal nucleus. While it was initially shown that CSD could trigger trigeminal activation (Moskowitz *et al.*, 1993), it has been suggested that this might be related to trauma rather than CSD (Ingvardsen *et al.*, 1997). This has been vigorously discussed (Ingvardsen *et al.*, 1998). More recently, two groups have demonstrated no link between CSD and trigeminal activation (Ebersberger *et al.*, 2001; Lambert *et al.*, 1999). The most recent experiments document an increase in fos expression in the trigeminal nucleus after CSD (Bolay *et al.*, 2002), but required six or more consecutive CSD events to elicit a significant effect. It is unusual to see multiple auras in humans; and aura itself may not be necessarily followed by pain in many older patients (Goadsby, 2001). It seems likely that there is some other crucial component to migraine beyond a simple reflex activation of nociceptive trigeminal fibres.

Clinical neurophysiological studies suggest that the cerebral cortex of migraineurs is hyperresponsive to external stimuli. Habituation of evoked potentials is reduced before attacks, suggesting periodic susceptibility (Afra *et al.*, 2000). This may be due to increased release of excitatory neurotransmitters, reduced intracortical inhibition, and abnormal function of neuronal Ca^{2+} channels and Na^+, K^+ pump ATPases (see below).

14.4 **The migraine threshold: role of genetics**

Migraine is known to run in families, suggesting genetic factors to be involved in the reduced trigger threshold for migraine attacks. Indeed, population-based surveys have shown that first-degree relatives of probands with migraine with (MA) or without aura (MO) have increased risks of migraine, both compared to first-degree relatives of probands without migraine (relative risk), and compared to the risk of migraine in the general population (population relative risk) (Kalfakis *et al.*, 1996; Mochi *et al.*, 1993; Russell and Olesen, 1995; Russell *et al.*, 1996; Stewart *et al.*, 1997). Twin studies showed significantly higher pairwise concordance rates for monozygotic twins than for dizygotic twin pairs (Gervil *et al.*, 1998; Ulrich *et al.*, 1999a). Both types of studies also strongly suggest that MO and MA are multifactorial disorders (Kalfakis *et al.*, 1996; Lalouel and Morton, 1981; Mochi *et al.*, 1993; Russell *et al.*, 1995; Ulrich *et al.*, 1997, 1999b).

In conclusion, multiple genetic factors seem to set the individual trigger threshold for migraine attacks, endogenous and exogenous factors may modulate this set point, and attacks involving physiological mechanisms are provoked by patient-specific trigger factors (Ferrari, 1998).

14.4.1 **Gene mapping approaches to multifactorial disorders**

The search for genetic risk factors for multifactorial paroxysmal diseases such as migraine is complicated by a number of clinical, genetic, and statistical problems (Ferrari *et al.*, 2003). Major clinical issues are how to determine whether or not a person is affected and how to distinguish likely gene carriers from possible phenocopies. While early onset and severe clinical course are traditionally regarded as indicators for a genetic background, it is unclear how one should deal with this in episodic disorders. Are the number of attacks or their severity indicators of the presence of genetic risk factors, or are these merely a consequence of the frequency and intensity of the exposure to environmental triggers?

Once the operational criteria for disease definition have been agreed upon, the genetic strategy will depend on the available patient and family material and on the presence of likely *candidate genes*. When family material is abundant and candidate genes are scarce, random genome screening for linkage will be the method of choice. There is, however, considerable debate about the preferred method of analysis (parametric or non-parametric) and the statistical thresholds that provide optimal distinction between truly positive linkage signals and background noise. Linkage findings may lead — after independent confirmation — to identification of *positional* candidate genes, as opposed to the *functional* candidates that originate from insights into the biochemical pathways underlying the disease. The involvement of such functional candidates may be evaluated not only via functional assays, but also by means of linkage tests in multiply affected families.

A third, less commonly practised method of identifying candidate genes for multifactorial disorders is to localize genes which cause rare Mendelian variants of that disorder. Such loci can then be evaluated as possible susceptibility loci, assuming that mutations, which convey susceptibility to a complex disease, are allelic to more serious gene defects leading to Mendelian segregation or are involved in the same biochemical pathways. Tentatively, one might call such candidate genes *phenotypic* candidates. Such rare variants usually have a clear inheritance pattern and candidate loci can be identified by using regular LOD (logarithm, to the base of 10, of the odds; a statistical estimate of whether two loci are likely to lie near each other on a chromosome) score analyses. This approach has proven to be successful in the search for genes implicated in migraine. Genes for familial hemiplegic migraine (FHM), a rare and severe Mendelial subtype of MA, proved to be involved in ('non-hemiplegic') MO and MA as well. Furthermore, the study of the functional consequences of mutations in these genes also improved our understanding of the mechanisms involved in the migraine attack, pain, and aura (see below).

The advantage of the analysis of functional and phenotypic candidates over a genome search for positional candidates is that the former approach will involve fewer statistical tests, and that consequently, a less stringent statistical correction for multiple testing is required. With respect to functional candidates, one may object that their number is a priori not strictly defined and that different investigators may favour different functional candidates. In contrast, for phenotypic candidates, the number of alternatives is usually very limited. How one should interpret a mildly significant linkage finding for a phenotypic candidate is largely dependent on how plausible a common genetic background is for the common and rare variants of a disease, and on independent confirmation.

A fourth approach is investigating *association with genetic markers*. The rationale of such studies is that genetic markers such as DNA polymorphisms may occur in disequilibrium with genes, various alleles of which may lead to differences of the phenotype.

Such linkage disequilibrium may have two causes: either the time that elapsed to separate the suspect genes from the tightly linked DNA polymorphism by recombination may not have been sufficient for the disequilibrium to disappear, or the marker allele itself influences the phenotype to be studied.

14.4.2 Familial hemiplegic migraine

Familial hemiplegic migraine (FHM) is a rare autosomal, dominantly inherited subtype of MA (Headache Classification Committee of The International Headache Society, 1988). Patients with FHM have attacks of MA which, in addition to the typical migraine aura and headache symptoms, are associated with hemiparesis and, in some families, also cerebellar ataxia and atrophy. Patients with FHM frequently also have attacks of 'non-hemiplegic' typical migraine with or without aura, and in families with FHM there are frequently also patients with 'non-hemiplegic' typical migraine. Attacks of FHM often resemble attacks of basilar migraine (Haan *et al.*, 1995) and, most importantly, the headache and aura symptoms of attacks of FHM are identical to those of MO and MA (apart from the hemiparesis) (Thomsen *et al.*, 2002). Finally, there are also 'sporadic cases' of hemiplegic migraine, whose family members only have 'non-hemiplegic' migraine (Bradshaw and Parson, 1965; Ducros *et al.*, 2001; Heyck, 1973; Terwindt *et al.*, 2002). In conclusion, FHM is part of the migraine spectrum, and genes for FHM are phenotypic and functional candidate genes for 'non-hemiplegic' typical MO and MA (Ferrari, 1998; Ferrari *et al.*, 2003).

14.4.2.1 Genes for FHM

Over 70% of the reported families with FHM, including all those with cerebellar ataxia, have been assigned to chromosome 19p13 (Haan *et al.*, 1994; Joutel *et al.*, 1993, 1994; Ophoff *et al.*, 1994; Teh *et al.*, 1995; Terwindt *et al.*, 1996). FHM linked to 19p13 is caused by missense mutations in the CACNA1A gene encoding the α_{1A} subunit of neuronal, voltage-gated P/Q type calcium channels ($Ca_v2.1$ channels) (Ophoff *et al.*, 1996). Approximately 15% of the reported FHM families have been assigned to chromosome 1q21–34 (Cevoli *et al.*, 2002; Ducros *et al.*, 1997; Gardner *et al.*, 1997; Marconi *et al.*, 2003). FHM linked to chromosome 1q23 is due to mutations in the ATP1A2 gene encoding the a2 subunit of a Na^+,K^+ pump ATPase (De Fusco *et al.*, 2003; Vanmolkot *et al.*, in press). Finally, in some families, linkage to either chromosome 1 or 19 could be excluded, indicating that there is at least a third gene for FHM (Ducros *et al.*, 1997).

14.4.2.2 The CACNA1A calcium channel α_{1A} subunit gene for FHM

The clinical spectrum of CACNA1A mutations in humans
Since the first discovery that missense mutations in the CACNA1A gene cause FHM linked to 19p13 (Ophoff *et al.*, 1996), a large variety and number of mutations in this gene have been associated with a wide spectrum of brain disorders (Fig. 14.2) (for review see Ferrari *et al.*, 2003). These range from pure episodic disorders with only

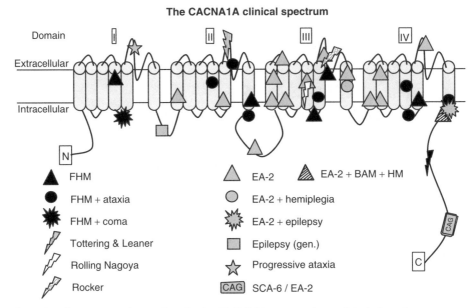

Fig.14.2 Full spectrum of mutations in the CACNA1A gene and associated phenotypes.

transient symptomatology, such as FHM (Ducros *et al.*, 1999, 2001; Kors *et al.*, in press; Ophoff *et al.*, 1996; Takahashi *et al.*, 2002; Wada *et al.*, 2002), episodic ataxia type 2 (EA-2) (Ophoff *et al.*, 1996), and epilepsy (Chioza *et al.*, 2001; Jouvenceau *et al.*, 2001), to chronic progressive brain abnormalities with permanent symptomatology, such as spino-cerebellar ataxia and progressive ataxia, combinations of FHM, and chronic ataxia (Battistini *et al.*, 1999; Ducros *et al.*, 1999, 2001; Kors *et al.*, in press; Ophoff *et al.*, 1996; Takahashi *et al.*, 2002; Wada *et al.*, 2002). At the far end of the CACNA1A clinical spectrum is a fatal disorder characterized by uninhibited cerebral oedema and fatal coma triggered by trivial head trauma (Fitzsimons and Wolfenden, 1985; Kors *et al.*, 2001). Some CACNA1A mutations were found in a few patients with sporadic hemiplegia (Ducros *et al.*, 2001; Terwindt *et al.*, 2002; Vahedi *et al.*, 2000), although in the majority of such patients no mutations were detected in the CACNA1A gene (Carrera *et al.*, 1999; Ducros *et al.*, 1999, 2001; Terwindt *et al.*, 2002).

The clinical spectrum of CACNA1A mutations in mice

There are also mice with spontaneous mutations in the orthologous CACNA1A mouse gene, or other subunit genes of the mouse P/Q type calcium channel, which are primarily characterized by paroxysmal symptoms such as episodic ataxia and epilepsy (Burgess *et al.*, 1997; Doyle *et al.*, 1997; Fletcher *et al.*, 1996; Zwingman *et al.*, 2001). Unlike FHM and EA-2, which are autosomal dominant traits, the mouse traits are recessive. *Tottering* mice have motor seizures and slowly progressive ataxia beginning around the third postnatal week; this phenotype is caused by a missense mutation resulting in a non-conservative (Pro600Leu) amino acid change near the second p-domain, a site putatively involved in channel formation. *Leaner* mice have absence spells (brief seizures) and are severely ataxic, often not surviving past weaning; this more severe phenotype is caused by a splice donor mutation, which results in truncation of the normal transcribed sequences and expression of multiple aberrant transcripts and a novel C-terminal sequence in the polypeptide. This has an analogous situation in humans: missense mutations cause FHM and truncating mutations cause EA-2.

Other spontaneous mice mutatants with a similar, primarily episodic phenotype, include the *Rocker* (Zwingman *et al.*, 2001) and *Rolling Nagoya* (Mori *et al.*, 2000) mice with mutations in the CACNA1A mouse gene, and the *Stargazer* and *Lethargic* mice (for review see Burgess and Noebels, 1999) which are caused by mutations in the γ and β4 subunits of mouse P/Q type calcium channels, respectively. In addition, two CACNA1A-null-mutant (knock-out) mice have been independently generated, displaying ataxia, dystonia, and lethality at about 4 weeks of age (Fletcher *et al.*, 2001; Jun *et al.*, 1999).

Involvement of the CACNA1A gene in migraine

Studies on the involvement of the CACNA1A gene in 'non-hemiplegic' migraine have produced inconclusive results, although the general impression is that the FHM 19p13 CACNA1A region is involved in at least some migraineurs. Two independent affected sib-pair analyses (May *et al.*, 1995; Terwindt *et al.*, 1996), one classical linkage study (Nyholt *et al.*, 1998*b*), and two mutation screen studies (Ducros *et al.*, 2001; Terwindt *et al.*, 1998*b*) suggest involvement of the FHM 19p13 region in 'non-hemiplegic' migraine in at least some migraineurs. May *et al.* (1995) found in 28 mainly German families with migraine, evidence for involvement of the FHM 19p13 region in 'non-hemiplegic' migraine with and without aura. There was, however, a major contribution of one large family. The results were inconclusive as to the magnitude of the involvement and the relative importance of migraine with and without aura.

In a second independent and larger affected sib-pair analysis, involving 36 extended Dutch families, involvement of the FHM 19p13 region in 'non-hemiplegic' migraine with aura was confirmed (maximum multipoint LOD score = 1.29; p≈0.013) (Terwindt *et al.*, 1996). There was no increased sharing for migraine without aura. The allele sharing increased (maximum multipoint LOD score = 1.69; $P <0.005$) when sib pairs were included with migraine with aura in one sib and migraine without aura in the other sib, and even further by combining the results of both studies (maximum multipoint LOD score = 2.27; $P <0.001$). The relative risk ratio for a sib (λ_s) to suffer from migraine with aura, defined as the increase in risk of the trait attributable to the 19p13 locus, was $\lambda_s = 2.4$. A classical linkage study in one large multigenerational family (but not in three others) demonstrated linkage of the FHM 19p13 region to both migraine with and without aura (Nyholt *et al.*, 1998*b*).

Finally, in total, seven members of FHM families have been described who had proven CACNA1A mutations but were suffering from typical 'non-hemiplegic' migraine with or without aura, and not from FHM (Ducros *et al.*, 2001; Terwindt *et al.*, 1998*b*).

A number of other genetic studies produced conflicting results as to the association of the CACNA1A region and migraine. Four classical linkage studies failed to show significant linkage of 'non-hemiplegic' MO or MA to the FHM 19p13 region (Baloh *et al.*, 1996; Hovatta *et al.*, 1994; Noble–Topham *et al.*, 2002; Nyholt *et al.*, 1998*b*). However, in none of these studies could linkage to 19p13 be excluded. The outcome of linkage studies is highly dependent on the chosen model for the penetrance, frequency, phenocopy rate, and other important assumptions. Similarly, although a few studies failed to identify mutations in the CACNA1A gene of migraineurs (Brugnoni *et al.*, 2002; Lea *et al.*, 2001), this does not exclude mutations in other parts of the gene (e.g. the promotor region). In the latter study, association was tested with two microsatellite markers within the CACNA1A gene, but no significant association was found. Again, this does not exclude involvement of CACNA1A in migraine because the gene is very large and positive associations are only found if the markers being used are in linkage disequilibrium (i.e. closely linked to the disease-causing mutation).

Finally, two studies did find linkage of MA to the 19p13 locus, but fine mapping suggested that an insulin receptor gene rather than the CACNA1A gene is associated with MA (Jones *et al.*, 2001; McCarthy *et al.*, 2001). Although interesting, these studies had some remarkable methodological peculiarities which will be discussed below.

$Ca_V2.1$ channels: localization and function

The CACNA1A gene encodes for the pore-forming α_{1A} ($Ca_V2.1$) subunit of neuronal voltage-gated P/Q type $Ca_V2.1$ calcium channels. Alternative splicing yields either P- or Q-type channels (Bourinet *et al.*, 1999). P/Q-type calcium channels are key protein structures in neuronal cell membranes (for review see Plomp *et al.*, 2001) which transduce electrical signals into a cellular influx of Ca^{2+}. The influx of Ca^{2+} acts as a second messenger in many processes such as regulation of excitability, transmitter release, gene regulation, and axonal growth. Ca^{2+} channels consist of a pore-forming, voltage-sensing α_1 subunit, and auxiliary β, $\alpha_2\delta$, and γ subunits. Several subtypes of heteromultimeric channels exist, which are discriminated using pharmacological and electrophysiological criteria (i.e. N, P/Q, L, R, and T types). The α_1 subunit consists of four homologous repeats (I to IV), each with six transmembrane segments (S1 to S6; see Fig. 14.1). The so-called P-loop between S5 and S6 is thought to form the inner lining of the ion pore. The S4 segments have been shown to be involved in voltage sensing.

$Ca_V2.1$ channels are located in presynaptic terminals and somatodendritic membranes throughout the brain (Westenbroek *et al.*, 1995), in particular in the cerebellum (Fletcher *et al.*, 1996; Volsen *et al.*, 1995; Westenbroek *et al.*, 1995), and play a prominent role in controlling both excitatory and inhibitory neurotransmitter release in the mature brain (Dunlap *et al.*, 1995; Iwasaki *et al.*, 2000; Matsushita *et al.*, 2002; Mintz *et al.*, 1995; Stephens *et al.*, 2001). In many central synapses they are preferentially located at the release sites and more effectively coupled to neurotransmitter release than other Ca^{2+} channel types (Mintz *et al.*, 1995; Qian and Noebels, 2001; Wu *et al.*, 1999). $Ca_V2.1$ channels are also important for other cellular functions, including spike generation, neural excitability, signal processing, and gene expression (Bayliss *et al.*, 1997; Eilers *et al.*, 1996; Fletcher *et al.*, 2001; Mori *et al.*, 2000; Pineda *et al.*, 1998; Sutton *et al.*, 1999). At the neuromuscular junction, $Ca_V2.1$ channels control the release of acetylcholine.

Functional consequences of CACNA1A mutations

FHM mutations   Fourteen different missense mutations in the CACNA1A gene have been associated with FHM (with or without associated symptoms such as ataxia or epilepsy). All result in substitutions of conserved amino acids in important functional regions including the pore lining and the voltage sensors (see Fig. 14.2) (Kors *et al.*, 2002; Pietrobon, 2002). Symptom variability among subjects and families with the same mutation indicate that other genetic and environmental factors also influence the phenotype.

The functional consequences of these FHM mutations on recombinant $Ca_V2.1$ channels have been investigated in heterologous expression systems (Hans *et al.*, 1999; Kraus *et al.*, 1998, 2000; Tottene *et al.*, 2002) and in neurons from $Ca_V2.1a_1^{-/-}$ mice expressing human $Ca_V2.1a_1$ subunits (Tottene *et al.*, 2002). There are recent reviews of these studies, as well as an excellent discussion of the functional interpretation for the pathogenesis of migraine (Pietrobon and Striessnig, 2003; Plomp *et al.*, 2001).

In summary, FHM mutations alter both the single channel biophysical properties and the density of functional channels in the membrane, depending on the mutations and cell models used. Two functional effects appear to be common to all FHM mutations: gain of function (increase of Ca^{2+} influx) at the single-channel level; and loss of function (decrease of maximal $Ca_V2.1$ current density) at the whole-cell (neuronal) level (Tottene *et al.*, 2002). Thus, the FHM synaptic phenotype will be a *gain-of-function* phenotype, characterized by increased action potential-evoked Ca^{2+} influx at the active zones (Borst and Sakmann, 1998) and increased neurotransmitter release in synapses where the Ca^{2+} sensor is not saturated.

The missense mutations in FHM suggest a molecular mechanism similar to that found in other human channelopathies. Both alleles are likely to be expressed with the allele harbouring the missense mutation resulting in loss or gain-of-function variants of the P/Q-type calcium channels. Such mutations have been described in the α subunit of the skeletal muscle sodium channel, resulting in hyperkalaemic periodic paralysis, paramyotonia congenita, and the sodium channel myotonias (Kullmann, 2002).

Episodic ataxia (EA-2) and SCA-6 mutations   The functional consequences of these mutations have been studied as well but the results discussion of these findings are beyond the scope of this chapter.

Spontaneous and knock-out CACNA1A mutations in mice   Tottering, leaner, and rolling Nagoya mice strains and their mutated P/Q-type channels have been studied in cerebellar cells and heterologous expression systems. The main effect appears to be reduction of calcium current density (Dove *et al.*, 1998; Lorenzon *et al.*, 1998; Mori *et al.*, 2000; Wakamori *et al.*, 1998).

The neuromuscular junction (NMJ) may be used to study the synaptic consequences of CACNA1A mutations since motor nerve terminals contain P-type calcium channels which control the release of acetylcholine. Transmitter release decreased during high-rate nerve stimulation in tottering NMJs *in vitro*, and spontaneous quantal transmitter release was doubled (Plomp *et al.*, 2000). NMJs of leaner and rolling Nagoya NMJs mice showed a reduction of about 30% and 60%, respectively, of low-rate stimulation-evoked acetylcholine release. Similar changes may occur at brain synapses in humans with mutated CACNA1A-encoded protein.

Interestingly, single-fibre electromyography studies in patients with EA-2 or migraine showed dysfunction of the NMJ (Ambrosini *et al.*, 2001; Jen *et al.*, 2001). Furthermore, P-type Ca^{2+} channels at the NMJ are the target of auto-antibodies causing the paralytic auto-immune disorder, Lambert–Eaton myasthenic syndrome and some of these patients also show ataxia and cerebellar degeneration.

In CACNA1A-null-mutant (knock-out) mice, total calcium current density was decreased in cerebellar cells. P/Q-type currents were abolished but were partly compensated for by R-, N-, and- L-type current. The relative contribution of N-type current to transmitter release at hippocampal synapses was increased. Cerebellar granule cells of heterozygous mice from one of the two null-mutants displayed a 50% reduction in P/Q-type current density (Fletcher *et al.*, 2001), whereas no reduction was observed in the other model (Jun *et al.*, 1999).

14.4.2.3 Are $Ca_V2.1$ channels involved in the pathogenesis of migraine?

Clinical and neurophysiological arguments
Migraine has remarkably many clinical characteristics in common with established brain and muscle channelopathies. These include a paroxysmal presentation with attacks which can be provoked by both endogenous and exogenous stimuli, which may last from minutes to hours or days, and which may come in a frequency ranging from once in a lifetime to one per day. Onset is usually at puberty, amelioration and complete remission may occur after age 40, and penetrance and expression is gender-related (Lehman–Horn and Ferrari 1997). Single-fibre EMG studies suggest abnormalities in migraine patients due to abnormal release of acetylcholine at the neuromuscular junction (Ambrosini *et al.*, 2001), reminiscent of the findings in *tottering* mice (Plomp *et al.*, 2000). Thus, there is some clinical, though still circumstantial, evidence supporting the notion that migraine might be a cerebral ion channelopathy.

Neurobiological arguments
$Ca_V2.1$ channels are expressed in all the structures involved in the pathogenesis of migraine and/or the expression of the migraine pain. In the cerebral cortex,

P/Q-type calcium channels play an important role in the initiation and spread of CSD. They contribute to the regulation of the firing behaviour of cortical neurons (Pineda et al., 1998). Release of glutamate from cortical neurons depends predominantly on P/Q-type channels (Qian and Noebels, 2001; Turner et al., 1992), whereas that of GABA depends primarily on N-type (Timmermann et al., 2002).

The $Ca_v2.1$ mutations of *leaner* and *tottering* mice reduce the channel open probability and shift the activation curve to more depolarized voltages (Dove et al., 1998; Wakamori et al., 1998). Glutamate release was markedly reduced in these mice without any change in GABA release (Ayata et al., 2000; Caddick et al., 1999; Jun et al., 1999). Furthermore, in these mice the threshold for initiating CSD was elevated, the velocity reduced, and the propagation often blocked (Ayata et al., 2000; Caddick et al., 1999; Jun et al., 1999).

Based on these observations and the findings that FHM $Ca_v2.1$ mutations show an synaptic phenotype opposite to that of the leaner and tottering mutations, we expect that the FHM $Ca_v2.1$ mutations will increase the cortical release of glutamate, will not affect the release of GABA, and thus will increase the neuronal cortical network excitability making the cortex more susceptible to CSD.

In the brainstem, $Ca_V2.1$ channels are localized in nuclei involved in the central control of nociception, including PAG, DRN, and nucleus raphae magnus (Craig et al., 1998; Hillman et al., 1991), and play an important role here in modulating Ca^{2+} influx and firing behaviour (Bayliss et al., 1997; Chieng, 2001; Connor et al., 1998; Ishibashi, 1995; Kim, 1997; Penington, 1995). In a rat model of trigeminovascular activation, blockade of P/Q-type channels in the ventrolateral PAG facilitated activation of cells in the trigeminal nucleus TNC to fire, suggesting a role of $Ca_V2.1$ channels in the descending pain inhibitory system that regulates the perception of pain (Knight et al., 2002). These brainstem areas are of particular interest because of the apparent overlap with the site of increased metabolic activity in PET scans during migraine attacks (Weiller et al., 1995). The gain-of-function synaptic FHM phenotype also predicts hyperexcitability of nociceptive trigeminovascular pathways as a result of enhanced release of vasoactive neuropeptides from perivascular nerve endings and, possibly, facilitation of sensitization of second order central trigeminal neurons. The precise effect on trigeminal nociception is, however, unknown. The hypothesis of a calcium channel dysfunction-mediated reduced local threshold for migraine onset seems not far fetched, but is still unproven.

Finally, within the trigeminovascular system, P/Q-type channels account for a large fraction of the Ca^{2+} current of dissociated trigeminal ganglion neurons (Borgland et al., 2001), and, together with N-type channels, control CGRP release from capsaicin-sensitive trigeminovascular afferents (Hong et al., 1999). The P/Q-type blocker, α-eudesmol, inhibits neurogenic vasodilation in facial skin and plasma extravasation in the dura mater following electrical stimulation of the trigeminal ganglion *in vivo* (Asakura et al., 2000) — one of the models for migraine pain.

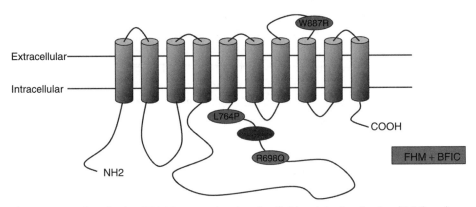

Fig. 14.3 Mutations in the ATP1A2 gene related to familial hemiplegic migraine (FHM) and benign familia infantile convulsions (BFIC).

In conclusion, there is mounting, though still indirect, evidence for involvement of P/Q-type calcium channels in the pathogenesis of migraine. Knock-in mouse models containing human FHM $Ca_V2.1$ mutations may prove instrumental in further elucidating the precise role of these ion channels in the episodic nature of migraine.

14.4.2.3 The ATP1A2 Na^+,K^+ pump ATPase $\alpha2$ subunit gene for FHM

The clinical spectrum of ATP1A2 mutations in human
FHM linked to 1q23 has recently been associated with mutations in the ATP1A2 gene encoding the $\alpha2$ subunit of a Na^+,K^+ pump ATPase (De Fusco *et al.*, 2003; Vanmolkot *et al.*, 2003). So far four different mutations have been identified (Fig. 14.3). One mutation also caused benign familial infantile convulsions in addition to FHM (Vanmolkot *et al.*, 2003).

Na^+,K^+-ATPases: biochemistry and function
The Na^+,K^+-ATPase is an integral plasma membrane enzyme that couples the hydrolysis of ATP to the counter-transport of Na^+ and K^+ across the membrane (Mobasheri *et al.*, 2000). As a key regulator of cellular ion homeostasis, it is important to a number of cellular functions, including control of cell volume and pH and the generation of action potentials. The Na^+, K^+-ATPase protein complex is composed of three heteromeric subunits — the α or catalytic subunit, the β or regulatory subunit, and the γ subunit, whose function is unknown.

There are four α subunit genes of which $\alpha1$–3 are expressed in the CNS (CNS). The $\alpha1$ isoform is ubiquitously expressed and serves as the 'housekeeping' form. The $\alpha2$ isoform is also expressed in muscle and adipose tissue (Mobasheri *et al.*, 2000); in the mouse CNS, expression of the $\alpha2$ isoform is primarily within the neurons during late gestation and the early neonatal stage but primarily in astrocytes in adult tissue (Mobasheri *et al.*, 2000). Only a small part of the α subunit is exposed on the extracellular side of the membrane. Both the amino and carboxyl termini are located intracellularly.

ATP1A2 mutations: functional consequences and possible relationship with migraine pathophysiology

All four ATP1A2 mutations which have been associated with FHM so far, appear to have a *haplo-insufficiency* effect (De Fusco *et al.*, 2003; Vanmolkot *et al.*, 2003). The Na^+,K^+-ATPase pump exchanges intracellular Na^+ for extracellular K^+. Loss of Na^+,K^+-ATPase function may therefore depolarize neurons and render them hyperexcitable. Furthermore, impaired clearance of K^+ by astrocytes, where expression of the α2 Na, K pump isoform is particularly high (Juhaszova and Blaustein, 1997), will increase extracellular K^+ and thus will facilitate CSD (Kraig *et al.*, 1983), the likely mechanism for migraine aura. Increase of intracellular Na^+ will enhance intracellular Ca^{2+} through decreased Na^+-Ca^+-exchanger function, which will also facilitate CSD (Kunkler and Kraig, 1998; Menna *et al.*, 2000), mimicking the effect of gain-of-function $Ca_V2.1$ mutants. In summary, both the calcium channel subunit and ATPase Na^+, K^+ pump FHM mutations seem to result in hyperexcitability of neuronal membranes, reduced threshold for CSD, and enhanced release of neurotransmitters.

The differential expression of the Na^+,K^+-ATPase α2 isoform over life may provide an attractive explanation for the different clinical effects of ATP1A2 mutations in the very young, infantile epilepsy caused by neuronal hyperexcitability, versus in adulthood, with FHM caused by a reduced threshold for CSD due to low reuptake of extracellular K^+ and neurotransmitters by glial cells (Vanmolkot *et al.*, 2003). This finding needs to be confirmed in future studies.

14.4.3 Linkage and association studies in migraine

Association studies have used polymorphisms of candidate genes and looked for over-representation of specific alleles in migraine samples from the general population. Many studies have provided significant or suggestive association; however, none of them have provided conclusive evidence of a specific risk allele for MA or MO.

14.4.4 The serotonin system

Serotonin is implicated in migraine pathophysiology (Sicuteri *et al.*, 1961). More than a dozen different 5-HT signal-mediating receptors have been described. Most of them belong to the metabotropic type of receptors, being composed of a single polypeptide which transmits its action through G-proteins. The only exception is the 5-HT$_3$ receptor type, which is an ionotropic receptor permeable to Na^+ and K^+ ions. Interestingly, this receptor is coded by one single gene on chromosome 11q22 and forms a homomeric complex composed of five copies of the same subunit — a relatively unique structure for neurotransmitter receptors.

Several studies investigated an association between 5-HT genes and migraine. Most of the studies were negative: no association was found with receptor type 5-HT$_{2A}$ (Buchwalder *et al.*, 1996; Monari *et al.*, 1997; Nyholt *et al.*, 1996), 5-HT$_{2C}$ (Buchwalder *et al.*, 1996; Burnet *et al.*, 1997), 5-HT$_{1D}$ (Monari *et al.*, 1997), 5-HT$_{1B}$ (Maassen VanDenBrink *et al.*, 1998; Monari *et al.*, 1997), human serotonin transporter gene (HSERT) (Monari *et al.*, 1997), and 5-HT$_{1F}$ (MaassenVanDenBrink *et al.*, 1998). On the other hand, a Danish–Scottish association study found an association of MO and MA with 5-HT-SERT HSERT (Ogilvie *et al.*, 1998), and Turkish studies found an association between a T102C polymorphism in the 5-HT$_{2A}$ receptor gene (Erdal *et al.*, 2001) and with the serotonin transporter, 2.10 allele (Yilmaz *et al.*, 2001). Finally, a short/short type polymorphism in the 5-HT transporter gene was associated with frequency of attacks in migraine patients, whereas the short/long and long/long types were not (Kotani *et al.*, 2002).

14.4.5 Dopamine D2 receptor gene

There are a number of observations supporting a role for dopamine in the pathophysiology of certain subtypes of migraine. Moreover, many symptoms, such as nausea, vomiting, and hypotension, suggest that brainstem dopaminergic neurotransmission is involved in the migraine attack. Further support for the involvement of the dopaminergic system in migraine has evolved from the finding that dopamine antagonists may be effective in the treatment of migraine symptoms.

Peroutka *et al.* studied the association of an intragenic polymorphism in dopamine D2 receptor (DRD2) in 129 unrelated MO (77) and MA (52) patients and 121 controls, and in MA patients with anxiety and depression (Peroutka *et al.*, 1997, 1998). They found an excess of a Nco I polymorphic allele in MA, with or without anxiety and depression, compared to controls and MO. Del Zompo and colleagues (1998) studied 50 nuclear families from the island of Sardinia, affected with MO, divided into non-dopaminergic (27) and dopaminergic (23) probands, and analyzed them by TDT (transmission disequilibrium test) to dopamine receptors D2, D3, and D4. The subgroup of dopaminergic migraineurs was selected based on the presence of both yawning and nausea immediately before or during the pain phase of migraine. No association was detected with intragenic polymorphisms in DR dopamine receptor gene D3 or D4 to MO. However, in the dopaminergic subgroup of migraine, an allelic association to DRD2 was detected. The association vanished if the DR dopamine receptor gene D2 polymorphism was analyzed in the entire set of MO individuals.

Both of these studies have their merits as well as methodological weaknesses. In the study by Peroutka and colleagues (1997) only scanty information was provided about patients' phenotypes and genetic background. On the other hand, the study by Del Zompo and colleagues (1998) had an almost optimal population design utilizing a genetic isolate and modern methodology, but subgrouping of patients resulted in quite small patient sets.

A German group found no association of MA with DRD2 Nco I (Dichgans *et al.*, 1998*a*), and another group did not find an association with the DRD2-141C Ins/Del polymorphism (Maude *et al.*, 2001). Thus it is not possible to make a definitive conclusion about the role of the DRD2 locus based on these studies. Sheperd and colleagues (2002) found no association between migraine and DRD1, 3, and 5.

14.4.6 Endothelin receptors

Endothelin has been suggested to be involved in migraine, and in a French population-based study it was observed that the G allele of the endothelin type A receptor (ETA-231 A/G) reduces the risk of migraine (Tzourio *et al.*, 2001). This could be an interesting link to the role of nitric oxide and elastase.

14.4.7 The X chromosome

An unequal sex distribution, with a female dominance, is a well-known finding in migraine (Russell *et al.*, 1992; Stewart *et al.*, 1992). There is also evidence of a higher frequency of migraneurs in first-degree relatives of male probands (Stewart *et al.*, 1997). These findings have stimulated studies of a possible involvement of X-chromosomal loci in migraine aetiology. Nyholt and colleagues (1998*a*) reported on a limited genome scan using 28 X-chromosomal markers. Using four large Australian migraine families, they found significant excess of allele sharing and suggestive evidence for linkage on a relatively large area on chromosome Xq. Although the clinical information provided was limited, families represented rather common migraine forms, with both MA and MO individuals. Interestingly, one family showed additional linkage to the 1Q31, which is near the FHM 1q21 locus. Further studies are necessary to confirm the role of X-chromosomal loci in the genetic predisposition to migraine.

14.4.8 Genome-wide scans

Recently, a genome-wide scan of MA has been published, using 50 medium-sized families from Finland (Wessman *et al.*, 2002). The families were selected based on strong representation of MA in all generations. Although MA was the overwhelmingly predominant phenotype, many families had some members with MO. In selecting families for this study, there was a strong bias towards severe phenotypes as the probands were identified from headache clinics, not from the general population or from general practitioner offices. A linkage for the MA phenotype to a rather broad region on chromosome 4q 24 was detected. This chromosomal area does not contain any known ion channel genes, which would be obvious candidates for predisposing sequence variants. However, there are several genes localized to this region that are known to be expressed in the CNS and are thus candidates for further research. This locus is waiting to be replicated in independent studies. The dissection of the phenotype of those families with strongest linkage to chromosome 4 is in progress.

An Italian study found significant linkage to chromosome 14q21.2-q22.3 in a large family with MO (Soragna *et al.*, in press), and a genome-wide scan in a Swedish family with MO and MA showed linkage to 6p12.2-p21.1 (Carlsson *et al.*, 2002).

Two studies focused on the dissection of the chromosome 19p area in MA (Jones *et al.*, 2001; McCarthy *et al.*, 2001). They suggest that the locus linked to MA is distinct from the FHM locus and that specific alleles in the insulin receptor gene would be associated with MA. In a set of 16 families, the maximum LOD score peaked at the insulin receptor locus. Surprisingly for a complex trait, the authors found that the λ-value, reflecting the locus homogeneity of the study sample, was 0.99. This would indicate that all families contribute to the linkage in this region. This is uncommon in any complex trait and has not been found in any other studies in any non-Mendelian disorder. McCarthy and colleagues (2001) found some evidence for association of MA with polymorphisms within the insulin receptor gene in two US populations from the San Francisco area. These associations could not be confirmed in an Australian control sample (only 1 SNP could be linked, but only for MO, not for MA) and an independent British control sample (no association whatsoever). Furthermore, there was no check for the Hardy–Weinberg equilibrium, nor correction for multiple testing. A confirmation of this potentially interesting finding would be welcome.

14.4.9 Other hereditary diseases frequently associated with migraine

Several hereditary diseases are associated with migraine, and can serve as a model to look for and study migraine genes (Haan *et al.*, 1997; Montagna, 2000). Cerebral autosomal dominant arteriopathy with subcortical infarcts and leukoencephalopathy (CADASIL) is characterized by recurrent subcortical ischaemic strokes, extensive white matter abnormalities on MRI, progressive subcortical dementia, and mood disorders with severe depressive episodes (Chabriat *et al.*, 1995*b*; Davous, 1998; Dichgans *et al.*, 1998*b*; Kalimo *et al.*, 2002). Up to one third of the patients have MA (Chabriat *et al.*, 1995*b*; Desmond *et al.*, 1999; Dichgans *et al.*, 1998*b*; Jung *et al.*, 1995; Verin *et al.*, 1995). In one CADASIL family, four of 10 MRI-affected members had co-occurrence with FHM, while one unaffected by MRI had FHM (Hutchinson *et al.*, 1995).

Initially, CADASIL and FHM were considered to be allelic, since the CADASIL locus was mapped to chromosome 19p12 (Tournier–Lasserve *et al.*, 1993). Further linkage studies revealed that the loci were separate (Dichgans *et al.*, 1996), and later, mutations in the Notch3 gene were found in CADASIL (Joutel *et al.*, 1996; Kalimo *et al.*, 2002; Markus *et al.*, 2002). Although CADASIL and FHM are genetically unrelated, the question remains why migraine with aura occurs so frequently in CADASIL. The relation of migraine and CADASIL is further underlined by the finding of families linked to the CADASIL locus, in which patients have MRI white matter lesions, attacks of MA, but without ischaemic stroke (Ceroni *et al.*, 2000; Chabriat *et al.*, 1995*a*).

Migraine was one of the prominent features in a large Dutch family with vascular retinopathy and Raynaud's phenomenon (Terwindt *et al.*, 1998*a*). The disease was subsequently linked to chromosome 3p21.1-p21.3 in this and two North American families (Ophoff *et al.*, 2001).

Mosewich and colleagues (1993) reported a family with a typical MELAS (mitochondrial myopathy, encephalopathy, lactic acidosis and stroke-like episodes) point mutation, with migraine, and not stroke-like episodes. Sano and colleagues (1996) reported a Japanese family with features from both MELAS and MERRF (mitochondrial disease with myoclonic epilepsy and ragged-red fibres), with migraine as one of the prominent symptoms. Migraine has been associated more often with MELAS and MERRF (Klopstock *et al.*, 1996). However, no point mutations nor large-scale deletion were found in 23 Germans with sporadic MA (Klopstock *et al.*, 1996), excluding a significant role for this mutation in Caucasians with migraine. A point mutation in mitochondrial nucleotide 11084 was found in 25% (13/53) of Japanese migraineurs, and in none of 39 normals or 60 tension-type headache sufferers (Shimomura *et al.*, 1995). Neither this, nor any other mutation, was detected in several other studies from different countries (Haan *et al.*, 1999; Russell *et al.*, 1997). Thus, mitochondrial mutations might explain some cases of migraine in Japanese, but do not play an important role worldwide.

14.5 Conclusions

Migraine is a complex neurobiological disorder that is best viewed as a disorder of sensory modulation. Basic laboratory science and brain imaging studies are beginning to provide an anatomical and physiological structure for the condition. Clearly, genetic factors are involved in migraine and, step by step, their contribution to the onset and episodic character of migraine attacks is being unravelled. The recent generation of transgenic knock-in mice carrying FHM $Ca_V2.1$ mutations will further elucidate the biochemical pathways in the early phases of the attack, providing potential novel targets for preventative treatments of migraine and related disorders.

Acknowledgements

The work of PJG has been supported by the Wellcome Trust and the Migraine Trust. PJG is a Wellcome Senior Research Fellow.

References

Adham N, Kao H–T, Schechter LE, Bard J, Olsen M, Urquhart D, *et al.* (1993) Cloning of another human serotonin receptor (5-HT$_{1F}$): a fifth 5-HT$_1$ receptor subtype coupled to the inhibition of adenylate cyclase. *Proceedings of the National Academy of Science (USA)* **90**:408–412.

Afra J, Sandor P, Schoenen J (2000) Habituation of visual and intensity dependence of cortical auditory evoked potentials tend to normalise just before and during migraine attacks. *Cephalalgia* **20**:347.

Afridi S, Goadsby PJ (2003) New onset migraine with a brainstem cavernous angioma. *Journal of Neurology, Neurosurgery and Psychiatry* **74**:680–682.

Akerman S, Kaube H, Goadsby PJ (2002) Vanilloid receptor 1 (VR1) evoked CGRP release plays a minor role in causing dural vessel dilation via the trigeminovascular system. *Cephalalgia* **22**: 572.

Ambrosini A, Maertens de Noordhout A, Schoenen J (2001) Neuromuscular transmission in migraine. A single-fiber EMG study in clinical groups. *Neurology* **56**:1038–1043.

Arbab MA–R, Delgado T, Wiklund L, Svendgaard NA (1988) Brain stem terminations of the trigeminal and upper spinal ganglia innervation of the cerebrovascular system: WGA-HRP transganglionic study. *Journal of Cerebral Blood Flow and Metabolism* **8**:54–63.

Arbab MA–R, Wiklund L, Svendgaard NA (1986) Origin and distribution of cerebral vascular innervation from superior cervical, trigeminal and spinal ganglia investigated with retrograde and anterograde WGA-HRP tracing in the rat. *Neuroscience* **19**:695–708.

Asakura K, Kanemasa T, Minagawa K, Kagawa K, Yagami T, Nakajima M, *et al.* (2000) α-Eudesmol, a P/Q-type Ca^{2+} channel blocker, inhibits neurogenic vasodilation and extravasation following electrical stimulation of trigeminal ganglion. *Brain Research* **873**:94–101.

Ayata C, Shimizu–Sasamata M, Lo EH, Noebels JL, Moskowitz MA (2000) Impaired neurotransmitter release and elevated threshold for cortical spreading depression in mice with mutations in the alpha 1A subunit of P/Q type calcium channels. *Neuroscience* **95**:639–645.

Bahra A, Matharu MS, Buchel C, Frackowiak RSJ, Goadsby PJ (2001) Brainstem activation specific to migraine headache. *The Lancet* **357**:1016–1017.

Baloh RW, Foster CA, Qing Yue MD, Nelson SF (1996) Familial migraine with vertigo and essential tremor. *Neurology* **46**:458–460.

Bartsch T, Goadsby PJ (2002) Stimulation of the greater occipital nerve induces increased central excitability of dural afferent input. *Brain* **125**:1496–1509.

Bartsch T, Akerman S, Goadsby PJ (2002) The ORL-1 (NOP_1) receptor ligand nociceptin/orphanin FQ (N/OFQ) inhibits neurogenic vasodilatation in the rat. *Neuropharmacology* **43**:991–998.

Battistini S, Stenirri S, Piatti M, Gelfi C, Righetti PG, Rocchi R, *et al.* (1999) A new CACNA1A gene mutation in acetazolamide-responsive familial hemiplegic migraine and ataxia. *Neurology* **53**:38–43.

Bayliss DA, Li YW, Talley EM (1997) Effects of serotonin on caudal raphe neurons: inhibition of N- and P/Q-type calcium channels and the afterhyperpolarization. *Journal of Neurophysiology* **77**:1362–1374.

Bland–Ward PA, Feniuk W, Humphrey PPA (2000) The adenosine A1 receptor agonist GR79236 inhibits evoked firing of trigeminal nucleus caudalis (TNC) neurons in the rat. *Cephalalgia* **20**:271.

Bolay H, Reuter U, Dunn AK, Huang Z, Boas DA, Moskowitz MA (2002) Intrinsic brain activity triggers trigeminal meningeal afferents in a migraine model. *Nature Medicine* **8**:136–142.

Borgland SL, Connor M, Christie MJ (2001) Nociceptin inhibits calcium channel currents in a subpopulation of small nociceptive trigeminal ganglion neurons in mouse. *Journal of Physiology* **536**:35–47.

Borst JG, Sakmann B (1998) Calcium current during a single action potential in a large presynaptic terminal of the rat brainstem. *Journal of Physiology* **506**:143–157.

Bouchelet I, Cohen Z, Case B, Hamel E (1996) Differential expression of sumatriptan-sensitive 5-hydroxytryptamine receptors in human trigeminal ganglia and cerebral blood vessels. *Molecular Pharmacology* **50**:219–223.

Bourinet E, Soong TW, Sutton K, Slaymaker S, Mathews E, Monteil A, *et al.* (1999) Splicing of alpha 1A subunit gene generates phenotypic variants of P- and Q-type calcium channels. *Nature Neuroscience* 2:407–415.

Bradshaw P, Parson M (1965) Hemiplegic migraine, a clinical study. *Quarterly Journal of Medicine* 34:65–85.

Branchek T, Archa JE (1997) Recent advances in migraine therapy. In: (ed. Robertson DW) *Central Nervous System Disease.* San Diego: Academic Press, pp. 1–10.

Brugnoni R, Leone M, Rigamonti A, Moranduzzo E, Cornelio F, Mantegazza R, *et al.* (2002) Is the CACNA1A gene involved in familial migraine with aura? *Neurological Science* 23:1–5.

Buchwalder A, Welch SK, Peroutka SJ (1996) Exclusion of 5 HT$_{2A}$ and 5 HT$_{2C}$ receptor genes as candidate genes for migraine. *Headache* 36:254–258.

Bures J, Buresova O, Krivanek J (1974) *The Mechanism and Applications of Leao's Spreading Depression of Electroencephalographic Activity.* New York: Academic Press.

Burgess DL, Noebels JL (1999) Single gene defects in mice: the role of voltage-dependent calcium channels in absence models. *Epilepsy Research* 36:111–122.

Burgess DL, Jones JM, Meister MH, Noebels JL (1997) Mutation of the Ca^{2+} channel ß subunit gene Cchb4 is associated with ataxia and seizures in the lethargic (lh) mouse. *Cell* 88:385–392.

Burnet PW, Harrison PJ, Goodwin GM, Battersby S, Ogilvie AD, Olesen J, *et al.* (1997) Allelic variation in the serotonin 5-HT2C receptor gene and migraine. *Neuroreport* 8:2651–2653.

Burstein R, Collins B, Jakubowksi M (2003) Defeating migraine pain with triptans: a race against developing allodynia. *Neurology* 60:A92-A93.

Burstein R, Cutrer MF, Yarnitsky D (2000*a*) The development of cutaneous allodynia during a migraine attack. *Brain* 123:1703–1709.

Burstein R, Yamamura H, Malick A, Strassman AM (1998) Chemical stimulation of the intracranial dura induces enhanced responses to facial stimulation in brain stem trigeminal neurons. *Journal of Neurophysiology* 79:964–982.

Burstein R, Yarnitsky D, Goor–Aryeh I, Ransil BJ, Bajwa ZH (2000*b*) An association between migraine and cutaneous allodynia. *Annals of Neurology* 47:614–624.

Buzzi MG, Sakas DE, Moskowitz MA (1989) Indomethacin and acetylsalicylic acid block neurogenic plasma protein extravasation in rat dura mater. *European Journal of Pharmacology* 165:251–258.

Caddick SJ, Wang C, Fletcher CF, Jenkins NA, Copeland NG, Hosford DA (1999) Excitatory but not inhibitory synaptic transmission is reduced in lethargic (Cacnb4(Lh)) and tottering (Cacna1atg) mouse thalami. *Journal of Neurophysiology* 81:2066–2074.

Carlsson A, Forsgren L, Nylander PO, Hellman U, Forsman–Semb K, Holmgren G, *et al.* (2002) Identification of a susceptibility locus for migraine with and without aura on 6p12.2-p21.1. *Neurology* 59:1804–1807.

Carrera P, Piatti M, Stenirri S, Grimaldi LM, Marchioni E, Curcio M, *et al.* (1999) Genetic heterogeneity in Italian families with familial hemiplegic migraine. *Neurology* 53:26–33.

Carruthers AM, Sellers LA, Jenkins DW, Jarvie EM, Feniuk W, Humphrey PP (2001) Adenosine A(1) receptor-mediated inhibition of protein kinase A-induced calcitonin gene-related peptide release from rat trigeminal neurons. *Molecular Pharmacology* 59:1533–1541.

Castro ME, Pascual J, Romon T, del Arco C, del Olmo E, Pazos A (1997) Differential distribution of [^{3}H]sumatriptan binding sites (5-HT$_{1B}$, 5-HT$_{1D}$ and 5-HT$_{1F}$ receptors) in human brain: focus on brainstem and spinal cord. *Neuropharmacology* 36:535–542.

Ceroni M, Poloni TE, Tonietti S, Fabozzi D, Uggetti C, Frediani F, *et al.* (2000)Migraine with aura and white matter abnormalities: notch3 mutation. *Neurology* 54:1869–1871.

Cevoli S, Pierangeli G, Monari L, Valentino ML, Bernardoni P, Mochi M, *et al.* (2002) Familial hemiplegic migraine: clinical features and probable linkage to chromosome 1 in an Italian family. *Neurological Science* **23**:7–10.

Chabriat H, Tournier–Lasserve E, Vahedi K, Leys D, Joutel A, Nibbio A, *et al.* (1995a) Autosomal dominant migraine with MRI white-matter abnormalities mapping to the CADASIL locus. *Neurology* **45**:1086–1091.

Chabriat H, Vahedi K, Iba–Zizen MT, Joutel A, Nibbio A, Nagy TG, *et al.* (1995b) Clinical spectrum of CADASIL: a study of 7 families. Lancet **346**:934–939.

Chioza B, Wilkie H, Nashef L, Blower J, McCormick D, Sham P, *et al.* (2001) Association between the alpha(1a) calcium channel gene CACNA1A and idiopathic generalized epilepsy. *Neurology* **56**:1245–1256.

Cohen ML, Schenck K (1999) 5-Hydroxytryptamine(1F) receptors do not participate in vasoconstriction: lack of vasoconstriction to LY344864, a selective serotonin(1F) receptor agonist in rabbit saphenous vein. *Journal of Pharmacology and Experimental Therapeutics* **290**:935–939.

Connor HE, Bertin L, Gillies S, Beattie DT, Ward P, The GR205171 Clinical Study Group (1998) Clinical evaluation of a novel, potent, CNS penetrating NK_1 receptor antagonist in the acute treatment of migraine. *Cephalalgia* **18**:392.

Craig PJ, McAinsh AD, McCormack AL, Smith W, Beattie RE, Priestley JV, *et al.* (1998) Distribution of the voltage-dependent calcium channel α_{1A} subunit throughout the mature rat brain and its relationship to neurotransmitter pathways. *Journal of Comparative Neurology* **397**:251–267.

Cumberbatch MJ, Hill RG, Hargreaves RJ (1997) Rizatriptan has central antinociceptive effects against durally evoked responses. *European Journal of Pharmacology* **328**:37–40.

Cumberbatch MJ, Hill RG, Hargreaves RJ (1998) Differential effects of the $5HT_{1B/1D}$ receptor agonist naratriptan on trigeminal versus spinal nociceptive responses. *Cephalalgia* **18**:659–664.

Cushing H (1904) The sensory distribution of the fifth cranial nerve. *Bulletin of the Johns Hopkins Hospital* **15**:213–232.

Data J, Britch K, Westergaard N, Weihnuller F, Harris S, Swarz H, *et al.* (1998) A double-blind study of ganaxolone in the acute treatment of migraine headaches with or without an aura in premenopausal females. *Headache* **38**:380.

Davous P (1998) CADASIL: a review with proposed diagnostic criteria. *European Journal of Neurology* **5**:219–233.

De Fusco M, Marconi R, Silvestri L, Atorino L, Rampoldi L, Morgante L, *et al.* (2003) Haploinsufficiency of ATP1A2 encoding the Na^+/K^+ pump $\alpha2$ subunit associated with familial hemiplegic migraine type 2. *Nature Genetics* **33**:192–196.

Del Zompo M, Cherchi A, Palmas MA, Ponti M, Bocchetta A, Gessa GL, *et al.* (1998) Association between dopamine receptor genes and migraine without aura in a Sardinian sample. *Neurology* **51**:781–786.

Desmond DW, Moroney JT, Lynch T, Chan S, Chin SS, Mohr JP (1999) The natural history of CADASIL: a pooled analysis of previously published cases. *Stroke* **30**:1230–1232.

Dichgans M, Forderreuther S, Dieterich M, Pfaffenrath V, Gasser T (1998a) The D2 receptor Nco1 allele: absence of allelic association with migraine with aura. *Neurology* **51**:928.

Dichgans M, Mayer M, Muller–Myhsok B, Straube A, Gasser T (1996) Identification of a key recombinant narrows the CADASIL gene region to 8 cM and argues against allelism of CADASIL and familial hemiplegic migraine. *Genomics* **32**:151–154.

Dichgans M, Mayer M, Uttner I, Bruning R, Muller–Hocker J, Rungger G, *et al.* (1998b) The phenotypic spectrum of CADASIL: clinical findings in 102 cases. *Annals of Neurology* **44**:731–739.

Diener HC, Tfelt–Hansen P, de Beukelaar F, Ferrari MD, Olesen J, Dahlof C, *et al.* (2001) The efficacy and safety of sc alniditan vs. sc sumatriptan in the acute treatment of migraine: a randomized, double-blind, placebo-controlled trial. *Cephalalgia* 21:672–679.

Diener H–C, The RPR100893 Study Group (2003) RPR100893, a substance-P antagonist, is not effective in the treatment of migraine attacks. *Cephalalgia* 23:183–185.

Dimitriadou V, Buzzi MG, Moskowitz MA, Theoharides TC (1991) Trigeminal sensory fiber stimulation induces morphological changes reflecting secretion in rat dura mater mast cells. *Neuroscience* 44:97–112.

Dimitriadou V, Buzzi MG, Theoharides TC, Moskowitz MA (1992) Ultrastructural evidence for neurogenically mediated changes in blood vessels of the rat dura mater and tongue following antidromic trigeminal stimulation. *Neuroscience* 48:187–203.

Dove LS, Abbott LC, Griffit WH (1998) Whole-cell and single-channel analysis of P-type calcium currents in cerebellar purkinje cells of leaner mutant mice. *Journal of Neuroscience* 18:7687–7699.

Doyle J, Ren XJ, Lennon G, Stubbs L (1997) Mutations in the CACNL1A4 calcium channel gene are associated with seizures, cerebellar degeneration, and ataxia in tottering and leaner mutant mice. *Mammalian Genome* 8:113–120.

Drummond PD, Gonski A, Lance JW (1983) Facial flushing after thermocoagulation of the gasserian ganglion. *Journal of Neurology, Neurosurgery and Psychiatry* 46:611–616.

Ducros A, Denier C, Joutel A, Cecillon M, Lescoat C, Vahedi K, *et al.* (2001) The clinical spectrum of familial hemiplegic migraine associated with mutations in a neuronal calcium channel. *New England Journal of Medicine* 345:17–24.

Ducros A, Denier C, Joutel A, Vahedi K, Michel A, Darcel F, *et al.* (1999) Recurrence of the T666M calcium channel CACNA1A gene mutation in familial hemiplegic migraine with progressive cerebellar ataxia. *American Journal of Human Genetics* 64:89–98.

Ducros A, Joutel A, Vahedi K, Cecillon M, Ferreir A, Bernard E, *et al.* (1997) Mapping of a second locus for familial hemiplegic migraine to 1q21-q23 and evidence of further heterogeneity. *Annals of Neurology* 42:885–890.

Dunlap K, Luebke JI, Turner TJ (1995) Exocytotic Ca2+ channels in mammalian central neurons. *Trends in the Neurosciences* 18:89–98.

Earl NL, McDonald SA, Lowy MT, 4991W93 Investigator Group (1999) Efficacy and tolerability of the neurogenic inflammation inhibitor, 4991W93, in the acute treatment of migraine. *Cephalalgia* 19:357.

Ebersberger A, Schaible H–G, Averbeck B, Richter F (2001) Is there a correlation between spreading depression, neurogenic inflammation, and nociception that might cause migraine headache? *Annals of Neurology* 41:7–13.

Edvinsson L, Mulder H, Goadsby PJ, Uddman R (1998) Calcitonin gene-related peptide and nitric oxide in the trigeminal ganglion: cerebral vasodilatation from trigeminal nerve stimulation involves mainly calcitonin gene-related peptide. *Journal of the Autonomic Nervous System* 70:15–22.

Eilers J, Plant T, Konnerth A (1996) Localized calcium signalling and neuronal integration in cerebellar Purkinje neurones. *Cell Calcium* 20:215–226.

Erdal ME, Herken H, Yilmaz M, Bayazit YA (2001) Association of the T102C polymorphism of 5-HT2A receptor gene with aura in migraine. *Journal of Neurological Science* 188: 99–101.

Fanciullacci M, Alessandri M, Figini M, Geppetti P, Michelacci S (1995) Increases in plasma calcitonin gene-related peptide from extracerebral circulation during nitroglycerin-induced cluster headache attack. *Pain* 60:119–123.

Feindel W, Penfield W, McNaughton F (1960) The tentorial nerves and localization of intracranial pain in man. *Neurology* **10**:555–563.

Ferrari MD (1998) Migraine. *Lancet* **351**:1043–1051.

Ferrari MD, Haan J, Palotie A (2003) Genetics of migraine. In: (eds. Olesen J, Tfelt–Hansen P, Welch KMA) *The Headaches*. Philadelphia: Lippincott Williams & Wilkins.

Fields HL, Basbaum AI (1994) Central nervous system mechanisms of pain modulation. In: (eds. Wall PD, Melzack R) *Textbook of Pain*. Edinburgh: Churchill-Livingstone, pp.243–257.

Fitzsimons RB, Wolfenden WH (1985) Migraine coma-meningitic migraine with cerebral edema associated with a new form of autosomal dominant cerebellar-ataxia. *Brain* **108**:555–557.

Fletcher CF, Lutz CM, O'Sullivan TN, Shaughnessy JD, Hawkes R, Frankel WN, *et al.* (1996) Absence epilepsy in tottering mutant mice is associated with calcium channel defects. *Cell* **87**:607–617.

Fletcher CF, Tottene A, Lennon VA, Wilson SM, Dubel SJ, Paylor R, *et al.* (2001) Dystonia and cerebellar atrophy in CACNA1A null mice lacking P/Q calcium channel activity. *FASEB Journal* **15**:1288–1290.

Fugelli A, Moret C, Fillion G (1997) Autoradiographic localization of 5-HT1E and 5-HT1F binding sites in rat brain: effect of serotonergic lesioning. *Journal of Receptor and Signal Transduction Research* **17**:631–645.

Gallai V, Sarchielli P, Floridi A, Franceschini M, Codini M, Trequattrini A, *et al.* (1995) Vasoactive peptides levels in the plasma of young migraine patients with and without aura assessed both interictally and ictally. *Cephalalgia* **15**:384–390.

Gardner K, Barmada M, Ptacek LJ, Hoffman EP (1997) A new locus for hemiplegic migraine maps to chromosome 1q31. *Neurology* **49**:1231–1238.

Gervil M, Ulrich V, Olesen J, Russell MB (1998) Screening for migraine in the general population: validation of a simple questionnaire. *Cephalalgia* **18**:342–348.

Giffin NJ, Kowacs F, Libri V, Williams P, Goadsby PJ, Kaube H (2003) Effect of adenosine A$_1$ receptor agonist GR79236 on trigeminal nociception with blink reflex recordings in healthy human subjects. *Cephalalgia* **23**:287–292.

Goadsby PJ (2000) The pharmacology of headache. *Progress in Neurobiology* **62**:509–525.

Goadsby PJ (2001) Migraine, aura and cortical spreading depression: why are we still talking about it? *Annals of Neurology* **49**:4–6.

Goadsby PJ (2002) Neurovascular headache and a midbrain vascular malformation — evidence for a role of the brainstem in chronic migraine. *Cephalalgia* **22**:107–111.

Goadsby PJ, Duckworth JW (1987) Effect of stimulation of trigeminal ganglion on regional cerebral blood flow in cats. *American Journal of Physiology* **253**:R270–R274.

Goadsby PJ, Duckworth JW (1989) Low frequency stimulation of the locus coeruleus reduces regional cerebral blood flow in the spinalized cat. *Brain Research* **476**:71–77.

Goadsby PJ, Edvinsson L (1994) Human *in vivo* evidence for trigeminovascular activation in cluster headache. *Brain* **117**:427–434.

Goadsby PJ, Edvinsson L (1996) Neuropeptide changes in a case of chronic paroxysmal hemicrania- evidence for trigemino-parasympathetic activation. *Cephalalgia* **16**:448–450.

Goadsby PJ, Gundlach AL (1991) Localization of [^{3}H]-dihydroergotamine binding sites in the cat central nervous system: relevance to migraine. *Annals of Neurology* **29**:91–94.

Goadsby PJ, Hoskin KL (1996) Inhibition of trigeminal neurons by intravenous administration of the serotonin (5HT)-1-D receptor agonist zolmitriptan (311C90): are brain stem sites a therapeutic target in migraine? *Pain* **67**:355–359.

Goadsby PJ, Hoskin KL (1997) The distribution of trigeminovascular afferents in the non-human primate brain *Macaca nemestrina*: a c-fos immunocytochemical study. *Journal of Anatomy* **190**:367–375.

Goadsby PJ, Hoskin KL (1999) Differential effects of low dose CP122,288 and eletriptan on Fos expression due to stimulation of the superior sagittal sinus in the cat. *Pain* **82**:15–22.

Goadsby PJ, Knight YE (1997*a*) Direct evidence for central sites of action of zolmitriptan (311C90): an autoradiographic study in cat. *Cephalalgia* **17**:153–158.

Goadsby PJ, Knight YE (1997*b*) Inhibition of trigeminal neurons after intravenous administration of naratriptan through an action at the serotonin ($5HT_{1B/1D}$) receptors. *British Journal of Pharmacology* **122**:918–922.

Goadsby PJ, Lipton RB (1997) A review of paroxysmal hemicranias, SUNCT syndrome and other short-lasting headaches with autonomic features, including new cases. *Brain* **120**:193–209.

Goadsby PJ, Zagami AS (1991) Stimulation of the superior sagittal sinus increases metabolic activity and blood flow in certain regions of the brainstem and upper cervical spinal cord of the cat. *Brain* **114**:1001–1011.

Goadsby PJ, Akerman S, Storer RJ (2001) Triptans can act post-synaptically in the trigeminal nucleus: a microiontophoretic study. *Cephalalgia* **21**:285–286.

Goadsby PJ, Edvinsson L, Ekman R (1988) Release of vasoactive peptides in the extracerebral circulation of man and the cat during activation of the trigeminovascular system. *Annals of Neurology* **23**:193–196.

Goadsby PJ, Edvinsson L, Ekman R (1990) Vasoactive peptide release in the extracerebral circulation of humans during migraine headache. *Annals of Neurology* **28**:183–187.

Goadsby PJ, Hoskin KL, Storer RJ, Edvinsson L, Connor HE (2002*a*) Adenosine (A1) receptor agonists inhibit trigeminovascular nociceptive transmission. *Brain* **125**:1392–1401.

Goadsby PJ, Kaube H, Hoskin K (1992) Nitric oxide synthesis couples cerebral blood flow and metabolism. *Brain Research* **595**:167–170.

Goadsby PJ, Knight YE, Hoskin KL, Butler P (1997) Stimulation of an intracranial trigeminally-innervated structure selectively increases cerebral blood flow. *Brain Research* **751**:247–252.

Goadsby PJ, Lambert GA, Lance JW (1982) Differential effects on the internal and external carotid circulation of the monkey evoked by locus coeruleus stimulation. *Brain Research* **249**:247–254.

Goadsby PJ, Lambert GA, Lance JW (1984) The peripheral pathway for extracranial vasodilatation in the cat. *Journal of the Autonomic Nervous System* **10**:145–155.

Goadsby PJ, Lambert GA, Lance JW (1985) The mechanism of cerebrovascular vasoconstriction in response to locus coeruleus stimulation. *Brain Research* **326**:213–217.

Goadsby PJ, Lipton RB, Ferrari MD (2002*b*) Migraine — current understanding and treatment. *New England Journal of Medicine* **346**:257–270.

Goadsby PJ, Zagami AS, Lambert GA (1991) Neural processing of craniovascular pain: a synthesis of the central structures involved in migraine. *Headache* **31**:365–371.

Goldstein DJ, Gossen D, Granier L (1999) Clinical experience with LY334370, a selective serotonin 1F receptor agonist (SSOFRA): absence of cardiovascular effects. *Cephalalgia* **39**:366–367.

Goldstein DJ, Roon KI, Offen WW, Ramadan NM, Phebus LA, Johnson KW, *et al.* (2001) Selective serotonin 1F (5-HT(1F)) receptor agonist LY334370 for acute migraine: a randomised controlled trial. *Lancet* **358**:1230–1234.

Goldstein DJ, Wang O, Saper JR, Stoltz R, Silberstein SD, Mathew NT (1997) Ineffectiveness of neurokinin-1 antagonist in acute migraine: a crossover study. *Cephalalgia* **17**:785–790.

Gunthorpe MJ, Benham CD, Randall A, Davis JB (2002) The diversity in the vanilloid (TRPV) receptor family of ion channels. *Trends in Pharmacological Science* **23**:183–191.

Haan J, Terwindt G, Ferrari MD (1997) Genetics of migraine. *Neurological Clinics* **15**:43–60.

Haan J, Terwindt GM, Bos PL, Ophoff RA, Frants RR, Ferrari MD, *et al.* (1994) Familial hemiplegic migraine in the Netherlands. *Clinical Neurology and Neurosurgery* **96**:244–249.

Haan J, Terwindt GM, Maassen JA, Hart LM, Frants RR, Ferrari MD (1999) Search for mitochondrial DNA mutations in migraine subgroups. *Cephalalgia* **19**:20–22.

Haan J, Terwindt GM, Ophoff RA, Bos PL, Frants RR, Ferrari MD, *et al.* (1995) Is familial hemiplegic migraine a hereditary form of basilar migraine? *Cephalalgia* **15**:477–481.

Haas DC, Kent PF, Friedman DI (1993) Headache caused by a single lesion of multiple sclerosis in the periaqueductal gray area. *Headache* **33**:452–455.

Hans M, Luvisetto S, Williams ME, Spagnolo M, Urrutia A, Tottene A, *et al.* (1999) Functional consequences of mutations in the human alpha(1A) calcium channel subunit linked to familial hemiplegic migraine. *Journal of Neuroscience* **19**:1610–1619.

Headache Classification Committee of The International Headache Society (1988) Classification and diagnostic criteria for headache disorders, cranial neuralgias and facial pain. *Cephalalgia* **8**:1–96.

Heyck H (1973) Varieties of hemiplegic migraine. *Headache* **13**:135–142.

Hillman D, Chen S, Aung TT, Cherksey B, Sugimori M, Llinas RR (1991) Localization of P-type calcium channels in the central nervous system. *Proceedings of the National Academy of Sciences (USA)* **88**.

Honey AC, Bland–Ward PA, Connor HE, Feniuk W, Humphrey PPA (2000) Study of an adenosine A1 receptor agonist on trigeminally evoked dural blood vessel dilation in the anaesthetized rat. *Cephalalgia* **22**:260–264.

Hong KW, Kim CD, Rhim BY, Lee WS (1999) Effect of omega-conotoxin GVIA and omega-agatoxin IVA on the capsaicin-sensitive calcitonin gene-related peptide release and autoregulatory vasodilation in rat pial arteries. *Journal of Cerebral Blood Flow Metabolism* **19**:53–60.

Hoskin KL, Bulmer DCE, Lasalandra M, Jonkman A, Goadsby PJ (2001) Fos expression in the midbrain periaqueductal grey after trigeminovascular stimulation. *Journal of Anatomy* **197**:29–35.

Hoskin KL, Kaube H, Goadsby PJ (1996) Central activation of the trigeminovascular pathway in the cat is inhibited by dihydroergotamine. A c-*Fos* and electrophysiology study. *Brain* **119**:249–256.

Hoskin KL, Zagami A, Goadsby PJ (1999) Stimulation of the middle meningeal artery leads to bilateral Fos expression in the trigeminocervical nucleus: a comparative study of monkey and cat. *Journal of Anatomy* **194**:579–588.

Hou M, Kanje M, Longmore J, Tajti J, Uddman R, Edvinsson L (2001*a*) 5-HT$_{1B}$ and 5-HT$_{1D}$ receptors in the human trigeminal ganglion: co-localization with calitonin gene-related peptide, substance P and nitric oxide synthase. *Brain Research* **909**:112–120.

Hou M, Tajti J, Uddman R, Edvinsson L (2001*b*) Demonstration of nociceptin positive cells and opioid-receptor like-1 in human trigeminal ganglion. *Cephalalgia* **21**:402.

Hou M, Uddman R, Tajti J, Kanje M, Edvinsson L (2002) Capsaicin receptor immunoreactivity in the human trigeminal ganglion. *Neuroscience Letters* **330**:223–226.

Hovatta I, Kallela M, Farkkila M, Peltonen L (1994) Familial migraine: exclusion of the susceptibility gene from the reported locus of familial hemiplegic migraine on 19p. *Genomics* **23**:707–709.

Hutchinson M, O'Riordan J, Javed M, Quinn E, Macerlaine D, Willcox T, *et al.* (1995) Familial hemiplegic migraine and autosomal dominant arteriopathy with leukoencephalopathy (CADASIL). *Annals of Neurology* **38**:817–824.

Ingvardsen BK, Laursen H, Olsen UB, Hansen AJ (1997) Possible mechanism of c-fos expression in trigeminal nucleus caudalis following spreading depression. *Pain* **72**:407–415.

Ingvardsen BK, Laursen H, Olsen UB, Hansen AJ (1998) Comment on Ingvardsen *et al.* (1997), *Pain*, **72**:407–415; Reply to Moskowitz *et al. Pain* **76**: 266–267.

Iwasaki S, Momiyama A, Uchitel OD, Takahashi T (2000) Developmental changes in calcium channel types mediating central synaptic transmission. *Journal of Neuroscience* **20**:59–65.

Jen J, Wan J, Graves M, Yu H, Mock AF, Coulin CJ, *et al.* (2001) Loss-of-function EA2 mutations are associated with impaired neuromuscular transmission. *Neurology* **57**:1843–1848.

Johnson KW, Schaus JM, Durkin MM, Audia JE, Kaldor SW, Flaugh ME, *et al.* (1997) 5-HT$_{1F}$ receptor agonists inhibit neurogenic dural inflammation in guinea pigs. *NeuroReport* **8**:2237–2240.

Jones KW, Ehm MG, Pericak–Vance MA, Haines JL, Boyd PR, Peroutka SJ (2001) Migraine with aura susceptibility locus on chromosome 19p13 is distinct from the familial hemiplegic migraine locus. *Genomics* **78**:150–154.

Joutel A, Bousser MG, Biousse V, Labauge P, Chabriat H, Nibbio A, *et al.* (1993) A gene for familial hemiplegic migraine maps to chromosome 19. *Nature Genetics* **5**:40–45.

Joutel A, Corpechot C, Ducros A, Vahedi K, Chabriat H, Mouton P, *et al.* (1996) Notch3 mutations in CADASIL, a hereditary adult-onset condition causing stroke and dementia. *Nature* **383**:707–710.

Joutel A, Ducros A, Vahedi K, Labauge P, Delrieu O, Pinsard N, *et al.* (1994) Genetic heterogeneity of familial hemiplegic migraine. *American Journal of Human Genetics* **55**:1166–1172.

Jouvenceau A, Eunson LH, Spauschus A, Ramesh V, Zuberi SM, Kullmann DM, *et al.* (2001) Human epilepsy associated with dysfunction of the brain P/Q-type calcium channel. *Lancet* **358**:801–807.

Juhaszova M, Blaustein MP (1997) Na$^+$ pump low and high ouabain affinity alpha subunit isoforms are differently distributed in cells. *Proceedings of the National Academy of Science (USA)* **94**:1800–1805.

Jun K, Piedras–Renteria ES, Smith SM, Wheeler DB, Lee SB, Lee TG, *et al.* (1999) Ablation of P/Q-type Ca(2+) channel currents, altered synaptic transmission, and progressive ataxia in mice lacking the alpha(1A)- subunit. *Proceedings of the National Academy of Science (USA)* **96**:15245–15250.

Jung HH, Bassetti C, Tournier–Lasserve E, Vahedi K, Arnaboldi M, Blatter Arifi V, *et al.* (1995) Cerebral autosomal dominant arteriopathy with subcortical infarcts and leukoencephalopathy: a clinicopathological and genetic study of a Swiss family. *Journal of Neurology, Neurosurgery and Psychiatry* **59**:138–143.

Kalfakis N, Panas M, Vassilopoulo D, Malliara Loulakaki S (1996) Migraine with aura: segregation analysis and heritability estimation. *Headache* **36**:320–322.

Kalimo H, Ruchoux MM, Viitanen M, Kalaria RN (2002) CADASIL: a common form of hereditary arteriopathy causing brain infarcts and dementia. *Brain Pathology* 12:371–384.

Kaube H, Hoskin KL, Goadsby PJ (1993*a*) Intravenous acetylsalicylic acid inhibits central trigeminal neurons in the dorsal horn of the upper cervical spinal cord in the cat. *Headache* **33**:541–550.

Kaube H, Hoskin KL, Goadsby PJ (1993*b*) Sumatriptan inhibits central trigeminal neurons only after blood-brain barrier disruption. *British Journal of Pharmacology* **109**:788–792.

Kaube H, Keay KA, Hoskin KL, Bandler R, Goadsby PJ (1993*c*) Expression of c-*Fos*-like immunoreactivity in the caudal medulla and upper cervical cord following stimulation of the superior sagittal sinus in the cat. *Brain Research* **629**:95–102.

Kerr FWL (1961) A mechanism to account for frontal headache in cases of posterior fossa tumous. *Journal of Neurosurgery* **18**:605–609.

Kerr FWL, Olafson RA (1961) Trigeminal and cervical volleys. *Archives of Neurology* **5**:69–76.

Klapper JA, Rosjo O, Charlesworth B, Jergensen AP, Soisson T (2002) Treatment of mild migraine with oral zolmitriptan 2.5mg provides high pain-free response rates in patients wih significant migraine-related disability. *Neurology* **58**:A416.

Klopstock T, May A, Seibel P, Papagiannuli E, Diener H–C, Reichmann H (1996) Mitochondrial DNA in migraine with aura. *Neurology* **46**:1735–1738.

Knight YE, Goadsby PJ (2001) The periaqueductal gray matter modulates trigeminovascular input: a role in migraine? *Neuroscience* **106**:793–800.

Knight YE, Bartsch T, Kaube H, Goadsby PJ (2002) P/Q-type calcium channel blockade in the PAG facilitates trigeminal nociception: a functional genetic link for migraine? *Journal of Neuroscience* **22**:1–6.

Knight YE, Edvinsson L, Goadsby PJ (1999) Blockade of CGRP release after superior sagittal sinus stimulation in cat: a comparison of avitriptan and CP122,288. *Neuropeptides* **33**:41–46.

Knight YE, Edvinsson L, Goadsby PJ (2001) 4991W93 inhibits release of calcitonin gene-related peptide in the cat but only at doses with 5HT$_{1B/1D}$ receptor agonist activity. *Neuropharmacology* **40**:520–525.

Kors EE, Haan J, Giffin NJ, Pazdera L, Schnittger C, Lennox GG, *et al.* (in press) Expanding the phenotypic spectrum of the CACNA1A gene T666M mutation: a description of five FHM families. *Archives of Neurology*.

Kors EE, Terwindt GM, Vermeulen FLMG, Fitzsimons RB, Jardine PE, Heywood P, *et al.* (2001) Delayed cerebral edema and fatal coma after minor head trauma: role of CACNA1A calcium channel subunit gene and relationship with familial hemiplegic migraine. *Annals of Neurology* **49**:753–760.

Kors EE, van den Maagdenberg AM, Plomp JJ, Frants RR, Ferrari MD (2002) Calcium channel mutations and migraine. *Current Opinion in Neurology* **15**:11–316.

Kotani K, Shimomura T, Shimomura F, Ikawa S, Nanba E (2002) A polymorphism in the serotonin transporter gene regulatory region and frequency of migraine attacks. *Headache* **42**:893–895.

Kraig RP, Ferreira–Filho CR, Nicholson C (1983) Alkaline and acid transients in cerebellar microenvironment. *Journal of Neurophysiology* **49**:831–850.

Kraig RP, Nicholson C (1978) Extracellular ionic variations during spreading depression. *Neuroscience* **3**:1045–1059.

Kraus RL, Sinnegger MJ, Glossmann H, Hering S, Striessnig J (1998) Familial hemiplegic migraine mutations change alpha(1A) Ca^{2+} channel kinetics. *Journal of Biological Chemistry* **273**:5586–5590.

Kraus RL, Sinnegger MJ, Koschak A, Glossmann H, Stenirri S, Carrera P, *et al.* (2000) Three new familial hemiplegic migraine mutants affect P/Q-type Ca(2+) channel kinetics. *Journal of Biological Chemistry* **275**:9239–9243.

Kullmann DM (2002) The neuronal channelopathies. *Brain* **125**:1177–1195.

Kunkler PE, Kraig RP (1998) Calcium waves precede electrophysiological changes of spreading depression in hippocampal organ cultures. *Journal of Neuroscience* **18**:3416–3426.

Lalouel JM, Morton NE (1981) Complex segregation analysis with pointers. *Human Hereditary* **31**:312–321.

Lambert GA, Goadsby PJ, Zagami AS, Duckworth JW (1988) Comparative effects of stimulation of the trigeminal ganglion and the superior sagittal sinus on cerebral blood flow and evoked potentials in the cat. *Brain Research* **453**:143–149.

Lambert GA, Michalicek J, Storer RJ, Zagami AS (1999) Effect of cortical spreading depression on activity of trigeminovascular sensory neurons. *Cephalalgia* **19**:631–638.

Lance JW, Goadsby PJ (1998) *Mechanism and Management of Headache.* London: Butterworth–Heinemann.

Lassen LH, Haderslev PA, Jacobsen VB, Iversen HK, Sperling B, Olesen J (2002) CGRP may play a causative role in migraine. *Cephalalgia* **22**:54–61.

Lauritzen M (1984) Long-lasting reduction of cortical blood flow of the rat brain after spreading depression with preserved autoregulation and impaired CO_2 response. *Journal of Cerebral Blood Flow and Metabolism* **4**:546–554.

Lauritzen M (1994) Pathophysiology of the migraine aura. The spreading depression theory. *Brain* **117**:199–210.

Lea RA, Curtain RP, Hutchins C, Brimage PJ, Griffiths LR (2001) Investigation of the CACNA1A gene as a candidate for typical migraine susceptibility. *American Journal of Medical Genetics* **105**:707–712.

Leysen JE, Gommeren W, Heylen L, Luyten WHML, Weyer IVD, Vanhoenacker P, et al. (1996) Alniditan, a new 5-hydroxytryptamine$_{1D}$ agonist and migraine-abortive agent: ligand-binding properties of human 5-hydroxytryptamine$_{1D\alpha}$, human 5-hydroxytryptamine$_{1D\beta}$, and calf 5-hydroxytryptamine$_{1D}$ receptors investigated with [^{3}H]-5-hydroxytryptamine and [^{3}H]alniditan. *Molecular Pharmacology* **50**:1567–1580.

Lipton RB, Goadsby PJ (2001) Acute management of migraine: clinical trials of triptans vs other agents. In: (eds. Olesen J, Ferrari MD, Humphrey PPA) *The Triptans: Novel Drugs in Migraine*. Oxford: Oxford University Press, pp. 285–296.

Liu–Chen L–Y, Gillespie SA, Norregaard TV, Moskowitz MA (1984) Co-localization of retrogradely transported wheat germ agglutinin and the putative neurotransmitter substance P within trigeminal ganglion cells projecting to cat middle cerebral. *Journal of Comparative Neurology* **225**:187–192.

Liu–Chen LY, Han DH, Moskowitz MA (1983a) Pia arachnoid contains substance P originating from trigeminal neurons. *Neuroscience* **9**:803–808.

Liu–Chen LY, Mayberg MR, Moskowitz MA (1983b) Immunohistochemical evidence for a substance P-containing trigeminovascular pathway to pial arteries in cats. *Brain Research* **268**:162–166.

Lorenzon NM, Lutz CM, Frankel WN, Beam KG (1998) Altered calcium channel currents in purkinje cells of neurological mutant mouse leaner. *Journal of Neuroscience* **18**:4482–4489.

MaassenVanDenBrink A, Vergouwe MN, Ophoff RA, Saxena PR, Ferrari MD, Frants RR (1998) 5-HT$_{1B}$ receptor polymorphism and clinical response to sumatriptan. *Headache* **38**:288–291.

Marconi R, De Fusco M, Aridon P, Plewnia K, Rossi M, Carapelli S, et al. (2003) Familial hemiplegic migraine type 2 is linked to 0.9Mb region on chromosome 1q23. *Annals of Neurology* **53**:376–381.

Markowitz S, Saito K, Moskowitz MA (1987) Neurogenically mediated leakage of plasma proteins occurs from blood vessels in dura mater but not brain. *Journal of Neuroscience* **7**:4129–4136.

Markowitz S, Saito K, Moskowitz MA (1988) Neurogenically mediated plasma extravasation in dura mater: effect of ergot alkaloids. A possible mechanism of action in vascular headache. *Cephalalgia* **8**:83–91.

Markus HS, Martin RJ, Simpson MA, Dong YB, Ali N, Crosby AH, et al. (2002) Diagnostic strategies in CADASIL. *Neurology* **59**:1134–1138.

Matharu MS, Bartsch T, Ward N, Frackowiak RSJ, Weiner RL, Goadsby PJ (2003) Central modulation in chronic migraine with implanted suboccipital stimulators. *Neurology* **60**:A404–A405.

Matsushita K, Wakamori M, Rhyu IJ, Arii T, Oda S, Mori Y, et al. (2002) Bidirectional alterations in cerebellar synaptic transmission of tottering and rolling Ca^{2+} channel mutant mice. *Journal of Neuroscience* **22**:4388–4398.

Maude S, Curtin J, Breen G, Collier D, Russell G, Shaw D, et al. (2001) The -141C Ins/Del polymorphism of the dopamin D2 receptor gene is not associated with either migraine or Parkinson's disease. *Psychiatric Genetics* **11**:49–51.

May A, Bahra A, Buchel C, Frackowiak RSJ, Goadsby PJ (1998a) Hypothalamic activation in cluster headache attacks. *Lancet* **352**:275–278.

May A, Bahra A, Buchel C, Turner R, Goadsby PJ (1999*a*) Functional MRI in spontaneous attacks of SUNCT: short-lasting neuralgiform headache with conjunctival injection and tearing. *Annals of Neurology* **46**:791–793.

May A, Buchel C, Bahra A, Goadsby PJ, Frackowiak RSJ (1999*b*) Intra-cranial vessels in trigeminal transmitted pain: a PET Study. *NeuroImage* **9**:453–460.

May A, Buchel C, Turner R, Goadsby PJ (2001) MR-angiography in facial and other pain: neurovascular mechanisms of trigeminal sensation. *Journal of Cerebral Blood Flow and Metabolism* **21**:1171–1176.

May A, Gijsman HJ, Wallnoefer A, Jones R, Diener HC, Ferrari MD (1996) Endothelin antagonist bosentan blocks neurogenic inflammation, but is not effective in aborting migraine attacks. *Pain* **67**:375–378.

May A, Kaube H, Buechel C, Eichten C, Rijntjes M, Jueptner M, *et al.* (1998*b*) Experimental cranial pain elicited by capsaicin: a PET-study. *Pain* **74**:61–66.

May A, Ophoff RA, Terwindt GM, Urban C, VanEijk R, Haan J, *et al.* (1995) Familial hemiplegic migraine locus on chromosome 19p13 is involved in common forms of migraine with and without aura. *Human Genetics* **96**:604–608.

May A, Shepheard S, Wessing A, Hargreaves RJ, Goadsby PJ, Diener HC (1998*c*) Retinal plasma extravasation can be evoked by trigeminal stimulation in rat but does not occur during migraine attacks. *Brain* **121**:1231–1237.

McCarthy LC, Hosford DA, Riley JH, Bird MI, White NJ, Hewett DR, *et al.* (2001) Single-nucleotide polymorphism alleles in the insulin receptor gene are associated with typical migraine. *Genomics* **78**:135–149.

McNaughton FL (1938) The innervation of the intracranial blood vessels and dural sinuses. *Proceedings of the Association for Research in Nervous and Mental Diseases* **18**:178–200.

McNaughton FL (1966) The innervation of the intracranial blood vessels and the dural sinuses. In: (eds. Cobb S, Frantz AM, Penfield W, Riley HA) *The Circulation of the Brain and Spinal Cord.* New York: Hafner Publishing Co. Inc, pp.178–200.

Menken M, Munsat TL, Toole JF (2000) The global burden of disease study — implications for neurology. *Archives of Neurology* **57**:418–420.

Menna G, Tong CK, Chesler M (2000) Extracellular pH changes and accompanying cation shifts during oabain-induced spreading depression. *Journal of Neurophysiology* **83**:1338–1345.

Mintz IM, Sabatini BL, Regehr WG (1995) Calcium control of transmitter release at a cerebellar synapse. *Neuron* **15**:675–688.

Mitsikostas DD, Sanchez del Rio M, Moskowitz MA, Waeber C (1999) Both 5-HT$_{1B}$ and 5-HT$_{1F}$ receptors modulate c-*fos* expression within rat trigeminal nucleus caudalis. *European Journal of Pharmacology* **369**:271–277.

Mobasheri A, Avila J, Cozar–Castellano I, Brownleader MD, Trevan M, Francis MJ, *et al.* (2000) Na$^+$, K$^+$-ATPase isozyme diversity; comparative biochemistry and physiological implications of novel functional interactions. *Bioscience Report* **20**:51–91.

Mochi M, Sangiorgi S, Cortelli P, Carelli V, Scapoli C, Crisci M, *et al.* Testing models for genetic determination in migraine. *Cephalalgia* **13**:389–394.

Monari L, Mochi M, Valentino ML, Arnaldi C, Cortelli P, De Monte A, *et al.* (1997) Searching for migraine genes: exclusion of 290 cM out of the whole human genome. *Italian Journal of Neurological Science* **18**:277–282.

Montagna P (2000) Molecular genetics of migraine headache: a review. *Cephalalgia* **20**:3–14.

Montell C, Birnbaumer L, Flockerzi V (2002) The TRP channels, a remarkably functional family. *Cell* **108**:595–598.

Mori Y, Wakamori M, Oda S, Fletcher CF, Sekiguchi N, Mori E, *et al.* (2000) Reduced voltage sensitivity of activation of P/Q-type Ca^{2+} channels is associated with the ataxic mouse mutation rolling Nagoya (tg(rol)). *Journal of Neuroscience* **20**:5654–5662.

Mosewich RK, Donat JR, DiMauro S, Ciafaloni E, Shanske S, Erasmus M, *et al.* (1993) The syndrome of mitochondrial encephalomyopathy, lactic acidosis, and strokelike episodes presenting without stroke. *Archives of Neurology* **50**:275–278.

Moskowitz MA, Cutrer FM (1993) Sumatriptan: a receptor-targeted treatment for migraine. *Annual Review of Medicine* **44**:145–154.

Moskowitz MA, Nozaki K, Kraig RP (1993) Neocortical spreading depression provokes the expression of C-fos protein-like immunoreactivity within the trigeminal nucleus caudalis via trigeminovascular mechanisms. *Journal of Neuroscience* **13**:1167–1177.

Noble–Topham SE, Dyment DA, Cader MZ, Ganapathy R, Brown JD, Rice GPA, *et al.* (2002) Migraine with aura is not linked to the FHM gene CACNA1A or the chromosomal region, 19p13. *Neurology* **59**:1099–1101.

Norman B, Panebianco D, Block GA (1998) A placebo-controlled, in-clinic study to explore the preliminary safety and efficacy of intravenous L-758,298 (a prodrug of the NK1 receptor antagonist L-754,030) in the acute treatment of migraine. *Cephalalgia* **18**:407.

Nyholt DR, Curtain RP, Gaffney PT, Brimage P, Goadsby PJ, Griffiths LR (1996) Migraine association and linkage analyses of the human 5-hydroxytryptamine ($5HT_{2A}$) receptor gene. *Cephalalgia* **16**:463–467.

Nyholt DR, Dawkins JL, Brimage PJ, Goadsby PJ, Nicholson GA, Griffiths LR (1998*a*) Evidence for an X-linked genetic component in familial typical migraine. *Human Molecular Genetics* **7**:459–463.

Nyholt DR, Lea RA, Goadsby PJ, Brimage PJ, Griffiths LR (1998*b*) Familial typical migraine: linkage to chromosome 19p13 and evidence for genetic heterogeneity. *Neurology* **50**:1428–1432.

Ogilvie AD, Russell MB, Dhall P, Battersby S, Ulrich V, Dale Smith CA, *et al.* (1998) Altered allelic distributions of the serotonin transporter gene in migraine without aura and migraine with aura. *Cephalalgia* **18**:23–26.

Olesen J (2001) Revision of the International Headache Classification. An interim report. *Cephalalgia* **21**:261.

Olesen J, Goadsby PJ (1999) *Cluster Headache and Related Conditions*, Vol 9. Oxford: Oxford University Press.

Olesen J, Tfelt–Hansen P, Welch KMA (2000) *The Headaches*. Philadelphia: Lippincott, Williams & Wilkins.

Ophoff RA, DeYoung J, Service SK, Joosse M, Caffo NA, Sandkuijl LA, *et al.* (2001) Hereditary vascular retinopathy, cerebroretinal vasculopathy, and hereditary endotheliopathy with retinopathy, nephropathy and stroke map to a single locus on chromosome 3p21.1-p21.3. *American Journal of Human Genetics* **69**:447–453.

Ophoff RA, Eijk Rv, Sandkuijl LA, Terwindt GM, Grubben CPM, Haan J, *et al.* (1994) Genetic heterogeneity of familial hemiplegic migraine. *Genomics* **22**:21–26.

Ophoff RA, Terwindt GM, Vergouwe MN, van Eijk R, Oefner PJ, Hoffman SMG, *et al.* (1996) Familial hemiplegic migraine and episodic ataxia type-2 are caused by mutations in the Ca^{2+} channel gene CACNL1A4. *Cell* **87**:543–552.

Paalzow G, Paalzow L (1973) The effects of caffeine and theophylline on nociceptive stimulation in the rat. *Acta Pharmacologia et Toxicologica* **32**:22–32.

Palmer KJ, Dalton J (2000) Drugs in development for migraine. *Drugs Research & Development* **2**:375–379.

Pascual J, Arco Cd, Romon T, Olmo Cd, Pazos A (1996) [^{3}H] Sumatriptan binding sites in human brain: regional-dependent labelling of 5HT$_{1D}$ and 5HT$_{1F}$ receptors. *European Journal of Pharmacology* **295**:271–274.

Penfield W, McNaughton FL (1940) Dural headache and the innervation of the dura mater. *Archives of Neurology and Psychiatry* **44**:43–75.

Peroutka SJ, Price SC, Wilhoit TL, Jones KW (1998) Comorbid migraine with aura, anxiety, and depression is associated with dopamine D2 receptor (DRD2) NcoI alleles. *Molecular Medicine* **4**:14–21.

Peroutka SJ, Wilhoit T, Jones K (1997) Clinical susceptibility to migraine aura is modified by dopamine D2 receptor (DRD2) NcoI alleles. *Neurology* **49**:201–206.

Phebus LA, Johnson KW, Zgombick JM, Gilbert PJ, Van Belle K, Mancuso V, *et al.* (1997) Characterization of LY334370 as a pharmacological tool to study 5HT$_{1F}$ receptors — binding affinities, brain penetration and activity in the neurogenic dural inflammation model of migraine. *Life Sciences* **61**:2117–2126.

Pietrobon D (2002) Calcium channels and channelopathies of the central nervous system. *Molecular Neurobiology* **25**:31–50.

Pietrobon D, Striessnig J (2003) Neurobiology of migraine. *Nature Review Neuroscience* **4**:386–398.

Pineda JC, Waters RS, Foehring RC (1998) Specificity in the interaction of HVA Ca^{2+} channel types with Ca^{2+}-dependent AHPs and firing behavior in neocortical pyramidal neurons. *Journal of Neurophysiology* **79**:2522–2534.

Plomp JJ, van den Maagdenberg AMJM, Molenaar PC, Frants RR, Ferrari MD (2001) Mutant P/Q-type calcium channel electrophysiology and migraine. *Current Opinion in Investigational Drugs* **2**:1250–1260.

Plomp JJ, Vergouwe MN, Van den Maagdenberg AM, Ferrari MD, Frants RR, Molenaar PC (2000) Abnormal transmitter release at neuromuscular junctions of mice carrying the *tottering* alpha-1-A Ca^{2+} channel mutation. *Brain* **123**:463–471.

Qian J, Noebels JL (2001) Presynaptic Ca^{2+} channels and neurotransmitter release at the terminal of a mouse cortical neuron. *Journal of Neuroscience* **21**:3721–3728.

Raskin NH, Hosobuchi Y, Lamb S (1987) Headache may arise from perturbation of brain. *Headache* **27**:416–420.

Rasmussen BK (1995) Epidemology of headache. *Cephalalgia* **15**:45–68.

Rasmussen BK, Jensen R, Schroll M (1991) Epidemiology of headache in the general population: a prevalence study. *Journal of Clinical Epidemiology* **44**:1147–1157.

Razzaque Z, Heald MA, Pickard JD, Maskell L, Beer MS, Hill RG, *et al.* (1999) Vasoconstriction in human isolated middle meningeal arteries: determining the contribution of 5-HT$_{1B}$- and 5-HT$_{1F}$-receptor activation. *British Journal of Clinical Pharmacology* **47**:75–82.

Roon KI, Olesen J, Diener HC, Ellis P, Hettiarachchi J, Poole PH, *et al.* (2000) No acute antimigraine efficacy of CP-122,288, a highly potent inhibitor of neurogenic inflammation: results of two randomized double-blind placebo-controlled clinical trials. *Annals of Neurology* **47**:238–241.

Russell MB, Diamant M, Norby S (1997) Genetic heterogeneity of migraine with and without aura in Danes cannot be explained by mutation in mtDNA nucleotide pair 11084. *Acta Neurologica Scandinavica* **96**:171–173.

Russell MB, Iselius L, Olesen J (1995) Investigation of the inheritance of migraine by complex segregation analysis. *Human Genetics* **96**:726–730.

Russell MB, Olesen J (1995) Increased familial risk and evidence of genetic factor in migraine. *British Medical Journal* **311**:541–544.

Russell MB, Rassmussen BK, Brennum J, Iversen HK, Jensen RA, Olesen J (1992) Presentation of a new instrument: the diagnostic headache diary. *Cephalalgia* **12**:369–374.

Russell MB, Rassmussen BK, Fenger K, Olesen J (1996) Migraine without aura and migraine with aura are distinct clinical entities: a study of four hundred and eight-four male and female migraineurs from the general population. *Cephalalgia* **16**:239–245.

Sano M, Ozawa M, Shiota S, Momose Y, Uchigata M, Goto Y (1996) The T-C(8356) mitochondrial DNA mutation in a Japanese family. *Journal of Neurology* **243**:441–444.

Sawynok J (1998) Adenosine receptor activation and nociception. *European Journal of Pharmacology* **347**:1–11.

Sawynok J (1999) Purines in pain management. *Current Opinion in Central and Peripheral Nervous System Investigational Drugs* **1**:27–38.

Sawynok J, Sweeney MI, White TD (1986) Classification of adenosine receptors mediating antinociception in the rat spinal cord. *British Journal of Pharmacology* **88**:923–930.

Schindler M, Harris CA, Hayes B, Papotti M, Humphrey PPA (2001) Immunohistochemical localization of adenosine A1 receptors in human brain regions. *Neuroscience Letters* **297**: 211–215.

Selby G, Lance JW (1960) Observations on 500 cases of migraine and allied vascular headache. *Journal of Neurology, Neurosurgery and Psychiatry* **23**:23–32.

Sheperd AG, Lea RA, Hutchins C, Jordan KL, Brimage PJ, Griffiths LR (2002) Dopamine receptor genes and migraine with and without aura: an association study. *Headache* **42**:346–351.

Shepheard S, Edvinsson L, Cumberbatch M, Williamson D, Mason G, Webb J, *et al.* (1999) Possible antimigraine mechanisms of action of the $5HT_{1F}$ receptor agonist LY334370. *Cephalalgia* **19**:851–858.

Shepheard SL, Williamson DJ, Williams J, Hill RG, Hargreaves RJ (1993) Comparison of the effects of sumatriptan and the NK1 antagonist CP-99,994 on plasma extravasation in the dura mater and c-fos mRNA expression in the trigeminal nucleus caudalis of rats. *Neuropharmacology* **34**:255–261.

Shimomura T, Kitano A, Merukawa H, Takahashi K (1995) Mutation in platelet mitochondrial gene in patients with migraine. *Cephalalgia* **15**:10.

Sicuteri F, Testi A, Anselmi B (1961) Biochemical investigations in headache: increase in hydroxyindoleacetic acid excretion during migraine attacks. *International Archives of Allergy* **19**:55–58.

Silberstein SD, Lipton RB, Goadsby PJ (2002) *Headache in Clinical Practice*. London: Martin Dunitz.

Sjolund K–F, Sollevi A, Segerdahl M, Hansson P, Lundeberg T (1996) Intrathecal and systemic R-phenylisopropy-adenosine reduces scratching behaviour in a rat mononeuropathy model. *NeuroReport* **7**:1856–1860.

Soragna D, Vettori A, Carraro G, Marchioni E, Vazza G, Bellini S, *et al.* (in press) A locus for migraine without aura maps on chromosome 14q21.2-q22.3. *American Journal of Human Genetics*

Stephens GJ, Morris NP, Fyffe RE, Robertson B *(2001)* The Cav2.1/alpha1A (P/Q-type) voltage-dependent calcium channel mediates inhibitory neurotransmission onto mouse cerebellar Purkinje cells. *European Journal of Neuroscience* **13**:1902–1912.

Stewart WF, Lipton RB, Celentano DD, Reed ML (1992) Prevalence of migraine headache in the United States: relation to age, income, race and other sociodemographic factors. *Journal of the American Medical Association* **267**:64–69.

Stewart WF, Staffa J, Lipton RB, Ottman R (1997) Familial risk of migraine: a population-based study. *Annals of Neurology* **41**:166–172.

Storer RJ, Goadsby PJ (1997) Microiontophoretic application of serotonin $(5HT)_{1B/1D}$ agonists inhibits trigeminal cell firing in the cat. *Brain* **120**:2171–2177.

Storer RJ, Akerman S, Connor HE, Goadsby PJ (2001*a*) 4991W93, a potent blocker of neurogenic plasma protein extravasation, inhibits trigeminal neurons at 5-hydroxytryptamine (5-HT$_{1B/1D}$) agonist doses. *Neuropharmacology* **40**:911–917.

Storer RJ, Akerman S, Goadsby PJ (2001*b*) GABA receptors modulate trigeminovascular nociceptive neurotransmission in the trigeminocervical complex. *British Journal of Pharmacology* **134**:896–904.

Storer RJ, Akerman S, Goadsby PJ (2001*c*) Opioid receptors modulate nociceptive neurotransmission in the trigeminocervical complex. *Cephalalgia* **21**:354.

Strassman AM, Raymond SA, Burstein R (1996) Sensitization of meningeal sensory neurons and the origin of headaches. *Nature* **384**:560–563.

Sutton KG, McRory JE, Guthrie H, Murphy TH, Snutch TP (1999) P/Q-type calcium channels mediate the activity-dependent feedback of syntaxin-1A. *Nature* **401**:800–804.

Takahashi T, Igarashi S, Kimura T, Hozumi I, Kawachi I, Onodera O, *et al.* (2002) Japanese cases of familial hemiplegic migraine with cerebellar ataxia carrying a T666M mutation in the CACNA1A gene. Journal of Neurology, Neurosurgery & Psychiatry **72**:676–677.

Teh BT, Silburn P, Lindblad K, Betz R, Boyle R, Schalling M, *et al.* (1995) Familial cerebellar periodic ataxia without myokymia maps to a 19-cM region on 19p13. *American Journal of Human Genetics* **56**:1443–1449.

Terwindt G, Kors E, Haan J, Vermeulen F, Van den Maagdenberg A, Frants R, *et al.* (2002) Mutation analysis of the CACNA1A calcium channel subunit gene in 27 patients with sporadic hemiplegic migraine. *Archives of Neurology* **59**:1016–1018.

Terwindt GM, Haan J, Ophoff RA, Groenen SMA, Storimans C, Lanser JBK, *et al.* (1998*a*) Clinical and genetic analysis of a large Dutch family with autosomal dominant vascular retinopathy, migraine and Raynaud's phenomenon. *Brain* **121**:303–316.

Terwindt GM, Ophoff RA, Haan J, Ferrari MD, The Dutch Migraine Genetics Research Group (1996) Familial hemiplegic migraine: a clinical comparison of families linked and unlinked to chromosome 19. *Cephalalgia* **16**:153–155.

Terwindt GM, Ophoff RA, Haan J, Vergouwe MN, van Eijk R, Frants RR, *et al.* (1998*b*) Variable clinical expression of mutations in the P/Q-type calcium channel gene in familial hemiplegic migraine. *Neurology* **50**:1105–1110.

Thomsen LL, Eriksen MK, Roemer SF, Andersen I, Olesen J, Russell MB (2002) A population-based study of familial hemiplegic migraine suggests revised diagnostic criteria. *Brain* **125**:1379–1391.

Timmermann DB, Westenbroek RE, Schousboe A, Catterall WA (2002) Distribution of high-voltage-activated calcium channels in cultured gamma-aminobutyric acidergic neurons from mouse cerebral cortex. *Journal of Neuroscience Research* **67**:48–61.

Tottene A, Tottene A, Fellin T, Pagnutti S, Luvisetto S, Striessnig J, *et al.* (2002) Familial hemiplegic migraine mutations increase Ca^{2+} influx through single human CaV2.1 channels and decrease maximal Ca$_V$2.1 current density in neurons. *Proceedings of the National Academy of Science (USA)* **99**:13284–13289.

Tournier–Lasserve E, Joutel A, Melki J, Weissenbach J, Lathrop GM, Chabriat H, *et al.* (1993) Cerebral autosomal dominant arteriopathy with subcortical infarcts and leukoencephalopathy maps to chromosome 19p12. *Nature Genetics* **3**:256–259.

Tran–Dinh YR, Thurel C, Cunin G, Serrie A, Seylaz J (1992) Cerebral vasodilation after the thermocoagulation of the trigeminal ganglion in humans. *Neurosurgery* **31**:658–662.

Turner TJ, Adams ME, Dunlap K (1992) Calcium channels coupled to glutamate release identified by omega-Aga-IVA. *Science* **258**:310–313.

Tzourio C, El Amrani M, Poirier O, Nicaud V, Bousser MG, Alperovitch A (2001) Association between migraine and endothelin type A receptor (ETA -231 A/G) gene polymorphism. *Neurology* **56**:1273–1277.

Uddman R, Edvinsson L, Ekman R, Kingman T, McCulloch J (1985) Innervation of the feline cerebral vasculature by nerve fibers containing calcitonin gene-related peptide: trigeminal origin and co-existence with substance P. *Neuroscience Letters* **62**:131–136.

Ulrich V, Gervil M, Kyvik KO, Olesen J, Russell MB (1999*a*) Evidence of a genetic factor in migraine with aura: a population based Danish twin study. *Annals of Neurology* **45**:242–246.

Ulrich V, Gervil M, Kyvik KO, Olesen J, Russell MB (1999*b*) The inheritance of migraine with aura estimated by means of structural equation modelling. *Journal of Medical Genetics* **36**:225–227.

Ulrich V, Russell MB, Østergaard S, Olesen J (1997) Analysis of 31 families with an apparently autosomal dominant transmission of migraine with aura in the nuclear families. *American Journal of Medical Genetics* **74**:395–397.

Vahedi K, Denier C, Ducros A, Bousson V, Levy C, Chabriat H, *et al.* (2000) CACNA1A gene *de novo* mutation causing hemiplegic migraine, coma, and cerebellar atrophy. *Neurology* **55**:1040–1042.

Vanmolkot KRJ, Kors EE, Hottenga JJ, Terwindt GM, Haan J, Hoefnagels WAJ, *et al.* (2003) Novel mutations in the Na$^+$,K$^+$-ATPase pump gene ATP1A2 associated with familial hemiplegic migraine and benign familial infantile convulsions. *Annals of Neurology* **54**:360–366.

Veloso F, Kumar K, Toth C (1998) Headache secondary to deep brain implantation. *Headache* **38**:507–515.

Verin M, Rolland Y, Landgraf F, Chabriat H, Bompais B, Michel A, *et al.* (1995) New phenotype of the cerebral autosomal dominant arteriopathy mapped to chromosome 19: migraine as the prominent clinical feature. *Journal of Neurology, Neurosurgery & Psychiatry* **59**:579–585.

Volsen SG, Day NC, McCormack AL, Smith W, Craig PJ, Beattie R, *et al.* (1995)The expression of neuronal voltage-dependent calcium channels in human cerebellum. *Brain Research Molecular Brain Research* **34**:271–282.

Wada T, Kobayashi N, Takahashi Y, Aoki T, Watanabe T, Saitoh S (2002) Wide clinical variability in a family with a CACNA1A T666m mutation: hemiplegic migraine, coma, and progressive ataxia. *Pediatric Neurology* **26**:47–50.

Waeber C, Moskowitz MA (1995) [^{3}H]sumatriptan labels both 5-HT$_{1D}$ and 5HT$_{1F}$ receptor bindings sites in the guinea pig brain: an autoradiographic study. *Naunyn–Schmiedeberg's Archives of Pharmacology* **352**:263–275.

Wainscott DB, Johnson KW, Phebus LA, Schaus JM, Nelson DL (1998) Human 5-HT1F receptor-stimulated [S-35]GTP gamma S binding: correlation with inhibition of guinea pig dural plasma protein extravasation. *European Journal of Pharmacology* **352**:117–124.

Wakamori M, Yamazaki K, Matsunodaira H, Teramoto T, Tanaka I, Niidome T, *et al.* (1998) Single tottering mutations responsible for the neuropathic phenotype of the P-Type calcium channel. *Journal of Biological Chemistry* **273**:34857–34867.

Waldenlind E, Ekbom K, Torhall J (1993) MR-angiography during spontaneous attacks of cluster headache: a case report. *Headache* **33**:291–295.

Weiller C, May A, Limmroth V, Juptner M, Kaube H, Schayck RV, *et al.* (1995) Brain stem activation in spontaneous human migraine attacks. *Nature Medicine* **1**:658–660.

Welch KM, Nagesh V, Aurora S, Gelman N (2001) Periaqueductal grey matter dysfunction in migraine: cause or the burden of illness? *Headache* **41**:629–637.

Wessman M, Kallela M, Kaunisto MA, Marttila P, Sobel E, Hartiala J, *et al.* (2002) A susceptibility locus for migraine with aura, on chromosome 4q24. *American Journal of Human Genetics* **70**:652–662.

Westenbroek RE, Sakurai T, Elliott EM, Hell JW, Starr TVB, Snutch TP, *et al.* (1995) Immunochemical identification and subcellular distribution of the alpha(1a) subunits of brain calcium channels. *Journal of Neuroscience* **15**:6403–6418.

Williamson DJ, Shepheard SL, Cook DA, Hargreaves RJ, Hill RG, Cumberbatch MJ (2001) Role of opioid receptors in neurogenic dural vasodilation and sensitization of trigeminal neurones in anaesthetized rats. *British Journal of Pharmacology* **133**:807–814.

Winner P, Mannix L, McNeal S, O'Quinn S, Metz A (2002) Treatment of migraine at the first sign of pain: prospective, double-blind, placebo-controlled, multicenter studies of sumatriptan 50mg and 200mg versus placebo. *Headache* **42**:401–402.

Wolff HG (1948) *Headache and Other Head Pain.* New York: Oxford University Press.

Wu LG, Westenbroek RE, Borst JG, Catterall WA, Sakmann B (1999) Calcium channel types with distinct presynaptic localization couple differentially to transmitter release in single calyx-type synapses. *Journal of Neuroscience* **19**:726–736.

Yilmaz M, Erdal ME, Herken H, Cataloluk O, Barlas O, Bayazi YA (2001) Significance of serotonin transporter gene polymorphism in migraine. *Journal of Neurological Science* **186**:27–30.

Zagami AS, Goadsby PJ (1991) Stimulation of the superior sagittal sinus increases metabolic activity in cat thalamus. In: (ed. Rose FC) *New Advances in Headache Research: 2.* London: Smith–Gordon and Co Ltd, pp. 169–171.

Zagami AS, Lambert GA (1991) Craniovascular application of capsaicin activates nociceptive thalamic neurons in the cat. *Neuroscience Letters* **121**:187–190.

Zagami AS, Goadsby PJ, Edvinsson L (1990) Stimulation of the superior sagittal sinus in the cat causes release of vasoactive peptides. *Neuropeptides* **16**:69–75.

Zwingman TA, Neumann PE, Noebels JL, Herrup K (2001) Rocker is a new variant of the voltage-dependent calcium channel gene CACNA1A. *Journal of Neuroscience* **21**:1169–1178.

Chapter 15

An integrative approach to the control of cancer pain

Patrick W. Mantyh and Tony L. Yaksh

15.1 Introduction

It is difficult to overestimate the negative impact that cancer pain has on a patient's quality of life. As advances in cancer detection and therapy are extending the life expectancy of cancer patients, there is increasing focus on improving their quality of life and, in particular, devising new therapies for cancer-associated pain. Many patients present with pain as the first sign of cancer, and 30–50% of all cancer patients will experience moderate to severe pain (Mercadante 1997; Mercadante and Arcuri 1998; Portenoy and Lesage 1999; Portenoy *et al.* 1999). Cancer-associated pain can occur at any time during the evolution of the disease, but the frequency and intensity of pain tend to increase with advancing stages of cancer so that in patients with metastatic or advanced cancer, 75–95% will experience significant, life-altering cancer-induced pain (Mercadante 1997; Mercadante and Arcuri 1998; Portenoy and Lesage 1999; Portenoy *et al.* 1999).

The treatment of cancer pain can involve a variety of modalities. Therapies targeted at decreasing tumor size are often effective and include radiation, chemotherapy, and surgery. However, these treatments can be burdensome to administer and are accompanied by significant adverse effects. Medications targeted at decreasing inflammation and pain, such as non-steroidal anti-inflammatory drugs or opiates, can also be very useful, but these too are frequently accompanied by significant unwanted side-effects.

The relative ineffectiveness of current treatments reflects the fact that therapies have not changed for decades (Coyle *et al.* 1990; Payne 1997; Payne *et al.* 1998; Hoskin 2000). Largely because of treatment-associated side-effects, 45% of cancer patients have inadequate and undermanaged pain control (de Wit *et al.* 2001; Meuser *et al.* 2001). A formidable obstacle to the development of new therapies is the fact that the current neurobiological basis for pharmacological treatments is largely empirical, and depends on scientific advances in painful conditions other than those induced by cancer.

Given the toll that cancer pain exacts from the patient, it is somewhat surprising that it was only recently that the first model of cancer pain was developed. In this mouse model, bone cancer pain is induced by injecting murine osteolytic sarcoma cells into the intramedullary space of the femur (Fig. 15.1) (Schwei *et al.* 1999). Critical to this model is ensuring that the tumor cells are confined within the marrow space of the injected femur and that they do not invade adjacent soft tissues, which would directly affect the joints of the muscle, making behavioral analysis problematic (Schwei *et al.* 1999; Honore *et al.* 2000*d*; Luger *et al.* 2001). Following injection, the tumor cells proliferate, and ongoing movement-evoked and mechanically evoked pain-related behaviors develop that increase in severity with time. These pain behaviors correlate with the progressive tumor-induced bone destruction that ensues, which appears to mimic the condition in patients with primary or metastatic bone cancer. These models have allowed us to gain mechanistic insights into how cancer pain is generated and how the sensory information it initiates is processed as it moves from sense organ to the cerebral cortex under a constantly changing molecular architecture. As detailed below, these insights promise to fundamentally change the way cancer pain is controlled.

15.2 Primary afferent sensory neurons

Primary afferent sensory neurons are the gateway by which sensory information from peripheral tissues is transmitted to the spinal cord and brain (Fig. 15.2), and these neurons innervate the skin and every internal organ of the body, including mineralized bone, marrow, and periosteum. The cell bodies of sensory fibers that innervate the head and body are housed in the trigeminal and dorsal root ganglia, respectively, and can be divided into two major categories: myelinated A fibers and smaller-diameter unmyelinated C fibers. Nearly all large-diameter myelinated A-β fibers normally conduct non-noxious stimuli applied to the skin, joints, and muscles, rather than noxious stimuli (Djouhri *et al.* 1998). In contrast, most small-diameter sensory fibers — unmyelinated C fibers and finely myelinated A fibers — are specialized sensory neurons known as nociceptors, whose major function is to detect environmental stimuli that are perceived as harmful and convert them into electrochemical signals that are then transmitted to the CNS.

Unlike primary sensory neurons involved in vision or olfaction, which are required to detect only one type of sensory stimulus (light or chemical odorants, respectively), individual primary sensory neurons of the pain pathway have the remarkable ability to detect a wide range of stimulus modalities, including those of a physical and chemical nature (Basbaum and Jessel 2000; Julius and Basbaum 2001). To accomplish this, nociceptors express an extremely diverse repertoire of transduction molecules that can sense forms of noxious stimulation (thermal, mechanical, and chemical), albeit with varying degrees of sensitivity.

The past few years have seen remarkable progress toward understanding the signaling mechanisms and specific molecules that nociceptors use to detect noxious stimuli. For example, the vanilloid receptor TRPV1 (formerly known as VR1), which is expressed by most nociceptors, detects heat (Kirschstein *et al.* 1999) and also appears

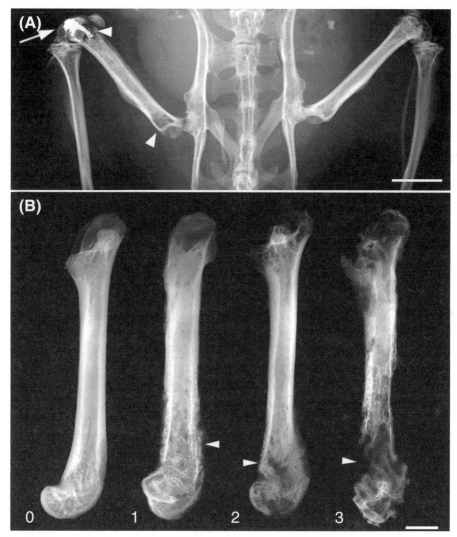

Fig. 15.1 Progressive destruction of mineralized bone in mice with bone cancer. **(A)** Low-power anterior-posterior radiograph of mouse pelvis and hindlimbs after a unilateral injection of sarcoma cells into the distal part of the femur and closure of the injection site with an amalgam plug (arrow), which prevents the tumor cells from growing outside the bone (Honore *et al.* 2000*a*). Radiographs of murine femora **(B)** show the progressive loss of mineralized bone caused by tumor growth. These images are representative of the stages of bone destruction in the murine femur. At week 1 there is a minor loss of bone near the distal head (arrow); at week 2, substantial loss of mineralized bone at both the proximal and distal (arrow) heads; and at week 3, loss of mineralized bone throughout the entire femur and fracture of distal head (arrow). Scale bar: 2 mm. (Modified from Schwei *et al.* 1999.)

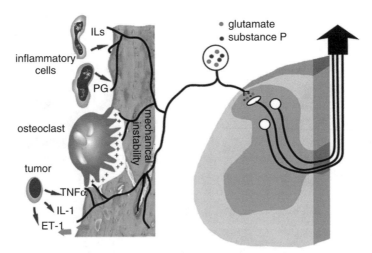

Fig. 15.2 Sensory neurons and detection of noxious stimuli due to tumor cells. Nociceptors use a diversity of signal-transduction mechanisms to detect noxious physiological stimuli, and many of these mechanisms may be involved in driving cancer pain. Thus, when nociceptors are exposed to products of tumor cells, tissue injury, or inflammation, their excitability is altered and this nociceptive information is relayed to the spinal cord and then to higher centers of the brain. Some of the mechanisms that appear to be involved in generating and maintaining cancer pain include activation of nociceptors by factors such as extracellular protons (+), endothelin-1 (ET-1), interleukins (ILs), prostaglandins (PG), and tumor necrosis factor (TNF).

to detect extracellular protons (Bevan and Geppetti 1994; Caterina *et al.* 2000; Welch *et al.* 2000) and lipid metabolites (Tominaga *et al.* 1998; Nagy and Rang 1999). In order to detect noxious mechanical stimuli, nociceptors express mechanically gated channels that initiate a signaling cascade upon excessive stretch (Price *et al.* 2001). The cells also express several purinergic receptors capable of sensing adenosine triphosphate (ATP), which may be released from cells upon excessive mechanical stimulation (Krishtal *et al.* 1988; Xu and Huang 2002).

To sense noxious chemical stimuli, nociceptors express a complex array of receptors capable of detecting inflammation-associated factors released from damaged tissue. These factors include protons (Bevan and Geppetti 1994; Caterina *et al.* 2000), endothelins (Nelson and Carducci 2000), prostaglandins (Alvarez and Fyffe 2000), bradykinin (Alvarez and Fyffe 2000), and nerve growth factor (McMahon 1996). Aside from providing promising targets for the development of more selective analgesics, identification of receptors expressed on the nociceptor surface has increased our understanding of how different tumors generate cancer pain in the peripheral tissues they invade and destroy.

In addition to expressing channels and receptors that detect tissue injury, sensory neurons are highly 'plastic', in that they can change their phenotype in the face of a sustained peripheral injury. Following tissue injury, sensory neuron subpopulations alter patterns of signaling peptide and growth factor expression (Woolf and Salter 2000). This change in phenotype of the sensory neuron in part underlies peripheral sensitization, whereby the activation threshold of nociceptors is lowered so that a stimulus that would normally be mildly noxious is perceived as highly noxious (hyperalgesia). Damage to peripheral tissues also activates previously 'silent' or 'sleeping' nociceptors, which then become highly responsive both to normally non-noxious stimuli (allodynia) and to noxious stimuli (hyperalgesia).

There are several examples of nociceptors that undergo peripheral sensitization in experimental cancer models (Schwei *et al.* 1999; Honore *et al.* 2000; Luger *et al.* 2001). In normal mice, the neurotransmitter, substance P, is synthesized by nociceptors and released in the spinal cord in response to a noxious (but not non-noxious) palpation of the femur. In mice with bone cancer, normally non-painful palpation of the affected femur induces the release of substance P from primary afferent fibers that terminate in the spinal cord. Substance P in turn binds to and activates the neurokinin-1 receptor that is expressed by a subset of spinal cord neurons (Mantyh *et al.* 1995*a*; Hunt and Mantyh 2001). Similarly, normally non-noxious palpation of tumor-bearing limbs of mice with bone cancer also induces the expression of c-fos protein in spinal cord neurons. In normal animals that do not have cancer, only noxious stimuli will induce this response (Hunt *et al.* 1987). Thus, peripheral sensitization of nociceptors appears to be involved in the generation and maintenance of bone cancer pain.

15.3 **Properties of tumors that excite nociceptors**

Tumor cells and tumor-associated cells that include macrophages, neutrophils, and T-lymphocytes secrete a wide variety of factors that sensitize or directly excite primary afferent neurons (see Fig. 15.2). These include prostaglandins (Nielsen *et al.* 1991; Galasko 1995), endothelins (Nelson and Carducci 2000; Davar 2001), interleukins 1 and 6 (Watkins *et al.* 1995; Leskovar *et al.* 2000; Opree and Kress 2000), epidermal growth factor (Stoscheck and King 1986), transforming growth factor (Poon *et al.* 2001; Roman *et al.* 2001), and platelet-derived growth factor (Daughaday and Deuel 1991; Radinsky 1991; Silver 1992). Receptors for many of these factors are expressed by primary afferent neurons. Each of these factors may play an important role in generating pain in particular forms of cancer, and therapies that block two of these factors, prostaglandins and endothelins, are currently approved for use in patients with other (non-cancer) indications.

Prostaglandins are pro-inflammatory lipids that are formed from arachidonic acid by the action of cyclooxygenase (COX) and other downstream synthetases. There are two distinct forms of the COX enzyme, COX-1 and COX-2. Prostaglandins are involved in the sensitization or direct excitation of nociceptors by binding to several prostanoid receptors (Vasko 1995). Many tumor cells and tumor-associated macrophages express high levels of COX-2 and produce large amounts of prostaglandins (Dubois *et al.* 1996; Molina *et al.* 1999; Kundu *et al.* 2001; Ohno *et al.* 2001; Shappell *et al.* 2001).

The COX enzymes are a major target of current medications, and COX inhibitors are commonly administered for reducing both inflammation and pain. A major problem with using COX inhibitors such as aspirin or ibuprofen to block cancer pain is that these compounds inhibit both COX-1 and COX-2, and inhibition of the constitutively expressed COX-1 can cause bleeding and ulcers. In contrast, the new COX-2 inhibitors or coxibs preferentially inhibit COX-2 and avoid many of the side-effects of COX-1 inhibition, which may allow their use in treating cancer pain. Other experiments have suggested that COX-2 is involved in angiogenesis and tumor growth (Masferrer *et al.* 2000; Moore and Simmons 2000), so in cancer patients, in addition to blocking cancer pain, COX-2 inhibitors may have the added advantage of reducing the growth and metastasis of the tumor. COX-2 antagonists show significant promise for alleviating at least some aspects of cancer pain, although clearly more research is required to fully define the actions of COX-2 in different types of cancer.

A second pharmacological target for treating cancer pain is the peptide, endothelin-1 (Fig. 15.3). Several tumors, including prostate cancer, express high levels of endothelins (Shankar *et al.* 1998; Kurbel *et al.* 1999; Nelson and Carducci 2000), and clinical studies have reported a correlation between the severity of the pain in patients with prostate cancer and plasma levels of endothelins (Nelson *et al.* 1995). Endothelins could contribute to cancer pain by directly sensitizing or exciting nociceptors, given that a subset of small unmyelinated primary afferent neurons express receptors for endothelin (Pomonis *et al.* 2001). Direct application of endothelin to peripheral nerves activates primary afferent fibers and induces pain behaviors (Davar *et al.* 1998). Like prostaglandins, endothelins that are released from tumor cells are also thought to be involved in regulating angiogenesis (Dawas *et al.* 1999) and tumor growth (Asham *et al.* 1998), suggesting again that endothelin antagonists may be useful not only in inhibiting cancer pain but in reducing the growth and metastasis of the tumor.

15.4 **Tumor-induced release of protons and acidosis**

Tumor cells become ischemic and undergo apoptosis as the tumor burden exceeds its vascular supply (Helmlinger *et al.* 2002). Local acidosis (a state where an accumulation of acid metabolites is present) is a hallmark of tissue injury (Reeh and Steen 1996; Julius and Basbaum 2001). In the past few years, the concept that sensory neurons can be directly excited by protons or acidosis has generated intense research and clinical interest. Studies have shown that subsets of sensory neurons express different acid-sensing ion channels (Olson *et al.* 1998; Julius and Basbaum 2001). The two major classes of acid-sensing ion channels expressed by nociceptors are TRPV1 (Caterina *et al.* 1997; Tominaga *et al.* 1998) and the acid-sensing ion channel-3 (ASIC-3) (Bassilana *et al.* 1997; Olson *et al.* 1998; Sutherland *et al.* 2000). Both of these channels are sensitized and excited by a decrease in pH. More specifically, TRPV1 is activated

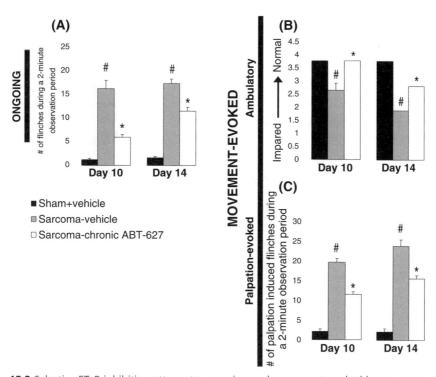

Fig. 15.3 Selective ET$_A$R inhibition attenuates ongoing and movement-evoked bone cancer pain behaviors. The number of spontaneous flinches of the cancerous limb over a 2-minute observation period was used as a measure of ongoing pain (**A**). Parameters of movement-evoked pain include assessment of the sarcoma-bearing limb during normal ambulation in an open field (**B**). Quantification of the number of flinches evoked by normally non-noxious palpation of the sarcoma bearing limb over a 2-minute observation period following palpation was used as a measure of palpation-evoked pain (**C**). All pain behaviors were significantly reduced 10 and 14 days after sarcoma injection with chronic administration of ABT-627 beginning at 6 days after sarcoma injection: bars, ± SEM. # P <0.05 versus sham; *P <0.05 versus sarcoma + vehicle group. Note that the ability of chronic ET$_A$R inhibition to attenuate ongoing pain was significantly reduced from day 10 to day 14 post sarcoma injection. (Modified from Peters *et al.* 2003.)

when the pH falls below 6.0, while the pH that activates ASIC-3 appears to be highly dependent on the coexpression of other ASIC channels in the same nociceptor (Lingueglia *et al.* 1997).

There are several mechanisms by which a decrease in pH could be involved in generating and maintaining cancer pain. As tumors grow, tumor-associated inflammatory cells invade the neoplastic tissue and release protons that generate local acidosis (Helmlinger *et al.* 2002). A second mechanism by which acidosis may occur is apoptosis of the tumor cells. Release of intracellular ions may generate an acidic environment that activates signaling by acid-sensing channels expressed by nociceptors.

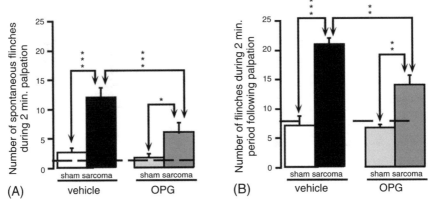

Fig. 15.4 Attenuation of bone cancer pain by osteoprotegerin (OPG). Histograms show that administration of OPG beginning 6 days after tumor implantation attenuated both **(A)** spontaneous and **(B)** palpation-evoked pain in mice at day 17 following tumor implantation (modified from Honore *et al.* 2000). OPG is a naturally occurring protein that is a secreted decoy receptor that inhibits osteoclast differentiation, proliferation, and hypertrophy, resulting in reduced osteoclast activity and bone resorption.

Tumor-induced release of protons and acidosis may be particularly important in the generation of bone cancer pain. In both osteolytic (bone-destroying) and osteoblastic (bone-forming) cancers there is a significant proliferation and hypertrophy of osteo-clasts (Clohisy *et al.* 2000*a,b*). Osteoclasts are terminally differentiated, multinucleated cells of the monocyte lineage that are uniquely designed to resorb bone by maintaining an extracellular microenvironment of acidic pH (4.0–5.0) at the interface between osteoclast and mineralized bone (Delaisse and Vaes 1992). Studies have shown significant expression of ASIC (Olson *et al.* 1998) and TRPV1 (Tominaga *et al.* 1998; Guo *et al.* 1999) in peptidergic afferent fibers, and we have localized peptidergic fibers in bone marrow and cortical bone (Mach *et al.* 2002). This evidence suggests that exposure of these sensory fibers to the osteoclast's acidic extracellular microenvironment could activate resident proton-sensitive ion channels, stimulating pain sensation.

Recent experiments in a murine model of bone cancer pain reported that osteoclasts play an essential role in cancer-induced bone loss and contribute to the etiology of bone cancer pain (Honore *et al.* 2000*a*; Luger *et al.* 2001). Recent work has shown that osteoprotegerin (Honore *et al.* 2000*a*) and a bisphosphonate (Fulfaro *et al.* 1998; Mannix *et al.* 2000), both of which are known to induce osteoclast apoptosis, are effective in decreasing osteoclast-induced bone cancer pain (Fig. 15.4). Similarly, TRPV1 or ASIC antagonists may be used to reduce pain in patients with soft tissue tumors or bone cancer by blocking excitation of the acid-sensitive channels on sensory neurons.

15.5 **Release of growth factors by tumor cells**

One of the most important discoveries in the past decade has been the demonstration that the biochemical and physiological status of sensory neurons is maintained and modified by factors derived from the innervated tissue. Changes in the periphery associated with inflammation, nerve injury, or tissue injury are mirrored by changes in the phenotype of sensory neurons (Honore *et al.* 2000c). After peripheral nerve injury, expression of a subset of neurotransmitters and receptors by damaged sensory neurons is altered in a highly predictable fashion. This is caused, in part, by a change in the tissue level of several growth factors released from the environment local to the injury site, including nerve growth factors (NGF) (Fu and Gordon 1997; Koltzenburg 1999; Fukuoka *et al.* 2001) and glial-derived neurotrophic factor (GDNF) (Boucher and McMahon 2001; Hoke *et al.* 2002). These neurochemical changes can be reversed in a receptor-specific fashion by intrathecal or peripheral application of NGF or GDNF (Bennett *et al.* 1996, 1998; Boucher *et al.* 2000; Ramer *et al.* 2000).

While the level of NGF expression reportedly correlates with the extent of pain in pancreatic cancer (Zhu *et al.* 1999; Schneider *et al.* 2001), relatively little is known about how other tumors affect the synthesis and release of growth factors. However, one certainty is that the repertoire of growth factors to which the sensory neuron is exposed will change as the developing tumor invades the peripheral tissue that the neuron innervates. Thus, in addition to a disruption of the growth factors normally released by the intact peripheral tissue, one can expect release of a variety of additional growth factors by tumor cells as well as by tumor-infiltrating macrophages, which can comprise up to 80% of the total tumor mass (Zhang *et al.* 2002). Activated macrophages synthesize and release high levels of several growth factors (Stoscheck and King 1986; Daughaday and Deuel 1991; Radinsky 1991; Silver 1992; Leon *et al.* 1994; Caroleo *et al.* 2001; Poon *et al.* 2001; Roman *et al.* 2001), and thus one would expect a significant change in the phenotype and response characteristics of the sensory neurons following tumor invasion of a peripheral organ.

While tumor growth alters the invaded tissue, it is also clear that the affected tissue also influences the phenotype of the invading tumor cell (Mundy 2002). Because the local environment can influence the molecules that tumor cells express and release, it follows that the same tumor in the same individual may be painful at one site of metastasis but not at another. Clinical observations reveal that pain from cancer can be quite perplexing because the size, location, or type of cancer tumor does not necessarily predict symptoms. Different patients with the same cancer may have vastly different symptoms. Kidney cancer may be painful in one person and asymptomatic in another. Metastases to bone in the same individual may cause pain at the site of a rib lesion, but not at that of a humeral lesion. Small cancer deposits in bone may be very painful, while large soft-tissue cancers may be painless (Mantyh *et al.* 2002). Important areas for future research include identification of tissue-specific mechanisms of cancer pain, comparing soft tissue with bone, as well as site-specific mechanisms, comparing flat bones (ribs) with tubular bones (femurs). It will also be of interest to determine patient-specific factors that influence disease progression and its relationship to pain perception.

15.6 Tumor-induced distension and destruction of sensory fibers

In general, previous reports have suggested that tumors are not highly innervated by sensory or sympathetic neurons (O'Connell *et al.* 1998; Seifert and Spitznas 2001; Terada and Matsunaga 2001). However, in many cancers, rapid tumor growth frequently entraps and injures nerves, causing mechanical injury, compression, or ischemia or direct proteolysis (Mercadante 1997). Proteolytic enzymes produced by the tumor can also injure sensory and sympathetic fibers, causing neuropathic pain.

The capacity of a tumor to injure and destroy peripheral nerve fibers has been directly observed in an experimental model of bone cancer. Following injection and containment of lytic murine sarcoma cells in the intramedullary of the mouse femur, tumor cells grow in the marrow space and disrupt innervating sensory fibers (Fig. 15.5 and 15.6). As the tumor cells grow, they first compress and then destroy both the hematopoietic cells of the marrow and the sensory fibers that normally innervate the marrow, mineralized bone, and periosteum (Schwei *et al.* 1999).

While the mechanisms by which any neuropathic pain is generated and maintained are still not well understood, several therapies that have proven useful in the control of other types of neuropathic pain may also be useful in treating tumor-induced neuropathic pain. For example, gabapentin, which was originally developed as an anticonvulsant but whose mechanism of action remains unknown, is effective in treating several forms of neuropathic pain and may also be useful in treating cancer-induced neuropathic pain (Ripamonti and Dickerson 2001).

15.7 Central sensitization in cancer pain

A critical question is whether the spinal cord and forebrain also undergo significant neurochemical changes as a chronic cancer pain state develops. The murine cancer pain model revealed extensive neurochemical reorganization within spinal cord segments that receive input from primary afferent neurons innervating the cancerous bone (Honore *et al.* 2000*d*; Luger *et al.* 2001). These changes included astrocyte hypertrophy (Fig. 15.7) and upregulation of the prohyperalgesic peptide, dynorphin. Spinal cord neurons that normally would only be activated by noxious stimuli were activated by non-noxious stimuli. These spinal cord changes were attenuated by blocking the tumor-induced tissue destruction and pain (Honore *et al.* 2000*a*; Luger *et al.* 2001). Together, these neurochemical changes suggest that cancer pain induces and is at least partially maintained by a state of central sensitization, in which an increased transmission of nociceptive information allows normally non-noxious input to be amplified and perceived as noxious stimuli.

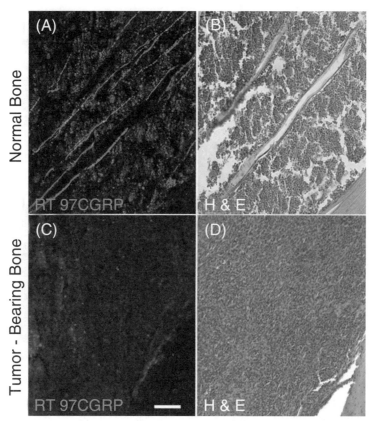

Fig. 15.5 Sensory nerve fibers in the marrow of the mouse femur are destroyed by invading sarcoma tumor cells. Confocal (A&C) images show calcitonin gene-related peptide (CGRP, green) and neurofilament-200 (RT-97, red) and serially adjacent sections (B&D) stained with hematoxylin and eosin (H&E, B&D) in the normal (A&B) and tumor-bearing (C&D) marrow. In the normal marrow, CGRP and RT-97 expressing sensory fibers are generally associated with the vasculature (A&B) whereas 14 days following injection and confinement of the tumor cells to the marrow space (C&D), few if any CGRP or RT-97 expressing sensory fibers can be detected. Scale bar: 150 μm.

Once nociceptive information has been transmitted to the spinal cord by primary afferent neurons, it can travel via multiple ascending 'pain' pathways that project from the spinal cord to higher centers of the brain. Classically, the main emphasis in examining the ascending conduction of pain has been placed on spinothalamic tract neurons. However, data from recent clinical studies have necessitated a reassessment of this position by showing significant attenuation of some forms of difficult to control visceral cancer pain following lesion of the axons of non-spinothalamic tract neurons (Willis *et al.* 1999; Nauta *et al.* 2000). Together these data suggest that one reason that

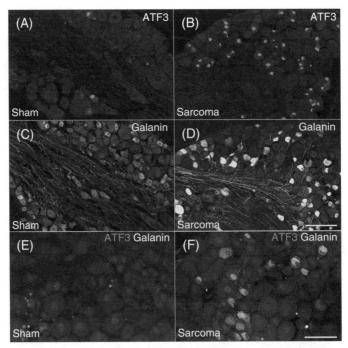

Fig. 15.6 Tumor-induced destruction of sensory nerve fibers in the tumor-bearing bone results in the up-regulation of activated transcription factor-3 and galanin in the cell body of sensory neurons that innervate the tumor-bearing femur. Neurons in the normal L2 dorsal root ganglia express low levels of both transcription factor-3 (ATF-3) **(A)** or the neuropeptide galanin **(C)**, whereas 14 days following injection and confinement of sarcoma cells to the marrow space there is a marked up-regulation of both ATF-3 and galanin in sensory neurons in the L2 dorsal root ganglia ipsilateral to the tumor-bearing bone. Many sensory neurons which show an up-regulation of galanin in response to tumor-induced destruction of sensory fibers in the bone also show up-regulation of ATF-3 in their nucleus (compare E vs. F). These data suggest that as tumor cells invade the bone, sensory nerve fibers that normally innervate the bone are destroyed, with a resulting generation of the neurochemical signature of neuropathy in sensory neurons that innervate the tumor-bearing bone. Scale bar: 100 μm. (Modified from Luger *et al.* forthcoming.)

cancer pain is frequently perceived as such an intense and disturbing pain is that it ascends to higher centers of the brain via multiple parallel neuronal pathways. Importantly for cancer patients, many of whom frequently experience anxiety or depression, it is clear that higher centers of the brain can modulate the ascending conduction of pain. Descending pathways that modulate the ascending conduction of cancer pain may play an important role in either enhancing or inhibiting the patient's perception of pain. The general mood and attention of the patient thus may be significant factors in determining the pain's intensity and degree of unpleasantness.

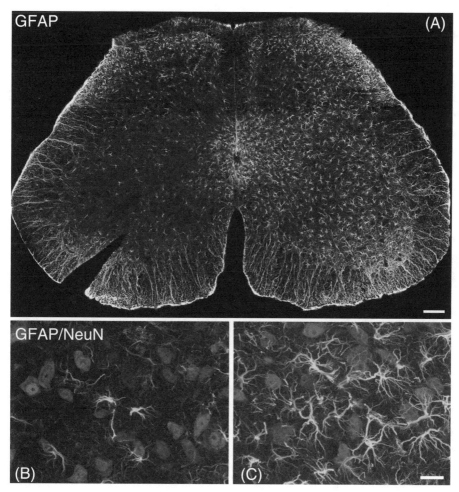

Fig. 15.7 Cancer-induced reorganization of the CNS. Chronic cancer pain not only sensitizes peripheral nociceptors, but also can induce significant neurochemical reorganization of the spinal cord. This reorganization may participate in the phenomenon of central sensitization (i.e. an increased responsiveness of spinal cord neurons involved in transmission of pain). (A) Confocal image of a coronal section of the mouse L4 spinal cord showing glial fibrillary acidic protein (GFAP) positive astrocytes (white) which have undergone hypertrophy on the side ipsilateral to the tumor-bearing bone. Panels B and C show higher magnification of the ipsilateral and contralateral dorsal horn seen in panel A, with colocalization of the neuron-specific antibody, NeuN. Note that while the astrocytes (spindle-shaped cells) have undergone a massive hypertrophy, there does not appear to be any significant loss of NeuN-positive neurons. Scale bars: A, 200 μm; B and C, 30 μm. (Modified from Schwei *et al.* 1999.)

15.8 **Changing factors may drive cancer pain with disease progression**

Cancer pain frequently becomes more severe as the disease progresses, and adequate control of cancer pain becomes more difficult to achieve without encountering significant unwanted side-effects (Payne 1998; Foley 1999; Portenoy and Lesage 1999). While tolerance may contribute to the escalation of the dose of analgesics required to control cancer pain, a compatible possibility is that with the progression of the disease, different factors assume a greater importance in driving cancer pain. For example, in the mouse model of bone cancer, as tumor cells first begin to proliferate, pain-related behaviors start to occur long before any significant bone destruction is evident. This pain may be due to prohyperalgesic factors such as prostaglandins and endothelin that are released by the growing tumor cells and subsequently activate nociceptors in the marrow. Pain at this stage might be attenuated by COX-2 inhibitors and endothelin antagonists. As the tumor continues to grow, sensory neurons innervating the marrow are compressed and destroyed, causing a neuropathic pain to develop that may best respond to treatment with drugs such as gabapentin that are known to attenuate non-cancer-induced neuropathic pain. When the tumor begins to induce proliferation and hypertrophy of osteoclasts, the pain due to excessive osteoclast activity might be largely blocked by anti-osteoclastogenic drugs such as bisphosphonates or osteoprotegerin (see Fig. 15.4). As the tumor cells completely fill the intramedullary space, tumor cells begin to die, generating an acidic environment; antagonists to TRPV1 or ASICs may attenuate the pain induced by this acidosis. Finally, as bone destruction compromises the mechanical strength of the bone, antagonists that block the mechanically gated channels and/or ATP receptors in the richly innervated periosteum may attenuate movement-evoked pain.

While the above pattern of tumor-induced tissue destruction and nociceptor activation may be unique to bone cancer, an evolving set of nociceptive events probably occurs in other cancers. This complex pattern may in part explain why cancer pain is frequently difficult to treat and why it is so heterogeneous in nature and severity. Changes in tumor-induced tissue injury, in nociceptor activation, and in the brain areas involved in transmitting these nociceptive signals as the disease progresses suggest that different therapies will be efficacious at particular stages of the disease. Understanding how tumor cells differentially excite nociceptors at different stages of the disease, and how the phenotype of nociceptors and CNS neurons involved in nociceptive transmission change as the disease progresses, should allow a mechanistic approach to designing more effective therapies to treat cancer pain.

15.9 **Future directions**

For the first time, animal models of cancer pain are now available that mirror the clinical picture of patients with cancer pain. Information generated from these models should elucidate the mechanisms that generate and maintain different types of cancer pain.

Many of these cancer models have been developed in mice and rats, but implantation of human tumors in immunocompromised rodent strains should allow examination of the pain that different human tumors generate. These animal models may also offer insight into one of the major conundrums of cancer pain: that the severity of cancer pain is so variable from patient to patient, from tumor to tumor, and even from site to site. Newer molecular techniques using microarrays and proteomics should reveal which specific features of different tumors are important in inducing cancer pain. Once we have determined the mechanisms by which the different types of cancer induce pain, we can identify molecular targets and develop mechanism-based therapies. Ultimately, the key will be to integrate information about tumor biology and the host's response to neoplasia with our understanding of how chronic pain is generated and maintained. These studies should improve the quality of life of all those who suffer from cancer pain.

Acknowledgements

Supported by grants from the National Institute of Neurologic Disorders and Stroke (NS23970) and the National Institute for Drug Abuse (DA11986), by the National Institute of Dental and Craniofacial Research Dentist Scientist Award (DSA) (DE00270) and training grant (DE07288), and a merit review from the Veterans Administration.

References

Alvarez FJ, Fyffe RE (2000) Nociceptors for the 21st century. *Curr Rev Pain* **4(6)**:451–458.

Asham EH, Loizidou M, Taylor I (1998) Endothelin-1 and tumour development. *Eur J Surg Oncol* **24(1)**:57–60.

Basbaum AI, Jessel TM (2000) The perception of pain. In: Kandel ER, Schwartz JH, Jessell TM (eds) *Principles of Neural Science*. New York: McGraw–Hill, pp. 472–490.

Bassilana F, Champigny G, Waldmann R, *et al.* (1997) The acid-sensitive ionic channel subunit ASIC and the mammalian degenerin MDEG form a heteromultimeric H^+-gated Na^+ channel with novel properties. *J Biol Chem* **272(46)**:28819–28822.

Bennett DL, French J, Priestley JV, McMahon SB (1996) NGF but not NT-3 or BDNF prevents the A fiber sprouting into lamina II of the spinal cord that occurs following axotomy. *Mol Cell Neurosci* **8(4)**:211–220.

Bennett DL, Michael GJ, Ramachandran N, *et al.* (1998) A distinct subgroup of small DRG cells express GDNF receptor components and GDNF is protective for these neurons after nerve injury. *J Neurosci* **18(8)**:3059–3072.

Bevan S, Geppetti P (1994) Protons: small stimulants of capsaicin-sensitive sensory nerves. *Trends Neurosci* **17(12)**:509–512.

Boucher TJ, McMahon SB (2001) Neurotrophic factors and neuropathic pain. *Curr Opin Pharmacol* **1(1)**:66–72.

Boucher TJ, Okuse K, Bennett DL, *et al.* (2000) Potent analgesic effects of GDNF in neuropathic pain states. *Science* **290(5489)**:124–127.

Caroleo MC, Costa N, Bracci–Laudiero L, Aloe L (2001) Human monocyte/macrophages activate by exposure to LPS overexpress NGF and NGF receptors. *J Neuroimmunol* **113(2)**:193–201.

Caterina MJ, Leffler A, Malmberg AB, *et al.* (2000) Impaired nociception and pain sensation in mice lacking the capsaicin receptor. *Science* **288(5464)**:306–313.

Caterina MJ, Schumacher MA, Tominaga M, *et al.* (1997) The capsaicin receptor: a heat-activated ion channel in the pain pathway. *Nature* **389(6653)**:816–824.

Clohisy DR, Perkins SL, Ramnaraine ML (2000*a*) Review of cellular mechanisms of tumor osteolysis. *Clin Orthop Res* **(373)**:104–114.

Clohisy DR, Ramnaraine ML, Scully S, *et al.* (2000*b*) Osteoprotegerin inhibits tumor-induced osteoclastogenesis and bone growth in osteopetrotic mice. *J Orthop Res* **18(6)**:967–976.

Clohisy DR, O'Keefe PF, Ramnaraine ML (2001) Pamidronate decreases tumor-induced osteoclastogenesis in mice. *J Orthop Res* **19(4)**:554–558.

Coyle NJ, Adelhardt KM, Foley KM, Portenoy RK (1990) Character of terminal illness in the advanced cancer patient: pain and other symptoms during the last four weeks of life. *J Pain Symptom Manage* **5(2)**:83–93.

Daughaday WH, Deuel TF (1991) Tumor secretion of growth factors. *Endocrinol Metab Clin North Am* **20(3)**:539–563.

Davar G (2001) Endothelin-1 and metastatic cancer pain. *Pain Med* **2(1)**:24–27.

Davar G, Hans G, Fareed MU, *et al.* (1998) Behavioral signs of acute pain produced by application of endothelin-1 to rat sciatic nerve. *Neuroreport* **9(10)**:2279–2283.

Dawas K, Laizidou M, Shankar A, *et al.* (1999) Angiogenesis in cancer: the role of endothelin-1. *Ann R Coll Surg Engl* **81**:306–310.

Delaisse J–M, Vaes G (1992) Mechanism of mineral solubilization and matrix degradation in osteoclastic bone resorption. In: Rifkin BR, Gay CV (eds) *Biology and Physiology of the Osteoclast.* Ann Arbor: CRC, pp. 289–314.

de Wit R, van Dam F, Loonstra S, *et al.* (2001) The Amsterdam Pain Management Index compared to eight frequently used outcome measures to evaluate the adequacy of pain treatment in cancer patients with chronic pain. *Pain* **91(3)**:339–349.

Djouhri L, Bleazard L, Lawson SN (1998) Association of somatic action potential shape with sensory receptive properties in guinea-pig dorsal root ganglion neurones. *J Physiol* **513(3)**:857–872.

Dubois RN, Radhika A, Reddy BS, Entingh AJ (1996) Increased cyclooxygenase-2 levels in carcinogen-induced rat colonic tumors. *Gastroenterology* **110(4)**:1259–1262.

Foley KM (1999) Advances in cancer pain. *Arch Neurol* **56(4)**:413–417.

Fu SY, Gordon T (1997) The cellular and molecular basis of peripheral nerve regeneration. *Mol Neurobiol* **14(1–2)**:67–116.

Fukuoka T, Kondo E, Dai Y, *et al.* (2001) Brain-derived neurotrophic factor increases in the uninjured dorsal root ganglion neurons in selective spinal nerve ligation model. *J Neurosci* **21(13)**:4891–4900.

Fulfaro F, Casuccio A, Ticozzi C, Ripamonti C (1998) The role of bisphosphonates in the treatment of painful metastatic bone disease: a review of phase III trials. *Pain* **78(3)**:157–169.

Galasko CS (1995) Diagnosis of skeletal metastases and assessment of response to treatment. *Clin Orthop* **(312)**:64–75.

Guo A, Vulchanova L, Wang J, *et al.* (1999) Immunocytochemical localization of the vanilloid receptor 1 (VR1): relationship to neuropeptides, the P2X3 purinoceptor and IB4 binding sites. *Eur J Neurosci* **11(3)**:946–958.

Helmlinger G, Sckell A, Dellian M, *et al.* (2002) Acid production in glycolysis-impaired tumors provides new insights into tumor metabolism. *Clin Cancer Res* **8(4)**:1284–1291.

Hoke A, Gordon T, Zochodne DW, Sulaiman OA (2002) A decline in glial cell-line-derived neurotrophic factor expression is associated with impaired regeneration after long-term Schwann cell denervation. *Exp Neurol* **173(1)**:77–85.

Honore P, Luger NM, Sabino MA, *et al.* (2000*a*) Osteoprotegerin blocks bone cancer-induced skeletal destruction, skeletal pain and pain-related neurochemical reorganization of the spinal cord. *Nat Med* **6(5)**:521–528.

Honore P, Menning PM, Rogers SD, *et al.* (2000*b*) Neurochemical plasticity in persistent inflammatory pain. *Prog Brain Res* **129**:357–363.

Honore P, Rogers SD, Schwei MJ, *et al.* (2000*c*) Murine models of inflammatory, neuropathic and cancer pain each generates a unique set of neurochemical changes in the spinal cord and sensory neurons. *Neuroscience* **98(3)**:585–598.

Honore P, Schwei J, Rogers SD, *et al.* (2000*d*) Cellular and neurochemical remodeling of the spinal cord in bone cancer pain. *Prog Brain Res* **129**:389–397.

Hoskin P (2000) In: Body J–J (ed) *Radiotherapy, Tumor Bone Diseases and Osteoporosis in Cancer Patients.* New York: Marcel Dekker, pp. 263–286.

Hunt SP, Mantyh PW (2001) The molecular dynamics of pain control. *Nat Rev Neurosci* **2(2)**:83–91.

Hunt SP, Pini A, Evan G (1987) Induction of c-fos-like protein in spinal cord neurons following sensory stimulation. *Nature* **328(6131)**:632–634.

Julius D, Basbaum AI (2001) Molecular mechanisms of nociception. *Nature* **413(6852)**:203–210.

Kirschstein T, Greffrath W, Busselberg D, Treede RD (1999) Inhibition of rapid heat responses in nociceptive primary sensory of rats by vanilloid receptor antagonists. *J Neurophysiol* **82(6)**:2853–2860.

Koltzenburg M (1999) The changing sensitivity in the life of the nociceptor. *Pain* (**Suppl 6**):S93–102.

Krishtal OA, Marchenko SM, Obukhov AG (1988) Cationic channels activated by extracellular ATP in rat sensory neurons. *Neuroscience* **27(3)**:995–1000.

Kundu N, Yang QY, Dorsey R, Fulton AM (2001) Increased cyclooxygenase-2 (COX-2) expression and activity in a murine model of metastatic breast cancer. *Int J Cancer* **93(5)**:681–686.

Kurbel S, Kurbel B, Kovacic D, *et al.* (1999) Endothelin-secreting tumors and the idea of the pseudoectopic hormone secretion in tumors. *Med Hypotheses* **52(4)**:329–333.

Leon A, Buriani A, Dal Toso R, *et al.* (1994) Mast cells synthesize, store, and release nerve growth factor. *Proc Natl Acad Sci USA* **91**:3739–3743.

Leskovar A, Moriarty LJ, Turek JJ, *et al.* (2000) The macrophage in acute neural injury: changes in cell numbers over time and levels of cytokine production in mammalian central and peripheral nervous systems. *J Exp Biol* **203**:1783–1795.

Lingueglia E, Weille JR, Bassilana F, *et al.* (1997) A modulatory subunit of acid sensing ion channels in brain and dorsal root ganglion cells. *J Biol Chem* **272**:29778–29783.

Luger NM, Honore P, Sabino MAC, *et al.* (2001) Osteoprotegerin diminishes advanced bone cancer pain. *Cancer Res* **61(10)**:4038–4047.

Luger NM, Keyser CP, Ghilardi JR, *et al.* (forthcoming) A neuropathic component to bone cancer pain.

Mach DB, Rogers SD, Sabino MC, *et al.* (2002) Origins of skeletal pain: sensory and sympathetic innervation of the mouse femur. *J Neurosci* **113(1)**:155–166.

Mannix K, Ahmedazai SH, Anderson H, *et al.* (2000) Using bisphosphonates to control the pain of bone metastases: evidence based guidelines for palliative care. *Palliat Med* **14**:455–461.

Mantyh PW, Allen CJ, Ghilardi JR, *et al.* (1995*b*) Rapid endocytosis of a G protein-coupled receptor: substance P evoked internalization of its receptor in the rat striatum in vivo. *Proc Natl Acad Sci USA* **92(7)**:2622–2626.

Mantyh PW, Clohisy DR, Koltzenburg M, Hunt SP (2002) Molecular mechanisms of cancer pain. *Nature Rev Cancer* **2(3)**:201–209.

Mantyh PW, DeMaster E, Malhotra A, *et al.* (1995*a*) Receptor endocytosis and dendrite reshaping in spinal neurons after somatosensory stimulation. *Science* **268(5217)**:1629–1632.

Masferrer JL, Leahy KM, Koki AT, *et al.* (2000) Antiangiogenic and antitumor activities of cyclooxygenase-2 inhibitors. *Cancer Res* **60**(5):1306–1311.

McMahon SB (1996) NGF as a mediator of inflammatory pain. *Philos Trans R Soc Lond B Biol Sci* **351**(1338):431–440.

Mercadante S (1997) Malignant bone pain: pathophysiology and treatment. *Pain* **69**(1–2):1–18.

Mercadante S, Arcuri E (1998) Breakthrough pain in cancer patients: pathophysiology and treatment. *Cancer Treat Rev* **24**(6):425–432.

Meuser T, Pietruck C, Radbruch L, *et al.* (2001) Symptoms during cancer pain treatment following WHO guidelines: a longitudinal follow-up study of symptom prevalence, severity and etiology. *Pain* **93**(3):247–257.

Molina MA, Sitja–Arnau M, Lemoine MG, *et al.* (1999) Increased cyclooxygenase-2 expression in human pancreatic carcinomas and cell lines: growth inhibition by nonsteroidal anti-inflammatory drugs. *Cancer Res* **59**(17):4356–4362.

Moore BC, Simmons DL (2000) COX-2 inhibition, apoptosis, and chemoprevention by nonsteroidal anti-inflammatory drugs. *Curr Med Chem* **7**(11):1131–1144.

Mundy GR (2002) Metastases to bone: causes, consequences, and therapeutic opportunities. *Nature Rev Cancer* **2**:584–593.

Nagy I, Rang H (1999) Noxious heat activates all capsaicin-sensitive and also a sub-population of capsaicin-insensitive dorsal root ganglion neurons. *Neuroscience* **88**(4):995–997.

Nauta HJW, Soukup VM, Fabian RH, *et al.* (2000) Punctate midline myelotomy for the relief of visceral cancer pain. *J Neurosurg* **92**(Suppl 2S):125–130.

Nelson JB, Carducci MA (2000) The role of endothelin-1 and endothelin receptor antagonists in prostate cancer. *BJU Int* **85**(Suppl 2):45–48.

Nelson JB, Hedican SP, George DJ, *et al.* (1995) Identification of endothelin-1 in the pathophysiology of metastatic adenocarcinoma of the prostate. *Nat Med* **1**(9):944–999.

Nielsen OS, Munro AJ, Tannock IF (1991) Bone metastases: pathophysiology and management policy. *J Clin Oncol* **9**(3):509–524.

O'Connell JX, Nanthakumar SS, Nielsen GP, Rosenberg AE (1998) Osteoid osteoma: the uniquely innervated bone tumor. *Modern Pathol* **11**(2):175–180.

Ohno R, Yoshinaga K, Fujita T, *et al.* (2001) Depth of invasion parallels increased cyclooxygenase-2 levels in patients with gastric carcinoma. *Cancer* **91**(10):1876–1881.

Olson TH, Riedl MS, Vulchanova L, *et al.* (1998) An acid sensing ion channel (ASIC) localizes to small primary afferent neurons in rats. *Neuroreport* **9**(6):1109–1113.

Opree A, Kress M (2000) Involvement of the proinflammatory cytokines tumor necrosis factor-alpha, IL-1 beta, and IL-6 but not IL-8 in the development of heat hyperalgesia: effects on heat-evoked calcitonin gene-related peptide release from rat skin. *J Neurosci* **20**(16):6289–6293.

Payne R (1997) Mechanisms and management of bone pain. *Cancer* **80**(Suppl 8):1608–1613.

Payne R (1998) Practice guidelines for cancer pain therapy. Issues pertinent to the revision of national guidelines. *Oncology* **12**(11A):169–175.

Payne R, Mathias SD, Pasta DJ, *et al.* (1998) Quality of life and cancer pain: satisfaction and side effects with transdermal fentanyl versus oral morphine. *J Clin Oncol* **16**(4):1588–1593.

Peters CM, Pomonis JD, *et al.* (forthcoming) Endothelin, endothelin receptors and the heterogeneity of bone cancer pain.

Pomonis JD, Rogers SD, Peters CM, *et al.* (2001) Expression and localization of endothelin receptors: implication for the involvement of peripheral glia in nociception. *J Neurosci* **21**(3):999–1006.

Poon RT, Fan ST, Wong J (2001) Clinical implications of circulating angiogenic factors in cancer patients. *J Clin Oncol* **19(4)**:1207–1225.

Portenoy RK, Lesage P (1999) Management of cancer pain. *Lancet* **353(9165)**:1695–1700.

Portenoy RKD, Payne D, Jacobsen P (1999) Breakthrough pain: characteristics and impact in patients with cancer pain. *Pain* **81(1–2)**:129–134.

Price MP, McIlwrath SL, Xie JH, *et al.* (2001) The DRASIC cation channel contributes to the detection of cutaneous touch and acid stimuli in mice. *Neuron* **32(6)**:1071–1083.

Radinsky R (1991) Growth factors and their receptors in metastasis. *Semin Cancer Biol* **2(3)**:169–177.

Ramer MS, Priestley JV, McMahon SB (2000) Functional regeneration of sensory axons into the adult spinal cord. *Nature* **403(6767)**:312–316.

Reeh PW, Steen KH (1996) Tissue acidosis in nociception and pain. *Prog Brain Res* **113**:143–151.

Ripamonti C, Dickerson ED (2001) Strategies for the treatment of cancer pain in the new millennium. *Drugs* **61(7)**:955–977.

Roman C, Saha D, Beauchamp R (2001) TGF-beta and colorectal carcinogenesis. *Microsc Res Tech* **52(4)**:450–457.

Schneider MB, Standop J, Ulrich A, *et al.* (2001) Expression of nerve growth factors in pancreatic neural tissue and pancreatic cancer. *J Histochem Cytochem* **49(10)**:1205–1210.

Schwei MJ, Honore P, Rogers SD, *et al.* (1999) Neurochemical and cellular reorganization of the spinal cord in a murine model of bone cancer pain. *J Neurosci* **19(24)**:10886–10897.

Seifert P, Spitznas M (2001) Tumours may be innervated. *Virchows Archiv* **438(3)**:228–231.

Shankar A, Loizidou M, Aliev G, *et al.* (1998) Raised endothelin 1 levels in patients with colorectal liver metastases. *Br J Surg* **85(4)**:502–506.

Shappell SB, Manning S, Boeglin WE, *et al.* (2001) Alterations in lipoxygenase and cyclooxygenase-2 catalytic activity and mRNA expression in prostate carcinoma. *Neoplasia* **3(4)**:287–303.

Silver BJ (1992) Platelet-derived growth factor in human malignancy. *Biofactors* **3(4)**:217–227.

Stoscheck CM, King Jr LE (1986) Role of epidermal growth factor in carcinogenesis. *Cancer Res* **46(3)**:1030–1037.

Sutherland S, Cook S, Ew M (2000) Chemical mediators of pain due to tissue damage and ischemia. *Prog Brain Res* **129**:21–38.

Terada T, Matsunaga Y (2001) S-100-positive nerve fibers in hepatocellular carcinoma and intrahepatic cholangiocarcinoma: an immunohistochemical study. *Pathol Int* **51(2)**:89–93.

Tominaga M, Caterina MJ, Malmberg AB, *et al.* (1998) The cloned capsaicin receptor integrates multiple pain-producing stimuli. *Neuron* **21(3)**:531–543.

Vasko MR (1995) Prostaglandin-induced neuropeptide release from spinal cord. *Prog Brain Res* **104**:367–380.

Watkins LR, Goehler LE, Relton J, *et al.* (1995) Mechanisms of tumor necrosis factor-alpha (TNF-alpha) hyperalgesia. *Brain Res* **692(1–2)**:244–250.

Welch JM, Simon SA, Reinhart PH (2000) The activation mechanism of rat vanilloid receptor 1 by capsaicin involves the pore domain and differs from the activation by either or heat. *Proc Natl Acad Sci USA* **97(25)**:13889–13894.

Willis WD, Al–Chaer ED, Quast MJ, Westlund KN (1999) A visceral pain pathway in the dorsal column of the spinal cord. *Proc Natl Acad Sci USA* **96(14)**:7675–7679.

Woolf CJ, Salter MW (2000) Neuronal plasticity: increasing the gain in pain. *Science* **288(5472)**:1765–1769.

Xu GY, Huang LYM (2002) Peripheral inflammation sensitizes P2X receptor-mediated responses in dorsal root ganglion neurons. *J Neurosci* **22(1)**:93–102.

Zhang F, Lu W, Dong Z (2002) Tumor-infiltrating macrophages are involved in suppressing growth and metastasis of human prostate cancer cells by INF-beta gene therapy in nude mice. PG-2942–51. *Clin Cancer Res* **8(9)**.

Zhu ZW, Friess H, diMola FF, *et al.* (1999) Nerve growth factor expression correlates with perineural invasion and pain in human pancreatic cancer. *J Clin Oncol* **17(8)**:2419–2428.

Index

Page references to **figures, tables and boxes** are shown in **bold**